2008
YEAR BOOK OF
PEDIATRICS®

The 2008 Year Book Series

Year Book of Anesthesiology and Pain Management™: Drs Chestnut, Abram, Black, Gravlee, Lee, Mathru, and Roizen

Year Book of Cardiology®: Drs Gersh, Cheitlin, Elliott, Graham, Sundt, and Waldo

Year Book of Critical Care Medicine®: Drs Dellinger, Parrillo, Balk, Bekes, Dorman, and Dries

Year Book of Dentistry®: Drs Olin, Belvedere, Davis, Henderson, Johnson, Ohrbach, Scott, Spencer, and Zakariasen

Year Book of Dermatology and Dermatologic Surgery™: Drs Thiers and Lang

Year Book of Diagnostic Radiology®: Drs Osborn, Abbara, Birdwell, Dalinka, Elster Gardiner, Levy, Oestreich, and Rosado de Christenson

Year Book of Emergency Medicine®: Drs Hamilton, Handly, Quintana, Werner, and Bruno

Year Book of Endocrinology®: Drs Mazzaferri, Bessesen, Clarke, Howard, Kennedy, Leahy, Meikle, Molitch, Rogol, and Schteingart

Year Book of Gastroenterology™: Drs Lichtenstein, Chang, Dempsey, Drebin, Jaffe, Katzka, Kochman, Makar, Morris, Osterman, Rombeau, and Shah

Year Book of Hand and Upper Limb Surgery®: Drs. Chang and Steinmann

Year Book of Medicine®: Drs Barkin, Berney, Frishman, Garrick, Loehrer, Phillips, and Khardori

Year Book of Neonatal and Perinatal Medicine®: Drs Fanaroff, Ehrenkranz, and Stevenson

Year Book of Neurology and Neurosurgery®: Drs Kim and Verma

Year Book of Obstetrics, Gynecology, and Women's Health®: Dr Shulman

Year Book of Oncology®: Drs Loehrer, Arceci, Glatstein, Gordon, Hanna, Morrow, and Thigpen

Year Book of Ophthalmology®: Drs Rapuano, Cohen, Eagle, Flanders, Hammersmith, Myers, Nelson, Penne, Sergott, Shields, Tipperman, and Vander

Year Book of Orthopedics®: Drs Morrey, Beauchamp, Huddleston, Peterson, Swiontkowski, and Trigg

Year Book of Otolaryngology-Head and Neck Surgery®: Drs Paparella, Gapany, and Keefe

Year Book of Pathology and Laboratory Medicine®: Drs Raab, Parwani, Bejarano, and Bissell

Year Book of Pediatrics®: Dr Stockman

Year Book of Plastic and Aesthetic Surgery™: Drs Miller, Bartlett, Garner, McKinney, Ruberg, Salisbury, and Smith

2008

The Year Book of PEDIATRICS®

Editor
James A. Stockman III, MD
President, The American Board of Pediatrics; Clinical Professor of Pediatrics, University of North Carolina Medical School at Chapel Hill, and Duke University Medical Center, Durham, North Carolina

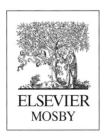

ELSEVIER
MOSBY

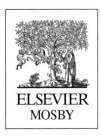

ELSEVIER
MOSBY

Vice President, Continuity: John A. Schrefer
Editor: Carla Holloway
Production Supervisor, Electronic Year Books: Donna M. Adamson
Electronic Article Manager: Jennifer C. Pitts
Illustrations and Permissions Coordinator: Linda Jones

2008 EDITION

Printed in the United States of America
Composition by Thomas Technology Solutions, Inc
Printing/binding by Sheridan Books, Inc.

Editorial Office:
Elsevier
Suite 1800
1600 John F. Kennedy Blvd.
Philadelphia, PA 19103-2899

International Standard Serial Number: 0084-3954
International Standard Book Number: 978-1-4160-5161-9

Table of Contents

Journals Represented

Journals represented in this YEAR BOOK are listed below.

Acta Paediatrica
Annals of Internal Medicine
Archives of Disease in Childhood
Archives of Disease in Childhood. Fetal and Neonatal Edition
Archives of Pediatrics and Adolescent Medicine
British Journal of Urology International
British Medical Journal
Clinical Pediatrics
Diabetes Care
Journal of Adolescent Health
Journal of Child Psychology and Psychiatry, and Allied Disciplines
Journal of Clinical Neuroscience
Journal of Developmental and Behavioral Pediatrics
Journal of Pediatric Gastroenterology and Nutrition
Journal of Pediatric Hematology/Oncology
Journal of Pediatric Ophthalmology and Strabismus
Journal of Pediatric Orthopaedics
Journal of Pediatric Orthopaedics Part B
Journal of Pediatric Surgery
Journal of Pediatrics
Journal of the American Academy of Child and Adolescent Psychiatry
Journal of the American Medical Association
Lancet
Neurology
New England Journal of Medicine
Otolaryngology - Head and Neck Surgery
Pediatric Cardiology
Pediatric Emergency Care
Pediatric Infectious Disease Journal
Pediatrics

STANDARD ABBREVIATIONS

The following terms are abbreviated in this edition: acquired immunodeficiency syndrome (AIDS), cardiopulmonary resuscitation (CPR), central nervous system (CNS), cerebrospinal fluid (CSF), computed tomography (CT), deoxyribonucleic acid (DNA), electrocardiography (ECG), health maintenance organization (HMO), human immunodeficiency virus (HIV), intensive care unit (ICU), intramuscular (IM), intravenous (IV), magnetic resonance (MR) imaging (MRI), ribonucleic acid (RNA), ultrasound (US), and ultraviolet (UV).

NOTE

To facilitate the use of the YEAR BOOK OF PEDIATRICS® as a reference tool, all illustrations and tables included in this publication are now identified as they appear in the original article. This change is meant to help the reader recognize that any illustration or table appearing in the YEAR BOOK OF PEDIATRICS® may be only one of many in the original article. For this reason, figure and table numbers will often appear to be out of sequence within the YEAR BOOK OF PEDIATRICS.®

Introduction

As one looks through this edition and past editions of the YEAR BOOK OF PEDIATRICS, one can see that some articles selected for inclusion in the YEAR BOOK, while not earthshaking, provide quite useful tips to assist the clinician in his or her daily practice. Other selections, however, serve as reports that may in time prove to be truly important and will likely be quoted for years to come. In this 2008 YEAR BOOK OF PEDIATRICS, in the former category are subjects such as the common flatfoot (see Chapter 12, Musculoskeletal), "googling" for a differential diagnosis (see Chapter 11, Miscellaneous), and how you can effectively treat head lice with a common household hair dryer (see Chapter 2, Allergy and Dermatology). Included in the latter category, you will find descriptions of the effects of maternal smoking during pregnancy on an offspring's cognitive ability (see Chapter 4, Child Development), the results of an international trial of the Edmonton Protocol using islet cell transplantation for type 1 diabetes (see Chapter 6, Endocrinology), and how the use of skin products containing lavender oil can be a serious cause of prepubertal gynecomastia (see Chapter 19, Therapeutics and Toxicology). Novel therapies, especially ones on the cutting edge, also capture this editor's imagination and are at increased risk for inclusion in the YEAR BOOK. Take, for example, reports on the use of oral fingolimod (FTY 720) for relapsing multiple sclerosis (see Chapter 13, Neurology and Psychiatry); AMG 531, a thrombopoiesis-stimulating protein, for chronic ITP (see Chapter 3, Blood); and activated drotrechogin alpha in children with severe sepsis (see Chapter 10, Infectious Diseases and Immunology).

Each year also sees reported the demise of some old faithful treatments. Witness, for example, the article in Chapter 2, Allergy and Dermatology, that dug the grave for duct tape as a treatment for the common wart . . . but you probably already tried the sticky stuff and knew that already, didn't you?

As you read through this YEAR BOOK OF PEDIATRICS, please do not give blanket acceptance to the conclusions of some of the studies reported or the durability, and perhaps reliability, of the editor's comments. Only time is the best judge of either of these. Take for example a read of the now 50-year-old 1958-1959 YEAR BOOK OF PEDIATRICS, edited by the always-masterful Sidney Gellis. Fifty years creates a long retrospectoscope indeed, and such a long interval illustrates how some editorial opinions would be better printed with ink that fades with time. In the Premature and Newborn chapter, it was recommended that given the risks of exchange transfusions at the time, it is best to wait until the bilirubin level rises to greater than 20 mg/100 mL before exchange transfusion is undertaken in tiny preterm babies, or it was suggested that the only practical solution for deciding when to perform an exchange transfusion is to wait for the "first signs of bilirubin encephalopathy" (1958-1959 YEAR BOOK OF PEDIATRICS, p 32). There was also a suggestion that a rise in bilirubin level to 20 mg/100 mL in the first 12 hours of life was the best predictor of a need for exchange transfusion (p 37). The 1958-1959 YEAR BOOK also commented liberally on the subject of staphylococcal infection in the newborn period and how the problem could be minimized by daily infant bathing with hexachlorophene (p 55), now known to be a serious cause of brain damage at this age.

Even as long as 50 years ago, the YEAR BOOK plucked the pithy pearls from the literature to help the busy pediatrician practice better medicine. Take the following from a commentary on page 95 of the 1958-1959 YEAR BOOK : "This is another of the many 'pearls' easily forgotten, but worth remembering . . . the triad association of hiatus hernia, mental deficiency, and sucrosuria appears too frequent to be merely coincidental." The latter "pearl" was almost as enduring as duct tape as a treatment for warts, as it was subsequently learned that the triad of findings was indeed a coincidence. It will be interesting to see in 2058 whether parents will be using hair dryers to rid their kids' scalps of lice.

Please do not get the sense that the 50-year-old YEAR BOOK OF PEDIATRICS was always off base with its commentaries. Take for example the insightful comment from Dr Gellis that unknowingly foreshadowed the development of collaborative office-based research (such as what we see now with the American Academy of Pediatrics' "PROSE" Network). Dr Gellis commented on a report by a private pediatrician who described a comparative study of temperatures taken orally, rectally, or axillary. He wrote "This paper illustrates well the fact that the busy practitioner can in this age of complicated technical research continue to make definite contributions to medical knowledge . . . the value of observation and documentation by the practicing physician remains of paramount importance" (1958-1959 YEAR BOOK OF PEDIATRICS, p 470). Each of us can indeed make a difference.

Hopefully the information contained in this year's YEAR BOOK OF PEDIATRICS will have a long half-life and, more importantly, that no one will be harmed by any recommendations that are later shown to be less than correct. Fortunately, the human body is fairly resilient and can handle most therapeutic misadventures. There is an old saying in this regard: *"A strong heart and a good set of kidneys are the best security against an ill-informed physician."* With these caveats in mind, read on and enjoy the 2008 YEAR BOOK OF PEDIATRICS.

J.A. Stockman III, MD

1 Adolescent Medicine

Adolescents' Reported Consequences of Having Oral Sex Versus Vaginal Sex
Brady SS, Halpern-Felsher BL (Univ of California San Francisco)
Pediatrics 119:229-236, 2007

Objective.—The present study examined whether adolescents' initial consequences of sexual activity differ according to type of sexual activity and gender.

Methods.—Surveys were administered to 618 adolescents recruited from 2 public high schools in the autumn of ninth grade (2002) and at 6-month intervals until the spring of tenth grade (2004). Analyses were limited to the 275 adolescents (44%) who reported engaging in oral sex and/or vaginal sex at any assessment. Participants were 14 years of age at study entry, 56% female, and of diverse socioeconomic and ethnic backgrounds.

Results.—In comparison with adolescents who engaged in oral sex and/or vaginal sex, adolescents who engaged only in oral sex were less likely to report experiencing a pregnancy or sexually transmitted infection, feeling guilty or used, having their relationship become worse, and getting into trouble with their parents as a result of sex. Adolescents who engaged only in oral sex were also less likely to report experiencing pleasure, feeling good about themselves, and having their relationship become better as a result of sex. Boys were more likely than girls to report feeling good about themselves, experiencing popularity, and experiencing a pregnancy or sexually transmitted infection as a result of sex, whereas girls were more likely than boys to report feeling bad about themselves and feeling used.

Conclusions.—Adolescents experience a range of social and emotional consequences after having sex. Our findings have implications for clinical practice and public health campaigns targeted toward youth.

▶ Oral sex, by virtue of its high prevalence among adolescents and its potential negative consequences, is both a medical and a public health issue. By the end of ninth grade, studies have shown that 1 of 5 adolescents has engaged in oral sex. Between the ages of 15 and 19 years, more than half of male and female adolescents have engaged in oral sex. More than 50% of predominantly heterosexual adolescents have had oral sex before their first experience of vaginal intercourse. Few adolescents who engage in oral sex are using barrier protection against sexually transmitted diseases. This is largely because adolescents expect that oral sex results in fewer physical health risks (eg, pregnancy or sexually transmitted infection) and social and emotional risks (eg, relationship becoming worse, gaining a bad reputation, or feeling guilty) in comparison with vaginal sex. No study, however, has identified the consequences of oral sex that adolescents actually experience nor has any study examined whether these consequences differ from those of vaginal sex, at least until this article by Brady et al appeared. The article involves surveys of more than 600 adolescents from 2 public schools; surveys were undertaken in the autumn of the 9th grade with 6-month interval follow-ups until the spring of the 10th grade. The results from the surveys generally support adolescents' expectations that oral sex is associated with fewer negative consequences in comparison with vaginal sex. Adolescents engaging in oral sex felt less guilty or "used" in comparison to their peers who had engaged in vaginal sex.

From the data presented in this article, one might be tempted to conclude that engagement in oral sex among adolescents is of less concern than involvement in other forms of sexual activity. This conclusion is not warranted. Engagement in oral sex is not without its negative consequences. Approximately one third of adolescents who had only oral sex reported negative feelings about their sexual behavior. Adolescents who had only oral sex were less likely than their peers with vaginal sexual experiences to report pleasure, feeling good about themselves, and having their relationship become better as a result of having had the oral sex. Thus, the decision to engage in this type of sexual activity may result in negative and emotional consequences or failure to experience anticipated positive consequences. Girls appear to be especially at risk of having these negative social and emotional feelings. Girls were nearly 2 times as likely as boys to report feeling bad about themselves as a result of their sexual behavior. In contrast, boys were twice as likely as girls to report positive social and emotional consequences of having sex, including gaining popularity and feeling good about themselves.

The data from this article are consistent with national statistics showing that large numbers of adolescents are engaging in oral sexual activity. In the sample surveyed, almost half of adolescents had engaged in oral and/or vaginal sex by the spring of the 10th grade. Of the sexually experienced adolescents in this study, one third of boys and one half of girls reported engaging only in oral sex at the first time they had a sexual experience.

The major implications of the findings of this study are that sexual education and health promotion interventions should focus on oral sex as well as vaginal sex and that interventions should focus on the social and emotional consequences that adolescents experience, as well as the physical health consequences of such sexual experiences. Needless to say, we are grateful that there is a discipline within pediatrics known as adolescent medicine in which professionals are specifically trained to deal with these types of issues to help us implement programs for teens that positively assist them in their early maturing years.

J. A. Stockman III, MD

Patterns of Oral Contraceptive Pill-taking and Condom Use among Adolescent Contraceptive Pill Users

Woods JL, Shew ML, Tu W, et al (Indiana Univ, Indianapolis)
J Adolesc Health 39:381-387, 2006

Purpose.—Imperfect oral contraceptive pill (OCP) regimen adherence may impair contraceptive effectiveness. The purpose of this study was to describe daily adherence patterns of OCP use, to analyze OCP protection on an event level basis, and to examine pill-taking and condom use during method transitions.

Methods.—Women (n = 123, ages 14–17 years) completed quarterly interviews to classify OCP method choice into four categories: stable, initiated, stopped, and discordant use. Within each OCP category, daily diaries were used to assess occurrence of coitus, condom use, and patterns of day-to-day OCP use (i.e., consecutive days of OCP use reported with no more than two consecutive days of nonuse). A coital event was OCP protected if pills were used on both the day of the coitus and the day preceding.

Results.—There were 123 participants who reported at least some OCP use in 210 diary periods (average diary length = 75.5 days). Fifty-three participants categorized as stable users reported 87 diary periods: the average interval of consecutive OCP use in this group was 32.5 days. Among stable users, only 45% of coital events were associated with both OCP and condom use. Over one-fifth of coital events in all groups were protected by no method of contraception.

Conclusion.—Dual use of OCP and barrier contraception remains an elusive goal. The time during OCP adoption or discontinuation is often unprotected by condoms. However, concurrent missed pills and condom nonuse increase pregnancy and infection risk even among stable OCP users. Understanding motivation for method usage may improve education and prevention techniques.

▶ This is a quite revealing report and shows the challenges we face in the care of teens when trying to counsel about effective contraception and protection against sexually transmitted diseases. If there is good news here, it is that this study shows many young women effectively manage the dual demands of pregnancy and sexually transmitted disease prevention. This means the use of oral contraceptives along with condoms. The challenging aspect of the report is that too many young women are at risk, especially during transitions into or out of periods of oral contraceptive use. Even for young women who are in a stable period of oral contraceptive use, some still have daily pill-taking patterns that are inconsistent in the prevention of pregnancy risk. When the pill is used correctly, failure rates with respect to pregnancy are under 1%. Nonetheless, imperfect use contributes to an average failure rate as high as 30%. Over 60% of contraception users switch their method of contraception at some point and, as this report shows, this is an especially risky transition for adequate protection against either pregnancy or sexually transmitted diseases.

We see from this study that about 50% of young women report imperfect pill use during a pill cycle. One in four women misses two or more pills during an oral contraceptive cycle. The overall proportion of unprotected coital events rises even higher when a woman is starting or stopping a particular form of contraception, including the use of the pill.

The Rickert VI report (Depo Now: preventing unintended pregnancies among adolescents and young adults) tells us about depot medroxyprogesterone acetate (DMPA), an injectable progestational agent that offers a highly effective, safe, convenient, and reversible method of contraception. Despite the World Health Organization's recommendation that the time of initiation of hormonal contraception need not be restricted to menstruation, most clinical protocols as well as product labeling require adolescent patients to wait until their next menses to receive agents such as DMPA. Thus, contraception in the form of condoms or, better still, abstinence is required in the interim. The reason for the delay has to do with the theoretical risks of hormonal contraception should a young lady be pregnant at the time of its administration, the risk being to the fetus. There is no evidence, however, to support this delay as a necessity.

J. A. Stockman III, MD

Depo Now: Preventing Unintended Pregnancies among Adolescents and Young Adults
Rickert VI, Tiezzi L, Lipshutz J, et al (Columbia Univ, New York)
J Adolesc Health 40:22-28, 2007

Purpose.—We compared the immediate administration of DMPA (Depo Now) to the immediate use of short-term hormonal methods that served as a "bridge method" until later DMPA initiation. We examined whether Depo Now, as compared to initiating with a bridge method (pills, transdermal patch, or vaginal ring), resulted in greater DMPA continuation at six months.

Methods.—Young women aged 14 to 26 years seeking to use DMPA were randomized (nonblinded) after meeting eligibility criteria to either the Depo Now (n = 101) or bridge method (n = 232) group. Depo Now subjects received their first injection of DMPA at the conclusion of their first visit provided each was medically suitable and had a negative urine pregnancy test regardless of menstrual cycle day. Those assigned to the bridge method group were allowed to choose their starting contraceptive method and it was provided at the first visit. All subjects were told to return to the clinic in 21 days to repeat the urine pregnancy test, and among those who were assigned to use a bridge method, to receive their first injection of DMPA. All subjects were followed to their third injection, or about 6 months later.

Results.—Those randomized to a bridge method were 1.8 (1.1, 2.9) times more likely than Depo Now subjects to return for their 21-day repeat pregnancy test, but only 55% (n = 125) of these young women actually received their first DMPA injection. Continuation rates at the third injection were 29.7% (n = 30) for those in the Depo Now group and 21.1% (n = 49) for those assigned to the bridge method ($p = .09$). Three factors were significantly associated with adherence to the third injection: randomized to Depo Now group, knowing more women who use DMPA, and returning to clinic for the 21-day repeat pregnancy test visit. Finally, 28 pregnancies were diagnosed during the study period, and those in the bridge method group were almost 4.0 (1.2, 13.4) times more likely to be diagnosed with a pregnancy than those in the Depo Now group.

Conclusions.—Immediate administration of DMPA is associated with improved adherence to DMPA continuation and fewer pregnancies.

▶ If one looks at teen pregnancy rates here in the United States, there is some good news. The incidence of teen pregnancy has been declining over the last decade or more. It is encouraging that less sexual activity accounts for some of this decrease. However, the majority of the decline among United States teens is attributable to the growing use of long-acting hormonal contraceptives, particularly depot medroxyprogesterone acetate (Depo-Provera, DMPA; Pfizer, New York, New York). A 2002 National Survey of Family Growth observed that as of that year, 21% of sexually experienced teens had used DMPA, a doubling of the rate of the use of this contraceptive method since 1995.[1] According to Steven-Simon et al, when comparing the use of Norplant, DMPA, oral contraceptives, and no contraception over a 6-month period, pregnancy rates respectively were at 0%, 4%, 14%, and 23%, respectively.[2]

So what do we know about DMPA? Long-acting hormonal contraceptives cause menstrual changes in all users. After initiating DMPA, users experience unpredictable spotting or light bleeding and, by 1 year of use (4 injections), some 70% of users will be amenorrheic. In contrast, the unpredictable spotting and/or light bleeding that accompany the use of agents such as Implanon persist as long as women use this contraceptive. Candid proactive counseling about these menstrual irregularities results in greater acceptance of DMPA and implant continuation. Be aware that during the use of DMPA, ovarian estradiol production declines, leading to decreases in bone mineral density. This side effect led the Food and Drug Administration to issue a Black Box warning regarding skeletal health and injectable contraception, a warning that has made some clinicians, patients, and parents reluctant to initiate or continue DMPA birth control. Fortunately, bone mineral density completely recovers after teens and adults discontinue the injections. Most studies have suggested that the use of DMPA is not linked to a later occurrence of osteoporosis or fracture. The Society for Adolescent Medicine has a position paper recommending continued prescription of DMPA for most adolescents. Likewise, the American College of Obstetricians and Gynecologists tell us that the advantages of DMPA likely outweigh the theoretical safety concerns regarding bone mineral density and fracture.

What we see in the report from New York City is an approach called "Quick Start" to contraceptive induction for teens. Quick Start refers to immediate, in-office initiation of oral contraceptive tablets in individuals with negative pregnancy tests, regardless of at what point they are in their menstrual cycle. This immediate initiation approach has been used with the vaginal contraceptive ring. When the alternative is to use DMPA, the authors actually prefer the

"Depo Now" approach, which allows patients with a negative pregnancy test to receive their first DMPA injection at the current office visit rather than return on their next menses for their injection. All patients were asked to return in 3 weeks for a repeat urine pregnancy test and for those randomized to a bridge contraceptive to receive their initial DMPA injection. All patients were far less likely to conceive during the study period in comparison to controls receiving delayed introduction of contraception until the onset of the next menses.

To read more about long-acting hormonal contraceptives and how they can be started, see the important editorial of Kaunitz.[3] Kaunitz believes that along with expediting the initial injection of agents such as DMPA, flexible approaches to follow-up injections will increase a patient's contraceptive success. Package labeling specifies that DMPA intramuscular injection patients return every 3 months for repeat injections. Some practices forbid follow-up injections occurring earlier than 12 or later than 14 weeks after the previous injection. In the real world of patient care, many women return for repeat injections outside this window. For example, if a DMPA user returns for an injection at 9, 10, or 11 weeks after her prior injection, immediate reinjection is more appropriate than not giving the injection in terms of overall likelihood of protection. Likewise, reinjection after a negative urine pregnancy test is also appropriate for DMPA users who present more than 14 weeks after their last injection, similar to the approach that you would use at the time of an initial visit.

Without saying, long-acting hormonal contraceptives represent the most important tool, other than abstinence, in our ongoing endeavor to prevent teen pregnancy. Clinicians who provide their adolescent patients ready access to injectable and implantable contraception and facilitate initiation and ongoing use of these methods will be taking an important step toward improving the health and well-being of their teenage patients, their families, and our society.

J. A. Stockman III, MD

References

1. Centers for Disease Control and Prevention. Teenagers in the United States: sexual activity, contraceptive use, and child bearing, 2002—a fact sheet for series 23, Number 24. CDC Web site. Available at: http://www.cdc.gov/nchs/data/series/sr_23/sr23_024FactSheet.pdf. Accessed May 28, 2007.
2. Stevens-Simon C, Kelly L, Kulick R. A village would be nice . . . but it takes a long-acting contraception to prevent repeat adolescent pregnancies. *Am J Prev Med.* 2001;21:60-65.
3. Kaunitz AM. Long-acting hormonal contraceptives—indispensable in preventing teen pregnancies. *J Adolesc Health.* 2007;40:1-3.

Has Age at Menarche Changed? Results from the National Health and Nutrition Examination Survey (NHANES) 1999–2004
McDowell MA, Brody DJ, Hughes JP (US Dept of Health and Human Services, Hyattsville, Md)
J Adolesc Health 40:227-231, 2007

Purpose.—To examine self-reported age at menarche in U.S. adults and the associations between age at menarche and race/ethnicity.

Methods.—Data from 1999–2004 National Health and Nutrition Examination Survey (NHANES) for 6788 females 20 years and over were analyzed. Self-reported age at first menses (in years) by birth year groups is reported overall and for Mexican Americans, non-Hispanic whites, and non-Hispanic blacks.

Results.—Mean age at menarche in the United States declined over time from 13.3 years (95% CI: 13.2–13.5) in the oldest age group, those born prior to 1920, to 12.4 years (95% C.I. 12.2–12.5 years) in the youngest group, born between 1980 and 1984. Declines in age at menarche were observed for all race/ethnicity groups. Non-Hispanic black females had the largest decline in mean age at menarche from 13.6 years (95% CI: 13.1–14.1) in women born prior to 1920, to 12.2 years (95% CI: 11.8–12.6) in the 1980–84 birth cohort. Mean age at menarche among non-Hispanic white females declined from 13.3 years (13.1–13.6) in the pre-1920 birth cohort to 12.5 years (12.3–12.8) in the 1980–84 birth cohort.

Conclusions.—Significant declines in the mean age of menarche for U.S. females occurred overall and for all race/ethnic groups examined. Mean age of menarche declined by .9 year overall in women born before 1920 compared to women born in 1980–84; the declines in the mean age at menarche ranged from .7 to 1.4 years depending on the race/ethnicity group.

▶ Here is another report summarizing recent findings documenting the decline in the age of menarche in the United States. The report of McDowell et al approaches the menarcheal age—secular trend question—in a novel though arguably less reliable way. Using the National Health and Nutrition Examination Survey (NHANES) data collected from 1999 to 2004, the authors analyzed self-reported age at first menses, determining the mean age of menarche for women now older than 80 years down to women 20 years old, grouped into 10-year cohorts. This technique has provided the first published data on Mexican-American women in the United States over an 80+-year span. Until recently, menarche studies did not include this ethnic group. They also report on non-Hispanic whites and blacks. Mean age for Mexican-American women decreased by 12 months from the pre-1920 cohort to the 1980 to 1984 cohort, and by almost 10 months for whites and by almost 15 months for blacks. All decreases were statistically significant.

One legitimately has to ask the question if the data are so clear about this decrease in age of menarche, why is there such a controversy about the validity of the data? Controversy over this subject has a long history. Because the menarcheal age varies according to the organism's response to environment (including diet), socioeconomic, social, climactic, genetic, and pre- and post-natal factors, among others, the age of menarche will always be in flux. Decades ago, when Tanner's well-known graph showing marked declines in menarcheal age from a number of western countries, including the United States, was published, an objection appeared in *Science*. This was back in 1981. In the United States, it had been thought that after the 1950s, the age of puberty and menarche had become stabilized. When the Pediatric Research in Office Settings (PROS) study from the American Academy of Pediatrics was published challenging this assumption, more controversy ensued. Since then, menarche data from NHANES have proven to be more accurate than the PROS data and have also showed consistent decline in age of menarche.

There currently are many theories about why the age of menarche is, in fact, changing. One of the major contributors seems to be the epidemic of overweight in our United States school children. The association between overweight and earlier age of puberty and menarche is supported by hundreds of studies going as far back as the 17th century. Sedentary lifestyle, growing up in a home without a father, being born small for gestational age, and having a diet high in protein and low in fiber have also been correlated with a decrease in the age of menarche.

The real issue regarding changes in age of menarche is whether it matters if girls are developing earlier. The answer is probably yes, it does. Early puberty is associated with a number of negative psychosocial and health outcomes. For example, the risk of breast cancer is increased with earlier menarche. Even though youngsters may be developing earlier physically, cognitive, and emotional maturity dose not keep pace with this. The disparity between physical maturity and social/emotional maturity grows even greater decade by decade.

It is well worth your time to read the excellent commentary on the subject of a decreasing age of menarche by Marsha Herman-Giddens.[1] Dr Herman-Giddens argues that somewhere in the 1960s the factors contributing to the decline in menarcheal age changed from positive ones, such as better nutrition and less infectious disease, to negative ones, such as overweight, physical activity decline, and chemical pollution. Thus, mean ages for pubertal characteristics do not necessarily denote a "normal" state. What is truly normal in an otherwise "normal" society remains to be seen. Presumably, age of menarche cannot contribute to decline indefinitely.

A few closing comments on the topic of menstruation. Menstrual suppression has been recommended for medical conditions such as endometriosis, but it is also being proposed as a lifestyle choice for women who dislike menstruation or find it inconvenient. For example, there are newer contraceptive methods that combine 84 days of active contraceptive pills (0.03mg ethinyl estradiol and 0.15mg levonorgestrel) with 7 days of placebo. Since menstrual flow occurs during the pill-free interval, a hormone-free interval every 3 months instead of the usual 21 days reduces the number of pill-induced periods from 13 to 4 annually. If you want to read more about this particular contraceptive, see the pharmaceutical Web site: http://www.seasonale.com. The contraceptive allowing menstruation just every 3 months is known as Seasonale, and it has been approved by the Food and Drug Administration. Unfortunately, long-term research was not required for approval of this agent.

You can decide how desirable it is or is not to have a "natural" cycle of menses. The case against menstruation was laid out in a book titled *Is Menstruation Obsolete?*[2] The authors argue that monthly menstruation throughout most of adult life is actually a modern development. In industrial societies, the average woman has few children and therefore may have 450 menstrual cycles throughout a lifetime. Women in hunter-gatherer cultures and other societies without birth control average just 160 periods because they are either pregnant or breast feeding much of the time and, the authors assert, exemplify what was natural in the prehistoric past when human bodies evolved and throughout most of human history. The authors suggest that monthly menstruation throughout adulthood is therefore at odds with what female bodies were designed to do and therefore is unnecessary and unnatural. To read more on this topic, see the interesting perspective of Paula Derry.[3] Dr Derry is a health psychologist who believes the argument that menstruation is obsolete is both illogical and unscientific. Even if prolonged monthly menstruation were unnatural and unhealthy, this is not an indicator that suppressing menstruation is actually any healthier. Menstrual suppression itself for many is an unnatural act requiring a drug that chronically overrides the physiological changes associated with the menstrual cycle, thereby creating an unnatural hormonal environment that is not found in nature, so says Dr Derry.

J. A. Stockman III, MD

References

1. Herman-Giddens ME. The decline in the age of menarche in the United States: should we be concerned? *J Adolesc Health*. 2007;40:201-203.
2. Coutinho EM, Segal SJ. *Is Menstruation Obsolete?*. Oxford, United Kingdom: Oxford University Press; 1999.
3. Derry PS. Is menstruation obsolete? *BMJ*. 2007;334:955.

Condom Use and the Risk of Genital Human Papillomavirus Infection in Young Women
Winer RL, Hughes JP, Feng Q, et al (Univ of Washington, Seattle)
N Engl J Med 354:2645-2654, 2006

Background.—To evaluate whether the use of male condoms reduces the risk of male-to-female transmission of human papillomavirus (HPV) infection, longitudinal studies explicitly designed to evaluate the temporal relationship between condom use and HPV infection are needed.

Methods.—We followed 82 female university students who reported their first intercourse with a male partner either during the study period or within two weeks before enrollment. Cervical and vulvovaginal samples for HPV

DNA testing and Papanicolaou testing were collected at gynecologic examinations every four months. Every two weeks, women used electronic diaries to record information about their daily sexual behavior. Cox proportional-hazards models were used to evaluate risk factors for HPV infection.

Results.—The incidence of genital HPV infection was 37.8 per 100 patient-years at risk among women whose partners used condoms for all instances of intercourse during the eight months before testing, as compared with 89.3 per 100 patient-years at risk in women whose partners used condoms less than 5 percent of the time (adjusted hazard ratio, 0.3; 95 percent confidence interval, 0.1 to 0.6, adjusted for the number of new partners and the number of previous partners of the male partner). Similar associations were observed when the analysis was restricted to high-risk and low-risk types of HPV and HPV types 6, 11, 16, and 18. In women reporting 100 percent condom use by their partners, no cervical squamous intraepithelial lesions were detected in 32 patient-years at risk, whereas 14 incident lesions were detected during 97 patient-years at risk among women whose partners did not use condoms or used them less consistently.

Conclusions.—Among newly sexually active women, consistent condom use by their partners appears to reduce the risk of cervical and vulvovaginal HPV infection.

▶ This report is a real standout. Prior studies have suggested that the use of condoms by men offer women little, if any, protection against genital HPV infection. The study of Winer et al, however, trumps all prior studies because of the solid way in which the study was designed and clearly suggests male condoms effectively reduce the risk of male-to-female genital HPV transmission. Specifically, women whose partners use condoms for all instances of vaginal intercourse during the previous 8 months are 70% less likely to acquire a new infection than were women whose partners use condoms less than 5% of the time; all other factors were taken into account. Even women whose partners use condoms just over 50% of the time experience a 50% risk reduction compared with those partners who use condoms less than 5% of the time. Also observed was an inverse association between frequency of condom use and the incidence of cervical squamous intraepithelial lesions. No such lesions were detected among women reporting 100% condom use by their partners during the previous 8 months, whereas there were 14 lesions detected (14.5 per 100 patient-years at risk) among women whose partners use condoms less consistently or never use condoms. It should be noted that the women recruited to this study were newly sexually active, reporting a yearly median number of instances of intercourse of 48 and a yearly median number of new partners of just one. These data suggest that starting off on the right foot can indeed help protect women beginning to engage in sexual activity.

Of course, for condoms to work they have to be used properly. A recent study has shown that many young people using condoms often do so in a way that is not properly protective. Of 1,373 teenagers, age 16 to 18 years, 375 reported engaging in vaginal sex using condoms. Of these, 108 were asked to keep a diary of sexual encounters over 6 months. In almost 10% of sexual encounters, a condom was applied after initial penetration, and in 2% of cases, a condom was removed early. In all, nearly a third of respondents recalled at least one episode of inadequate use. The teens were more likely to rely on other methods of contraception; intriguingly, young men who reported a close maternal relationship in their early teenage years were more likely to use condoms efficiently.[1] Explain that one!

While on the subject of condoms, one of the oldest condoms ever discovered by archeologists was on display at the Tyrolean County Museum in Innsbruck, Austria, as part of an exhibition titled the "Cultural History of Sex." Dating from about 1650, it was shown with 4 other condom fragments from the same date, all found in a cesspit at Dudley Castle in England. Curators gathered objects from 60 sites in 9 different countries for the display, which ran throughout the summer of 2006. The collection included several ancient condoms, most of which were made from animal intestines. The collection also included a reusable condom made from pig intestine and dated 1813. This was found in Lund in Sweden. It was discovered with a user's manual, written in Latin, recommending that the user immerse the condom in warm milk before engaging in intercourse "to avoid diseases when sleeping with prostitutes."[2]

J. A. Stockman III, MD

References

1. Hatherall B, Ingham R, Stone N, McEachran J. How, not just if, condoms are used: the timing of condom application and removal during vaginal sex among young people in England. *Sex Transm Infect.* 2007;83:68-70.
2. Leidig M. Condom from Cromwell's time goes on display. *BMJ.* 2006;333:10.

Improving women's experience during speculum examinations at routine gynaecological visits: randomised clinical trial

Seehusen DA, Johnson DR, Earwood JS, et al (Eisenhower Army Med Ctr, Fort Gordon, Ga; Augusta State Univ, Ga)
BMJ 333:171-174, 2006

Objectives.—To determine if a standardised method of leg positioning without stirrups reduces the physical discomfort and sense of vulnerability and increases the sense of control among women undergoing speculum examination as part of a routine gynaecological examination.

Design.—Randomised clinical trial.

Setting.—Family medicine outpatient clinic.

Patients.—197 adult women undergoing routine gynaecological examination and cervical smear.

Intervention.—Examination with or without stirrups.

Main Outcome Measures.—Women's perceived levels of physical discomfort, sense of vulnerability, and sense of control during the examination, measured on 100 mm visual analogue scales.

Results.—Women undergoing examination without stirrups had a reduction in mean sense of vulnerability from 23.6 to 13.1 (95% confidence interval of the difference − 16.6 to − 4.4). Mean physical discomfort was reduced from 30.4 to 17.2 (− 19.7 to − 6.8). There was no significant reduction in sense of loss of control.

Conclusion.—Women should be able to have gynaecological examinations without using stirrups to reduce the stress associated with speculum examinations.

▶ Here in the United States, we are trained to perform gynecologic examinations on women in the dorsal lithotomy position using stirrups, whereas in countries such as the United Kingdom, Australia, and New Zealand, speculum examinations are performed without stirrups using the dorsal or lateral positions. The pelvic examination using a vaginal speculum is something all medical students are trained to do, and in certain areas of pediatric practice, this is a routine examination. ER physicians do such examinations frequently and some physicians in office practice, depending on the type of practice one has, would also do this.

The article from Georgia raises the possibility that the routine use of stirrups may not be best for patients, and that other positioning options should be considered. When this editor first read the report, my initial reaction was probably similar to others reading this report and that is, how would such an examination actually work? Indeed, it does work as attested to by tens of thousands of physicians who perform nonstirrup vaginal examinations throughout most of the rest of the world. It would seem that women who have speculum examinations without stirrups report less discomfort and feelings of vulnerability than do women who have examinations with stirrups. The study from Georgia seems to be of high quality with adequate randomization, reasonable inclusion and exclusion criteria, and adequate follow-up by the investigators who recorded and reported the outcome measures. If there is a problem with the report, it is that the patient population was a somewhat homogenous one, coming from among those in the military. Nonetheless, the report raises the question of whether physicians who routinely perform speculum examinations should consider changing their practice to offer a more patient-centered option without stirrups. It is fairly clear that a significant proportion of women do not like to have a pelvic examination performed, much less one where their feet are restricted in stirrups. A sense of vulnerability or defenselessness is one of the reasons why many women dislike a pelvic examination. Once a woman's feet are placed in stirrups, getting out is neither quick nor easy. Stirrups suspend the feet in the air and greatly reduce the ability to maneuver, which may give women a sense of being unable to protect themselves from potential danger. Women undergoing an examination without stirrups are much freer to adjust the position of their feet and hips during the examination.

It permits considerable internal or external rotation of the hips and knees as well as supination of the feet, allowing for greater comfort.

Old practices change slowly in medicine. I suspect that pediatricians are more likely than other providers to change their practice when it is clear that patients are more comfortable with an alternative. Last, be aware that a recent report has shown that the widespread practice of not lubricating plastic vaginal speculums because of fears of interfering with bacteriologic sample processing has been shown to be invalid. A water-based lubricant, Aquagel, was shown to have no effect on colony counts when different dilutions of *Neisseria gonorrhoeae* were cultured, nor did the gel alter the results of standard assays for *Chlamydia* spp. Without lubrication, plastic speculums are more difficult to insert and may cause more discomfort.[1]

J. A. Stockman III, MD

Reference

1. Kozakis L, Vuddamalay J, Munday P. Plastic specula: can we ease the passage? *Sex Transm Infect.* 2006;82:263-264.

Cervicitis: To Treat or Not To Treat? The Role of Patient Preferences and Decision Analysis

Sheeder J, Stevens-Simon C, Lezotte D, et al (Univ of Colorado, Denver)
J Adolesc Health 39:887-892, 2006

Purpose.—Mucopurulent cervicitis is neither a sensitive nor a specific indicator of antibiotic sensitive infection. This analysis examines the positive and negative ramifications of treating cervicitis empirically as a Chlamydial (CT) infection. It begins where prior analyses leave off, with the number of cases of pelvic inflammatory disease (PID) prevented.

Methods.—Three treatments were compared: 1) treat empirically/refer partner; 2) test, treat, and base partner treatment on results; 3) test, base treatment on results. The outcomes were the physical sequelae of PID and the psychological sequelae of being diagnosed with CT in a hypothetical cohort of 500 teenagers with cervicitis, among whom the prevalence of CT averaged 33%, but ranged between 10% and 70%.

Results.—At a CT prevalence of 33%, Treatments 1 and 2 prevented three times as many cases of PID-related physical sequelae (n = 14) as Treatment 3 (n = 5). However, to prevent these 14 cases of physical sequelae, with Treatment 1, 163 teens needlessly suffer the psychological sequelae of a false CT diagnosis and with Treatment 2, 101 do so. The ratio of physical sequelae prevented to psychological sequelae caused, changed in relationship to the prevalence of CT, but was always numerically most favorable with Treatment 3. Moreover, it was the only therapeutic approach for which overall morbidity never exceeded the PID-related physical morbidity incurred in the absence of treatment.

Conclusions.—By including the effects of over diagnosing and treating CT, we have demonstrated how the risks and benefits of empiric and nonempiric cervicitis therapy vary in relationship to CT prevalence. Failure to consider both the physical and the psychological aspects of patient well-being may mean that well-intentioned policies to reduce physical morbidity do not result in an overall improvement in health of teenagers.

▶ The authors of this report do us a service by defining mucopurulent cervicitis. It is a clinical syndrome characterized by erythema, edema, friability of the ectocervix, and purulent endocervical exudate. The 2 most common bacterial causes are *Chlamydia trachomatis* and *Neisseria gonorrhoeae*. Fewer than a third of women, however, with mucopurulent cervicitis will have *C trachomatis* or *N gonorrhoeae*. Also curious is that mucopurulent cervicitis often persists for weeks after documented eradication of these pathogens. It can be caused by other infectious and noninfectious agents. In practice, the question arises as to whether all individuals with mucopurulent cervicitis should be empirically treated for *Chlamydia* or *Neisseria*. Teenagers with mucopurulent cervicitis are especially apt to be treated empirically because they have a higher prevalence rate of sexually transmitted diseases and are especially vulnerable to the adverse reproductive consequences of having an untreated sexually transmitted disease. They also tend to be noncompliant with follow-up. However, taken together, the low positive predictive value of mucopurulent cervicitis for *C trachomatis* and *N gonorrhoeae* infections, the futility of treating index cases if their sexual networks are not treated, the adverse psychological effects of being diagnosed with a sexually transmitted disease, and the serious public health problem caused by the indiscriminate use of antibiotics all raise serious concerns about the wisdom of empirically treating this common gynecologic problem as a sexually transmitted disease.

Should all patients with mucopurulent cervicitis therefore be treated empirically? Decision analysis has been used to evaluate the financial cost of such an approach. PID, the most common sequela of *C trachomatis* and gonococcal cervicitis, develops in 10% to 40% of untreated women, but only 3% to 5% of treated women. Almost half of women who develop PID also develop costly complications ranging from chronic pelvic pain to ectopic pregnancy and infertility. Thus, most decision analyses favor empiric treatment of cervicitis. Unfortunately, these statistics deal with largely an adult population—thus the value of the report abstracted, which focuses on the adolescent population. The results of the study show that if all 500 patients with cervicitis were treated empirically with azithromycin and instructed to have their sexual partners treated, about 335 females would be overtreated, having no sexually transmitted disease as the cause of their problem. If you include treated partners, a total of 544 individuals would have been told they had a sexually transmitted disease when in fact they did not. Thus, a few hundred teenagers would have needlessly suffered the psychological sequelae of being told they had a sexually transmitted disease.

It is difficult to draw firm conclusions from this study since the actual prevalence of sexually transmitted diseases as a cause of cervicitis depends more precisely on the population of patients that you are serving. Nonetheless, the analysis provides a novel contribution, as it illustrates that there are significant costs as well as benefits to empirically treating mucopurulent cervicitis as a sexually transmitted disease. This is because most teenagers with this common physical finding do not have a treatable lower genital tract infection, and being diagnosed with a sexually transmitted disease can have damaging psychological effects. Mucopurulent cervicitis is a widely accepted trigger for sexually transmitted disease testing. However, there is far less consensus concerning how best to operationalize the Centers for Disease Control and Prevention's vague recommendation to treat cervicitis empirically if "the likelihood of infection with *Chlamydia* or gonorrhea is high, or the patient is unlikely to return for treatment." The study suggests that this is because there is no single optimal therapeutic approach. The authors have demonstrated the magnitude of the risk of developing physical and psychological sequelae depending upon the prevalence of *Chlamydia*, yet they are unable to select an "optimal" approach.

If there is any bottom line here, it is that despite the intuitive appeal of empiric therapy, the data from this analysis demonstrate that health care providers who fail to consider the negative ramifications of this therapeutic approach are apt to become victims of inadvertent consequences. The data from the report suggest that in most scenarios, empiric treatment of a teen increases overall morbidity if one includes both physical as well as psychological morbidity. Failure to consider the consequences of overtreatment may mean that well-intentioned policies to reduce physical morbidity do not lead to overall improvements in a teen's well-being.

What was not discussed in this report is empiric therapy, but without implying that a teen has a sexually transmitted disease, at least until the confirmatory reports determine whether the teen does indeed have either a chlamydial or gonococcal infection. This would seem to be the middle ground.

While on the topic of sexually transmitted infections, the history of research in this area, particularly having to do with syphilis, shows very little caution in the first studies of transmission of such diseases. It was William Wallace who first demonstrated the transmissibility of syphilis, for example, back in 1836. At that time, the infectivity of syphilis in its secondary stage was doubted by the medical community. Wallace set out to prove that the infection could be transmitted. By means of an inoculation of the "secretions from the exanthematic sores" of two patients with secondary syphilis into three "healthy subjects" and careful documentation by clinical observation, he was able to show the transmissibility of secondary syphilis during its incubation period. Wallace subsequently treated the inoculated patients with mercury and "cured them" of syphilis. These inoculations, of course, were indefensible even at that time. They were done on otherwise healthy people who were probably unaware of the nature of the experiments. Also unfortunate was the fact that his experiments were thought to be legitimate enough to be published in *The Lancet* in 1837.[1] Less than half a century after Wallace carried out his infamous experiments, in 1881, Robert Cory self-inoculated himself with syphilis by means of "lymph" obtained from a vaccination vesicle of a syphilitic infant.[2] Wallace clearly was a villain while Cory has been praised throughout history as a largely forgotten hero in the syphilis saga.

J. A. Stockman III, MD

References

1. Wallace W. Clinical lectures and remarks delivered on diseases of the skin, venereal diseases, and surgical cases, at the skin infirmary and at Jervis Street Hospital Dublin. *Lancet*. 1837;2:534-540.
2. Mortimer P. Robert Cory and the vaccine syphilis controversy: a forgotten hero? *Lancet*. 2006;367:1112-1115.

Fluoxetine After Weight Restoration in Anorexia Nervosa: A Randomized Controlled Trial

Walsh BT, Kaplan AS, Attia E, et al (Columbia Univ, New York; Univ of Toronto)
JAMA 295:2605-2612, 2006

Context.—Antidepressant medication is frequently prescribed for patients with anorexia nervosa.

Objective.—To determine whether fluoxetine can promote recovery and prolong time-to-relapse among patients with anorexia nervosa following weight restoration.

Design, Setting, and Participants.—Randomized, double-blind, placebo-controlled trial. From January 2000 until May 2005, 93 patients with anorexia nervosa received intensive inpatient or day-program treatment at the New York State Psychiatric Institute or Toronto General Hospital. Participants regained weight to a minimum body mass index (calculated as weight in kilograms divided by the square of height in meters) of 19.0 and were then eligible to participate in the randomized phase of the trial.

Interventions.—Participants were randomly assigned to receive fluoxetine or placebo and were treated for up to 1 year as outpatients in double-blind fashion. All patients also received individual cognitive behavioral therapy.

Main Outcome Measures.—The primary outcome measures were time-to-relapse and the proportion of patients successfully completing 1 year of treatment.

Results.—Forty-nine patients were assigned to fluoxetine and 44 to placebo. Similar percentages of patients assigned to fluoxetine and to placebo maintained a body mass index of at least 18.5 and remained in the study for 52 weeks (fluoxetine, 26.5%; placebo, 31.5%; $P = .57$). In a Cox proportional hazards analysis, with prerandomization body mass index, site, and diagnostic subtype as covariates, there was no significant difference between fluoxetine and placebo in time-to-relapse (hazard ratio, 1.12; 95% CI, 0.65-2.01; $P = .64$).

Conclusions.—This study failed to demonstrate any benefit from fluoxetine in the treatment of patients with anorexia nervosa following weight restoration. Future efforts should focus on developing new models to understand the persistence of this illness and on exploring new psychological and pharmacological treatment approaches.

▶ Recently there has been much interest in the use of serotonin reuptake inhibitors for acute treatment and relapse prevention in those affected with anorexia nervosa. Trials of acute treatment for those still at low weight with fluoxetine have failed to demonstrate clinical benefit. Trials of fluoxetine for anorexia nervosa relapse prevention have also shown mixed results. The study of Walsh et al reports the results of a placebo-controlled trial of fluoxetine in the relapse prevention treatment of anorexia nervosa. Participants were 93 women, including teenagers, who were completing multimodal inpatient or day hospital treatment and had weight restoration to a body mass index of at least 19. These patients were randomly assigned to either placebo or fluoxetine, with a total dosage goal of 60 mg/d. A total of 12 months of treatment was provided during which time all subjects received cognitive behavioral therapy. Relapse was defined as a weight loss to a body mass index of less than 16.5 or the development of medical complications or imminent suicide risk or the onset of severe psychiatric disorder.

Unfortunately, the data from this randomized trial do not support the efficacy of fluoxetine in relapse prevention for anorexia nervosa. In addition, premature study termination, mainly because of treatment failures and patient-initiated withdrawals was common, but the rate of premature termination did not differ between fluoxetine- and placebo-treated patients.

So what do we learn? What, if any, current role is there for medication treatment in anorexia nervosa? What we do learn is that there is little role for fluoxetine in the management of eating disorders. This does not mean that fluoxetine has no role. The drug does have well-established efficacy in bulimia nervosa.[1] It has been studied widely enough in obsessive-compulsive disorders to receive US Food and Drug Administration indication for that use. Given the seemingly close relationship of anorexia nervosa to this illness, it was reasonable to assume that fluoxetine might provide some benefit for patients affected with anorexia nervosa. The authors do speculate that providing the drug later in the course of therapy (that is, a longer period after hospitalization and weight restoration) might have yielded different results. Although this may be true, the clinical data to support this do not exist, at least at this point in time. Meanwhile, the search goes on to help teenagers and young adults who recover from anorexia nervosa to stay in recovery.

See the Pernick et al report (Disordered eating among a multi-racial/ethnic sample of female high-school athletes) that gives us some perspective on the frequency of eating disorders among differing racial and ethnic groups.

J. A. Stockman III, MD

Reference

1. Goldstein DJ, Wilson MG, Thompson VL, Potvin JH, Rampey AH Jr. Long-term fluoxetine treatment of bulimia nervosa. Fluoxetine Bulimia Nervosa Research Group. *Br J Psychiatry.* 1995;166:660-666.

Disordered eating among a multi-racial/ethnic sample of female high-school athletes

Pernick Y, Nichols JF, Rauh MJ, et al (San Diego State Univ, Calif; Rocky Mountain Univ of Health Professions, Provo, Utah; Washington Univ, St Louis)
J Adolesc Health 38:689-695, 2006

Purpose.—To determine the prevalence of disordered eating (DE) attitudes and behaviors in a multi-racial/ethnic sample of female high-school athletes.

Methods.—The Eating Disorders Examination Questionnaire (EDE-Q) was administered to 453 suburban female high-school athletes (277 Caucasian, 103 Latina, and 73 African American; aged 15.7 ± 1.2 years) during their competitive season.

Results.—The prevalence of DE in the total sample was 19.6%; among the three ethnic groups, prevalence estimates were 19.2%, 18.4%, and 23.3% for African Americans, Caucasians, and Latinas, respectively. The prevalence estimates of binge eating (12.6%) and vomiting (7.8%) were significantly higher in Latinas as compared to African Americans (5.5%, 1.4%) and Caucasians (5.4%, 2.2%; χ^2 $p < .05$). The prevalence of diuretic and laxative use was low among all athletes (< 3%), with no differences by ethnicity ($p > .05$). After adjusting for body mass index (BMI) and sport, analysis of covariance (ANCOVA) with Bonferroni post-hoc pair-wise comparisons indicated that Caucasian and Latina athletes scored higher than African Americans on all EDE-Q subscales except eating restraint, which was higher only in Caucasians compared to African Americans ($p = .001$– .046).

Conclusions.—Caucasian and Latina female high-school athletes may be at greater risk for eating disorders than their African American peers. Furthermore, Latina athletes may be particularly at risk for binge-eating disorder. Culturally-sensitive behavioral interventions targeted specifically for high-school athletes are needed to reduce the risk of eating disorders and associated long-term health consequences in this population.

The prevalence of unwanted and unlawful sexual experiences reported by Danish adolescents: Results from a national youth survey in 2002

Helweg-Larsen K, Larsen HB (Natl Inst of Public Health, Copenhagen; Univ of Copenhagen)
Acta Paediatr 95:1270-1276, 2006

Aim.—To obtain current data about child sexual abuse in Denmark and to assess abused children's own perception of early sexual experiences, which are unlawful according to the Danish Penal Code.

Methods.—Multimedia computer-based self-administered questionnaires (CASI) were completed by a national representative sample of 15–16-y-olds. Child sexual abuse was defined according to the penal code and measured by questions defining specific sexual activities, the relationship between the older person and the child, and the youth's own perception of the incident.

Results.—Among 5829 respondents, 11% reported unlawful sexual experiences, 7% of boys and 16% of girls. Only 1% of boys and 4% of girls felt that they "definitely" or "maybe" had been sexually abused.

Conclusion.—A relatively high percentage of Danish adolescents have early, unlawful sexual experiences. However, young people's own perception of sexual abuse tends to differ from that of the authorities, or their tolerance of abusive incidents is high. Gender differences were found in factors predicting perception of abuse (Tables 1, 3, 4, and 5).

▶ If things in the United States are anywhere nearly like what they are in Denmark, we are in real trouble. Chances are we are. This editor is unaware of any other report like this one. Most data providing information on childhood sexual abuse are derived from reported cases. The study from Denmark, however, does something different. It actually asked high school-aged children

---

TABLE 1.—Detailed Questions on Sexual Experiences

Request of participation in sexual activity
Photographed partly or totally nude
Watched a person masturbating
Presented pornographic magazines or movies
Kissed or caressed against his/her will
Touched in a sexual way over his/her clothes
Have touched the older person's genitals over his/her clothes
Touched with attempts made to undress
The older person undressed in preparation for sexual contact
Touched and caressed naked, including oral sex
Have touched or caressed another person who was naked, including oral sex
Attempts at intercourse
Completed intercourse
Attempts at anal intercourse

(Courtesy of Helweg-Larsen K, Larsen HB. The prevalence of unwanted and unlawful sexual experiences reported by Danish adolescents: results from a national youth survey in 2002. *Acta Paediatr.* 2006;95:1270-1276. Published by Taylor & Francis, Ltd. at http://www.tandf.cc.uk/journals/jsp.htm.)

TABLE 3.—Number and Distribution of the Character of Sexual
Abuse, by Sex (*n* = 657)

	Boys	Girls	Total
No physical contact	28 (14.4%)	32 (6.9%)	60 (9.1%)
Physical contact, but no intercourse	44 (22.6%)	161 (34.8%)	205 (31.2%)
Attempted or completed intercourse	123 (63.1%)	269 (58.2%)	392 (59.7%)
All cases of CSA	195 (100%)	462 (100%)	657 (100%)

(Courtesy of Helweg-Larsen K, Larsen HB. The prevalence of unwanted and unlawful sexual experiences reported by Danish adolescents: results from a national youth survey in 2002. *Acta Paediatr.* 2006;95:1270-1276. Published by Taylor & Francis, Ltd. at http://www.tandf.cc.uk/journals/jsp.htm.)

about any sexual experiences before the age of 15 years, ones with a person "much older" than the child, without defining any exact age difference. Those who answered the question affirmatively then answered a 14-item scale on different specific sexual activities ranging from noncontact sexual activities to intercourse (Table 1). In Denmark, the Danish Penal Code criminalizes sexual activity with a child younger than 15 years, regardless of consent. A sexual relationship between an adolescent younger than 18 years and a coach, teacher, or guardian is also criminalized. Tables 3 through 5 show the extent of the problem, at least in Denmark.

If there is one major understanding from the results of this study, it is that there is a considerable difference between the self-reported prevalence of sexual contact with an older person and the proportion of teens that perceive these incidents as sexual abuse. Less than half of teens recognize these experiences as sexual abuse. Had the survey included only a single question about whether the youngster had been sexually abused before 15 years of age, it is probable that only a small proportion of early sexual experiences as defined by the penal code as being criminal would have been reported.

Clearly, the youth among us is a vulnerable population. Most surveys have presented an inaccurate picture of the prevalence of sexual abuse against young children. Unfortunately, only a minor part of these cases is perceived as sexual abuse by youngsters, and therefore relatively few are disclosed to police or to parents. Lots of education is needed here. Unfortunately, many media, such as television, do not help educate our teens about violence. For ex-

TABLE 4.—Age of the Child at First Incident of Sexual Abuse, by the Older Person's Age
Group (*n* = 657)

Child's Age at First Incident (y)	Age of Older Person (y)				
	15-17	18-30	31-50	51+	Total
2-11	22 (30%)	22 (30%)	21 (29%)	8 (11%)	73 (100%)
12-14	360 (62%)	164 (28%)	38 (7%)	14 (3%)	576 (100%)
Missing	3 (37%)	0	4 (50%)	1 (13%)	8 (100%)
All age groups	385 (59%)	186 (28%)	63 (10%)	23 (3%)	657 (100%)

(Courtesy of Helweg-Larsen K, Larsen HB. The prevalence of unwanted and unlawful sexual experiences reported by Danish adolescents: results from a national youth survey in 2002. *Acta Paediatr.* 2006;95:1270-1276. Published by Taylor & Francis, Ltd. at http://www.tandf.cc.uk/journals/jsp.htm.)

TABLE 5.—Relationship Between the Child and the Older Person by the Respondent's Perception of the Sexual Abuse (*n* = 656)

Relationship	Not Perceived as Sexual Abuse		Perceived as Sexual Abuse		Total	
	Boys	Girls	Boys	Girls	Boys	Girls
Friend	75 (47%)	177 (54%)	5 (15%)	27 (20%)	80 (42%)	204 (44%)
Distant acquaintance	41 (25%)	84 (25%)	5 (15%)	41 (31%)	46 (24%)	125 (27%)
Stranger or unidentified person	17 (11%)	33 (10%)	11 (33%)	25 (19%)	28 (15%)	58 (13%)
Teacher, coach, employer, etc.	11 (7%)	20 (6%)	8 (24%)	4 (3%)	19 (9%)	24 (5%)
Family member; biological parent, grandparent, brother, cousin	16 (10%)	15 (5%)	4 (12%)	26 (20%)	20 (10%)	41 (9%)
Stepfather	1	1	0	9 (7%)	1	10 (2%)
All	161 (100%)	330 (100%)	33 (100%)	132 (100%)	194 (100%)	462 (100%)

(Courtesy of Helweg-Larsen K, Larsen HB. The prevalence of unwanted and unlawful sexual experiences reported by Danish adolescents: results from a national youth survey in 2002. *Acta Paediatr.* 2006;95:1270-1276. Published by Taylor & Francis, Ltd. at http://www.tandf.cc.uk/journals/isp.htm.)

ample, it has recently been shown that watching wrestling on television is hardly a harmless passing of time for a teen. Teenage fans of television wrestling are more likely to engage in "date fighting" (violence between people in a sexual relationship), fighting in general, and the carrying of weapons. Interestingly, this association is stronger for girls than it is for boys.[1] This problem is exacerbated by alcohol or drug usage. Clearly wrestling, drugs, and a touch of the "nip" are a prescription for violence.

J. A. Stockman III, MD

Reference

1. DuRant RH, Champion H, Wolfson M. The relationship between watching professional wrestling on television and engaging in date fighting among high school students. *Pediatrics*. 2006;118: e265-e272.

Deaths in juvenile justice residential facilities

Gallagher CA, Dobrin A (George Mason Univ, Fairfax, Va; Florida Atlantic Univ, Davie)
J Adolesc Health 38:662-668, 2006

Purpose.—To provide the first national description of death in juvenile justice residential facilities.

Methods.—Data come from recent censuses of all public and private juvenile justice facilities in the United States. Death rates for the custody population are adjusted for length at risk, and are compared to death rates of adolescents in the general population. Multivariate modeling is used to identify facility-level risk factors related to deaths.

Results.—Adjusting for the number of days at risk, adolescents in juvenile justice facilities have lower risks of death by accident and homicide, but considerably higher risks of death from suicide and illness (200% and 50%, respectively). Facilities with larger Black populations, those that lock sleeping room doors, and facilities designed to screen young persons for future placements all had significantly higher odds of experiencing a death.

Conclusions.—The higher rates of death from suicide or illness suggest either (a) juvenile justice facilities host very high risk adolescents who would have died on the outside, (b) the facility environment itself increases the risk of death relative to the adolescents' environment outside the facility, particularly in the case of deaths from suicide, (c) placement in a juvenile justice facility may be indicative of a time of crisis in adolescents' lives in terms of physical or mental health and thus the risk of death increases, or most realistically, (d) some combination of the above. That deaths are more likely in facilities with larger Black populations warrants significant future investigation. Finally, the policy of locking sleeping room doors should be seriously evaluated in light of the strong association found with suicide.

▶ Many thanks are due to the editor of the *Journal of Adolescent Health* for the decision to devote a significant portion of one issue of the journal to the topic of juveniles who are incarcerated. In the report of Gallagher et al, we see just how high risk an environment juvenile justice residential facilities are for this vulnerable population. Teenagers entering such facilities are more likely to have been previously abused and to have current physical health, mental health, substance abuse, and/or educational problems compared with children and teenagers outside the system. The risk of death for young people in juvenile justice facilities runs almost 10% higher than the death rate for the general population of teenagers aged 15 to 19 years when adjusted for numbers of days of risk exposure. Although the death rate from accidental injury and homicide turns out to be lower for young people in juvenile justice facilities, placement in such a facility dramatically increases the risk of suicide and deaths from illness and natural causes. Reception in diagnostic centers in particular is significantly more likely to be associated with suicides, deaths from illness, and deaths in general. Also, the larger a facility, the more likely it is that a youngster will die in that facility. This suggests that converting large facilities into smaller ones might reduce the risk of death in young people in juvenile justice detention center. The strongest relationship between dying in a juvenile facility was found between locked sleeping rooms and the odds of suicide. Whether this relates to an increased opportunity for committing suicide without intervention, or whether this phenomenon is merely picking up on the general increase in risk in the more secure facilities studied was not established.

One final comment, and an important one. In addition to the substantially higher risk of death from suicide and illness, perhaps the most alarming result in this study is the positive relationship between the percentage of the population in a juvenile justice facility that is black and the risk of suicide. It is not clear why this association exists. It very well may be due to worse conditions of confinement in facilities with larger percentages of black teenagers.

J. A. Stockman III, MD

Changes in Adolescents' Sources of Cigarettes

Robinson LA, Dalton WT III, Nicholson LM (Univ of Memphis, Tenn)
J Adolesc Health 39:861-867, 2006

Purpose.—No previous research has tracked changes in teen sources for tobacco. Such information might help public health officials to target tobacco control efforts more precisely. This investigation used a two-year longitudinal design to determine (1) how adolescents' sources change and (2) whether the timing of smoking onset and duration of tobacco use predict the number and types of sources accessed.

Methods.—A survey assessing usual sources of cigarettes and related variables was administered to 4461 seventh-graders annually. Of the target population, 79% provided baseline data, and 64.2% participated in all surveys.

Results.—At baseline, 30% of the 1144 smokers got cigarettes from peers, compared with 11% using stores, 6% using vending machines, and 17% who stole them. Age of smoking onset did not predict the number or types of sources teens accessed. We did, however, find a significant effect of duration of smoking, showing that more practiced smokers were more likely to get cigarettes both from stores and from their friends. Further, the longer students smoked, the more likely they were to have friends who smoked.

Conclusions.—Our results indicated that the means through which teens got their first cigarettes were similar, regardless of when smoking onset occurred. In contrast, as teens became more established smokers, they increased the number of sources they used and relied more on *both* stores and peers. Once adolescents become smokers, they form a social network of fellow smokers who support their habit, making it even more difficult to quit.

▶ Efforts to reduce teen smoking have targeted 2 areas. First, tobacco prevention programs have been developed for a variety of communities, schools, and homes. Most data from such programs have revealed significant benefits, but these benefits tend to slip over time. The second approach has been the focus on the supply side of the problem—that is, to identify the sources of cigarettes through which teens obtain tobacco products. Knowledge of these sources can inform health initiatives and legislation designed to restrict the flow of cigarettes to underage consumers. Considerable research has explored these sources that teens use for obtaining tobacco. Unfortunately, findings from these studies are surprisingly inconsistent. For example, the proportion of teens who report "borrowing" cigarettes has ranged from as low as 22% among high school students to 99% depending on what study one reads. Estimates of the proportion of teens who buy cigarettes in stores have been even more diverse, ranging from a low of 6% among middle school students to 90% in the middle teen years.

The study reported from the Department of Psychology, the University of Memphis, actually tracked students by measuring shifts in the number and type of sources of cigarettes used by adolescent smokers through annual follow-up assessments. Two important questions were asked: whether the number and types of sources used by teens differed, depending on when they started smoking, and whether the number and types of sources changed as teens became established smokers. Consistent with other studies, the results indicated that social sources are the primary method through which young teens obtain cigarettes. A solid third of seventh graders acknowledged getting tobacco from friends, and another 17% reported "taking cigarettes without an adult's knowledge." To say this differently, they snuck into their mother's purse or father's stash. Parents are often inadvertently the first source of tobacco products for young teens. Young teens do not take the chance attempting to buy cigarettes in a store (only 11% in this series did so). As teenage smokers become more experienced, they do become more comfortable buying cigarettes over the counter. Unfortunately, this study shows that after 3 years of smoking, continuous smokers appear to have more friends who are also tobacco users than did teens who had either not started smoking or who only recently began to smoke. This pattern suggests that once teens become smokers, they will bond with other smokers, embedding themselves in a tobacco-friendly network. Look at any company that has a nonsmoking policy, and you will also see the latter being true in adults. Working smokers tend to walk during breaks with their smoking friends. Smokers structure their social system to support their tobacco use.

It is important to learn from this report that the very social structure in which teens move makes it almost impossible for them to want to stop smoking. They are mired in a cohort of friends who light up, and unless they want to potentially lose those friends, they will continue smoking. How to break up this dynamic would be the topic for a very interesting study.

This commentary closes with a few additional comments regarding smoking. A recent report from the *Canadian Medical Association Journal* shows that nicotine dependence develops very soon after the first puff.[1] Young novice smokers may not realize that once they experience cravings, it is almost too late to stop progression to daily tobacco use and that the likelihood of dependence is greatly increased. Interventions designed to help young people stop smoking should incorporate the information that even one puff may be one puff too many for some, if not most. Last, do not think that the use of "light" cigarettes is any better than smoking regular cigarettes. Smokers who have used light cigarettes are 54% less likely to cease smoking than smokers who had only smoked full-strength cigarettes. Your guess is as good as anyone as to why these data are what they are, but they have been confirmed in a study of over 32,000 adults.[2]

J. A. Stockman III, MD

References

1. Gervais A, O'Loughlin J, Meshefedjian G, Bancej C, Tremblay M. Milestones in the natural course of onset of cigarette use among adolescents. *CMAJ*. 2006;175: 255-261.
2. Tindle HA, Rigotti NA, Davis RB, Barbeau EM, Kawachi I, Shiffman S. Cessation among smokers of "light" cigarettes: results from the 2000 national health interview survey. *Am J Public Health*. 2006;96:1498-1504.

2 Allergy and Dermatology

Timing of Solid Food Introduction in Relation to Atopic Dermatitis and Atopic Sensitization: Results From a Prospective Birth Cohort Study
Zutavern A, for the LISA Study Group (Inst of Epidemiology, Neuherberg, Germany; et al)
Pediatrics 117:401-411, 2006

Objective.—Prophylactic feeding guidelines recommend a delayed introduction of solid foods for the prevention of atopic diseases. Scientific evidence for this is scarce. This study investigates whether a delayed introduction of solids (past 4 months or 6 months) is protective against the development of atopic dermatitis (AD) and atopic sensitization when considering reverse causality.

Methods.—Data from 2612 infants in an ongoing birth cohort study were analyzed at 2 years of age. Information on diet and on symptoms and diagnoses of AD was collected semiannually, and information on specific immunoglobulin E levels was collected at 2 years of age.

Results.—Solid food introduction past the first 4 months of life decreased the odds of symptomatic AD but not for doctor-diagnosed AD, combined doctor-diagnosed and symptomatic AD, or atopic sensitization. Postponing the introduction beyond the sixth month of life was not protective in relation to either definition of AD or atopic sensitization. There was also no evidence for a protective effect of a delayed introduction of solids on AD and atopic sensitization in children of atopic parents. There was clear evidence for reverse causality between early skin or allergic symptoms and the introduction of solids.

Conclusions.—This study does not find evidence supporting a delayed introduction of solids beyond the sixth month of life for the prevention of AD and atopic sensitization. We cannot rule out that delaying the introduction of solids for the first 4 months of life might offer some protection. Measures to avoid reverse causality have to be considered in the conduction, analysis, and interpretation of cohort studies on the topic.

Timing of Initial Exposure to Cereal Grains and the Risk of Wheat Allergy

Poole JA, Barriga K, Leung DYM, et al (Natl Jewish Med and Research Ctr, Denver; Univ of Colorado, Denver)
Pediatrics 117:2175-2182, 2006

Objective.—Early exposure to solid foods in infancy has been associated with the development of allergy. The aim of this study was to examine the association between cereal-grain exposures (wheat, barley, rye, oats) in the infant diet and development of wheat allergy.

Methods.—A total of 1612 children were enrolled at birth and followed to the mean age of 4.7 years. Questionnaire data and dietary exposures were obtained at 3, 6, 9, 15, and 24 months and annually thereafter. The main outcome measure was parent report of wheat allergy. Children with celiac disease autoimmunity detected by tissue transglutaminase autoantibodies were excluded. Wheat-specific immunoglobulin E levels on children reported to have wheat allergy were obtained.

Results.—Sixteen children (1%) reported wheat allergy. Children who were first exposed to cereals after 6 months of age had an increased risk of wheat allergy compared with children first exposed to cereals before 6 months of age (after controlling for confounders including a family history of allergic disorders and history of food allergy before 6 months of age). All 4 children with detectable wheat-specific immunoglobulin E were first exposed to cereal grains after 6 months. A first-degree relative with asthma, eczema, or hives was also independently associated with an increased risk of wheat-allergy development.

Conclusions.—Delaying initial exposure to cereal grains until after 6 months may increase the risk of developing wheat allergy. These results do not support delaying introduction of cereal grains for the protection of food allergy.

▶ This report and the Zutavern et al report (Timing of solid food introduction in relation to atopic dermatitis and atopic sensitization: results from a prospective birth cohort study) give us important information about the relationship between introduction of certain types of food and the subsequent development of allergies. With respect to the study of Poole et al, we see that delaying initial exposure to cereal grains until after 6 months may actually increase the risk of developing wheat allergy.

The history surrounding dietary introductions and the risk of the development of food allergy is quite sorted. The European Society for Pediatric Allergology and Clinical Immunology and the European Society for Pediatric Gastroenterology, Hepatology, and Nutrition (joint European committees) and the American Academy of Pediatrics have recommended exclusive breastfeeding in early infancy for the primary prevention of allergic disease, partly on the basis of evidence from earlier, somewhat flawed studies. If one looks carefully at the literature, however, evidence to support delaying the introduction of solids for food-allergy prevention is quite lacking.

Given that allergic disorders can be serious conditions, means to prevent their development would be ideal. Previous studies have focused on eczema and asthma, but these are relatively complex disorders and are not always associated with allergy. No study to date has prospectively evaluated the time of specific dietary exposures with the development of specific food allergies. Here in the United States, the most common solid food first introduced into the infant's diet is rice cereal, followed by the cereal grains (oats, barley, wheat, and rye). Clinically significant cross-reactivity exists across these cereal grains. It is for this reason that an assessment of the role of cereal-grain exposure and the development of wheat allergy is important in better understanding the association between solid food introduction and possible food-allergy development. This was the aim of the study reported above.

What we learn from this study is that delaying the introduction of cereal grains until after 6 months does not protect against the development of wheat allergy and may actually increase the risk of a child developing wheat allergy even after controlling for a family history of allergy, breastfeeding duration, prior food allergy, and introduction of rice cereal. These data therefore fly in the face of the theory that delayed introduction of foods is necessary given that an infant's gut-mucosal barrier is immature in the first half-year of life. A possible explanation for the new findings may be the induction of immune tolerance. It is also possible that when cereal grains are introduced late, they are introduced in greater amounts and that a large antigen load may result in T-cell activation instead of anergy or tolerance.

There was one other finding from this study of note. The investigators did not observe a protective effect of breastfeeding on allergy prevention. In a recent review of breastfeeding and allergy prevention, the protective effect of exclusive breast feeding for at least 4 months was found with atopic dermatitis and wheezing and was primarily in children with a family history of atopy.[1] The population studied here was not defined by a family history of allergy. In addition, allergic disorders such as eczema and asthma likely benefit from the immunoregulatory properties of breast milk versus the development of a food allergy, which may be more related to the allergenicity of the food protein and not related to breastfeeding.

See the Zutavern et al report (Timing of solid food introduction in relation to atopic dermatitis and atopic sensitization: results from a prospective birth cohort study) that indicates that delayed solid food introduction beyond the sixth month of life is also not protective, in this case, for atopic dermatitis and atopic sensitization, findings that are consistent with the findings that have examined wheat allergy sensitization.

We will close this commentary with a clinical scenario correlated with dermatologic problems, to see how you would handle the following cases. An 18-year-old, 12th grade student presents with a 1 month history of ichthyosis-like dermatosis, which symmetrically involves the lower limbs, elbows, and hands. Blood tests demonstrate iron-deficiency anemia, lymphopenia, and neutropenia. The patient also has an unsteady gait, urinary retention, signs of intracranial hypertension, a cerebellar syndrome, pyramidal signs in all limbs without weakness, and mental sluggishness. The results of cerebral and spinal magnetic resonance imaging, electroencephalography, and cerebrospinal fluid analysis are normal. Simultaneous with this teen's presentation is that of her twin sister, who has similar but less severe skin lesions in the same distribution along with an unsteady gait. Her physical examination shows only slightly increased reflexes. There is no family history of neurologic or dermatologic disease or consanguinity. Any idea as to what is going on here?

It turns out that after several days of hospitalization, health care workers accidentally discovered a bag of mothballs in the patient's hospital room. Both sisters were encouraged by classmates to use mothballs as a recreational drug. The first patient had been "bagging" (inhaling) mothball fumes daily for 10 minutes for the previous 4 to 6 months. She had also chewed half a mothball per day for 2 months. Her biological abnormalities improved after she was mothball-free for 2 months. Clinical evaluation at 6 months showed a total recovery. At 3 months, her twin sister, who had sniffed mothballs for 5 to 10 minutes a day for only a few weeks, had recovered completely.

Recognize that mothballs contain paradichlorobenzene (PDB) as the only active substance. PDB is derived from aromatic hydrocarbons, which form one of the families of volatile substances that are commonly abused. Most physicians are not aware of the phenomenon of self-intoxication with PDB. It is easy to abuse PDB since mothballs and other household products containing PDB (insect repellants, air fresheners, toilet bowl and diaper-pail deodorizers, and fungicides) are legal and are readily available. Needless to say, the incidence of PDB bagging is probably underestimated. The association of an ichthyosis-like dermatosis and neurologic signs may be the hallmark of such abuse.[2]

J. A. Stockman III, MD

References

1. Friedman NJ, Zeiger RS. The role of breast feeding in the development of allergies and asthma. *J Allergy Clin Immunol.* 2005;115:1238-1248.
2. Feuillet L, Mallet S, Spadari M. Twin girls with neurocutaneous symptoms caused by mothball intoxication. *N Engl J Med.* 2006;355:423-424.

A mixture of prebiotic oligosaccharides reduces the incidence of atopic dermatitis during the first six months of age
Moro G, Arslanoglu S, Stahl B, et al (Macedonio Melloni Maternity Hosp, Milan, Italy; Numico Research Germany, Friedrichsdorf; Charité Campus Virchow Klinikum, Berlin; et al)
Arch Dis Child 91:814-819, 2006

Background.—Oligosaccharides may alter postnatal immune development by influencing the constitution of gastrointestinal bacterial flora.

Aims.—To investigate the effect of a prebiotic mixture of galacto- and long chain fructo-oligosaccharides on the incidence of atopic dermatitis (AD) during the first six months of life in formula fed infants at high risk of atopy.

Methods.—Prospective, double-blind, randomised, placebo controlled trial; 259 infants at risk for atopy were enrolled. A total of 102 infants in the prebiotic group and 104 infants in the placebo group completed the study. If bottle feeding was started, the infant was randomly assigned to one of two hydrolysed protein formula groups (0.8 g/100 ml prebiotics or maltodextrine as placebo). All infants were examined for clinical evidence of atopic dermatitis. In a subgroup of 98 infants, faecal flora was analysed.

Results.—Ten infants (9.8%; 95 CI 5.4–17.1%) in the intervention group and 24 infants (23.1%; 95 CI 16.0–32.1%) in the control group developed AD. The severity of the dermatitis was not affected by diet. Prebiotic supplements were associated with a significantly higher number of faecal bifidobacteria compared with controls but there was no significant difference in lactobacilli counts.

Conclusion.—Results show for the first time a beneficial effect of prebiotics on the development of atopic dermatitis in a high risk population of infants. Although the mechanism of this effect requires further investigation, it appears likely that oligosaccharides modulate postnatal immune development by altering bowel flora and have a potential role in primary allergy prevention during infancy.

▶ Atopic dermatitis is usually the first manifestation of allergy during early infancy. It has been reported that atopic dermatitis is associated with a delayed maturation of immune responses during infancy, with raised total IgE and specific IgE to dietary antigens in the serum. Infants with early-onset allergic disease are also at increased risk of other manifestation of allergic disease, a phenomenon described in the literature as the "allergic march." The intestinal flora is part of a complex ecosystem, and many of its constituent bacteria remain unidentified. However, there is strong evidence that the intestinal flora influences the postnatal development of the immune system. Breastfeeding remains the single most important "intervention" to prevent the development of atopy. Unfortunately, many infants are not breastfed, thus the theoretic benefits of a "prebiotic" diet during early infancy.

A prebiotic formula is a formula that reproduces intestinal flora similar to the type found in infants who are breastfed. A common prebiotic formula based on analysis of human milk oligosaccharides is a prebiotic mixture of 90% short-chain galacto-oligosaccharides and 10% long-chain fructo-oligosaccharides. Such a prebiotic formula has been shown to produce intestinal flora similar to that found in breastfed infants.

What we see in this study is that the cumulative incidence of atopic dermatitis during the first 6 months of life can be significantly reduced by supplementation of a hypoallergenic formula with a prebiotic formula mixture. The majority of the infants investigated had a maternal history of atopy. Over the course of 6 months, just 9.8% of infants developed atopic dermatitis in the prebiotic group compared with 23.1% in the control group, a highly significant difference. These authors are to be congratulated for conducting a double-blind trial in an important area of concern. Evidence is accumulating that human milk oligosaccharides can influence the immune system not only via intestinal flora, but also by direct interaction with immune cells. These substances have been shown to affect the cytokine production and activation of human cord blood–derived T cells in vitro. Thus, this study and others clearly underscore the fact that intestinal flora plays an important role in postnatal development of the immune system, and that dietary prebiotics will stimulate an intestinal flora largely mimicking the flora seen in breastfed infants. It may be awhile before formula manufacturers here in the United States wake up to the data we are seeing emerge from overseas, but when that awakening occurs, perhaps our infants will be better served.

To close this commentary, consider this case scenario. A 17-year-old in your practice asks you for some career guidance. Specifically, he wants to know whether he may lead a normal, healthy life should he throw his lot in with his father, who is a North Carolina commercial fisherman. The question is, what can you tell him about the medical risks, short-term and long-term, associated with the occupation of commercial fishing off the eastern seaboard of the United States?

North Carolina is usually ranked among the nation's top 10 seafood producing states and has approximately 4,000 to 7,000 active full-time commercial fisherman harvesting catches from 4,000 miles of marine and estuarine shoreline. Situated where the cold-water Labrador Current meets the warm tropical waters of the Gulf Stream, North Carolina waters offer an especially wide and diverse variety of seafood.

So much for the education related to the coastal waters of the state where this editor lives. As bucolic as fishing might be in this area, commercial fishing is well known to be one of the most hazardous of all occupations. A significant proportion of work-related health problems in this industry affect the skin, and if there is one risk that this 17-year-old might encounter throughout his life, it is disorders of the skin.

So what are the skin conditions that fishermen have to deal with? The skin of fishermen is often exposed to high levels of wetness; to a variety of potential cutaneous pathogens; to estuarine and marine flora and fauna that can bite, sting, shock or otherwise cause contact/irritant skin reactions; to multiple types of trauma; and to extremes of heat and cold. A recent study tells us just how common skin problems are among fishermen in North Carolina who fish commercially.[1] By the time fishermen are in their early 50s, 60% have actinic keratosis. Some 15% will have evidence on physical examination of actinic cheilitis. Almost 10% have one or more basal cell carcinomas. Some 6% have an active squamous cell carcinoma. Four percent have a history of melanoma. Virtually all have been bitten or stung by an aquatic predator. Some 15% have had a fish shock. Some 60% have had a significant cutaneous bacterial infection from handling fish/crustaceans with spines, sharp shells, etc. The largest number of the latter cases are described as "fish poison," "shrimp poison," "crab poison," or "scallop poison." These are common names for the usually transient and self-limited cellulitis known as erysipeloid due to the organism, *Erysipelothrix rhusiopathiae*. While most of these skin infections are mild and transient, *Erysipelothrix rhusiopathiae* can disseminate and cause endocarditis as well as other sequelae. Abscess formation is also quite common. Some 4% of fishermen have reported seeking medical attention for infection with *Mycobacterium marinum* infection. This slow-growing aquatic organism causes granuloma formation and is associated with tumorous or verrucoid lesions enlarging over many weeks to months. It usually follows traumatic injury to the skin.

A couple of final comments about the risks of being a coastal fisherman pertaining to bites and stings: the most serious or extensive injuries that fishermen suffer with respect to stings usually come from jellyfish. Nettles falling from nets can lead to extensive and severe stings in some individuals. One in four commercial fishermen have reported being stung by jellyfish in the eyes, a phenomenon resulting in temporary blindness, blistering of the eyes, severe conjunctivitis and eye pain. One in 10 fishermen reported at least one serious sting by a Portuguese man-of-war, with one individual reporting such a severe sting to his chest and face that he went into shock. Some fish have specialized cells known as electrocytes, which are capable of producing an electric current strong enough to shock individuals coming into contact with them. Fish known to cause electric shocks off the middle Atlantic and northern southern states include the stargazer and the torpedo ray. It is not fun to be shocked, but there are no serious sequelae reported.

After you explain all of these interesting medical problems, in addition to the traumatic ones and the environmental risks associated with fishing, you can be quite sure the teen you have spoken with may very well be looking for a job at the local Burger King.

J. A. Stockman III, MD

Reference

1. Burke WA, Griffith DC, Scott CM, Howell ER. Skin problems related to the occupation of commercial fishing in North Carolina. *NC Med J*. 2006;67:260-265.

Trends in Sunburns, Sun Protection Practices, and Attitudes Toward Sun Exposure Protection and Tanning Among US Adolescents, 1998–2004

Cokkinides V, Weinstock M, Glanz K, et al (American Cancer Society, Atlanta, Ga; VA Med Centre Providence, RI; Brown Univ, Providence, RI; et al)
Pediatrics 118:853-864, 2006

Background.—Sun exposure in childhood is an important risk factor for developing skin cancer as an adult. Despite extensive efforts to reduce sun exposure among the young, there are no population-based data on trends in sunburns and sun protection practices in the young. The aim of this study was to describe nationally representative trend data on sunburns, sun protection, and attitudes related to sun exposure among US youth.

Methods.—Cross-sectional telephone surveys of youth aged 11 to 18 years in 1998 (N = 1196) and in 2004 (N = 1613) were conducted using a

2-stage sampling process to draw population-based samples. The surveys asked identical questions about sun protection, number of sunburns experienced, and attitudes toward sun exposure. Time trends were evaluated using pooled logistic regression analysis.

Results.—In 2004, 69% of subjects reported having been sunburned during the summer, not significantly less than in 1998 (72%). There was a significant decrease in the percentage of those aged 11 to 15 years who reported sunburns and a nonsignificant increase among the 16- to 18-year-olds. The proportion of youth who reported regular sunscreen use increased significantly from 31% to 39%. Little change occurred in other recommended sun protection practices.

Conclusions.—A small reduction in sunburn frequency and modest increases in sun protection practices were observed among youth between 1998 and 2004, despite widespread sun protection campaigns. Nevertheless, the decrease in sunburns among younger teens may be cause for optimism regarding future trends. Overall, there was rather limited progress in improving sun protection practices and reducing sunburns among US youth between 1998 and 2004.

▶ You would think that here in the United States we would have gotten the message, not only for ourselves, but for our children, with respect to the dangers of sunbathing. We include only melanoma in cancer center registry statistics published each year here in the United States, but more than 1 million cases of basal cell and squamous cell carcinomas are also likely to be diagnosed. The latter two skin problems occur at a frequency rate that is some 18 times greater than melanoma. Both basal cell and squamous cell skin cancers (also known as keratinocyte carcinomas) are highly treatable, but they do account for considerable morbidity and health care expenditures. In most instances, all three skin malignancies are the result of excessive exposure to sun.

So are we winning or losing the battle of decreasing sun exposure in our offspring? The data from this report show that there are significant trends of decreasing prevalence of sunburns among younger teens, and that it is likely that this age-specific trend may relate in part to greater parent influence in early adolescence, and possibly as well as in younger children. Several studies indicate that parent vigilance and parent use of sun protection are related to a greater sun protection practice and reduced likelihood of sunburn experiences in their children. Unfortunately, among older teens the problem still continues to exist to the same, if not to a greater, degree. This study did find an increase in the numbers of days spent at the beach among older teens.

We here in the United States have not been as aggressive as those in certain countries, such as Australia. Australia has served as a model for initiating a national (in scope) comprehensive skin cancer prevention program, which has used systematic population-based tracking of disease and behavioral modification as a methodology to reduce skin exposure. More than 35 years ago, Australia adopted a national health care policy that made skin cancer prevention a public health priority. The public educational campaign known as Slip! Slop! Slap! (slip on a shirt, slop on some sunscreen, and slap on a hat) and the SunSmart program have gone a long way to modify sun exposure practices in the Australian population. We need to be as aggressive as the land down under.

One final observation about sun exposure and sunburn, this among Swedish toddlers. Sweden is experiencing the same problem we have here in the United States. There, one fifth of toddlers experience at least 1 severe sunburn before they exit toddlerhood. More than one third of all toddlers have been abroad on a vacation to a sunny resort. Also, 35% of all toddlers' parents spend 2 or more hours in the sun during peak exposure times (11:00 AM–3:00 PM) on a typical work-free day in the summer, and almost 10% of all parents have their children exposed to the sun for a similar amount of time, putting these kids at great risk as they age.[1]

J. A. Stockman III, MD

Reference

1. Bränström R, Kristjansson S, Dal H, Rodvall Y. Sun exposure and sunburn among Swedish toddlers. *Eur J Cancer*. 2006;42:1441-1447.

The significance of cutaneous spider naevi in children
Finn SM, Rowland M, Lawlor F, et al (Univ College Dublin)
Arch Dis Child 91:604-605, 2006

Background.—Cutaneous spider naevi are commonly considered to be a clinical sign of chronic liver disease. Little is known about their occurrence in children.

Aim.—To evaluate the occurrence of spider naevi in children with and without liver disease.

Methods.—The presence of spider naevi was investigated in 460 children, 34 of whom had chronic liver disease.

Results.—Of children without liver involvement, 38% had at least one spider naevus. The prevalence of spider naevi increased with age. Of control patients aged 5 to 15 years, 2.5% had more than five spiders present. Although eight of 10 children with cirrhosis had at least one spider naevus, only four of 34 children with chronic liver disease had five or more spiders present. Most spiders were on the hands and very few were >5 mm in size.

Conclusions.—Children with liver disease rarely have large numbers of spider naevi. Although the finding of five or more spider naevi is more common in liver disease, many normal children also have one or more of these lesions.

▶ This is truly a great report. All of us see in our practice children with spider nevi. Many of us have scratched our heads, puzzled by whether these little vascular lesions mean anything. When on internal medicine services in medical school, we learned that such skin signs are a marker of patients with liver disease, particularly cirrhosis. What this report shows is that somewhere between 1% and 2% of all normal children have greater than 5 spider nevi when the skin is carefully examined. Youngsters with liver disease of all sorts have about 5 times the probability of having this many spider nevi, but the majority of children with established chronic liver disease, in fact, do not have large numbers. The bottom line is that multiple nevi may be present in otherwise well children without liver disease, and most children with chronic liver disease appear to have few or no spider nevi. Thus, we probably can relax when we see these things as we go about our business performing routine physical examinations.

Because there is not much more to say about spider nevi, we will extend this commentary by asking you two questions pertaining to things cold. First, recall the popular seasonal film, "Christmas Story" in which the young boy elects to lick a pole with his tongue in freezing weather, the tongue instantly becoming attached? The question is, in reality, just how long does it take the surface of the skin to freeze when in contact with various substances?

The answer here is fairly straightforward. Touching very cold surfaces with bare skin causes pain, numbness, and tissue damage remarkably quickly. In a recent scientific study, a series of experiments in volunteers provided data for the construction of a model to establish safe temperature limits for cold touchable surfaces. It turns out that what matters most is the thermal conductivity of the material of which the surface is made. Skin temperature falls to 0°C within 20 seconds on contact with aluminum or steel at 4°C, but even at much, much lower temperatures, skin surface temperature never falls as low as this on contact with either wood or fabric materials such as nylon.[1]

Here is the second, and the last, question. You are a practitioner in Kentucky, and you see a college freshman who presents with tender erythematous subcutaneous plaques and nodules on her thighs. It is February, and she reports crops of new lesions throughout the winter months. On physical examination, the individual lesions resemble erythema nodosum, although her lower legs seem to be completely spared. You ask about any unusual exposure she may have had. The only thing that she relates is the fact that she, in her spare college time, likes to ride race horses, even in the winter. Your diagnosis?

If you answered with the diagnosis "equestrian cold panniculitis," you have appropriately recognized this occupational skin disease. It results from inflammation in the subcutaneous fat and is not immunologically mediated, but is a consequence of a combination of cold weather and tight-fitting jodhpurs, which cause restrictive blood flow to the skin in areas most exposed to the cold during riding. The treatment of equestrian cold panniculitis is to give the horses a break in winter and/or to wear looser-fitting clothing. Jodhpurs may look great, if you have the right body shape, but they are a no-no when the thermometer dips low.[2]

J. A. Stockman III, MD

References

1. Geng Q, Holmer I, Hartog DE et al. Temperature limit values for touching cold surfaces with the fingertip. *Ann Occup Hyg.* 2006;50:851-862.
2. Mehta A. Equestrian cold panniculitis. *BMJ.* 2006;333:558.

Azithromycin Does Not Cure Pityriasis Rosea

Amer A, Fischer H (Wayne State Univ, Detroit; Children's Hosp of Michigan, Detroit)
Pediatrics 117:1702-1705, 2006

Objectives.—Pityriasis rosea (PR) is a common skin disorder in children. Its cause is unknown. A recent publication reported a 73% cure rate in patients with PR after treatment with erythromycin. To duplicate this result using a drug with fewer adverse effects and greater biological half-life, we set out to study the effect of azithromycin on PR. Azithromycin is an azalide antibiotic with a spectrum of antimicrobial activity very similar to that of erythromycin.

Design.—We randomly assigned 49 children with PR to receive either azithromycin (12 mg/kg per day, up to a maximum of 500 mg/day) for 5 days or a similar-appearing placebo. Study physicians were blinded to patients' treatment type. Two pediatricians had to agree on the diagnosis of PR before patients could be enrolled. Subjects were seen at follow-up visits 1, 2, and 4 weeks after starting treatment.

Outcome Measures.—We measured the appearance of new lesions and resolution of lesions.

Results.—Rates of cure and of partial resolution were similar in the azithromycin and placebo groups.

Conclusion.—Azithromycin does not cure PR.

▶ The title of this article says it all! Whether you treat PR or not, the skin lesions will persist 4 to 10 weeks. Several organisms have been considered as potential etiologic agents of this skin condition, but to date no one has documented any specific cause. Despite suggestions in the literature that antibiotics might shorten the course of the problem, no consistent results have been found in clinical trials and now we see that azithromycin is no better than no treatment at all.

J. A. Stockman III, MD

Efficacy of Duct Tape vs Placebo in the Treatment of Verruca Vulgaris (Warts) in Primary School Children

de Haen M, Spigt MG, van Uden CJT, et al (Maastricht Univ, The Netherlands; Univ Hosp Maastricht, The Netherlands; Regional Public Health Inst, Maastricht, The Netherlands)
Arch Pediatr Adolesc Med 160:1121-1125, 2006

Objective.—To determine the efficacy of duct tape compared with placebo in the treatment of verruca vulgaris.

Design and Setting.—A randomized placebo-controlled trial in 3 primary schools in Maastricht, the Netherlands.

Participants.—One hundred three children aged 4 to 12 years with verruca vulgaris.

Interventions.—Duct tape applied to the wart or placebo, a corn pad (protection ring for clavi), applied around the wart for 1 night a week. Both treatments were applied for a period of 6 weeks. Patients were blinded to the hypothesis of the study.

Main Outcome Measurement.—Complete resolution of the treated wart.

Results.—After 6 weeks, the wart had disappeared in 16% of the children in the duct tape group compared with 6% in the placebo group ($P = .12$). The estimated effect of duct tape compared with placebo on diameter reduction of the treated wart was 1.0 mm ($P = .02$, 95% confidence interval, -1.7 to -0.1). After 6 weeks, in 7 children (21%) in the duct tape group, a surrounding wart had disappeared compared with 9 children (27%) in the placebo group ($P = .79$). Fifteen percent of the children in the duct tape group reported adverse effects such as erythema, eczema, and wounds compared with 0 in the placebo group ($P = .14$).

Conclusion.—In a 6-week trial, duct tape had a modest but nonsignificant effect on wart resolution and diameter reduction when compared with placebo in a cohort of primary school children.

▶ Ever since the report that appeared in 2002 showing the effectiveness of duct tape versus cryotherapy in the treatment of the common wart, primary care providers have gravitated to the use of duct tape in droves.[1] This report, however, from The Netherlands, throws a wet blanket on the duct tape approach to the management of the common wart. Considering the serious discomfort of cryotherapy and the awkwardness of applying salicylic acid for a long time, the simple application of duct tape is a very attractive as well as cheap alternative. Unfortunately, the study of Focht et al[1] was not the most rigorous in the world in terms of being randomized and blinded, defects addressed by and large in the more recent study from The Netherlands. The overseas study shows that duct tape has no significantly better effect on the resolution of warts than placebo. The majority of children and families even reported that duct tape just would not stick, and 15% reported problems with erythema.

By now, most clinicians have already formed their own opinion about the value of duct tape for the removal of the common wart. Perhaps more studies are needed. Perhaps those overseas do not have the kind of sticky duct tape that we have here in the United States. 3M rules. We need more innovative approaches. I, for one, would suggest putting a dab of "gorilla glue" on a wart before applying the duct tape. That would make a very interesting study.

J. A. Stockman III, MD

Reference

1. Focht DR III, Spicer C, Fairchok MP. The efficacy of duct tape vs cryotherapy in the treatment of verruca vulgaris (the common wart). *Arch Pediatr Adolesc Med.* 2002;156:971-974.

Treatment of Pemphigus Vulgaris with Rituximab and Intravenous Immune Globulin

Ahmed AR, Spigelman Z, Cavacini LA, et al (New England Baptist Hosp, Boston; Harvard School of Dental Medicine, Boston; Harvard Med School, Boston; et al)

N Engl J Med 355:1772-1779, 2006

Background.—Pemphigus vulgaris is a potentially fatal autoimmune mucocutaneous blistering disease. Conventional therapy consists of high-dose corticosteroids, immunosuppressive agents, and intravenous immune globulin.

Methods.—We studied patients with refractory pemphigus vulgaris involving 30% or more of their body-surface area, three or more mucosal sites, or both who had inadequate responses to conventional therapy and intravenous immune globulin. We treated the patients with two cycles of rituximab (375 mg per square meter of body-surface area) once weekly for 3 weeks and intravenous immune globulin (2 g per kilogram of body weight) in the fourth week. This induction therapy was followed by a monthly infusion of rituximab and intravenous immune globulin for 4 consecutive months. Titers of serum antibodies against keratinocytes and numbers of peripheral-blood B cells were monitored.

Results.—Of 11 patients, 9 had rapid resolution of lesions and a clinical remission lasting 22 to 37 months (mean, 31.1). All immunosuppressive therapy, including prednisone, could be discontinued before ending rituximab treatment in all patients. Two patients were treated with rituximab only during recurrences and had sustained remissions. Titers of IgG4 antikeratinocyte antibodies correlated with disease activity. Peripheral-blood B cells became undetectable shortly after initiating rituximab therapy but subsequently returned to normal values. Side effects that have been associated with rituximab were not observed, nor were infections.

Conclusions.—The combination of rituximab and intravenous immune globulin is effective in patients with refractory pemphigus vulgaris.

▶ Pemphigus is a disease that can affect youngsters and is potentially fatal. It is a blistering mucocutaneous autoimmune disease involving the skin and the oral cavity and other mucosal sites. The lesions of pemphigus are characterized by intraepidermal vesicles with acantholysis and an intact basal layer. Serum samples from affected individuals contain antibodies against desmoglein 3, and these antibodies have been shown to be part of the pathogenesis of pemphigus. Individuals with pemphigus have been treated largely with systemic corticosteroids. Most are given high doses of steroids plus immunosuppressive agents. This combination often needs to be given over long periods and can result in immunosuppression, a common cause of death in patients with the disorder. An alternative to steroids and immunosuppressive agents in nonresponding patients or in those who have had severe side effects from such therapy is IV immunoglobulin. There are failures with this approach as well.

The report of Ahmed et al gives us information on 11 patients with severe pemphigus vulgaris who were resistant to steroids plus immunosuppressive agents and IV immunoglobulin. These patients were treated with rituximab, a human monoclonal antibody against the B-cell antigen CD20 that depletes antibody-producing B cells. Complete remission of the disease was observed in 9 of the 11 patients, and eventually complete control of the disease was achieved in all 11 patients. All patients ultimately were able to discontinue their treatment.

Treatment with rituximab has been used for other autoimmune diseases. In the study involving patients with pemphigus, there were no clinically significant side effects of therapy. The cytokine-release syndrome can develop in patients receiving rituximab for lymphoma and is most common in patients with bulky adenopathy or bone marrow involvement. Although none of the patients with the dermatologic disorder had these serious side effects, the long-term consequences of rituximab therapy in patients with autoimmune diseases remain largely unknown. Given the potentially lethal nature of refractory pemphigus, however, it does seem reasonable to use rituximab when other forms of therapy have been ineffective.

For more on the topic of pemphigus, bullous impetigo, and the staphylococcal scalded skin syndrome and how they interrelate pathophysiologically, see the excellent review by Stanley and Amagai.[1]

This commentary having to do with things dermatologic closes with a who-dun-it-type question. You are seeing a teenage girl who presents to the emergency room with a painful, cold, pale hand. The only significant history is that 36 hours before she had her arm tattooed. On physical examination her hand is cold and edematous, with paraesthesias and a capillary refill of 4 seconds. The radial pulse is not palpable, but is able to be detected on Doppler ultrasound examination. The skin examination shows a recently placed tattoo that circumscribes her forearm ("ring" tattoo). What is your diagnosis here?

What you are seeing is what is know as a "tattoo tourniquet syndrome." Tattoo pigments can have a constrictive effect and can act as a tourniquet. In the patient described, the symptoms resolved after keeping the patient's arm raised overnight. It appears that deep tattooing may have similar effects to full thickness burns, and escharotomy may be needed if the tattoo circumscribes a compromised limb.[2]

J. A. Stockman III, MD

References

1. Stanley JR, Amagai M. Pemphigus, bullous impetigo, and the staphylococcal scalded-skin syndrome. *N Engl J Med*. 2006;355:1800-1808.
2. Briant-Evans TW. Editorial note. *BMJ*. 2006;333:52.

An Effective Nonchemical Treatment for Head Lice: A Lot of Hot Air

Goates BM, Atkin JS, Wilding KG, et al (Univ of Utah, Salt Lake City)
Pediatrics 118:1962-1970, 2006

Objectives.—Head lice (*Pediculus humanus capitis*) are a major irritant to children and their parents around the world. Each year millions of children are infested with head lice, a condition known as pediculosis, which is responsible for tens of millions of lost school days. Head lice have evolved resistance to many of the currently used pediculicides; therefore, an effective new treatment for head lice is needed. In this study we examined the effectiveness of several methods that use hot air to kill head lice and their eggs.

Methods.—We tested 6 different treatment methods on a total of 169 infested individuals. Each method delivers hot air to the scalp in a different way. We evaluated how well these methods kill lice and their eggs in situ. We also performed follow-up inspections to evaluate whether the sixth, most successful, method can cure head louse infestations.

Results.—All 6 methods resulted in high egg mortality ($\geq 88\%$), but they showed more-variable success in killing hatched lice. The most successful method, which used a custom-built machine called the LouseBuster, resulted in nearly 100% mortality of eggs and 80% mortality of hatched lice. The LouseBuster was effective in killing lice and their eggs when operated at a comfortable temperature, slightly cooler than a standard blow-dryer. Virtually all subjects were cured of head lice when examined 1 week after treatment with the LouseBuster. There were no adverse effects of treatment.

Conclusions.—Our findings demonstrate that one 30-minute application of hot air has the potential to eradicate head lice infestations. In summary, hot air is an effective, safe treatment and one to which lice are unlikely to evolve resistance.

▶ Before this report appeared, this editor did not realize that there are estimated to be up to 12 million cases of head lice occurring here in the United States each year. It is also estimated that children in the United States miss some 12 million to 24 million days of school as a consequence of having lice. That is a lot of itchy scalp. Although head lice do not produce any illness per se, they are physically and psychologically unpleasant for the youngster and, needless to say, exasperating for parents and schools. Before this report appeared, there were 3 general approaches for managing head lice infestation: chemical shampoos, specialized louse combs, and a whole variety of "home remedies." Each approach has had its problems. Shampoos, largely consisting of pyrethroids or lindane, are not very effective at killing louse eggs. An additional treatment with shampoo is necessary 1 week after the first treatment to kill lice from newly hatched eggs. Many parents are wary of such shampoos, given the fact that they contain fairly potent insecticides, particularly lindane. None are safe for patients who happen to have asthma. Louse combs are great, but effective combing may require many hours over several days, and most patients do not have the time or patience to truly eradicate all the lice and eggs. As far as home remedies are concerned, they consist of a variety of oddball things, such as application of bug sprays and mayonnaise. In some locales, the application of kerosine is popular. There is no evidence that these home remedies are truly effective, and you better not light a match when using some of them.

So what is a parent to do? This article suggests that one can just blow some hot air on the problem and voilà, you can have a cure rate as good as any other form of therapy. Nearly 60 years ago, Buxton did, in fact, point out that body lice, *Pediculus humanus corporis*, which are closely related to head lice, die when exposed to 51°C air for 5 minutes.[1] More recently, Kobayashi et al reported that body lice can be killed in vitro with air from a blow-dryer at 50°C for 5 minutes, and that body louse eggs fail to hatch in vitro after exposure to hot air at 55°C for 90 seconds.[2]

The ability of hot air to kill body lice is what suggested to Goates et al that perhaps hot air might kill head lice. They carried out the first experiment in the published literature and demonstrated that exposure to a large volume of hot air can result in 98% mortality of eggs and 80% mortality of hatched lice. They further showed that simply blowing hot air on lice is sufficient to eliminate viable head lice from virtually all subjects when restudied 1 week after treatment. If you can stand a single 30-minute hot air blow to your hair, you will have kicked this little critter. Recognize, however, that the most successful hairdryer was one that the investigators had custom built for the study. Chances are that one will find the LouseBuster soon at your local Walmart.

J. A. Stockman III, MD

References

1. Buxton PA. *The Louse*. Baltimore, MD: Williams & Wilkins; 1946.
2. Kobayashi M, Hiraoka T, Mihara M. Thermotolerance of human body louse, *Pediculus humanus corporis*: II. Preliminary evaluation of hot air for killing adults and eggs. *Jpn J Sanit Zool*. 1995;46:83-86.

Redarkening of Port-Wine Stains 10 Years after Pulsed-Dye–Laser Treatment

Huikeshoven M, Koster PHL, de Borgie CAJM, et al (Univ of Amsterdam)
N Engl J Med 356:1235-1240, 2007

Background.—Although pulsed-dye–laser therapy is currently the gold standard for the treatment of port-wine stains, few objective data are available on its long-term efficacy. Using objective color measurements, we performed a 10-year follow-up of a previously conducted prospective clinical study of the treatment of port-wine stains with a pulsed-dye laser.

Methods.—We invited the patients to undergo repeated color measurements performed by the same procedures as in the previous study. The results at long-term follow-up were compared with color measurements obtained before treatment and after completion of an average of five laser treatments of the complete port-wine stain. A questionnaire was used to investigate pa-

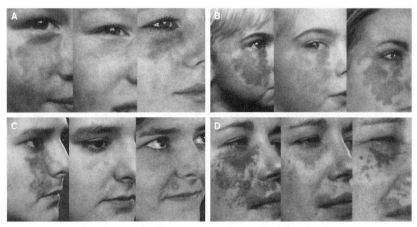

FIGURE 1.—Redarkening of port-wine stains after pulsed-dye–laser treatment. Recent photographs of the patients are included, along with the illustrations used in the previous study. Each panel shows a patient before treatment (left), after six treatments of the complete port-wine stain (middle), and at follow-up 9 years (Panel A) or 10 years (Panels B, C, and D) after five treatments (right). In all four patients, redarkening of the stain can be observed when the right-hand photograph is compared with the middle photograph. (Reprinted by permission from Huikeshoven M, Koster PHL, de Borgie CAJM, et al. Redarkening of port-wine stains 10 years after pulsed-dye–laser treatment. *N Engl J Med*. 356:1235-1240. Copyright 2007, Massachusetts Medical Society. All rights reserved.)

tients' satisfaction with the treatment and their perception of long-term changes in the stain.

Results.—Of the 89 patients from whom color measurements were obtained in the previous study, 51 were included in this study. The patients had received a median of seven additional treatment sessions since the last color measurement, which had been made after an average of five treatments. The median length of follow-up was 9.5 years. On average, the stain when measured at follow-up was significantly darker than it was when measured after the last of the initial five laser treatments (P=0.001), but it was still significantly lighter than it was when measured before treatment (P<0.001). Fifty-nine percent of patients were satisfied with the overall treatment result. Six percent of patients reported that the stain had become lighter since their last treatment, 59% that it was unchanged, and 35% that it had become darker.

Conclusions.—Using objective color measurements, we observed significant redarkening of port-wine stains at long-term follow-up after pulsed-dye–laser therapy. Patients should be informed about the possibility of redarkening before beginning treatment (Fig 1).

▶ One of the great unknowns in medicine is how long laser treatment of port-wine stains would last for permanent removal of the birthmark. These stains are capillary malformations and are fairly common, affecting about 3 of 1000 newborns. Although a benign skin disorder, port-wine stains can be a cosmetic problem for youngsters and adults. Since the initial report by Tan et al almost 20 years ago, port-wine stains have been managed by pulsed–dye-laser therapy.[1] This report of Huikeshoven et al indicates that port-wine stains can recur after pulsed–dye-laser treatment. Other studies have suggested a 50% recurrence rate at 5 years after laser therapy. Some studies up through about 7 years of follow-up have found lesser rates of recurrence. As can be seen in this report from Amsterdam, at an average length of follow-up of 9.5 years, most previously treated port-wine stains were, in fact, darkening. Nonetheless, the majority of patients still were satisfied with the overall treatment result.

It is not exactly clear why port-wine stains might darken after a long time after therapy. It has been suggested that blood vessels that have not been completely eradicated may become ectatic. It is also possible that there is neoangiogenesis of capillary structures in deeper parts of the port-wine stain that were not treatable with the pulsed–dye-laser because of its limited penetration depth.

Although the majority of patients with port-wine stains who had later darkening of the stain remain satisfied with the results, a small subset of patients appear to be sufficiently unhappy that they are undergoing additional treatments years after the initial therapy was offered. Despite the mixed long-term results, pulsed–dye-laser therapy is likely to stay the gold standard for treatment of port-wine stains because it has a persistent beneficial effect in a significant portion of patients. Nonetheless, as the authors of this report suggest, all patients and their families should be informed about the possibility of redarkening of the stain years after treatment.

We will close this commentary with a quiz. Have you ever heard of the Irukandji syndrome? The Irukandji syndrome is a painful and unpleasant consequence of being stung by certain jellyfish. The sting itself leaves few local signs, but 20 minutes later, back pain, nausea, abdominal pain, sweating, and hypertension along with tachycardia and a fear of impending death may develop. The syndrome has been reported in the Caribbean and the Pacific, but until now only two jellyfish (*Carukia barneisi* and an unnamed species) have been identified. The nature of the venom is unknown, but recent identification of another 5 species of *Cubozoan* jellyfish that sting can cause the same syndrome extends the number of jellyfish that can be a cause of the Irukandji syndrome.[2]

J. A. Stockman III, MD

References

1. Tan OT, Sherwood K, Gilchrist BA. Treatment of children with port-wine stains using flashlamp-pulsed tunable dye laser. *N Engl J Med.* 1989;320:416-421.
2. Little M, Pereira P, Carrette T, Seymour J. Jellyfish responsible for Irukandji syndrome. *QJM.* 2006;99:425-427.

3 Blood

Transmission of Human Herpesvirus 8 by Blood Transfusion

Hladik W, Dollard SC, Mermin J, et al (Ctrs for Disease Control and Prevention, Entebbe, Uganda; Ctrs for Disease Control and Prevention, Atlanta, Ga; Mulago Hosp, Kampala, Uganda; et al)
N Engl J Med 355:1331-1338, 2006

Background.—Whether human herpesvirus 8 (HHV-8) is transmissible by blood transfusion remains undetermined. We evaluated the risk of HHV-8 transmission by blood transfusion in Uganda, where HHV-8 is endemic.

Methods.—We enrolled patients in Kampala, Uganda, who had received blood transfusions between December 2000 and October 2001. Pretransfusion and multiple post-transfusion blood specimens from up to nine visits over a 6-month period were tested for HHV-8 antibody. We calculated the excess risk of seroconversion over time among recipients of HHV-8–seropositive blood as compared with recipients of seronegative blood.

Results.—Of the 1811 transfusion recipients enrolled, 991 were HHV-8–seronegative before transfusion and completed the requisite follow-up, 43% of whom received HHV-8–seropositive blood and 57% of whom received seronegative blood. HHV-8 seroconversion occurred in 41 of the 991 recipients. The risk of seroconversion was significantly higher among recipients of HHV-8–seropositive blood than among recipients of seronegative blood (excess risk, 2.8%; P<0.05), and the increase in risk was seen mainly among patients in whom seroconversion occurred 3 to 10 weeks after transfusion (excess risk, 2.7%; P=0.005), a result consistent with the transmission of the virus by transfusion. Blood units stored for up to 4 days were more often associated with seroconversion than those stored for more than 4 days (excess risk, 4.2%; P<0.05).

Conclusions.—This study provides strong evidence that HHV-8 is transmitted by blood transfusion. The risk may be diminished as the period of blood storage increases.

▶ The more we learn about newer agents transmitted via blood transfusion, the more inclined all of us should be to decline a transfusion whenever possible and to donate one's own blood for elective surgery. Before 2002, we were not aware, for example, that West Nile virus could be transmitted by blood components. In that year alone, 7 transfusion-related deaths secondary to West Nile virus were described. Fortunately, it did not take too terribly long before nucleic acid amplification technology was adapted for the detection of this virus. The Food and Drug Administration and Health Canada have mandated screening of donated blood for West Nile virus nucleic acid.

It was the problem of transfusion associated HIV infection that woke us all up in the mid 1980s to the need for maintaining vigilance when it came to blood safety. Over the next 20 years, the overall risk of transfusion-transmitted infection has become quite small. Screening is performed by a combination of history taking about risk factors for several parenterally or sexually transmitted viruses, including hepatitis B and C viruses, HIV types 1 and 2, and human T-cell lymphotrophic viruses type I and II. In addition to this, donors are asked about risk factors for malaria, babesiosis, and Chagas' disease. Before blood is transfused into at-risk patients, a cytomegalovirus (CMV) screening is performed or blood undergoes leukocyte reduction (CMV resides in white blood cells). In addition to this, a number of other serologic tests or nucleic acid screenings are performed.

Viruses are not the only infectious agents that can be transmitted in blood. Since March 2004, all platelet components in the United States have been screened for the presence of bacteria because as many as 1 in 3000 random-donor platelet concentrates have been reported to be contaminated by gram-positive and gram-negative bacteria. Bacterial sepsis has turned out to be the most common transfusion-related infectious complication secondary to the administration of platelets. Between 2001 and 2003, an average of 11.7 deaths from bacterial sepsis per year in the United States were reported to the Food and Drug Administration.

These are not the only hazards affecting blood safety. Hepatitis G virus, SEN virus, and TT virus can be transmitted by transfusion and can cause posttransfusion hepatitis. Add to these, HHV-8, simian foamy virus, the coronavirus of the severe acute respiratory syndrome, and the prion that causes variant Creutzfeldt-Jakob disease, and the story continues. Parvovirus B19, enterovirus, and leishmania all have the potential for transmission by blood component therapy.

The report abstracted by Hladik et al offers strong evidence that HHV-8 can be transmitted via transfusion, particularly in parts of the world that have a high prevalence of this viral infection. HHV-8–seropositive blood can cause a HV-like illness similar to CMV. The infection is life long with periodic reactivations during which the virus may circulate in peripheral blood white cells and be transmissible through transfusion. This virus is known to cause Kaposi's sarcoma in immunocompromised individuals.

So the issue with HHV-8 is what to do about it. Unfortunately, no suitable screening assay is currently available for detecting antibody against this virus and there is no nucleic acid screening. As is true of CMV, depleting blood component products of white blood cells might prevent transmission of HHV-8, but the efficacy of leukocyte depletion in this regard has not been established.

In Europe, various technologies are under evaluation by using pathogen-reduction methodologies that include methylene-blue or solvent-detergent treatments to eradicate infectious pathogens. Exposure of blood component products to UVA light can also be helpful. Such technologies have been shown to be effective against most transfusion-transmitted bacteria, viruses, and parasites, but are ineffective against pathologic prions, intracellular pathogens, spore-forming bacteria, and nonenveloped viruses, and viruses that present in exceedingly high concentrations in blood. These techniques sometimes partially destroy blood components, resulting in lessened therapeutic efficacy and necessitating the transfusion of greater quantities of blood component therapy, thus exposing patients to even more blood from more donors.

To learn more about the continuing risk of transfusion-transmitted diseases, see the superb editorial on this topic by Blachman and Vamvakas.[1]

J. A. Stockman III, MD

Reference

1. Blajchman MA, Vamvakas EC. The continuing risk of transfusion-transmitted infections. *N Engl J Med.* 2006;355:1303-1305.

Doppler Ultrasonography versus Amniocentesis to Predict Fetal Anemia
Oepkes D, for the DIAMOND Study Group (Leiden Univ, The Netherlands; et al)
N Engl J Med 355:156-164, 2006

Background.—Pregnancies complicated by Rh alloimmunization have been evaluated with the use of serial invasive amniocentesis to determine bilirubin levels by measuring in the amniotic fluid the change in optical density at a wavelength of 450 nm (ΔOD_{450}); however, this procedure carries risks. Noninvasive Doppler ultrasonographic measurement of the peak velocity of systolic blood flow in the middle cerebral artery also predicts severe fetal anemia, but this test has not been rigorously evaluated in comparison with amniotic-fluid ΔOD_{450}.

Methods.—We performed a prospective, international, multicenter study including women with RhD-, Rhc-, RhE-, or Fy^a-alloimmunized pregnancies with indirect antiglobulin titers of at least 1:64 and antigen-positive fetuses to assess whether Doppler ultrasonographic measurement of the peak systolic velocity of blood flow in the middle cerebral artery was at least as sensitive and accurate as measurement of amniotic-fluid ΔOD_{450} for diagnosing severe fetal anemia. The results of the two tests were compared with the incidence of fetal anemia, as determined by measurement of hemoglobin levels in fetal blood.

Results.—Of 165 fetuses, 74 had severe anemia. For the detection of severe fetal anemia, Doppler ultrasonography of the middle cerebral artery had a sensitivity of 88 percent (95 percent confidence interval, 78 to 93 percent), a specificity of 82 percent (95 percent confidence interval, 73 to 89 percent), and an accuracy of 85 percent (95 percent confidence interval, 79 to 90 percent). Amniotic-fluid ΔOD_{450} had a sensitivity of 76 percent (95 percent confidence interval, 65 to 84 percent), a specificity of 77 percent (95 percent confidence interval, 67 to 84 percent), and an accuracy of 76 percent (95 percent confidence interval, 69 to 82 percent). Doppler ultrasonography was more sensitive, by 12 percentage points (95 percent confidence interval, 0.3 to 24.0), and more accurate, by 9 percentage points (95 percent confidence interval, 1.1 to 15.9), than measurement of amniotic-fluid ΔOD_{450}.

Conclusions.—Doppler measurement of the peak velocity of systolic blood flow in the middle cerebral artery can safely replace invasive testing in the management of Rh-alloimmunized pregnancies.

▶ As time passes, we are finding better ways to detect fetal anemia in babies affected by RhD disease. Back in 1961, Liley reported the use of amniocentesis to measure levels of amniotic-fluid bilirubin as an indirect measure of the destruction of red blood cells. The values obtained were plotted on a three-zone Liley curve, a normative curve for gestations of greater than 27 weeks. The values in zone 1 indicated minimal fetal hemolytic disease, whereas values in zone 3 indicated severe disease with the potential for fetal death without intervention. The advent of ultrasonographically directed access to the fetal umbilical cord (cordocentesis) permitted direct assessment of fetal hematocrit. The rub with cordocentesis to measure something as simple as a hematocrit is that it is a highly invasive technique.

Attempts to identify noninvasive (ultrasonographic) measures that would accurately detect fetal anemia were initially limited by high false-negative rates. Mari and coworkers are credited with introducing noninvasive measurements of the peak velocity of blood flow in the fetal middle cerebral artery with the use of Doppler ultrasonography to detect fetal anemia.[1] The theory behind the techniques described by Mari et al is straightforward. In the anemic fetus, low blood viscosity and increased cardiac output contribute to an increased blood velocity in the middle cerebral artery. Blood flows in excess of 1.5 × normal have a sensitivity of 100% and a specificity of 86% in detecting moderate or severe fetal anemia. Other laboratories have shown a sensitivity of 88% and a specificity of 87% for the detection of moderate or severe anemia.

In the study abstracted, Oepkes et al report the results of a prospective study involving 10 centers comparing Doppler ultrasonography and amniocentesis in 165 fetuses with maternal red-cell alloimmunization, of which 74 were observed to be severely anemic. The sensitivity of Doppler values in the middle cerebral artery above 1.5 multiples of the median was 88%, and the specificity was 82% for severe anemia. This sensitivity was observed to be statistically superior to that of amniocentesis using the Liley curve (sensitivity 76%), but similar to that of amniocentesis with the use of the Queenan method (sensitivity 81%). Please note that an important distinction between the study of Oepkes et al and Mari et al has to do with the definition of fetal anemia. Oepkes et al define significant anemia as more than 5 SD from the mean hemoglobin for the corresponding gestational age, whereas Mari et al used hemoglobins at or below 0.65 multiples of the median. Thus, the definition of Oepkes et al represents a hemoglobin that is 5% to 10% higher than that definition used by Mari et al. If one reviews the data of Oepkes et al using the definitions of Mari et al, the sensitivity reported would actually be better than the data shown by Mari et al.

The data of these two major studies using noninvasive technology support the hypothesis that Doppler values in the middle cerebral artery may largely replace amniocentesis in the management of red-cell alloimmunization in pregnancy, but there are some exceptions. Early experiences indicated the need for dual testing until a perinatal center had in fact mastered the technique of Doppler measurement in the middle cerebral artery. Such measurements are not and should not be left to those who are not expert in the technique. In addition, referral to a perinatal center with experience in the use of Doppler measurement may not be practical for weekly testing. Nonetheless, the data reported by Oepkes et al, combined with other evidence supporting the use of Doppler measure in the middle cerebral artery as superior to amniocentesis in assessing red-cell alloimmunization in pregnancy, suggest that the time has come to put our needles aside when evaluating affected fetuses.

While on the topic of blood and the fetus, the American Academy of Pediatrics (AAP) has recently issued a revised policy on cord blood banking.[2] The policy encourages parents to donate their newborn's cord blood to public cord banks, where it is available to those most in need. It definitively discourages parents from using private cord banks, which can cost thousands of dollars, noting that the chances of a child ever needing their own cord blood are extremely low. Private cord blood banking is recommended for parents who have an older child with a disorder such as a genetic immune deficiency that may be treatable with a transplant of cord blood stem cells. Thus far, more than 5500 unrelated cord blood stem cell transplants have been accomplished and the one-year survival rate of such transplants runs from 40% to 80%, depending on the underlying disorder necessitating the transplant. The cord blood stem cell transplant, if from an HLA-matched sibling, shows a survival rate of somewhere from 75% to 90% (one-year survival rates). There is a shortage of banked cord blood from minority donors, making it less likely that minority patients will find a match in a public cord blood bank. As a result, everyone now recommends that there should be targeted efforts to recruit African-American, Hispanic, American Indian, and Alaskan natives to donate their newborn's cord blood to public cord blood banks. The AAP current policy advises care providers to inform parents that cord blood donated to public banks will be screened for genetic and infectious diseases, and that parents will be notified if any diseases are identified. Parents should also be told that publically banked cord blood may not be available for future private use by the family. Physicians recruiting patients for private cord blood banking services should also disclose any financial interest or other potential conflicts of interest to parents.

Most people are familiar with Sir Richard Branson, owner of the Virgin Group, who has recently formed an entity known as the Virgin Health Bank that will provide parents with a facility to store their child's umbilical cord blood in two portions—one as a private sample for the sole use of the child and his or her family and the second as a public sample, available free of charge to anyone requiring stem cell transplantation. It is expected that about 80% of each sample will be placed in the public bank, and 20% held in the private bank, although this will depend on the individual cord blood sample, stem cell expansion, and whether the cells meet the regulatory requirements for the international transplantation registry. For a fee of £1500, parents can buy processing services and a 20-year storage of umbilical cord blood. These private banks have been widely criticized by health care staff and medical associations for approaching parents at a vulnerable time, making far-fetched references to future regenerative use in diseases such as Parkinson's disease, diabetes, and heart disease while concealing the true likelihood for personal use for current indications, which is somewhere between 1 in 1000 and 1 in 200,0000. What makes the Virgin Health Bank different is this dual public/private approach in which a portion of the sample will be available for public use anywhere in the world, at no cost. Additionally, Branson has pledged to donate 50% of the proceeds from Virgin Health Bank to initiatives involved in realizing the potential of cord blood stem cells. It is hard to criticize Sir Richard for his thinking on this topic.

J. A. Stockman III, MD

References

1. Mari G, Deter RL, Carpenter RL, et al. Noninvasive diagnosis by Doppler ultrasonography of fetal anemia due to maternal red-cell alloimmunization. *N Engl J Med*. 2000;342:9-14.
2. American Academy of Pediatrics Section on Hematology/Oncology; American Academy of Pediatrics Section on Allergy/Immunology, Lubin BH, Shearer WT. Cord blood banking for potential future transplantation. *Pediatrics*. 2007; 119:165-170.

Clinical Manifestations of Hemoglobin Chico at High Altitude

Starkey CR, Davies L, Hoyer JD, et al (Univ of New Mexico, Albuquerque; Mayo Clinic, Rochester, Minn)
J Pediatr Hematol Oncol 28:760-762, 2006

Summary.—Hemoglobin Chico is a rare hemoglobinopathy characterized by low oxygen affinity and a right-shifted oxygen dissociation curve. Detailed clinical evaluations of affected individuals have not been previously reported. We therefore report on the clinical features of Hemoglobin Chico in a Latino male living at high altitude, who desired to participate in school sports. As a young boy with asthma, he had the unusual finding of growth delay and digital clubbing which improved with asthma control. At 16 years of age, he had mild anemia and a decreased pulse oximetry (83%) but sufficient pulmonary reserve to participate in physically demanding activities.

► The youngster who is the focus of this report presented in a very interesting way with his hematologic disorder. He was a Latino boy with a past medical history of multiple hospitalizations related to reactive airway disease. He was treated at the University of New Mexico Hospital in Albuquerque. He had multiple low oxygen saturations assessed with pulse oximetry. This was initially attributed to living with poorly controlled asthma at an altitude of 5395 feet above sea level. He also had an unexplained mild normochromic normocytic anemia. Even with adequate management of his asthma, the patient had a persistently low pulse oximetry and the etiology of his anemia remained elusive. Although well appearing, his pulse oximetry ran in the low 80% range. Ultimately, a hemoglobin electrophoresis was performed. This revealed Hb Chico. A review of the family history showed that the patient was related to an extended family with this same hemoglobinopathy, who resided in California.

Most pediatricians are not familiar with Hemoglobin Chico. It is a hemoglobinopathy characterized by a substitution of the amino acid lysine at position 66 of the beta chain by threonine. This substitution causes a decrease in oxygen affinity of hemoglobin, resulting in a right-shifted hemoglobin oxygen dissociation curve. In a sense, such hemoglobinopathies produce a "super hemoglobin" that readily releases oxygen to tissues. In fact, Hemoglobin Chico releases oxygen twice as readily as normal hemoglobin. Patients with hemoglobinopathies related to a right-shifted hemoglobin oxygen dissociation curve release oxygen so well that they sometimes look bluish because of their low oxygen saturations.

Hemoglobin Chico is a rare hemoglobinopathy and was first identified in a mildly anemic but otherwise asymptomatic 3-year-old boy and 4 additional family members in three generations in Chico, California. This was back in 1987.[1]

One final comment about subjects who have hemoglobinopathies causing a right-shifted hemoglobin oxygen dissociation curve: Oxygen is released so well from these abnormal hemoglobins that the patient does not need the same level of hemoglobin as a normal person. The relative abundance of tissue oxygenation causes a secondary compensatory decrease in erythropoietin production causing a decreased rate of erythropoiesis and the development of a "physiologic anemia."

Remember the principles related to the pathophysiology caused by these rare hemoglobins associated with decreased oxygen affinity. Patients with them generally are healthy, but often blue, and with a mild anemia that evades routine diagnostic testing, until one thinks of the possible correct diagnosis.

J. A. Stockman III, MD

Reference

1. Shih DT, Jones RT, Shih MF, Jones MF, Koler RD, Howard J. Hemoglobin Chico [beta 66(E10)Lys-Thr]: a new variant with decreased oxygen affinity. *Hemoglobin.* 1987;11:453-464.

N-Terminal Pro-Brain Natriuretic Peptide Levels and Risk of Death in Sickle Cell Disease

Machado RF, for the MSH Investigators (NIH, Bethesda, Md; et al)
JAMA 296:310-318, 2006

Context.—Thirty percent of patients with sickle cell disease (SCD) develop pulmonary hypertension, a major risk factor for death in this population. A validated blood biomarker of pulmonary hypertension in SCD could provide important prognostic and diagnostic information and allow the exploration of the prevalence of pulmonary hypertension in participants in the 1996 Multicenter Study of Hydroxyurea in Sickle Cell Anemia (MSH) Patients' Follow-up Study. Levels of N-terminal pro-brain natriuretic peptide (NT-proBNP) provide such information in patients with idiopathic pulmonary arterial hypertension.

Objective.—To determine the relationship between NT-proBNP levels and severity of pulmonary hypertension and prospective mortality in patients with SCD.

Design, Setting, and Participants.—NT-proBNP levels were measured in 230 participants in the National Institutes of Health (NIH) Sickle Cell Disease–Pulmonary Hypertension Screening Study (enrollment between February 2001 and March 2005) and in 121 samples from patients enrolled starting in 1996 in the MSH Patients' Follow-up Study. A threshold level predictive of high pulmonary artery pressure and mortality was identified in the NIH Sickle Cell Disease–Pulmonary Hypertension Screening Study and used to define an a priori analytical plan to determine the prevalence and associated mortality of pulmonary hypertension in the MSH follow-up study.

Main Outcome Measures.—Severity of pulmonary hypertension and risk of all-cause mortality.

Results.—NT-proBNP levels were higher in patients with sickle cell pulmonary hypertension and correlated directly with tricuspid regurgitant jet velocity in the NIH cohort ($R = 0.50$, $P<.001$). An NT-proBNP level of 160 pg/mL or greater had a 78% positive predictive value for the diagnosis of pulmonary hypertension and was an independent predictor of mortality (21 deaths at 31 months' median follow-up; risk ratio, 5.1; 95% confidence interval, 2.1-12.5; $P<.001$; 19.5% absolute increase in risk of death). In the MSH cohort, 30% of patients had an NT-proBNP level of 160 pg/mL or greater. An NT-proBNP level of 160 pg/mL or greater in the MSH cohort was independently associated with mortality by Cox proportional hazards regression analysis (24 deaths at 47 months' median follow-up; risk ratio, 2.87; 95% confidence interval, 1.2-6.6; $P = .02$; 11.9% absolute increase in risk of death).

Conclusions.—Pulmonary hypertension, as indicated by an NT-proBNP level of 160 pg/mL or greater, was very common in patients in the NIH study and in the MSH cohort. The MSH analysis suggests that rates of vaso-occlusive pain episodes in these patients were unrelated to risk of death; this risk was largely determined by occult hemolytic anemia–associated pulmonary hypertension.

▶ In patients with SCD, pulmonary hypertension is associated with a high mortality rate and has been linked to anemia, high hemolytic rates, iron overload, and systemic vasculopathy.

You would think that pulmonary hypertension in a patient with SCD might result from repetitive episodes of the acute chest syndrome and repetitive cycles of pulmonary vascular vaso-occlusion. This does not appear to be the case. Unexpectedly, data have shown that pulmonary pressures do not appear to be associated with rates of vaso-occlusive pain crises, acute chest syndrome, or leukocytosis. This lack of association is consistent with a higher prevalence of pulmonary hypertension in other hereditary hemolytic anemias such as thalassemia intermedia, for example, in which vaso-occlusive crises and acute chest syndrome are absent. A pathogenic link between pulmonary hypertension and hemolytic anemia is also consistent with the role of intravascular hemolysis and the development of endothelial dysfunction and vasculopathy.

So, what is the link between hemolytic anemia and the development of pulmonary hypertension? The linkage between pulmonary hypertension and hemolytic anemia may be brain natriuretic peptide (BNP). BNP is a hormone released in response to cardiomyocyte stretch, and high levels reflect cardiac chamber volume and pressure overload. The importance of BNP has been demonstrated in several cardiovascular disorders. For example, in patients with pulmonary arterial hypertension, BNP levels correlate with the severity of pulmonary artery pressure elevation and with right ventricular dysfunction. The study reported suggests that in patients with SCD, an elevated BNP level largely reflects the severity of right ventricular dysfunction associated with pulmonary arterial hypertension rather than left ventricular filling abnormalities and is strongly associated with advanced stage, renal insufficiency, iron overload, and hemolytic anemia and not with repetitive episodes of acute chest syndrome. These data suggest that the number of episodes of vaso-occlusive crisis or acute chest syndrome are not associated with pulmonary hypertension, and that pulmonary hypertension represents the single largest determinant of prospective risk of death in the SCD population. BNP levels have been shown to correlate with functional capacity, severity of pulmonary hypertension, and prognosis in patients with pulmonary arterial hypertension. The same appears to be true in patients with SCD.

The most apparent central process in the development of pulmonary hypertension in patients with SCD is their hemolytic anemia. There is a theory as to what is going on here. As a result of hemolysis, hemoglobin is released into plasma, where it reacts and destroys nitric oxide, resulting in the state of intrinsic resistance to nitric oxide–dependent vasodilatation. In addition, hemolysis also releases erythrocyte arginase into plasma, which depletes L-arginine, the substrate for nitric oxide synthesis, by its conversion to ornithine. The association between markers of hemolytic anemia and BNP levels provides further epidemiologic evidence for a mechanistic link between hemolysis and pulmonary hypertension. Hemolysis and impaired nitric oxide bioavailability are likely also to increase the risk of intravascular thrombosis. Hemolysis leads to the accumulation of plasma and tissue redox-active heme and iron, which contributes to the generation of reactive oxygen species that can exacerbate ischemia-reperfusion injury, thrombosis, and endothelial and smooth muscle proliferative responses. There are a number of clinical complications of SCD that are associated with low hemoglobin levels, including not only pulmonary hypertension, but also priapism and leg ulcers, which suggests that there may exist a clinical subtype of SCD also caused by chronic hemolytic anemia.

Chances are you are going to hear a lot more about BNP and hemolytic anemia. Because BNP levels can be readily measured, they may become markers that will be recognized as a major risk factor for morbidity and mortality in patients with SCD. If the data from this report are true, the trick will be to find ways to interfere with the various pathogenetic mechanisms that are being described.

J. A. Stockman III, MD

Right ventricular abnormalities in sickle cell anemia: Evidence of a progressive increase in pulmonary vascular resistance
Qureshi N, Joyce JJ, Qi N, et al (UCLA, Los Angeles; Children's Hosp and Research Ctr at Oakland, Calif; Univ of Florida, Jacksonville)
J Pediatr 149:23-27, 2006

Objective.—To assess the effects of sickle cell anemia (SCA) on the right ventricle (RV).

Study Design.—Echocardiograms of 32 children with SCA were compared with age-matched healthy controls. RV measurements included diastolic area index, fractional area change, free-wall mass index, ejection time corrected for heart rate (ET_c), and tricuspid regurgitation (TR) gradient.

Results.—SCA subjects had elevated RV ETc (mean ± standard deviation, $0.369 ± 0.030$ sec vs $0.351 ± 0.022$ sec; P < .01), diastolic area index ($19.9 ± 2.4$ cm^2/m^2 vs $13.2 ± 2.1$ cm^2/m^2; $P < .01$) and free-wall mass index ($33.2 ± 4.4$ g/m^2 vs $23.9 ± 4.3$ g/m^2; $P < .01$), whereas RV fractional area change ($37 ± 8\%$ vs $36 ± 4\%$) was not different from controls. Although RV diastolic area index in SCA paralleled the normal range over time, RV free-wall mass index continued to gradually rise throughout childhood ($r = .42$; $P < .05$). TR gradients > 2.5 m/sec, consistent with pulmonary hypertension, were found in 5 (16%) of SCA subjects, all older than 9 years.

Conclusions.—RV preload and systolic function do not worsen during childhood in SCA; however, RV mass index and the prevalence of pulmonary hypertension increase consistent with rising pulmonary vascular resistance.

▶ The Machado et al (N-terminal pro-brain natriuretic peptide levels and risk of death in sickle cell disease), deals with natriuretic factor as part of the pathophysiology of pulmonary hypertension in patients with sickle cell disease. This report of Qureshi et al adds to our knowledge about this problem by addressing right ventricular abnormalities in sickle cell disease in patients aged 6 months to 21 years. By using this as a marker of pulmonary hypertension, some 16% of this population had evidence of pulmonary hypertension. The data suggest that early diagnosis might be possible, offering the potential for developing both preventative and therapeutic strategies.

There seems to be some correlation between age and the onset of pulmonary hypertension, suggesting that more specific studies are needed to determine at what age screening with echocardiography is warranted. Given the relatively modest cost of echocardiography and the long-term consequences of the development of pulmonary hypertension, it would seem that liberal use of ultrasound is warranted in the routine surveillance of patients with sickle cell disease being followed in centers created for this purpose. In fact, the Section on Hematology-Oncology, Committee on Genetics of the American Academy of Pediatrics, does recommend routine screening echocardiograms as an integral component of surveillance health supervision of children with SCA.[1] Specific attention to right ventricular function, however, is not part of the standard recommendations and probably should be.

J. A. Stockman III, MD

Reference

1. Section on Hematology-Oncology, Committee on Genetics, American Academy of Pediatrics. Health supervision for children with sickle cell disease. *Pediatrics.* 2002;109:526-535.

Daytime pulse oximeter measurements do not predict incidence of pain and acute chest syndrome episodes in sickle cell anemia
Uong EC, Boyd JH, DeBaun MR (Washington Univ, St Louis)
J Pediatr 149:707-709, 2006

Background.—Relationships have been postulated between oxygen saturation (SpO_2) values and acute chest syndrome (ACS) episodes in children with sickle cell anemia (SCA). However, the results of tests comparing the two have often proved inconclusive. Infants with SCA were evaluated to determine if the baseline daytime SpO_2 reading can predict subsequent rates of pain and ACS episodes.

Methods.—One hundred thirty African American children with hemoglobin SS (HbSS) who had pulse oximetry data available and who were less than 6 months of age were analyzed prospectively. They received annual checkups and monitoring of clinical episodes over a mean of 13 years. The mean age of the children at final follow-up was 9.8 years, with a range of 4.8 to 15.7 years.

Results.—The range of SpO_2 varied from 75% to 100%, with a mean of 94.1% and a median of 95%. The SpO_2 measurements showed no relationship to pain rate. None of the specific SpO_2 values were associated with increased pain rates. Similarly, SpO_2 measurements showed no association with ACS rate, even after controlling for age, white blood cell count, hematocrit, and fetal hemoglobin levels. No SpO_2 measurement was related to an increased ACS incidence rate. Statistical analysis verified a single SpO_2 measurement was not related to preceding pain episodes or ACS.

Conclusions.—No relationship existed between SpO_2 values and the SCA-related morbidity occurring subsequently. Daytime SpO_2 measurements were thus not predictive of SCA morbidity, but this finding does not indicate whether a relationship exists between pain rate and nocturnal SpO_2 values. Evaluation of a possible relationship between daytime and nocturnal SpO_2 values is needed.

▶ Today, most sickle cell programs routinely measure oxygen saturation by pulse oximetry (SpO_2) during well-child visits for all patients. Back in 1993,

Rackoff et al[1] developed a nomogram using measurements of SpO_2 and baseline hemoglobin level to derive the partial pressure of oxygen in arterial blood and to determine whether this value was suggestive of an acute pulmonary process. We see in this report that a large proportion of otherwise well-appearing children with sickle cell disease are walking around with an SpO_2 less than 96%. The cause of this low SpO_2 in asymptomatic children with sickle cell disease is not completely understood. It is important to know whether baseline SpO_2 has clinical significance or predictive value for the development of future sickle cell complications.

What we also learn from this report is the complete lack of an association between a single baseline SpO_2 measurement obtained by pulse oximetry and the subsequent occurrence of pain or acute chest syndrome over a mean follow-up period of 3 years. However, this does not mean that clinicians can be unconcerned that baseline hypoxemia is detrimental to children and adolescents with sickle cell disease. The relative contributions of daytime and nighttime SpO_2, how to best measure daytime SpO_2, and how to assess its effects on the course of disease remain to be determined.

J. A. Stockman III, MD

Reference

1. Rackoff WR, Kunkel N, Silber JH, Asakura T, Ohene-Frempong K. Pulse oximetry and factors associated with hemoglobin oxygen desaturation in children with sickle cell disease. *Blood.* 1993;81:3422-3427.

Impact of acute chest syndrome on lung function of children with sickle cell disease

Sylvester KP, Patey RA, Mulligan P, et al (King's College, London)
J Pediatr 149:17-22, 2006

Objective.—To test the hypothesis that children with sickle cell disease (SCD) who experienced an acute chest syndrome (ACS) hospitalization episode would have worse lung function than children with SCD without ACS episodes.

Study Design.—Forced expiratory volume in 1 second (FEV_1); forced vital capacity (FVC); FEV_1/FVC ratio; peak expiratory flow (PEF); forced expiratory flow at 25% (FEF_{25}), 50% (FEF_{50}), and 75% (FEF_{75}) of FVC; airway resistance (Raw); and lung volumes were compared in 20 children with ACS and 20 aged-matched children without ACS (median age, 11 years; range, 6 to 16 years). Fourteen age-matched pairs were assessed before and after bronchodilator use.

Results.—The mean Raw ($P = .03$), TLC ($P = .01$), and RV ($P = .003$) were significantly higher in the group with ACS than in the group without ACS. There were no significant differences in the changes in lung function test results in response to bronchodilator administration between the 2 groups, but the children with ACS had a lower FEF_{25} ($P = .04$) and FEF_{75}

(P = .03) pre-bronchodilator use and a lower mean FEV_1/FVC ratio (P = .03) and FEF_{75} (P = .03) post-bronchodilator use.

Conclusions.—Children with SCD who experienced an ACS hospitalization episode had significant differences in lung function compared with those who did not experience ACS episodes. Our results are compatible with the hypothesis that ACS episodes predispose children to increased airway obstruction.

▶ These British investigators examined the pulmonary function of some 20 children with SCD who had a previous episode of ACS. They observe increases in mean airway resistance, total lung capacity, and residual volume in those who have experienced an ACS episode. These data are consistent with previous studies that have identified that both an obstructive and restrictive pattern of lung function is common in subjects with SCD. Airway hyperresponsiveness has also been described in this population.

There is no question that we need more research to better define ways to achieve better outcomes for children and adults with SCD. It was 30 years ago that the first major legislation concerning SCD was passed. This resulted in development of comprehensive sickle cell centers. We are now at another watershed moment in the treatment of this illness with the passage in October 2004 of the Sickle Cell Treatment Act, designed to substantially expand specialized sickle cell treatment programs. Unfortunately, despite major advances in SCD treatments that have occurred over the past 3 decades, important gaps exist in both the equity of government and private philanthropic support for research and in the uniform provision of high quality clinical care. Back in 1970, the life expectancy for a subject with SCD was just 10 to 12 years. The development of sickle cell centers was a key factor in the extension of life expectancy to 20 to 22 years by the time of the mid-1980s. By the 1990s, with the introduction of prophylactic penicillin, survivorship increased to 35 years. By the turn of the century with various other therapies (hydroxyurea, bone marrow transplantation, stroke prevention, and the introduction of the pneumococcal vaccine) survivorship has increased to an average life expectancy of 40 to 45 years. Hopefully, the passage of the Sickle Cell Treatment Act providing funding for 40 SCD treatment centers, the establishment of a national coordinating center, and federal matching funds for genetic counseling and education will add to this increase in life expectancy.

To read more about SCD and questions of equity and quality, see the superb review by Smith et al.[1] No one likes to pit one disease against another in terms of governmental research funding or private philanthropy, but the data are clear when it comes to SCD. For example, a comparison of funding for this disease and cystic fibrosis shows remarkable discrepancies. The studies of the prevalence of SCD here in the United States indicate that about 80,000 individuals are affected in comparison to 30,000 individuals with cystic fibrosis. The NIH spends about $90 million (in 2004) on sickle cell disease versus $128 million on cystic fibrosis. This equates to approximately $1125 spent on each patient with SCD versus $4267 on each patient with cystic fibrosis. With respect to private philanthropic dollars, the Sickle Cell Disease Association of America is about the only source of private philanthropic dollars for SCD accounting for fundraising of less than half a million dollars a year (or $6.00 per subject with sickle cell disease) versus private philanthropy from the Cystic Fibrosis Foundation, which generates in excess of $150 million a year (somewhat over $5000 per patient with cystic fibrosis).

J. A. Stockman III, MD

Reference

1. Smith LA, Oyeku SO, Homer C, Zuckerman B. Sickle cell disease: a question of equity and quality. *Pediatrics*. 2006;117:1763-1770.

Exchange blood transfusion compared with simple transfusion for first overt stroke is associated with a lower risk of subsequent stroke: A retrospective cohort study of 137 children with sickle cell anemia
Hulbert ML, Scothorn DJ, Panepinto JA, et al (Washington Univ, St Louis; Univ of Texas, Dallas; Med College of Wisconsin, Milwaukee; et al)
J Pediatr 149:710-712, 2006

Background.—Children with sickle cell disease who suffer stroke can undergo either simple or exchange transfusion. The benefits and risks associated with each of these methods have not been assessed sufficiently, particularly in relation to outcomes. A retrospective approach was used to determine which is most effective as an initial treatment: simple or exchange transfusion.

Methods.—All 137 patients included in the study had sickle cell anemia (SCA) and had undergone transfusion therapy for at least 5 years after having a stroke. The initial stroke had occurred between ages 1.4 and 14 years (mean age, 6.3 years). Follow-up extended for 5 to 24 years, with a mean of 10.1 years. Exchange transfusion was accomplished with either manual exchange or automated erythrocytapheresis. The stroke-free survival times for patients receiving simple or exchange transfusions were compared.

Results.—Thirty-one of the 137 patients (23%) suffered recurrent stroke while they were receiving blood transfusion therapy. Most patients received exchange transfusion as the initial therapy after stroke, with increasing percentages from 0 of 4 having a stroke before 1980 to 37 of 43 having a stroke after 1990. Recurrent strokes developed in 57% of the patients who received simple transfusion therapy, but only 21% of those who received exchange transfusion therapy. The incidence of recurrent stroke among patients treated with simple transfusion was 5-fold greater than the incidence in patients with exchange transfusion treatments. The relative risk for a second stroke was diminished in patients who were given both acute and chronic exchange transfusions.

Conclusions.—Exchange transfusion is now the most common treatment given to children with SCA who suffer a stroke. The use of an initial exchange transfusion is linked to a reduced risk for developing a second stroke in these children. Thus exchange transfusion treatment may prevent recurrent stroke in pediatric SCA patients.

▶ This report provides much needed insight into secondary stroke prevention in children with sickle cell disease. Although not a randomized trial on the prevention of secondary stroke, this study does support the hypothesis that an initial exchange transfusion after a first stroke may prevent recurrent strokes better than an initial simple transfusion. Exchange transfusion is a more efficient way than simple transfusion to acutely reduce the proportion of circulating sickle hemoglobin. The technique can be performed manually or by automated erythrocytapheresis. The latter procedure can precisely target the desired final hematocrit and desired percentage of hemoglobins while maintaining a stable blood volume; total transfusion time is shorter than for simple transfusion, even though the volume of blood used is larger. The problem with automated exchange transfusion procedures includes the long setup time (as long as 4 to 6 hours in some institutions), the need for two large-bore intravenous lines or an apheresis catheter, and exposure of the patient to an increased number of donors. The study does document that exchange transfusion is quickly becoming the predominant initial treatment for acute stroke in patients with sickle cell disease.

Many sickle cell centers are also using exchange transfusion as the treatment of choice for their chronic transfusion regimens. This approach removes senescent red cells before they are taken out of the circulation by the body, unlike standard hypertransfusion programs. The approach therefore somewhat minimizes the iron overload problem associated with chronic transfusions. An advantage associated with chronic exchange transfusion may be more effective maintenance of the target hemoglobin S level at less than 30%, which is considered the standard of care for secondary stroke prevention.

See the Strouse et al report (Primary hemorrhagic stroke in children with sickle cell disease is associated with recent transfusion and use of corticosteroids), which tells us about the risk factors for primary hemorrhagic stroke in children with sickle cell disease.

J. A. Stockman III, MD

Primary Hemorrhagic Stroke in Children With Sickle Cell Disease Is Associated With Recent Transfusion and Use of Corticosteroids
Strouse JJ, Hulbert ML, DeBaun MR, et al (Johns Hopkins Univ, Baltimore, Md; Washington Univ, St Louis)
Pediatrics 118:1916-1924, 2006

Objectives.—Primary hemorrhagic stroke is an uncommon complication of sickle cell disease, with reported mortality rates of 24% to 65%. Most reported cases are in adults; little is known about its occurrence in children. Proposed risk factors include previous ischemic stroke, aneurysms, low steady-state hemoglobin, high steady-state leukocyte count, acute chest syndrome, and hypertransfusion. We performed a retrospective case-control study to evaluate risk and prognostic factors for primary hemorrhagic stroke among children with sickle cell disease.

Patients and Methods.—Case subjects (sickle cell disease and primary hemorrhagic stroke) and control subjects (sickle cell disease and ischemic stroke) were identified at 2 children's hospitals from January 1979 to December 2004 by reviewing divisional records and the discharge databases.

Results.—We identified 15 case subjects (mean age: 10.4 ± 1.3 years) and 29 control subjects (mean age: 5.2 ± 0.4 years). An increased risk of hemorrhagic stroke was associated with a history of hypertension and recent (in the last 14 days) transfusion, treatment with corticosteroids, and possibly nonsteroidal antiinflammatory drugs. Average blood pressures at well visits (adjusted for age and gender) were similar between the 2 groups, suggesting that hypertension was intermittent.

Conclusions.—In this group of children with sickle cell disease, hemorrhagic stroke was associated with a history of hypertension or antecedent events including transfusion or treatment with corticosteroids. Improved understanding of risk and prognostic factors, especially those that are modifiable, may help prevent this devastating complication in children with sickle cell disease.

▶ The incidence of hemorrhagic stroke is greatly increased in patients with sickle cell anemia compared with the general population. In the Cooperative Study of Sickle Cell Disease, the incidence of hemorrhagic stroke ranges from 0.17 per 100 patient years for children younger than 10 years to 0.44 per 100 years for patients aged 20 to 29 years.[1] Hemorrhage accounts for more than one quarter of all strokes in patients under 20 years of age and is defined as including intraparenchymal, subarachnoid, and intraventricular hemorrhage. Hemorrhagic stroke accounts for almost all of the initial mortality associated with stroke and sickle cell disease. Approximately 3% of children with sickle cell anemia (HbSS) will have a hemorrhagic stroke by 20 years of age, and 25% to 50% of these patients will die within 2 weeks of the event. There is a nearly 250-fold increase in the risk of hemorrhagic stroke in patients with sickle cell disease compared with the general population of children.

The typical presentation of a hemorrhagic stroke includes severe headache, nuchal rigidity, coma, and focal neurologic deficits. The spinal fluid is often bloody and xanthochromic. There have been many proposed risk factors for hemorrhagic stroke, but only a few have been rigorously evaluated and none have been looked at exclusively in children. The Cooperative Study of Sickle Cell Disease has now identified three significant risk factors for first hemorrhagic stroke in children and adults with sickle cell disease: age, low steady-state hemoglobin concentration, and high steady-state leukocyte count. Other proposed risk factors include previous ischemic stroke, moyamoya disease, cerebral aneurysm, acute chest syndrome, acute hypertension, and hypertransfusion. In the study abstracted, the investigators also identified a very strong association with recent blood transfusion and treatment with corticosteroids.

Exactly why recent transfusion or steriod use might incur a higher risk of hemorrhagic stroke remains speculative because these management techniques are often used in patients with other risk factors. The relationship between hemorrhagic stroke and transfusion may reflect a deleterious effect of transfusion on the viscosity of blood or the regulation of cerebral blood flow. Several investigators have postulated an effect of transfusion on blood pressure or other hemodynamic parameters through vasoactive substances in stored blood. Steroids may be a factor as a result of their ability to increase blood pressure. An increase in blood pressure is more detrimental in patients with sickle cell disease. The higher systolic blood pressure at presentation in many patients with primary hemorrhagic stroke supports the contribution of elevated blood pressure to risk of hemorrhagic stroke. Steroid use may also be a proxy for more severe disease related to sickle cell disease, the latter being the root cause of the hemorrhagic stroke.

Unfortunately there is no established specific therapy for acute hemorrhagic stroke in sickle cell disease once a stroke is established. Death usually occurs within days of diagnosis and is related to the mass effect of the hemorrhage causing tonsillar herniation or vasospasm. Invasive monitoring and treatment of increased intracranial pressure should be routine. All children should be carefully studied to be sure that an aneurysm is not the cause of the bleeding, because this may be treatable with surgery. One interesting observation in this study is that none of the patients who survived a primary hemorrhagic stroke had a recurrent neurologic event or died during nearly 30 years of follow-up, suggesting that this group may be at a lower risk for recurrent events or death. This differs from patients with a history of ischemic stroke, who usually have recurrent events unless properly managed.

Before leaving the topic of stroke, a query unrelated to sickle cell disease: what is meant by the term "economy class stroke" and what is now thought to be a major cause of the problem? If you are not familiar with the term "economy class" syndrome, this usually refers to the development of a deep venous thrombosis resulting from sitting still for several hours while on an airliner, while driving a car for lengthy periods, or while sitting on a train. More recently, it has been recognized that similar periods of inactivity may increase one's risk of stroke. In an observational study, 43 of 338 patients with a first cerebral ischemic event had spent at least 4 hours traveling in a sitting position in the four preceding weeks of a stroke. Forty-five percent of patients who were investigated further were found to have a patent foramen ovale, compared with just 11% of stroke patients who had not spent 4 hours or more traveling recently. The former group also had fewer known risk factors for stroke such as smoking, hypertension, atrial fibrillation, and diabetes, and were more likely to have signs related to the posterior cerebral artery. Paradoxical embolism is the suggested cause, although this could not be proven in all cases. The risk of "economy class stroke" appears to apply not only to plane travel, but to travel in buses, cars, and trains. Needless to say, the prevention of the problem of economy class stroke is to move around as much as one can during periods of prolonged travel.[2]

J. A. Stockman III, MD

References

1. Ohene-Frempong K, Weiner SJ, Sleeper LA, et al. Cerebrovascular accidents in sickle cell disease: rates and risk factors. *Blood*. 1998;91:288-294.

2. Heckmann JG, Stadter M, Reulbach U, Duetsch M, Nixdorff U, Ringwald J. Increased frequency of cardioembolism and patent foramen ovale in patients with stroke and a positive travel history suggesting economy class stroke syndrome. *Heart.* 2006;92: 1265-1268.

AMG 531, a Thrombopoiesis-Stimulating Protein, for Chronic ITP

Bussel JB, Kuter DJ, George JN, et al (New York Presbyterian Hosp; Massachusetts Gen Hosp, Boston; Univ of Oklahoma, Oklahoma City; et al)
N Engl J Med 355:1672-1681, 2006

Background.—Most current treatments for chronic immune thrombocytopenic purpura (ITP) act by decreasing platelet destruction. In a phase 1-2 study, we administered a thrombopoiesis-stimulating protein, AMG 531, to patients with ITP.

Methods.—In phase 1, 24 patients who had received at least one treatment for ITP were assigned to escalating-dose cohorts of 4 patients each and given two identical doses of AMG 531 (0.2 to 10 µg per kilogram of body weight). In phase 2, 21 patients were randomly assigned to receive six weekly subcutaneous injections of AMG 531 (1, 3, or 6 µg per kilogram) or placebo. The primary objective was to assess the safety of AMG 531; the secondary objective was to evaluate platelet counts during and after treatment.

Results.—No major adverse events that could be attributed directly to AMG 531 occurred during the treatment period; 4 of 41 patients had transient post-treatment worsening of thrombocytopenia. In phase 1, a platelet count that was within the targeted range (50,000 to 450,000 per cubic millimeter) and at least twice the baseline count was achieved in 4 of 12 patients given 3, 6, or 10 µg of AMG 531 per kilogram. Overall, a platelet count of at least 50,000 per cubic millimeter was achieved in 7 of 12 patients, including 3 with counts exceeding 450,000 per cubic millimeter. Increases in the platelet count were dose-dependent; mean peak counts were 163,000, 309,000, and 746,000 per cubic millimeter with 3, 6, and 10 µg of AMG 531 per kilogram [corrected], respectively. In phase 2, the targeted platelet range was achieved in 10 of 16 patients treated with 1 or 3 µg of AMG 531 per kilogram per week for 6 weeks. Mean peak counts were 135,000, 241,000, and 81,000 per cubic millimeter in the groups that received the 1-µg dose, the 3-µg dose, and placebo, respectively.

Conclusions.—AMG 531 caused no major adverse events and increased platelet counts in patients with ITP.

▶ By now, most of us have come to accept the fact that multiple mechanisms cause thrombocytopenia in children (and adults) with ITP. The disorder is likely to be a heterogeneous one. Over 50 years ago, Harrington first demonstrated that a factor in plasma from patients with ITP induced thrombocytopenia in normal subjects. Subsequent studies identified this factor as an autoantibody against glycoproteins in the platelet membrane. Additional mechanisms that lead to platelet destruction involve the activation of helper T cells and cytotoxic T cells. The initiating event for ITP still remains unknown.

The major issue pediatricians face when presented with a youngster with ITP is whether or not to treat. The decision to treat is based on the platelet count, the degree of bleeding, and the patient's lifestyle. Many if not most patients with ITP require no therapy, only careful monitoring. Because severe bleeding is uncommon with platelet counts that exceed 30,000 per cubic millimeter, treatments are often initiated when platelet counts fall well below this number. Most current treatments are aimed at interfering with antibody-mediated platelet destruction by inhibiting the function of macrophage Fc receptors, decreasing antibody production, or both. Corticosteroids are the backbone of the initial treatment and are effective in 50% to 80% of cases. Other effective treatments include intravenous immunoglobulin and Rh(D) immune globulin (for patients who are Rh-positive). Sustained remission with any of these agents, however, is uncommon if the disease is not going away by itself. Splenectomy is the traditional second-line treatment for patients who do not have a response to steroids or who do not have a sustained remission with any form of therapy. In most cases, splenectomy can be curative. The relapse rate post splenectomy is approximately 15% to 25%. Needless to say, there are some risks associated with splenectomy, including a lifelong increased risk of bacterial sepsis.

In the last decade or so, we have seen a number of additional therapies becoming available for patients who either decline splenectomy or for whom splenectomy has not been effective. Rituximab, the monoclonal antibody against CD20 B-cells, has an overall response rate of 25% to 50%, and when it works, it really works. Other agents that have induced responses when used as third-line treatments include Rh(D) immune globulin, intravenous immune globulin, azathioprine, cyclophosphamide, danazol, vinca alkaloids, dapsone, combination chemotherapy, cyclosporine, and mycophenolate mofetil. Most pediatric hematologists have not had a great deal of experience with some of these therapies. All these therapies, except for Rh(D) immune globulin, may prove useful in patients who have been splenectomized.

In the report abstracted, Bussel et al report on a phase 1-2 study of AMG 531, administered subcutaneously for 3 to 6 weeks in 41 adults with chronic ITP in whom one or more prior therapies had failed. Most of these patients had undergone splenectomy, and many required corticosteroid therapy. In the past 10 years, this new class of drugs known as thrombopoietic agents has emerged. Spawned by the cloning of thrombopoietin, the ligand for the Mpl receptor expressed by megacaryocytes, and platelets, these agents induce the growth and maturation of megacaryocytes and result in elevated platelet counts in healthy volunteers. On the basis of the observation that platelet production is impaired in most patients with ITP, small pilot studies have evaluated the use of human thrombopoietin with encouraging results. Unfortunately, antibodies formed against thrombopoietin and this agent therefore has been withdrawn from further clinical investigation. Non-immunogenic thrombopoietic peptides and small, non-peptide molecules have subsequently been developed, including one such agent, AMG 531. The latter is composed of an immunoglobulin domain fragment linked to two identical peptide chains that bind and activate the Mpl receptor.

What we learn from the report of Bussel et al is that increases in platelet count to satisfactory levels will occur within 8 days in most patients treated with AMG 531. The overall response rate was found to be 68%. Short-term complications appear to be minimal with the administration of AMG 531.

Thus we now have a promising new therapeutic strategy for ITP if the latter is refractory to second- and third-line therapies. The exact role of AMG 531 obviously remains to be seen and further clinical trials of longer duration are needed. Nonetheless, the outlook for patients with chronic ITP refractory to other forms of therapy has now improved just a notch with the introduction of AMG 531.

J. A. Stockman III, MD

The Genotype of the Original Wiskott Phenotype

Binder V, Albert MH, Kabus M, et al (Ludwig Maximillians Univ, Munich; Technical Univ Munich; Technical Univ Dresden, Germany)
N Engl J Med 355:1790-1793, 2006

Background.—The Wiskott–Aldrich syndrome is now known as an X-linked hereditary disorder associated with combined immunodeficiency, thrombocytopenia, small platelets, eczema, and an increased risk of autoimmune disorders and cancers. It is caused by mutations in the gene (*WAS*) for the Wiskott–Aldrich syndrome protein (WASP). Mutations in the *WAS* gene result in truncated or absent WASP in cells of the hematopoietic system, but there is no strict correlation between the mutant genotype and expression of WASP or the phenotype of the syndrome. This syndrome can be cured through hematopoietic stem-cell transplantation. This study recruited members of the family first described by Wiskott in 1937 in order to identify the hypothesized mutation in *WAS* that caused the severe phenotype of the Wiskott–Aldrich syndrome in the three brothers first described by Wiskott.

Methods.—Genetic testing was performed in three generations of the kindred. Genomic DNA was extracted from peripheral white cells. A *WAS* mutation was ruled out in 400 controls by means of denaturing high-performance liquid chromatography with the Wave system.

Results.—Genetic testing for the mutation revealed a deletion of two nucleotides at positions 73 and 74 in *WAS* exon 1. This mutation is not listed in WASPbase, an Internet-based database of *WAS* mutations. The deletion results in a frame shift that starts with amino acid 25; the shifted reading frame is open for another 11 amino acids before it results in a stop codon. Further characterization of this 73–74delAC mutation was sought in 400 control subjects, and none was found to carry the mutation. Thus it is improbable that the mutation is a polymorphic variant in the normal population. The mutation was identified in three generations of the pedigree.

Conclusions.—A new frame shift mutation in exon 1 of *WAS* was identified in family members of the patients originally described by Wiskott in 1937. This mutation is likely the hypothesized genotype that caused the severe form of the syndrome in the three brothers described by Wiskott.

▶ The Wiskott–Aldrich syndrome is a well-recognized triad of eczema, bleeding diathesis, and recurrent infections occurring in boys. Although it is rare with an estimated incidence of less than 1 in 100,000 births, the syndrome offers rich historical, clinical, and scientific lessons. Alfred Wiskott (1898-1978), a German authority on childhood pneumonias, first described the clinical syndrome in 1937, noting that it affected three brothers but not their sisters. In 1954, Robert Aldrich (1917-1998) and colleagues published an independent description of a large Dutch kindred in which segregation analysis showed X-linked recessive inheritance. By the mid-1960s, additional cases had been recognized, and the clinical syndrome became known by the names of both pediatricians. In the mid-1990s, the disease-causing gene was identified; initially of unknown function, it was called *WAS*, for the Wiskott-Aldrich syndrome. More than 10 years later, some 160 or more different *WAS* mutations spanning all 12 exons of the gene had been found in more than 270 unrelated families and functional domains of the Wiskott-Aldrich protein (WASP) have been identified.

The report of Binder et al describes the identification of a unique null mutation—a dinucleotide deletion in *WAS* exon 1—carried by relatives of the boys Wiskott described, solving the 70-year-old mystery of the fatal illness of the three brothers. This in a way is an intellectually satisfying conclusion to Wiskott's original story of the syndrome. Even more satisfying is the author's report of a successful cure, by transplantation of bone marrow from a matched, unrelated donor, of the affected boy in the current generation of the family—the original brother's first cousin twice removed. Thus, in the span of two generations, a previously undescribed fatal condition has become treatable. This history of the syndrome is enriched by the fact that this condition, along with severe combined immunodeficiency (SCID), stimulated the earliest development of bone marrow transplantation for the treatment of immunodeficiency. The first reports on the results of bone marrow transplantation in the Wiskott–Aldrich syndrome and SCID were published back-to-back in *The Lancet* by the teams of Bortin et al and Good et al, respectively, back in 1968.

As time has passed, we have learned a few other things about the Wiskott–Aldrich syndrome. Female carriers of X-linked disorders are generally asymptomatic, but affected carriers with symptomatic Wiskott–Aldrich syndrome have been discovered. Some of these women have unbalanced X-chromosome activation. Also, researchers have discovered missense *WAS* mutations with variant phenotypes associated with either mild disease or unexpected isolated neutropenia.

The prevalence of the Wiskott–Aldrich syndrome is such that the average pediatrician just may see a case appearing in his or her practice if one lives long enough. In a typical case of severe Wiskott–Aldrich syndrome, petechiae, bruising, and bloody diarrhea may develop in the first days of life owing to thrombocytopenia associated with small platelets. Prolonged bleeding after circumcision often leads to the discovery of the thrombocytopenia. Eczema, which may be severe, ensues, and throughout childhood there may be frequent episodes of otitis media, pneumonia, and diarrhea. Sepsis or meningitis may occur. Such severe cases will require bone marrow transplantation. Although the syndrome was originally described by pediatricians, the wide spectrum of its clinical manifestations and complications makes it important for specialists to recognize several disciplines, including hematology, oncology, immunology, infectious diseases, rheumatology, and genetics. The management of the disorder requires a multidisciplinary approach that begins with molecular confirmation of the clinical diagnosis. The determination of the specific disease-causing mutation is the basis for genetic counseling, prenatal diagnosis, and, in some cases, prediction of the severity of the disease. In affected individuals, more than 50% of the mutations described to date have been unique and thus the type of genetic testing described by Binder et al will continue to provide needed critical information for genetic counseling.

For more on the topic of the Wiskott–Aldrich syndrome, see the superb commentary by Puck and Candotti.[1]

J. A. Stockman III, MD

Reference

1. Puck JM, Candotti F. Lessons from the Wiskott–Aldrich syndrome. *N Engl J Med.* 2006;355:1759-1761.

Evaluation of Prolonged aPTT Values in the Pediatric Population
Shah MD, O'Riordan MA, Alexander SW (Univ Hosps of Cleveland, Ohio)
Clin Pediatr (Phila) 45:347-353, 2006

Background.—Bleeding symptoms, including epistaxis, menorrhagia, and easy bruising, are common findings in children. These patients are often evaluated by performing specific laboratory investigations to screen for abnormalities in hemostasis. Laboratory screening is often performed in asymptomatic children in an effort to anticipate perioperative bleeding complications. A prolonged activated partial thromboplastin time (aPTT) during these screenings often prompts referral to pediatric hematologists for further investigations. However, a prolonged aPTT may be attributed to several different etiologies, some of which are not associated with an increased risk of bleeding. Presently there is insufficient information in the literature regarding the utility of an aPTT level in assessing clinically significant bleeding disorders in the general pediatric population. The purpose of the present study was to assess the likelihood of significant bleeding disorders in children with prolonged aPTTs.

Methods.—A retrospective chart review was conducted on all pediatric patients with prolonged aPTTs referred to an outpatient hematology clinic at a single tertiary care institution. The primary outcome variables were the presence or absence of a clinically significant bleeding disorder. Statistical analyses included χ^2 analysis or Fisher's exact test, sample t tests, and Wilcoxon rank sum tests.

Results.—The study group comprised 90 subjects, including 38 boys and 52 girls, with a median age of 8 years at initial evaluation. The most common symptoms identified by subjects were epistaxis (38%) and easy bruising (38%). Other symptoms included pallor (12%), menorrhagia (11%), prolonged postoperative bleeding (10%), hematochezia/melena (9%), tooth eruption or dental procedure–associated bleeding (8%), bleeding with circumcision (4%), hematuria (3%), and hematemesis and hemarthrosis (each 2%). Overall, 81% of subjects had at least one reported bleeding symptom. Despite extensive diagnostic investigations, 48% of the study subjects had no identifiable coagulation defect.

Conclusions.—In the absence of symptoms and a negative family history, the diagnosis of a bleeding disorder was unlikely in a patient with a prolonged aPTT (negative predictive value, 80%). However, a prolonged aPTT was predictive of a bleeding disorder in the presence of both clinical symptoms and a documented family history (positive predictive value, 62%). The scope of laboratory investigations in any child with a prolonged aPTT should be tempered by the clinical presentation and associated family and personal histories of the patient. However, the appropriate use of clinical assessment strategies may reduce the incidence of unnecessary testing in pediatric patients.

▶ The evaluation of a child with a prolonged aPTT is a common event for both the generalist pediatrician as well as the pediatric hematologist. The aPTT is frequently requested as part of preoperative screening, particularly before tonsillectomy and adenoidectomy. In a child who has an abnormal aPTT who has no personal or family history of a bleeding disorder, the conundrum is clear. Does the long aPTT represent abnormalities in factor VIII, IX, or XI? Does it represent a previously undiagnosed von Willebrand disease? This is what this report attempts to address.

What we learn is that if a child is shown to have a long aPTT but no personal or family history of a bleeding disorder, chances are excellent that there is nothing significantly wrong with that child, and that child will not experience any bleeding problem resulting from injury or surgery. On the other hand, a prolonged aPTT and any history suggestive of a bleeding diathesis (eg, recurrent or severe epistaxis, menorrhagia, ecchymoses inconsistent with supposed trauma, or unexplained postsurgical bleeding) do warrant a more detailed hematologic evaluation. The child without significant history most likely does not require extensive coagulation factor studies. In most instances, if further evaluation is undertaken, a lupus anticoagulant or anticardiolipin antibodies will account for the prolonged aPTTs in a large majority of children. These coagulation inhibitors are usually transient, often resulting from recent infections, and are generally clinically insignificant. The greatest likelihood is that if the aPTT level is repeated in a month or two, it will have returned to normal.

If there is any bottom line to this report, it is that history is critical in determining how extensive an evaluation should be undertaken for a possible coagulation disorder. If the history is positive, even a normal screening aPTT means little. Normal aPTTs are commonly seen in mild von Willebrand cases. Any significant bleeding history should be more fully evaluated beyond simply doing an aPTT. On the other hand, in the absence of any significant history, a mildly elevated aPTT may simply require follow-up rather than putting a child through a template of "required" coagulation tests. All too often, however, the pediatric hematologist feels "obliged" to do more than may actually be necessary when evaluating mildly abnormal screening tests in otherwise well children with negative histories. That is a wasteful shame.

J. A. Stockman III, MD

Pediatric reference intervals for uncommon bleeding and thrombotic disorders
Flanders MM, Phansalkar AR, Crist RA, et al (Univ of Utah, Salt Lake City)
J Pediatr 149:275-277, 2006

Background.—Most of the pediatric coagulation reference intervals in use currently are based on a study by Andrew et al in 1992 (Andrew M, Vegh P, Johnston M, Bowker J, Ofosu F, Mitchell L. Maturation of the hemostatic system during childhood. *Blood.* 1992;80:1998-2005). There have been significant changes in coagulation reagents and instruments since that study, and therefore the older reference intervals may not be applicable. A recently published report provided pediatric reference intervals for seven coagulation assays associated with common bleeding disorders for children 7 to 17 years of age. The purpose of the present study was to determine pediatric reference intervals and median values for coagulation assays associated with uncommon bleeding and thrombotic disorders, including factors II, V, VII, X, fibrinogen, α–2-antiplasmin (AP), antithrombin (AT) plasminogen, protein C (PC), and protein S (PS).

Methods.—Blood was obtained for reference interval studies from 887 healthy children 7 through 17 years of age with nearly equal numbers collected for each year of age. None of the subjects had a history of bleeding or thrombotic disorders, and none were taking any medications in the 2 weeks before collection of the blood specimens. Pediatric reference intervals and medians were determined for ages 7 to 9, 10 to 11, 12 to 13, 14 to 15, and 16 to 17, with a minimum of 75 and a maximum of 245 patients per group. In addition, 120 persons were used for adult reference intervals with a mean age of 33 years and a range from 20 to 55 years. All reference intervals were established nonparametrically by ordering results from lowest to highest and excluding the lowest and highest 2.5% of the results.

Results.—The median values for the extrinsic factors II, VII, and X showed statistically significant differences from adult medians for each age group. The lower and upper reference limits were lower than those observed for adults throughout late childhood and adolescence. However, by 16 to 17 years of age, the confidence intervals of factors II, VII, and X overlap those of adults. Pediatric mean values for AT, plasminogen, and PC showed significant differences from adults. The lower limit of pediatric AT levels was significantly higher than that of adults; however, by 16 to 17 years of age, AT levels decreased slightly, and lower and upper reference limits showed no statistical difference between children and adults. PC levels are consistently lower than adults, but PS levels in girls are consistently higher than adults. In boys, PS levels are higher than adults in the 16- to 17-year-old group. AP median values showed statistical differences from adults in early and middle childhood, but there were no statistically significant differences at age 14 and beyond.

Conclusions.—This study identified significant differences between adult and pediatric reference intervals, and these findings are supportive of the use of these age-related reference intervals in the diagnosis of pediatric bleeding and thrombotic disorders.

▶ It is uncommon that one sees hematology reference data in pediatric journals, largely because the information is not a common part of general pediatric practice. The information contained in this report, however, is. Most pediatric coagulation reference data used in current practice are based on studies from more than a decade and a half ago. Since coagulation reagents and instrumentation have changed fairly dramatically over that interval, older reference intervals may very well no longer apply to the pediatric population. What you see in this report are the most up-to-date results for coagulation values in the healthy normal pediatric population. There are significant changes over time in these values as children age. Pediatric values are definitely different than adult reference values. For example, for coagulation factors II, VII and X, lower and upper reference limits in children are definitively lower than those observed for adults. It is only by age 16 to 17 years that truly adult values are seen. With respect to fibrinogen levels, these are comparable to adult median values by adolescence. Some values, such as antithrombin, turn out to be significantly higher in children and adolescents than in adults.

Chances are that many laboratories that pediatricians use for doing coagulation studies use adult reference data. It is up to us to be sure that the proper reference tables are used in order to properly interpret coagulation studies as they return to our offices.

J. A. Stockman III, MD

Cystic fibrosis as a risk factor for recurrent venous thrombosis at a pediatric tertiary care hospital
Raffini LJ, Raybagkar D, Blumenstein MS, et al (Univ of Pennsylvania, Philadelphia)
J Pediatr 148:659-664, 2006

Objective.—To evaluate risk factors for recurrent thrombosis in pediatric patients.

Study Design.—This prospective observational cohort study enrolled 120 patients with acute venous thromboembolism from January 2003 to April 2005. Data collection included medical and family history, radiologic and laboratory studies, therapy, and follow-up.

Results.—The overall prevalence of recurrent thrombosis in our cohort was 19/120 (15.8%). Patients with recurrence were older, with a median age of 14.8 years (range 2 weeks-23.6 years), compared with 10.1 years (range newborn 23.4 years) in patients without recurrence ($P = .03$). Six of the 19 patients with recurrent thrombosis had cystic fibrosis (CF), compared with

0/101 without recurrence ($P < .001$). Five of these 6 patients were colonized with *Burkholderia cepacia* in their sputum. Central venous catheters were associated with most, but not all, of the thromboses in patients with CF.

Conclusions.—In this study, patients with CF had a high risk of recurrent venous thrombosis, as well as a high prevalence of colonization with *B cepacia*. The cause of this risk has not been defined. This observation may have important implications for thromboprophylaxis, particularly in the setting of central venous catheters.

▶ This is a fascinating report. At the Children's Hospital of Philadelphia (CHOP), a study was undertaken to determine what risk factors might exist for the occurrence of recurrent venous thrombosis in the pediatric population. Out of the blue came CF as such a risk factor. In the CHOP registry of 284 patients with CF, there were 401 hospital admissions and 162 patients for pulmonary exacerbation during the timeframe of the prospective thrombosis study. It turns out that subjects with CF who were not infected with *Burkholderia cepacia* had a risk of symptomatic venous thrombosis of just 3.7%. Those colonized with *B cepacia* had a 27% risk of developing a venous thrombosis.

B cepacia is a potent stimulator of inflammation, and respiratory colonization is associated with a decreased survival rate in patients with cystic fibrosis. It should be noted that the patients with CF in this report, both those colonized with *B cepacia* and those who were not, had central venous catheters for antibiotic use. For whatever reason, colonization with this particular bacterium caused these catheters to develop thrombi, which in fact turned out to be potentially life threatening, because emboli to the lungs in a patient with preexisting pulmonary compromise might wreak havoc.

Chances are that many children with CF who have central venous catheters will have asymptomatic thromboses. Currently, there are no published studies looking for asymptomatic central venous catheter associated thromboses in patients with CF. We badly need more information on this topic. From what we know right now, it is difficult to recommend routine anticoagulation prophylaxis for all patients with CF who require a central venous catheter for IV therapy. As we learn more this recommendation might change. Patients at high risk who have had a prior venous thrombosis, and perhaps those with *B cepacia*, might in fact benefit from prophylactic anticoagulation when central venous catheters are in place. At CHOP, the policy is that patients with CF who have had a prior central venous catheter–related venous thrombosis will in fact receive full anticoagulation with all future catheter placements. Such an approach is not a perfect one, however, because several patients so managed did in fact develop second thrombotic events.

If there is a message from this report, it is that any patient with CF with a central venous catheter should be considered at risk for the development of a venous thrombosis. This risk will be multiplied several-fold if they are infected with *B cepacia*.

It is interesting that patients with CF might be at increased risk for thrombosis because this disorder is classically associated with vitamin K deficiency due to malabsorption of vitamin K. Obviously, the children who experience the problem with thromboses were being well managed in terms of vitamin supplementation and did not suffer from low levels of vitamin K. While on the topic of vitamin K, do you know how the discovery of this vitamin came about? In 1943, the Nobel Prize in Physiology or Medicine was equally divided between Henrik Dam (1895-1976), Polytechnic Institute, Copenhagen, Denmark, and Edward Doisy (1893-1986), Saint Louis University, St. Louis, Missouri, for the discovery of vitamin K and its chemical nature. Indeed, Dr. Dam is credited for most of the discovery. His discovery of the new vitamin was almost an "incidental finding." In 1928, Dam started a project to find out whether chickens were able to synthesize cholesterol. Newly-hatched chickens were fed on a diet that was practically free of sterols and poor in fat, but supplemented with vitamins A and B. In 1929, he proved that chickens could produce their own cholesterol; however, he observed that some of the chickens developed subcutaneous hemorrhages. To continue his investigations on sterol metabolism, Dam then went to the biochemist Schoenheimer in Frieberg, Germany, where he stayed until the fall of 1933. After his return to Copenhagen, Dam started a systematic and comprehensive series of investigations to explain the bleeding phenomenon observed in chickens fed on a poor diet in fat and free of cholesterol. In 1934, after having found that the chicken bleeding was preventable with a diet supplemented with green leaves, tomatoes and hog liver, he postulated that the bleeding was caused by a deficiency of some fat-soluble factor. In a letter to *Nature* in 1935, the name vitamin K was proposed for this factor. The letter K was considered suitable, as it had not been given to any other vitamin.[1]

One final tidbit: the word "coagulation" in the English language comes from the Scandinavian word "Koaguation," in which the first letter "K" relates to one of the reasons why the newly found vitamin was named K.

J. A. Stockman III, MD

Reference

1. Zetterström R. H.C.P. Dam (1895-1976) and E.A. Doisy (1893-1986): the discovery of antihaemorrhagic vitamin and its impact on neonatal health. *Acta Paediatr.* 2006;95:642-644.

4 Child Development

Cigarette smoking during pregnancy and hyperactive-distractible pre-schooler's: A follow-up study

Linnet KM, Obel C, Bonde E, et al (Aarhus Univ, Skejby Sygehus, Denmark; Hvidovre Hosp, Copenhagen)

Acta Paediatr 95:694-700, 2006

Aim.—To study the association between intrauterine exposure to tobacco smoke and behavioural disorders in preschool children, primarily symptoms of inattention, hyperactivity and impulsivity but also hostile-aggressive and anxious-fearful symptoms.

Methods.—We conducted a follow-up study in 1355 singletons born to Danish-speaking mothers. Information on smoking habits during pregnancy and other lifestyle factors was obtained from self-administered questionnaires filled in during second and third trimester. Approximately 3.5 years later, the parents provided information on their child's behaviour using the self-administered Preschool Behaviour Questionnaire. The children were categorized into three not mutually exclusive behaviour groups: hyperactive—distractible (13.6%), hostile–aggressive (4.6%), and anxious-fearful (6.4%) children.

Results.—Compared with children of non-smokers, children born to women who smoked 10 or more cigarettes per day had a 60% increased risk of hyperactivity and distractibility perceived by the parents (OR 1.6; 95% CI 1.0–2.3; $P < 0.05$). The results were adjusted for maternal lifestyle factors and socioeconomic characteristics. Additional adjustment for perinatal factors and parental psychiatric hospitalization did not change the results substantially (OR 1.7; 95% CI 1.1–2.6). We found no statistically significant association between maternal smoking in pregnancy and hostile–aggressive and anxious-fearful behaviour in the offspring.

Conclusion.—Exposure to tobacco smoke in utero was associated with hyperactive-distractible behaviour in preschool children.

▶ It was more than 30 years ago that the first descriptions appeared showing an inverse association between maternal smoking during pregnancy and lower intelligence in products of that pregnancy. These descriptions have appeared not only here in the United States, but also from Denmark, the United Kingdom, Canada, Australia, New Zealand, and Finland. If one takes together the findings of all studies, there is a 3- to 7-point deficit in the IQ scores of children born to mothers who smoke relative to those born to mothers who do not. There also seems to be a dose-dependent relationship between the amount of smoking and the IQ deficit. In most, but not all studies, this inverse maternal smoking—offspring IQ gradient holds after adjustment for a range of social and biologic covariates that attempt to capture characteristics of the parents. These covariates include socioeconomic status, adiposity, alcohol consumption, illicit drug use, and factors related to the home environment such as emotional support and the quality of childcare.

The Batty et al report (Effect of maternal smoking during pregnancy on offspring's cognitive ability: empirical evidence for complete confounding in the US National Longitudinal Survey of Youth) further explores the relationship between maternal smoking during pregnancy and offsprings, a study that suggests that previous studies have not adequately adjusted for maternal education and/or IQ. This study did show a 2.87 lower IQ in children born to smoking mothers (≥1 pack of cigarettes per day) in comparison to nonsmoking mothers. However, of this 2.8 IQ point difference, 0.27 IQ points could be accounted for by the fact that smoking mothers had less formal education. Also, when maternal IQ was taken into account, some 1.51 IQ points of the 2.87 IQ point differential could be accounted for by the fact that smoking mothers tend to be somewhat less smart than their nonsmoking peers. These findings suggest that previous studies have not correctly adjusted for maternal education and/or IQ differences in mothers and have generally tended to overestimate the association of maternal smoking with the offspring's cognitive ability. This does not mean that maternal smoking during pregnancy does not affect an infant's IQ, simply that the effect may not be quite as dramatic as previously thought.

The data of Linnet et al suggest that increased activity level, inattention and impulsiveness in 3- to 4-year-old children may also be a consequence of cigarette smoking. As importantly, these signs and symptoms tend to be associated with oppositional, aggressive, and hyperactive behavior during school years, low academic achievement, and the need for special educational services. The data from this report suggest that compared with the children of nonsmokers, children born to mothers who smoked 10 or more cigarettes a day during pregnancy experience a 60% increased risk of being hyperactive or being distractible during their preschool years. Unfortunately, it is not clear that this study, one performed in Australia, adequately matched personality characteristics and IQs of smoking and nonsmoking mothers. Nonetheless, where there is smoke, there is fire and it is reasonable to assume that you have to be awfully dumb to fire up when you are pregnant.

This commentary closes with a recent observation from *Science News* that tells us a fair amount about the roles that actors play who smoke. Any actor who smokes in a film probably should be considered a bad actor, but we now know the statistics on the roles they play. Smokers in films here in the United States are more likely to be villainous or poor than heroic or wealthy, according to a study recently reported. Investigators in New York City recorded the smoking habits of the five main characters in each of 447 films made during the 1990s, including such hits as *Independence Day* and *There's Something*

About Mary. Excluded were science fiction and animated films because they typically are not intended to represent reality.

So what did the parts played by smoking actors look like? Overall, 48% of cinematic smokers appeared to be from a low socioeconomic class while 23% seemed to be middle class, and 11% appeared to be upper class. When compared with "controls" in the same films, these statistics deviated from what one would expect. Only 21% of protagonists smoked compared with 36% of their adversaries. If one looks at all actors in all films reviewed, it is apparent that in R-rated and independent films, the prevalence of smoking among populations seen on screen is significantly higher than in the United States population as a whole.[1]

J. A. Stockman III, MD

Reference

1. Seppa N. Movies put smoking in bad light. *Sci News*. 2005;168:158.

Effect of Maternal Smoking During Pregnancy on Offspring's Cognitive Ability: Empirical Evidence for Complete Confounding in the US National Longitudinal Survey of Youth
Batty GD, Der G, Deary IJ (Univ of Glasgow, UK; Univ of Edinburgh, UK)
Pediatrics 118:943-950, 2006

Background.—Numerous studies have reported that maternal cigarette smoking during pregnancy is related to lower IQ scores in the offspring. Confounding is a crucial issue in interpreting this association.

Methods.—In the US National Longitudinal Survey of Youth 1979, IQ was ascertained serially during childhood using the Peabody Individual Achievement Test, the total score for which comprises results on 3 subtests: mathematics, reading comprehension, and reading recognition. Maternal IQ was assessed by using the Armed Forces Qualification Test. There were 5578 offspring (born to 3145 mothers) with complete information for maternal smoking habits, total Peabody Individual Achievement Test score, and covariates.

Results.—The offspring of mothers who smoked ≥1 pack of cigarettes per day during pregnancy had an IQ score (Peabody Individual Achievement Test total) that was, on average, 2.87 points lower than children born to nonsmoking mothers. Separate control for maternal education (0.27-IQ-point decrement) and, to a lesser degree, maternal IQ (1.51-IQ-point decrement) led to marked attenuation of the maternal-smoking–offspring-IQ relation. A similar pattern of results was seen when Peabody Individual Achievement Test subtest results were the outcomes of interest. The only exception was the Peabody Individual Achievement Test mathematics score, in which adjusting for maternal IQ essentially led to complete attenuation of the maternal-smoking–offspring-IQ gradient (0.66-IQ-point decrement). The impact of controlling for physical, behavioral, and other social indices was much less pronounced than for maternal education or IQ.

Conclusions.—These findings suggest that previous studies that did not adjust for maternal education and/or IQ may have overestimated the association of maternal smoking with offspring cognitive ability.

Iron Deficiency in Infancy and Mother-Child Interaction at 5 Years

Corapci F, Radan AE, Lozoff B (Univ of Michigan, Ann Arbor; Univ of Costa Rica, San Jose)

J Dev Behav Pediatr 27:371-378, 2006

Five-year-old Costa Rican children, who had either chronic, severe iron deficiency or good iron status in infancy, were observed with their mothers during a structured interaction task in a laboratory setting and everyday interactions in their home. Child affect and behavior as well as the quality of mother-child interaction of the formerly chronic iron-deficient children (n = 40) were compared to those with good iron status in infancy (n = 102). Children who had chronic iron deficiency in infancy were more likely to display lower levels of physical activity, positive affect, and verbalization during the structured task at 5 years, despite iron therapy that corrected their iron deficiency anemia in infancy. Mother-child reciprocity during the structured task (e.g., eye contact, shared positive affect, turn taking) was more likely to be lower in the chronic iron deficiency group compared to the good iron group. Mothers of children in the chronic iron deficiency group showed less responsivity in both settings. These results show that children with chronic, severe iron deficiency in infancy continue at behavioral disadvantage relative to their peers at school entry. Sustained differences in mother-child interaction might contribute to the long-lasting behavioral and developmental alterations reported in children with chronic, severe iron deficiency in infancy.

▶ There are many non-hematologic manifestations to iron deficiency anemia. No longer does anyone question evidence of chronic, severe iron deficiency and its association with poor mental, motor, and social/emotional functioning in comparison to children with good iron status. The more subtle forms of iron deficiency, including those not associated with anemia have been more suspect, however, in this regard. Although there is growing empirical evidence regarding altered affect and behavior in infants with chronic and severe iron deficiency, research on parent-child interaction has been limited. Before the report abstracted appeared, only 2 studies of iron-deficient infants have examined the quality of caregiving using direct observation of mothers and infants. During play observation in a clinical testing room in a Guatemala study, mothers of infants with chronic, severe iron deficiency were less likely to spend time at a distance from them, less likely to break close contact, and more likely to reestablish close contact when the baby moved away.[1] In a study of the effects of iron deficiency on behavior and development, 12- to 23-month-old

Costa Rican infants and their mothers were observed during free play, during mental and motor testing, and in the home. Infants with chronic, severe iron deficiency maintained closer contact with their mothers during play as well as motor testing and showed less pleasure and delight.[2] Observations in the home showed that these infants were more likely to be carried by their mothers and that the babies themselves smiled and laughed less than their peers.

In the present study, 5-year-old Costa Rican children who either had chronic, severe iron deficiency or good iron status in infancy were observed. The chronic iron deficiency group consisted of children with moderate iron deficiency in infancy and those with hemoglobin levels greater than 10g/L. Despite correction of iron deficiency anemia with treatment and excellent iron stores by 5 years of age, children who were previously iron deficient were more likely to display lower levels of physical activity, positive affect, and verbalization during a structured interaction task, compared with children with good iron status in infancy. There was a persistent difference in affect and behavior as well as altered mother-child interaction. These sustained differences in maternal behavior may contribute to the long-lasting effects of early chronic severe iron deficiency on a child's behavior and development. Iron therapy alone is not enough to handle this problem. Additional interventions may be needed to prevent long-term effects.

Congratulations should be directed to Dr Betsy Lozoff. She has written expansively about the non-hematologic manifestations of iron deficiency over several decades. Those who were naysayers about the relationship between iron deficiency and behavioral disturbances should pack their tents. Dr Lozoff's data are rock solid.

J. A. Stockman III, MD

References

1. Lozoff B, Klein NK, Prabucki KM. Iron-deficient anemic infants at play. *J Dev Behav Pediatr.* 1986;7:152-158.
2. Lozoff B, Klein NK, Nelson EC, McClish DK, Manuel M, Chacon ME. Behavior of infants with iron-deficiency anemia. *Child Dev.* 1998;69:24-36.

Behavioural and emotional problems in very preterm and very low birthweight infants at age 5 years

Reijneveld SA, de Kleine MJK, van Baar AL, et al (Univ of Groningen, The Netherlands; Maxima Med Centre, Veldhoven, The Netherlands; Tilburg Univ, The Netherlands; et al)
Arch Dis Child Fetal Neonatal Ed 91:F423-F428, 2006

Background.—Children born very preterm (VP; <32 weeks' gestation) or with very low birth weight (VLBW, <1500 g; hereafter called VP/VLBW) are at risk for behavioural and emotional problems during school age and adolescence. At school entrance these problems may hamper academic functioning, but evidence on their occurrence at this age in VP/VLBW children is lacking.

Aim.—To provide information on academic functioning of VP/VLBW children and to examine the association of behavioural and emotional problems with other developmental problems assessed by paediatricians.

Design, Setting and Participants.—A cohort of 431 VP/VLBW children aged 5 years (response rate 76.1%) was compared with two large national samples of children of the same age (n = 6007, response rate 86.9%).

Outcome Measures.—Behavioural and emotional problems measured by the Child Behavior Checklist (CBCL), and paediatrician assessment of other developmental domains among VP/VLBW children.

Results.—The prevalence rate of a CBCL total problems score in the clinical range was higher among VP/VLBW children than among children of the same age from the general population (13.2% v 8.7%, odds ratio 1.60 (95% confidence interval 1.18 to 2.17)). Mean differences were largest for social and attention problems. Moreover, they were larger in children with paediatrician-diagnosed developmental problems at 5 years, and somewhat larger in children with severe perinatal problems.

Conclusion.—At school entrance, VP/VLBW children are more likely to have behavioural and emotional problems that are detrimental for academic functioning. Targeted and timely help is needed to support them and their parents in overcoming these problems and in enabling them to be socially successful.

▶ The development of infants born prematurely is of great interest in the field of neonatology. The focus has primarily been on the development of very and extremely prematurely born children and has shifted from a narrow spectrum of neurologic outcomes towards a wider interest in the overall psychological development of the children. Some studies have focused on intellectual development by using measures of general intellectual ability. A recent meta-analysis has found the mean intellectual capacity of prematurely born children to be 10.9 IQ points lower than that of children born at term.[1]

We see in this report that it is not only a decrement in IQ that these children suffer, but also a proclivity to behavioral and emotional problems. The data show that these children are 50% more likely to have behavioral and emotional issues. One in four youngsters born prematurely will show such difficulties. We need to be prepared to meet this relatively common problem head on and to prepare parents to deal with it. Routine screenings for developmental and behavioral issues are a mandatory part of follow-up. Schools need to be aware as well.

The Esbjørn et al report (Intellectual development in a Danish cohort of prematurely born preschool children: specific or general difficulties?) tells us a great deal about the intellectual development of children who are born preterm. The findings of Esbjørn et al confirm global cognitive deficits in a national sample of 5-year-old children born prematurely. The investigators administered a standardized IQ test as well as assessments of more specific skills (memory, executive function, motor ability). Parent education was controlled for in this study. The results provide solid evidence for global and clinically significant deficits in cognitive ability in a recent birth cohort of these children and underscore the importance of assessing high-risk children before or soon after school entry.

One closing comment about intelligence: researchers have found that young children with a thinner cortex that subsequently thickens during later childhood tend to have higher IQs than those who have a thick cortex from early childhood onward. The most intelligent children, in particular, have an unusually plastic cortex, with an initial phase of cortical increase followed by equally vigorous cortical thinning during late adolescence.[2]

J. A. Stockman III, MD

References

1. Bhutta AT, Cleves MA, Casey PH. Cognitive and behavioral outcomes of school-aged children who were born preterm: a meta-analysis. *JAMA.* 2002;288:728-737.
2. Shaw P, Greenstein D, Lerch J, et al. Intellectual ability and cortical development in children and adolescents. *Nature.* 2006;440:676-679.

Intellectual Development in a Danish Cohort of Prematurely Born Preschool Children: Specific or General Difficulties?
Esbjørn BH, Hansen BM, Greisen G, et al (Univ of Copenhagen; Rigshospitalet, Copenhagen)
J Dev Behav Pediatr 27:477-484, 2006

A national cohort of extremely low birth weight (ELBW) and/or extremely preterm (EPT) children and a term control group was followed up at the age of 5 years. The primary objective was to investigate whether premature birth had a global impact on cognitive functions or affected specific functions only. Assessment tools were Wechsler Preschool and Primary Scale of Intelligence–Revised (WPPSI-R), Movement Assessment Battery for Children (M-ABC), and subtests from the Neuropsychological Assessment 4–7 years (NEPSY). The mean Full Scale IQ (FSIQ) and M-ABC score of the index children were 1.1 and 1.2 SDs lower than that of the control children (p < .001). Most WPPSI-R subtests showed medium to large differences between index and control children, suggesting a global impact of premature birth on cognitive functions. For both unadjusted and FSIQ adjusted means, no significant group differences on tests of memory or executive function were observed (p >.1), suggesting little impact of premature birth on these specific functions. In this sample, cognitive difficulties in 5-year-old ELBW and/or EPT children tended to be associated with general intellectual difficulties rather than with specific dysfunctions; however, the implications of this finding are ambiguous due to substantial attrition on the NEPSY subtests.

▶ The commentary for the Reijneveld et al abstract (Behavioural and emotional problems in very preterm and very low birthweight infants at age 5 years) discussed intellectual development in relationship to prematurity and because there is little more to say on this topic at this point, we simply ask a question, what is the evidence that genius breeds genius?

One way to look at this question is to examine Nobel laureates and discover what their families were like. That the unusual capacity designated as genius is born, not made, that it is an inherited capacity, is a long-held tenet. In fact, contemporary researchers cite Francis Galton's work on hereditary genius as proof of this contention, despite the lack of any definitive support for Galton's research. Galton basically showed that people of higher accomplishment are generally born of a parent of similar high accomplishment whose occupation is pretty much in the same arena. The rub with Galton's work is that it was done in England, and his findings may very well be unduly influenced by the British practice of primogeniture and by his exclusion of persons who were simply well respected (for example, jurists and military commanders) in the same genius category. Nonetheless, Galton's studies are the foundation for what emerged as the science of behavioral genetics. His influences and conclusions still persist.[1]

A more contemporary examination of genius is the recent set of findings of Rothenberg, who has examined Nobel laureates and their families. A while ago, Rothenberg assessed outstanding literary prize Nobel laureate winners and found that less than one percent had parents in the same occupation. When he compared the outstanding literary prize winner group with an independently selected and matching group of distinguished persons in a wide variety of fields, occupational inheritance was significantly absent.[2] More recently, Rothenberg examined family background and genius among Nobel laureates in science. He collected data on 435 of all 488 Nobel laureates in chemistry, physics, medicine and physiology from 1901 through 2003 and compared them with a matching group of more than 500 distinguished nonscientists for incidence of occupational inheritance. Also examined were more than 500 high IQ non-prize winners. Again, he found no correlation between a parent's occupation and that of their genius offspring.[3] Rather, it was observed that creative achievement in science (as well as in literature and presumably in other fields) is associated with a family background constellation including the work and aspirations of a parent or parents and creative orientation of a parent or parents. This constellation, which may involve genetic transmission, very likely instills strong motivation for creative achievement that blossoms in a youngster who may have a higher than expected IQ.

Among Nobel laureates, less than 1% have the same occupation as a parent or parents. With respect to the average "Joe" here in the United States, the general incidence of all types of occupational inheritance, at least as assessed by the Bureau of Census, is that 21% of all men follow the same occupation as their fathers, something akin to apples not falling far from their trees.

J.A. Stockman III, MD

References

1. Galton F. *Hereditary Genius.* London: Macmillan; 1869.
2. Rothenberg A, Wyshak G. Family background and genius. *Can J Psychiatry.* 2004;49:185-191.
3. Rothenberg A. Family background and genius II: Nobel laureates in science. *Can J Psychiatry.* 2005;50:918-925.

Effect of breast feeding on intelligence in children: prospective study, sibling pairs analysis, and meta-analysis
Der G, Batty GD, Deary IJ (Univ of Edinburgh, UK)
BMJ 333:945-948, 2006

Objective.—To assess the importance of maternal intelligence, and the effect of controlling for it and other important confounders, in the link between breast feeding and children's intelligence.

Design.—Examination of the effect of breast feeding on cognitive ability and the impact of a range of potential confounders, in particular maternal IQ, within a national database. Additional analyses compared pairs of siblings from the sample who were and were not breast fed. The results are considered in the context of other studies that have also controlled for parental intelligence via meta-analysis.

Setting.—1979 US national longitudinal survey of youth.

Subjects.—Data on 5475 children, the offspring of 3161 mothers in the longitudinal survey.

Main Outcome Measure.—IQ in children measured by Peabody individual achievement test.

Results.—The mother's IQ was more highly predictive of breast feeding status than were her race, education, age, poverty status, smoking, the home environment, or the child's birth weight or birth order. One standard deviation advantage in maternal IQ more than doubled the odds of breast feeding. Before adjustment, breast feeding was associated with an increase of around 4 points in mental ability. Adjustment for maternal intelligence accounted for most of this effect. When fully adjusted for a range of relevant confounders, the effect was small (0.52) and non-significant (95% confidence interval -0.19 to 1.23). The results of the sibling comparisons and meta-analysis corroborated these findings.

Conclusions.—Breast feeding has little or no effect on intelligence in children. While breast feeding has many advantages for the child and mother, enhancement of the child's intelligence is unlikely to be among them.

▶ One more theory about the advantages of breastfeeding bites the dust. Fortunately, there are scores of other reasons to breastfeed, although hiking up the intelligence of one's baby no longer is among them. Many prior studies have suggested that children who were breastfed performed better in tests of intellectual competence than those who were not. This association was seen for full-term babies, and it was also quite strong for those who were also born preterm or at a low birth weight. This IQ advantage from early studies of preterm infants, however, was fairly small (roughly equal to 3 or 4 IQ points), but in a world of competitive advantages, 3 or 4 points is not all that bad. However, what was unclear from prior studies was whether the difference in intelligence reflected a direct nutritional advantage or a difference in socioenvironmental factors that are more favorable among women who breast feed. The latter seems to be the case.

Women who breastfeed do seem to be more likely to provide their children with a more enriched and cognitively stimulating environment than those who do not breastfeed, which could contribute to their children's better cognitive performance. This report by Der and colleagues demonstrates the importance of controlling for maternal IQ by showing that the association of breastfeeding with cognitive performance in children drops from 4.7 IQ points to just 0.5 points after adjusting for a mother's cognitive competence and other socioenvironmental measures. The study included 5475 children from a national longitudinal survey of youth, and it identified maternal IQ as the main variable that accounts for the association between breastfeeding and childhood IQ. The report also suggests that mothers with a higher IQ are more likely to breastfeed. The data of Der and colleagues do not support a direct nutritional benefit for childhood IQ in full-term infants.

Other benefits of breastfeeding—such as the effect of colostrum on the immune system, emotional benefits that may promote more secure infant–mother attachment, and the effects of omega-3 fatty acids on cognitive and visual development in preterm and low birth weight infants—are all well established. We should still recommend breastfeeding for all of its good purposes, but if a woman cannot breastfeed, she should not be shamed into thinking that she is depriving her baby of any IQ points. It just is not so.

J. A. Stockman III, MD

Association between sleep position and early motor development
Majnemer A, Barr RG (McGill Univ, Montreal; Univ of British Columbia, Vancouver, Canada)
J Pediatr 149:623-629, 2006

Objective.—To compare motor performance in infants sleeping in prone versus supine positions.

Study Design.—Healthy 4-month-olds (supine: n = 71, prone: n = 12) and 6-month-olds (supine: n = 50, prone: n = 22) were evaluated with the Alberta Infant Motor Scale (AIMS) and Peabody Developmental Motor Scale (PDMS), and parents completed a positioning diary. Infants were reassessed at 15 months.

Results.—At 4 months, motor scores were lower in the supine group and were less likely to achieve prone extension ($P < .05$). At 6 months, there were wide discrepancies on the AIMS (supine: 44.5 ± 21.6, prone: 60.0 ± 18.8, $P = .005$) and the gross motor PDMS (supine: 85.7 ± 7.6, prone: 90.2 ± 9.5, $P = .03$). Motor delays were documented in 22% of babies sleeping supine. Prone sleep–positioned infants were more likely to sit and roll. Daily exposure to awake prone positioning was predictive of motor performance in infants sleeping supine. At 15 months, sleep position continued to predict motor performance.

Conclusions.—Infants sleeping supine may exhibit early motor lags, associated with less time in prone while awake. This has implications for accurate interpretation of assessment of infants at risk and prevention of inappropriate referrals. Rate of infant motor development appears influenced by extrinsic factors such as positioning practices.

▶ This report considers tone and motor skills affected by sleep in infants, and several important findings that were observed related to complications of supine sleeping among 155 babies in Quebec. During a home visit, motor skills were evaluated using the Alberta Infant Motor Scale and the Peabody Developmental Motor Scale. Of the 4-month-old infants, 16% usually slept prone; of the 6-month-old infants, 30% usually slept prone. There were statistical if not clinically significant differences in motor skills among the 4-month-old infants who usually slept prone versus those who slept supine. Among the 6-month-old infants with presumably 2 more months of habitual prone or supine positioning, the differences were more significant. Eleven of the 50 supine-sleeping infants who were 6 months old were "below the clinical cutoff for the identification of gross motor delay," and more than half were one standard deviation below the mean for gross motor scores. Prone-sleeping infants rolled over and sat independently more often at 6 months of age, and, in particular, failure to spend quality tummy time was associated with slower gross motor development among supine-sleeping infants. By 15 months of age, prone-sleeping infants were more likely to walk alone and walk up stairs. Importantly, characterization of the motor development differences was observed to be based on clinical examination rather than parent recall.

In many respects, these findings are not all that exciting or new. The real issue, however, is whether there will be long-term persistence of these early motor lags in otherwise normally developing infants. Further study is necessary in this regard. It is likely, however, that with time these lags will fade and that no differences will be seen between prone- versus supine-sleeping infants. In a world of unintended consequences, however, the recommendation to sleep supine to prevent SIDS might have unintended consequences resulting from delayed developmental milestones. Further studies are needed to establish whether there are long-term effects of infant positioning on the quality and timing of global development. In no way should the results of this study be taken as a précis for changing the recommendation to promote supine sleep positioning for young infants. We need to be aware, however, of how positioning can affect early motor development to prevent needless referrals for investigation of motor delay. In other words, perhaps we should have differing developmental milestones for babies who sleep prone versus supine. Parents will need to be aware of this and told that motor milestones are likely to emerge somewhat later than expected if their infant is rarely exposed to the prone sleeping position. The middle ground, of course, is to suggest that when a baby is awake, he or she should be placed prone to allow development to these milestones. The rub with this recommendation is that it may be unnecessary if long-term studies show no true adverse outcome from supine positioning.

J. A. Stockman III, MD

Maternal seafood consumption in pregnancy and neurodevelopmental outcomes in childhood (ALSPAC study): an observational cohort study

Hibbeln JR, Davis JM, Steer C, et al (US NIH, Bethesda, Md; Univ of Illinois at Chicago; Univ of Bristol, England)
Lancet 369:578-585, 2007

Background.—Seafood is the predominant source of omega-3 fatty acids, which are essential for optimum neural development. However, in the USA, women are advised to limit their seafood intake during pregnancy to 340 g per week. We used the Avon Longitudinal Study of Parents and Children (ALSPAC) to assess the possible benefits and hazards to a child's development of different levels of maternal seafood intake during pregnancy.

Methods.—11,875 pregnant women completed a food frequency questionnaire assessing seafood consumption at 32 weeks' gestation. Multivariable logistic regression models including 28 potential confounders assessing social disadvantage, perinatal, and dietary items were used to compare developmental, behavioural, and cognitive outcomes of the children from age 6 months to 8 years in women consuming none, some (1–340 g per week), and >340 g per week.

Findings.—After adjustment, maternal seafood intake during pregnancy of less than 340 g per week was associated with increased risk of their children being in the lowest quartile for verbal intelligence quotient (IQ) (no seafood consumption, odds ratio [OR] 1.48, 95% CI 1.16–1.90; some, 1.09, 0.92–1.29; overall trend, p=0.004), compared with mothers who consumed more than 340 g per week. Low maternal seafood intake was also associated with increased risk of suboptimum outcomes for prosocial behaviour, fine motor, communication, and social development scores. For each outcome measure, the lower the intake of seafood during pregnancy, the higher the risk of suboptimum developmental outcome.

Interpretation.—Maternal seafood consumption of less than 340 g per week in pregnancy did not protect children from adverse outcomes; rather, we recorded beneficial effects on child development with maternal seafood intakes of more than 340 g per week, suggesting that advice to limit seafood consumption could actually be detrimental. These results show that risks from the loss of nutrients were greater than the risks of harm from exposure to trace contaminants in 340 g seafood eaten weekly.

▶ We have heard a lot about whether women who are pregnant should or should not eat fish during pregnancy. Clearly the fetal brain grows rapidly in size and complexity during gestation and could be easily affected by things in the diet. At birth, the brain accounts for about 25% of the basal metabolic rate and about 50% of the body's lipid. This lipid content is predominantly polyunsaturated long-chain fatty acids, some of which are essential fatty acids. These fatty acids are the precursors of prostaglandins and are incorporated into cell membranes and have many other roles in the CNS. The fetal and neonatal brain receives its essential fatty acids either preformed or by synthesis from precursors. Two of the most important essential fatty acids are docosahexaenoic acid and arachidonic acid. Although the developing brain needs large quantities of these nutrients, especially docosahexaenoic acid, the human body cannot synthesize adequate quantities from precursors. Consequently, these are mostly obtained from the diet, which makes adequate maternal nutrition very important to the development of the fetal brain. Fish and seafood contain large amounts of essential fatty acids as does breast milk. The fatty acid content of a mother's breast milk is largely determined by her diet. With this as a background, you can see how important the findings of the report of Hibbeln et al are. These investigators conclude that higher maternal fish consumption results in children showing better neurologic function than children whose mothers ate low amounts or no fish during pregnancy. These results highlight the importance of including fish in the maternal diet during pregnancy and lend support to the popular opinion that fish is indeed "brain food."

The rub with fish eating, of course, is that all fish contain some amount of methylmercury in their flesh while at the same time they contain nutrients essential to brain development, including essential fatty acids, iodine, choline, and iron. Although there is much worry about prenatal exposure to methylmercury, the only confirmed cases of prenatal human poisoning by methylmercury from fish consumption occurred in Minamata and Niigata, Japan in the 1950s and 1960s after mass industrial pollution of nearby water. A subsequent epidemiologic study of mercury poisoning in Iraq suggests that a risk might be present at exposure of around 10 parts per million as measured by maternal hair analysis. Individuals consuming fish can achieve these concentrations. However, in Iraq, exposure was from seed grain treated with methylmercury, not from fish consumption.[1] Some studies have, however, suggested that maternal exposure to mercury in the form of fish eating could produce problems in one's offspring. These differing findings have led to a public concern and also to misperceptions. One study here in the United States has shown that two thirds of Americans believe that every year 1000 to 100,000 US children are poisoned by mercury from eating fish.[2] In fact there has never been even 1 child with prenatal mercury poisoning identified as a result of the consumption of fish outside of Japan, as noted above.

So here is the dilemma: should fish consumption be restricted to lower methylmercury exposure or should it be encouraged to allow babies in utero to get the nutrients necessary for neurodevelopment? An editorial that appeared this past year in *The Lancet*[3] reminds us that the Food and Drug Administration and Environmental Protection Agency in 2004 published an advisory recommending that people should restrict their consumption of specific fish that accumulate higher concentrations of methylmercury, but the same editorial questions whether such advisories are in the public's interest, given the information regarding health benefits from eating fish described by Hibbeln et al.

Before leaving the topic of mercury in the diet, here are a couple of other facts. If you do decide that you want to add some fatty fish to your diet, recognize that the major fatty fishes include salmon, herring, sardines, and mackerel. The leanest fish that we can eat include cod, tuna, and sweet water fish. The later do not contain much in the way of contaminated mercury. Shrimp, lobster, and crayfish are pretty fatty, but not included in the category of healthy fish because they technically neither swim nor contain all the good stuff in terms of polyunsaturated fatty acids. It does appear that the ingestion of fatty fish will reduce the occurrence of renal cell carcinoma, particularly in women.[4] Women who consume one or more servings of fatty fish per week, while at increased risk for mercury problems, will have a statistically significant 44% decreased risk of the development of renal cell carcinoma compared with women who do not consume any fish. Lean fish do not provide a similar level of protection.

J. A. Stockman III, MD

References

1. Cox C, Clarkson TW, Marsh DO, Amin-Zaki L, Tikriti S, Myers GG. Dose-response analysis of infants prenatally exposed to methyl mercury: an application of a single compartment model to single-strand hair analysis. *Environ Res.* 1989;49:318-332.
2. The Center for Consumer Freedom. 61% of Americans mistakenly believe fish causes "mercury poisoning" in children. August 3, 2006. Available at: http://www.consumerfreedom.com/pressrelease_detail.cfm/release/16. Accessed December 26, 2006.
3. Myers GJ, Davidson PW. Maternal fish consumption benefits children's development [editorial]. *Lancet.* 2007;369:537-538.
4. Wolk A, Larsson SC, Johansson JE, Ekman P. Long-term fatty fish consumption and renal cell carcinoma incidence in women. *JAMA.* 2006;296:1371-1376.

Neurodevelopment and Cognition in Children after Enterovirus 71 Infection

Chang L-Y, Huang L-M, Gau SS-F, et al (Natl Taiwan Univ, Taipei; Chang Gung Univ, Taoyuan, Taiwan)
N Engl J Med 356:1226-1234, 2007

Background.—Enterovirus 71 is a common cause of hand, foot, and mouth disease and encephalitis in Asia and elsewhere. The long-term neurologic and psychiatric effects of this viral infection on the central nervous system (CNS) are not well understood.

Methods.—We conducted long-term follow-up of 142 children after enterovirus 71 infection with CNS involvement—61 who had aseptic meningitis, 53 who had severe CNS involvement, and 28 who had cardiopulmonary failure after CNS involvement. At a median follow-up of 2.9 years (range, 1.0 to 7.4) after infection, the children received physical and neurologic examinations. We administered the Denver Developmental Screening Test (DDST II) to children 6 years of age or younger and the Wechsler intelligence test to children 4 years of age or older.

Results.—Nine of the 16 patients with a poliomyelitis-like syndrome (56%) and 1 of the 5 patients with encephalomyelitis (20%) had sequelae involving limb weakness and atrophy. Eighteen of the 28 patients with cardiopulmonary failure after CNS involvement (64%) had limb weakness and atrophy, 17 (61%) required tube feeding, and 16 (57%) required ventilator support. Among patients who underwent DDST II assessment, delayed neurodevelopment was found in only 1 of 20 patients (5%) with severe CNS involvement and in 21 of 28 patients (75%) with cardiopulmonary failure (P<0.001 for the overall comparison). Children with cardiopulmonary failure after CNS involvement scored lower on intelligence tests than did children with CNS involvement alone (P=0.003).

Conclusions.—Enterovirus 71 infection with CNS involvement and cardiopulmonary failure may be associated with neurologic sequelae, delayed neurodevelopment, and reduced cognitive functioning. Children with CNS involvement without cardiopulmonary failure did well on neurodevelopment tests.

▶ You would have thought that by now we would have seen data on the long-term follow-up of youngsters who have experienced an enteroviral infection producing hand, foot, and mouth disease associated with encephalitis (enterovirus 71 [EV71]). Outbreaks have occurred from time to time here in the United States and elsewhere in the world. In 1998, an especially pervasive outbreak occurred in Taiwan caused by EV71. During that epidemic, almost all who experienced cardiopulmonary failure died. Obviously, since EV71 is an important cause of viral encephalitis, many other patients survived, and the importance of this report is that it catalogs the problems these youngsters have had over time. The report prospectively identified all patients with EV71 infection who have been treated at 1 Taiwan hospital between 1998 and 2003, the period during which the presence of EV71 infection was confirmed on the basis of positive viral isolation of EV71, positive EV71 immunoglobulin M (IgM), or an increase by a factor of 4 in the EV71 neutralizing antibody serotiter. Of some 232 children with CNS involvement, just over 10% died of cardiopulmonary failure and brainstem encephalitis during the acute phase of infection. Another 6% died from deep coma or aspiration pneumonia during the convalescent stage. Of the remaining patients with CNS involvement, most were able to be enrolled in the Taiwan study. It was observed that patients who had EV71 infection with CNS involvement had an increased likelihood of long-term neurologic sequelae, as well as delayed neurodevelopment. This was a function of the clinical severity of the CNS involvement. Presumably the neurologic problems were a direct consequence of EV71 invasion of various parts of the brain.

Among the cognitive problems these youngsters experienced were higher rates of learning and behavioral problems at school age. Some of the patients studied had an excess likelihood of having attention deficit hyperactivity disorder. A careful analysis of the data from Taiwan shows that patients who had CNS involvement with EV71 generally did well if they did not have cardiopulmonary complications as part of the course of their illness.

We still see this infection with CNS involvement from time to time here in the United States and thanks to our friends in Taiwan, we now know that we have to pay careful attention to long-term follow up of affected youngsters.

J. A. Stockman III, MD

Beliefs about the appropriate age for initiating toilet training: Are there racial and socioeconomic differences?

Horn IB, Brenner R, Rao M, et al (Children's Natl Med Ctr, Washington, DC; Children's Research Inst, Washington, DC; George Washington Univ, Washington, DC; et al)

J Pediatr 149:165-168, 2006

Objective.—To examine racial and socioeconomic differences in parental beliefs about the appropriate age at which to initiate toilet training.

Study Design.—A cross-sectional survey of 779 parents visiting child health providers in 3 clinical sites in Washington, DC and the surrounding metropolitan area completed a self-report survey. The main outcome variable was parental beliefs about the appropriate age at which to initiate toilet training. Using multiple linear regression, differences in beliefs were assessed in relation to race, family income, parental education, parental age, and age of the oldest and youngest children.

Results.—Among respondents, parents felt that the average age at which toilet training should be initiated was 20.6 months (±7.6 months), with a range of 6 to 48 months. Caucasian parents believed that toilet training should be initiated at a significantly later age (25.4 months) compared with both African-American parents (18.2 months) and parents of other races (19.4 months). In the multiple regression model, factors predicting belief in when to initiate toilet training were Caucasian race and higher income.

Conclusions.—Race and income were independent predictors of belief in age at which to initiate toilet training. More research is needed to determine what factors contribute to toilet training practices in diverse populations.

▶ This report gives us some insights as to parents' beliefs about the appropriate age for toilet training their children. The data represent the United States profile as of 2006 and show that the results are very different than a century or more ago in terms of when parents initiate toilet training. We see that Caucasian parents believe toilet training should be initiated at a later age (25.4 months) compared with both African-American parents (18.2 months) and parents of other races (19.4 months). Looking back in time, Holt's classic *Textbook of Pediatrics*, written in 1884, recommended that the goal of training regular bowel habits be completed by 3 months of age. If simply placing the infant on the pot were an insufficient stimulus to get the training going, then the judicious use of sticks, soap slivers, lubricants, enemas, stool softeners, laxatives, or cathartics could be used to facilitate the training. What was going on here was fairly obvious. The Victorian period was a part of history when there was a significant worship of cleanliness, with children being "trained" as early as 1 month of age being fairly common. Indeed, the practice in the United States at that time went all the way back to the Colonial era. The relation between cleanliness and godliness was not simply a popular religious association but was firmly rooted in the belief that "cleanliness of body was ever deemed to proceed from a due reverence to God."[1] This view was further reinforced in the early 20th century by the new science of behavioral psychology.

Watson[2] recommended that conditioned response training for daytime continence begin at 3 to 5 weeks of age. It was not until 1930 that things began to change. This was when Gesell wrote his 1930 parenting book *The Guidance of Mental Growth in Infant and Child.*[3] Gesell suggested that it is more physiologically reasonable to begin toilet training between 15 and 18 months of age.

Currently, the vast majority of American children complete toilet training between 30 and 36 months of age. An editorial that accompanied the report of Horn et al suggests that there is an explanation for the difference between the previous recommendations going back over a century for earlier training and the present achievement age. In that editorial, Dr Accardo[4] suggests that there are 3 approaches to training: (1) toilet training that begins in the first weeks of life is a reflex conditioning of the mother; (2) training started around 18 months of age is a reflex conditioning of the child; and (3) training that is completed closer to the third birthday is more dependent on social imitative learning in which the child decides to imitate "the way the big people do it" pretty much on his or her own without any conscious adult teaching/training. If the data of Horn et al are correct, it would appear that African-American mothers prefer the second approach, whereas Caucasian families lean more towards the third approach. Why this difference exists is at best speculative.

J. A. Stockman III, MD

References

1. Bacon F. *Advancement of Learning.* Facsimile Ed edition. Whitefish, MT: Kessinger; 1997.
2. Watson JB. *Psychological Care of the Infant and Child.* New York, NY: WW Norton; 1928.
3. Gesell A, Ilg FL. *Infant and Child in the Culture of Today.* New York, NY: Harper & Brothers; 1943.
4. Accardo P. Who's training whom? *J Pediatr.* 2006;149:151-152.

5 Dentistry and Otolaryngology (ENT)

Association between allergic rhinitis, bottle feeding, non-nutritive sucking habits, and malocclusion in the primary dentition
Vázquez-Nava F, Quezada-Castillo JA, Oviedo-Treviño S, et al (Autonomous Univ of Tamaulipas, Tampico-Madero City, Tamp, Mexico)
Arch Dis Child 91:836-840, 2006

Aim.—To determine the association between allergic rhinitis, bottle feeding, non-nutritive sucking habits, and malocclusion in the primary dentition.

Methods.—Data were collected on 1160 children aged 4–5 years, who had been longitudinally followed since the age of 4 months, when they were admitted to nurseries in a suburban area of Tampico-Madero, Mexico. Periodically, physical examinations were conducted and a questionnaire was given to their parents or tutors.

Results.—Malocclusion was detected in 640 of the children (51.03% had anterior open bite and 7.5% had posterior cross-bite). Allergic rhinitis alone (adjusted odds ratio = 2.87; 95% CI 1.57 to 5.25) or together with non-nutritive sucking habits (adjusted odds ratio = 3.31; 95% CI 1.55 to 7.09) had an effect on anterior open bite. Bottle feeding alone (adjusted odds ratio = 1.95; 95% CI 1.07 to 3.54) or together with allergic rhinitis (adjusted odds ratio = 3.96; 95% CI 1.80 to 8.74) had an effect on posterior cross-bite. Posterior cross-bite was more frequent in children with allergic rhinitis and non-nutritive sucking habits (10.4%).

Conclusions.—Allergic rhinitis alone or together with non-nutritive sucking habits is related to anterior open bite. Non-nutritive sucking habits together with allergic rhinitis seem to be the most important factor for development of posterior open bite in children under the age of 5 years.

▶ Pediatricians have generally not paid as much attention as they should to the causes of dental problems, including malocclusion. This large study from Mexico warns us, however, of the problems that can occur with malocclusion, problems that are the result of issues developing on a pediatrician's watch. The data on 1160 children in Mexico show that allergic rhinitis, bottle feeding, and nonnutritive sucking habits (ie, pacifier use) during the first 12 months of life favor malocclusion, particularly anterior open bite.

The theory behind how bottle feeding and nonnutritive sucking habits favor the development of malocclusion relates to different participation of the craniofacial muscle complexes in comparison with infants who are breast-feeding. An infant's tongue moves like a piston, exerting a force against the palate. Over time this alters the harmonious development of the dental arcades. It is generally accepted that breastfeeding during the first year of life contributes to a more harmonious development of the craniofacial complex. The mechanism proposed relies on the infant placing the mother's areola and nipple in his mouth and using his lips to squeeze rather than to suck. Allergic rhinitis produces malocclusion via a different mechanism. Malocclusion resulting from the presence of allergic rhinitis relates to the fact that children will breathe through their mouth instead of their nose. Mouth breathing favors an open anterior bite.

Because breastfeeding is one of the major ways to prevent the onset of allergies, it would seem that if you want to have an infant grow into adulthood with a "harmonious" facial structure, breastfeeding would be the way to go. Breast is almost always best.

This commentary obviously has to do with dental issues and will conclude with a diagnostic challenge for the reader. You are seeing a teenager who has a 5 week history of inflammatory skin lesions on her palms and soles. Physical examination reveals multiple pustules, vesicles and scaly erythema disseminated; clinically, the findings are typical of palmoplantar pustulosis. The rest of the physical examination is normal and basic laboratory studies are unrevealing. The only additional history you obtain is that during the past year this teen has been treated for multiple dental caries with dental metal restorations. What do you suspect the diagnosis is?

If you surmise that there is a possible relationship between this patient's palmoplantar pustulosis and a dental metal allergy, you would be correct. A patient presented virtually identically to this patient a year or two ago in Japan. Her health care providers did patch testing on her forearm using standard metal patch tests including aluminum chloride, chromium sulfate, cobalt chloride, copper sulfate, ferric chloride, gold chloride, indium trichloride, iridium tetrachloride, manganese chloride, mercury bichloride, nickel sulfate, platinum chloride, palladium chloride, potassium dichloride, stannous chloride, silver bromide, and zinc chloride. This test panel includes virtually all the usual metals that can find their way into fillings and metal restorations. After 48 hours, the skin tests produced a pronounced positive reaction with zinc; all other tests were negative.[1] Further testing was undertaken. Drug lymphocyte stimulating tests revealed a very strong reaction to zinc sulfate. Analysis of her dental fillings showed that they contained gold, indium, silver, palladium, copper, tin, and zinc. All of her dental fillings were completely removed and replaced with a zinc-free compound. Without any further therapy, the patient's palmoplantar pustulosis resolved over a period of a few weeks.

If you are not familiar with palmoplantar pustulosis, it does occur in children and is a chronic skin disease characterized by sterile intraepidermal pustules associated with erythematous scaling on the palms and soles. Its cause is not completely known, although an association with thyroid disease, smoking, and focal infections such as tonsillitis has been suggested. Recently, metal allergy, including to nickel, iron, and cobalt has been reported to be associated with this problem.[2]

J. A. Stockman III, MD

References

1. Yanagi T, Shimizu T, Abe R, Shimizu H. Zinc dental fillings and palmoplantar pustulosis. *Lancet.* 2005;366:1050.
2. Nakamura K, Imakado S, Takizawa M, et al. Exacerbation of pustulosis palmaris et plantaris after topical application of metals accompanied by elevated levels of leukotriene B4 in pustules. *J Am Acad Dermatol.* 2000;42:1021-1025.

Controlled Delivery of High vs Low Humidity vs Mist Therapy for Croup in Emergency Departments: A Randomized Controlled Trial
Scolnik D, Coates AL, Stephens D, et al (Hosp for Sick Children, Toronto; Univ of Toronto)
JAMA 295:1274-1280, 2006

Context.—Children with croup are often treated with humidity even though this is not scientifically based, consumes time, and can be harmful. Although humidity using the traditional blow-by technique is similar to room air and no water droplets reach the nasopharynx, particles sized for laryngeal deposition (5-10 µm) could be beneficial.

Objective.—To determine whether a significant difference in the clinical Westley croup score exists in children with moderate to severe croup who were admitted to the emergency department and who received either 100% humidity or 40% humidity via nebulizer or blow-by humidity.

Design and Setting.—A randomized, single-blind, controlled trial conducted between 2001 and 2004 in a tertiary care pediatric emergency department.

Participants.—A convenience sample of 140 previously healthy children 3 months to 10 years of age with Westley croup score of more than 1 or 2 or higher (scoring system range, 0-17); 21 families refused participation.

Intervention.—Thirty-minute administration of humidity using traditional blow-by technique (commonly used placebo, n = 48), controlled delivery of 40% humidity (optimally delivered placebo, n = 46), or 100% humidity (n = 46) with water particles of mass median diameter 6.21 µm.

Main Outcome Measure.—A priori defined change in the Westley croup score from baseline to 30 and 60 minutes in the 3 groups.

Results.—Groups were comparable before treatment. At 30 minutes the difference in the improvement in the croup score between the blow-by and low-humidity groups was 0.03 (95% confidence interval [CI], −0.72 to 0.66), between low- and high-humidity groups, 0.16 (95% CI, −0.86 to 0.53), and between blow-by and high-humidity groups, 0.19 (95% CI, −0.87 to 0.49). Results were similar at 60 minutes. Differences between groups in pulse and respiratory rates and oxygen saturation changes were insignificant, as were proportions of excellent responders; proportions with croup score of 0 at study conclusion; and proportions receiving dexamethasone, epinephrine, or requiring additional medical care or hospitalization.

Conclusions.—One hundred percent humidity with particles specifically sized to deposit in the larynx failed to result in greater improvement than 40% humidity or humidity by blow-by technique. This study does not support the use of humidity for moderate croup for patients treated in the emergency department.

▶ Here is a quiz for you. A child presents with croup. Should you use a vehicle that humidifies the air and produces particle sizes of A) smaller than 5 μm; B) 5 to 10 μm; or C) > 10 μm?

The answer to the above, based on the data from this study, is that it seems to make no difference. Theoretically, particle sizes larger than 10 μm in diameter of water deposit in the nose and mouth. Particle sizes smaller than 5 μm reach the lower airway, but may cause bronchospasm. Particles of 5 to 10 μm in diameter have the greatest probability of reaching the larynx, making this particle size the most theoretically appropriate choice for croup therapy. Unfortunately, as we see in this report of Scolnik et al, in children with moderate to severe croup, 100% humidity, even when delivered in water particle size designed to deposit in the larynx, does not result in greater clinical improvement than either controlled delivery of 40% humidity (optimally delivered placebo) or humidity delivered using the blow-by method (commonly used placebo). The differences in all secondary outcomes between these three groups of humidity delivery were both clinically and statistically insignificant.

Mist has been used as croup therapy since the 19th century. Humidity has long been a treatment for croup, using kettles, blow-by humidity, croup tents, facemasks, and the venerable shower stall. Humidity is still used, despite lack of scientific evidence. Furthermore, humidification therapy with droplets suspended in inhaled gas (blow-by technique) is not without problems. Its use has led to hot water scalds, pulmonary changes, impairment of the mucociliary apparatus, bronchospasm in children prone to wheezing, and hyponatremia in newborns. These harmful side effects underscore the need to establish whether humidification therapy has important enough positive effects in croup treatment to justify its ongoing use.

It is difficult to say what impact the results of this study will have, if any, on our discussions with parents of children presenting with croup or who call on the phone with symptoms consistent with a diagnosis of croup. Chances are that the venerable mainstays of therapy will remain venerable, including exposure to humidity. Change does not come easily.

While on the topic of upper airway obstruction, see how you would deal with the following case scenario. You are seeing a 17-year-old in your office who is complaining of fever and difficulty swallowing. The young lady recently emigrated from Somalia. On physical examination you notice a small red mass protruding upward from the base of the tongue and absence of the uvula, almost as if the uvula had been removed and was stuck to the back of her tongue. If you had not known otherwise, you would have diagnosed an edematous epiglottis and made a diagnosis of supraglottitis had it not been for the missing uvula. What is the real diagnosis here?

The correct answer is that this youngster is likely to indeed have epiglottitis/supraglottitis. The absence of the uvula is easily explained given this youngster's nationality. It is common practice in Somalian communities to cut off the uvula in the first week of life in the belief that it promotes future good health and prevents weakness. Many in the United States are not familiar with this custom, but should be, just in case.[1]

J. A. Stockman III, MD

Reference

1. Maskell SC. Supraglottitis and absence of the uvula in a Somalian woman. *BMJ.* 2006;333:662.

Language Ability after Early Detection of Permanent Childhood Hearing Impairment

Kennedy CR, McCann DC, Campbell MJ, et al (Univ of Southampton, England; Univ of Sheffield, England; Univ College London; et al)
N Engl J Med 354:2131-2141, 2006

Background.—Children with bilateral permanent hearing impairment often have impaired language and speech abilities. However, the effects of universal newborn screening for permanent bilateral childhood hearing impairment and the effects of confirmation of hearing impairment by nine months of age on subsequent verbal abilities are uncertain.

Methods.—We studied 120 children with bilateral permanent hearing impairment identified from a large birth cohort in southern England, at a mean of 7.9 years of age. Of the 120 children, 61 were born during periods with universal newborn screening and 57 had hearing impairment that was confirmed by nine months of age. The primary outcomes were language as compared with nonverbal ability and speech expressed as z scores (the number of standard deviations by which the score differed from the mean score among 63 age-matched children with normal hearing), adjusted for the severity of the hearing impairment and for maternal education.

Results.—Confirmation of hearing impairment by nine months of age was associated with higher adjusted mean z scores for language as compared with nonverbal ability (adjusted mean difference for receptive language, 0.82; 95 percent confidence interval, 0.31 to 1.33; and adjusted mean difference for expressive language, 0.70; 95 percent confidence interval, 0.13 to 1.26). Birth during periods with universal newborn screening was also associated with higher adjusted z scores for receptive language as compared with nonverbal ability (adjusted mean difference, 0.60; 95 percent confidence interval, 0.07 to 1.13), although the z scores for expressive language as compared with nonverbal ability were not significantly higher. Speech scores did not differ significantly between those who were exposed to newborn screening or early confirmation and those who were not.

Conclusions.—Early detection of childhood hearing impairment was associated with higher scores for language but not for speech in midchildhood.

▶ If anyone is due credit for the initiation of screening of newborns for hearing deficits in this country, it is the audiologist, Marion Downs. As long ago as 1964, she showed that severe- to profound-hearing loss could be reliably detected by behavioral hearing screening of neonates. She found such losses in 17 of 17,000 newborn infants, a figure identical to contemporary estimates for severe to profound bilateral hearing loss. For every such infant, 1 or 2 are born with lesser but clinically significant degrees of hearing loss. Despite the early accomplishments of Dr Downs, it was not for another 2 decades or more that hearing screening became standard. Before the implementation of universal newborn hearing screening—beginning in Rhode Island in 1989, Hawaii in 1990, and Colorado in 1993—2 important developments were required. The first was the application of objective in noninvasive physiologic tests for hearing loss that could be administered by nonprofessional personnel. The second was the demonstration that the early detection of hearing loss influences the educational outcome of affected infants. By the early 1990s, both these requisites had been met and the endorsement of universal newborn hearing screening by the National Institutes of Health Consensus Development Conference in 1993 led to the gradual spread of programs throughout the country during the last 10 years.

When universal hearing screening programs were initially implemented, the test failure rates ranged from 2% to 4%. Among newborn infants failing the screening test, 85% to 90% were later determined later to have normal hearing. This was considered to be an acceptable performance standard for all well-established screening programs, nonetheless, the high proportion of infants with normal hearing who failed screening led to criticism that unwarranted parenteral anxiety elicited by the test failure would outweigh the benefits of the program. With time, the testing characteristics of these programs have improved dramatically, and many hospitals now have failure rates of less than 0.5%, only about half of which is due to infants who actually have normal hearing. With hearing screening in place now in the nursery, the average age at which hearing loss is confirmed has dropped from 24 to 30 months to just 2 to 3 months. Infants in whom remediation is begun within 6 months are better able to maintain language and social and emotional development that is commensurate with their physical development in striking contrast to those whose hearing loss is first detected after 6 months of age.

Most current data suggest that about 93% of infants here in the United States are being screened in the newborn period for hearing loss. Early detection and intervention programs have been established in every state in the Union, but are not mandated in all states. Contrast this with the extraordinarily successful newborn screening program that has been implemented in Poland. As of 2 years ago, 99% of all infants in that country are screened before leaving the hospital. Recognize also, however, that existing universal screening programs to identify hearing defects in newborn infants are not universally bulletproof. Some forms of early-onset hearing loss are not apparent at birth. The Joint Committee on Infant Hearing has identified a series of 10 risk indicators that should prompt the primary care clinician to continue to monitor hearing status even if the results of newborn screening are normal. To see what these risk factors are, see the superb editorial of Morton and Nance.[1] The prevalence of detectable hearing loss at birth runs 186 cases per 100,000, but by 4 years of age this prevalence has increased to 270 per 100,000. Some of this increase is due to congenital causes of hearing loss that are not detectable at birth, but would be detectable by conducting molecular tests on all infants for the several important genetic causes of hearing loss. Soon we may be adding such genetic screening to the type of hearing loss screening we are currently performing in our nurseries.

J. A. Stockman III, MD

Reference

1. Morton CC, Nance WE. Newborn hearing screening—a silent revolution. *New Engl J Med*. 2006;354:2151-2164.

Direct Detection of Bacterial Biofilms on the Middle-Ear Mucosa of Children With Chronic Otitis Media

Hall-Stoodley L, Hu FZ, Gieseke A, et al (Allegheny-Singer Research Inst, Pittsburgh, Pa; Drexel Univ, Pittsburgh, Pa; Max Planck Inst for Marine Microbiology, Bremen, Germany; et al)
JAMA 296:202-211, 2006

Context.—Chronic otitis media (OM) is a common pediatric infectious disease. Previous studies demonstrating that metabolically active bacteria exist in culture-negative pediatric middle-ear effusions and that experimental infection with *Haemophilus influenzae* in the chinchilla model of otitis media results in the formation of adherent mucosal biofilms suggest that chronic OM may result from a mucosal biofilm infection.

Objective.—To test the hypothesis that chronic OM in humans is biofilm-related.

Design, Setting, and Patients.—Middle-ear mucosa (MEM) biopsy specimens were obtained from 26 children (mean age, 2.5 [range, 0.5-14] years) undergoing tympanostomy tube placement for treatment of otitis media with effusion (OME) and recurrent OM and were analyzed using microbiological culture, polymerase chain reaction (PCR)-based diagnostics, direct microscopic examination, fluorescence in situ hybridization, and immunostaining. Uninfected (control) MEM specimens were obtained from 3 children and 5 adults undergoing cochlear implantation. Patients were enrolled between February 2004 and April 2005 from a single US tertiary referral otolaryngology practice.

Main Outcome Measures.—Confocal laser scanning microscopic (CLSM) images were obtained from MEM biopsy specimens and were evaluated for biofilm morphology using generic stains and species-specific probes for *H influenzae*, *Streptococcus pneumoniae*, and *Moraxella catarrhalis*. Effusions, when present, were evaluated by PCR and culture for evidence of pathogen-specific nucleic acid sequences and bacterial growth, respectively.

Results.—Of the 26 children undergoing tympanostomy tube placement, 13 (50%) had OME, 20 (77%) had recurrent OM, and 7 (27%) had both diagnoses; 27 of 52 (52%) of the ears had effusions, 24 of 24 effusions were PCR-positive for at least 1 OM pathogen, and 6 (22%) of 27 effusions were culture-positive for any pathogen. Mucosal biofilms were visualized by CLSM on 46 (92%) of 50 MEM specimens from children with OME and recurrent OM using generic and pathogen-specific probes. Biofilms were not observed on 8 control MEM specimens obtained from the patients undergoing cochlear implantation.

Conclusion.—Direct detection of biofilms on MEM biopsy specimens from children with OME and recurrent OM supports the hypothesis that these chronic middle-ear disorders are biofilm-related.

▶ Evidence that otitis media with effusion (OME) is associated with persistent bacterial infection in the absence of culture, combined with its recalcitrance to antibiotic treatment has led to the development of the biofilm hypothesis. Biofilms consist of aggregated bacteria, usually adherent to a surface, surrounded by an extracellular matrix, and have been implicated in several chronic bacterial infections. Laboratory studies have been able to demonstrate isolates of *H influenzae* in biofilms of MEM in the chinchilla. However, no studies have directly examined human MEM for biofilms and that is what this report from Germany, Pennsylvania, and Wisconsin has done.

We learn from this report that highly sophisticated imaging studies do reveal clusters of bacteria on MEM of patients with both OME and recurrent OM. The study is clearly supportive of a biofilm cause for chronic OM. The findings suggest that recurrent OM is actually a chronic disease with episodic acute exacerbations. The findings also may help to explain the lack of antibiotic efficacy for this disorder in so many patients, given that biofilm-associated bacteria are more antibiotic resistant than are bacterial cells in suspension. This resistance may stem from the fact that oxygen and nutrient limitations within biofilms induce metabolic quiescence, which in turn reduces antibiotic effectiveness. If nothing else, the biofilm provides a physical barrier that enhances pathogen resistance to host defenses such as opsonization, lysis by complement and phagocytosis.

This editor has a hunch. That hunch is that some day OME will be treated by a yet-to-be-described technique, purely mechanical in nature that physically disrupts a biofilm. I do not know what this technique may turn out to be. Maybe it is something as simple as an ear vibrator. Perhaps it will be high-frequency US. The theory is straightforward. You have to shake these bacterial critters loose for antibiotics to do anything effective.

J. A. Stockman III, MD

Predictors of Pain and/or Fever at 3 to 7 Days for Children With Acute Otitis Media Not Treated Initially With Antibiotics: A Meta-analysis of Individual Patient Data

Rovers MM, Glasziou P, Appelman CL, et al (Univ Med Ctr Utrecht, The Netherlands; Univ of Oxford, England; Univ of Texas Med Branch, Galveston; et al)
Pediatrics 119:579-585, 2007

Objective.—The goal was to determine the predictors of a prolonged course for children with acute otitis media.

Methods.—A meta-analysis of data with the observation groups of 6 randomized, controlled trials was performed. Participants were 824 children, 6 months to 12 years of age, with acute otitis media. The primary outcome was a prolonged course of acute otitis media, which was defined as fever and/or pain at 3 to 7 days.

Results.—Of the 824 included children, 303 had pain and/or fever at 3 to 7 days. Independent predictors of a prolonged course were age of <2 years and bilateral acute otitis media. The absolute risk of pain and/or fever at 3 to 7 days for children <2 years of age with bilateral acute otitis media (20% of all children) was 55%, and that for children ≥2 years of age with unilateral acute otitis media (47% of all children) was 25%.

Conclusions.—The risk of a prolonged course was 2 times higher for children <2 years of age with bilateral acute otitis media than for children ≥ 2 years of age with unilateral acute otitis media. Clinicians can use these features (ie, age of <2 years and bilateral acute otitis media) to inform parents more explicitly about the expected course of their child's otitis media and to explain which features should prompt parents to contact their clinician for reexamination of the child.

► Thanks to our friends from The Netherlands, United Kingdom, Canada, and those in Galveston,TX for adding to our understanding about the natural course of otitis media when not treated with antibiotics. Most systematic reviews suggest that there is, at best, only a marginal benefit for antibiotic use as part of the management of acute otitis media. One study, for example, suggested that an estimated 8 to 17 children would need to be treated for every 1 child to benefit in earlier resolution of symptoms. The prescription of antibiotics could increase antibiotic resistance, increase revisit rates, and increase the likelihood of seeking medical care for future illnesses, the latter phenomenon in recent times being called "medicalisation."[1] Unfortunately, we have had few tools to discriminate the child who will have a mild, self-limiting episode of acute otitis media from those at greater risk for a prolonged course. It would be useful to have such tools, even if we decide not to use antibiotics, to properly educate parents about how long their child will likely have 1 or more signs and symptoms of this infection.

What we see in this study are prognostic indicators for length of symptoms related to acute otitis media in children who are not treated with antibiotics. The data were accumulated from 6 prior randomized clinical trials. Age less than 2 years and the presence of bilateral acute otitis media are independent predictors of a prolonged course of acute otitis media. The absolute risk of pain and/or fever at 3 to 7 days for children less than 2 years old with bilateral acute otitis media is 55%, whereas the risk for children older than 2 years with unilateral acute otitis media is less than half this (25%). These data can be used to educate parents about the expected course of their child's acute otitis media and can help influence whether a child should be seen back if his or her clinical course is out of the ordinary.

See the Poehling et al report (Reduction of frequent otitis media and pressure-equalizing tube insertions in children after introduction of pneumococcal conjugate vaccine), which tells us how effective the pneumococcal conjugate vaccine has been in reducing episodes of otitis media and the need for pressure-equalizing tube insertions.

J. A. Stockman III, MD

Reference

1. Metzl JM, Herzig RM. Medicalisation in the 21st century: introduction. *Lancet.* 2007;369:697-698.

Reduction of Frequent Otitis Media and Pressure-Equalizing Tube Insertions in Children After Introduction of Pneumococcal Conjugate Vaccine

Poehling KA, Szilagyi PG, Grijalva CG, et al (Vanderbilt Univ Med Ctr, Nashville, Tenn; Univ of Rochester School of Medicine and Dentistry, NY; Ctrs for Disease Control and Prevention, Atlanta, Ga)
Pediatrics 119:707-715, 2007

Objective.—*Streptococcus pneumoniae* is an important cause of otitis media in children. In this study we estimated the effect of routine childhood immunization with heptavalent pneumococcal conjugate vaccine on frequent otitis media (3 episodes in 6 months or 4 episodes in 1 year) and pressure-equalizing tube insertions.

Patients and Methods.—The study population included all children who were enrolled at birth in TennCare or selected upstate New York commercial insurance plans as of July 1998 and continuously followed until 5 years old, loss of health plan enrollment, study outcome, or end of the study. We compared the risk of developing frequent otitis media or having pressure-equalizing tube insertion for 4 birth cohorts (1998–1999, 1999–2000, 2000–2001, and 2001–2002) by using Cox regression analysis. We used data from the National Immunization Survey to estimate the heptavalent pneumococcal conjugate vaccine uptake for children in these 4 birth cohorts in Tennessee and New York.

Results.—The proportion of children in Tennessee and New York who received at least 3 doses of heptavalent pneumococcal conjugate vaccine by 2 years of age increased from ≤1% for the 1998–1999 birth cohort to ~75% for the 2000–2001 birth cohort. By age 2 years, 29% of Tennessee and New York children born in 2000–2001 had developed frequent otitis media, and 6% of each of these birth cohorts had pressure-equalizing tubes inserted.

Comparing the 2000–2001 birth cohort to the 1998–1999 birth cohort, frequent otitis media declined by 17% and 28%, and pressure-equalizing tube insertions declined by 16% and 23% for Tennessee and New York children, respectively. For the 2000–2001 to the 2001–2002 birth cohort, frequent otitis media and pressure-equalizing tubes remained stable in New York but increased in Tennessee.

Conclusions.—After heptavalent pneumococcal conjugate vaccine introduction, children were less likely to develop frequent otitis media or have pressure-equalizing tube insertions.

Antibiotics for acute otitis media: a meta-analysis with individual patient data

Rovers MM, Glasziou P, Appelman CL, et al (Univ Med Centre Utrecht, The Netherlands; Univ of Oxford, England; Univ of Texas, Galveston; et al)
Lancet 368:1429-1435, 2006

Background.—Individual trials to test effectiveness of antibiotics in children with acute otitis media have been too small for valid subgroup analyses. We aimed to identify subgroups of children who would and would not benefit more than others from treatment with antibiotics.

Methods.—We did a meta-analysis of data from six randomised trials of the effects of antibiotics in children with acute otitis media. Individual patient data from 1643 children aged from 6 months to 12 years were validated and re-analysed. We defined the primary outcome as an extended course of acute otitis media, consisting of pain, fever, or both at 3–7 days.

Findings.—Significant effect modifications were noted for otorrhoea, and for age and bilateral acute otitis media. In children younger than 2 years of age with bilateral acute otitis media, 55% of controls and 30% on antibiotics still had pain, fever, or both at 3–7 days, with a rate difference between these groups of −25% (95% CI −36% to −14%), resulting in a number-needed-to-treat (NNT) of four children. We identified no significant differences for age alone. In children with otorrhoea the rate difference and NNT, respectively, were −36% (−53% to −19%) and three, whereas in children without otorrhoea the equivalent values were −14% (−23% to −5%) and eight.

Interpretation.—Antibiotics seem to be most beneficial in children younger than 2 years of age with bilateral acute otitis media, and in children with both acute otitis media and otorrhoea. For most other children with mild disease an observational policy seems justified.

▶ Acute otitis media remains the most common reason that antibiotics are prescribed in children, even though the effect of such treatment is surprisingly restricted. In many children, acute otitis media resolves spontaneously. These factors have led to the policy widely practiced overseas of not prescribing antibiotics on the first visit, but rather to treat the child with adequate pain relief and start watchful waiting. The main problem has been to identify those children who will most likely benefit from antibiotics. To address this question, Rovers et al did a meta-analysis of individual patients' data, combining the data from 6 randomized trials that assessed the effectiveness of antibiotics in acute otitis media. Some 1643 children age 6 months to 12 years with acute otitis media were included. The study allowed identification of subgroups that would benefit most from treatment.

The results of the Rovers et al study seem fairly straightforward. Antibiotics were most beneficial in children younger than 2 years with bilateral acute otitis media and in children with acute otitis media and a draining ear. The data also suggest that observation without antibiotic treatment would be justified for most other children, which would be more than half of the children who had acute otitis media develop. Thus, implementing the results of this meta-analysis in current practice would suggest that more than half of children with acute otitis media could be treated with watchful waiting. The resulting reduction in the use of antibiotics would have vast financial implications and would considerably reduce the adverse effects of antibiotic use, such as diarrhea and the generation of antibiotic resistance.

What everyone wonders about, and worries about, is that if antibiotics are not given initially to manage acute otitis media, will we be putting children at an increased risk of mastoiditis, a rare, but serious complication of ear infection. Please note that in the 1643 children included in the Rovers et al study, none had mastoiditis develop. Also note that a diagnosis of acute otitis media in a child with fever does not exclude the presence of other bacterial diseases, including pneumonia, sepsis, or meningitis. These must be excluded by whatever means appropriate if one entertains watchful waiting.

See the Plasschaert et al report (Trends in doctor consultations, antibiotic prescription, and specialist referrals for otitis media in children: 1995–2003) that tells us the trends that have occurred over the last decade in terms of physician consultation, antibiotic prescription writing, and referrals to subspecialists for otitis media in children.

J. A. Stockman III, MD

Trends in Doctor Consultations, Antibiotic Prescription, and Specialist Referrals for Otitis Media in Children: 1995–2003
Plasschaert AIO, Rovers MM, Schilder AGM, et al (Univ Med Ctr, Utrecht, The Netherlands)
Pediatrics 117:1879-1886, 2006

Background.—Reported trends regarding the incidence of otitis media and antibiotic prescription rates are inconsistent.

Objective.—Our goal was to assess changes in incidence of consultation rates, antibiotic prescription, and referral rates for otitis media in children over the years 1995–2003.

Methods.—A cohort study including all children aged 0 to 13 years within the research database of the Netherlands University Medical Center Utrecht Primary Care Network covering the period 1995–2003. Otitis media diagnoses were recorded according to the International Classification of Primary Care codes and antibiotic prescription according to the Anatomic Therapeutic Chemical Classification System codes. Otitis media incidence rates were calculated as episodes per 1000 person-years. Antibiotic prescription and referral rates were calculated per 100 otitis media episodes.

Results.—From 1995 to 2003, the overall general practitioner consultation rates for acute otitis media and otitis media with effusion declined by 9% and 34%, respectively. In children aged 2 to 6 years and those aged 6 to 13 years, the incidence rates of acute otitis media and otitis media with effusion declined by 15% and 41% and 40% and 48%, respectively. In children <2 years of age, the incidence rates of acute otitis media and otitis media with effusion increased by 46% and 66%, respectively. Antibiotic prescription rates for acute otitis media and otitis media with effusion increased by 45% and 25%, respectively. The referral rate for acute otitis media did not change, whereas the referral rate for otitis media with effusion increased by 45%.

Conclusions.—Consultation rates for otitis media have changed considerably over the last decade, and so have antibiotic prescriptions and specialist referrals. The rising antibiotic prescription rate for otitis media causes concern, because this may induce increasing medical costs and antibiotic resistance.

▶ Population-based studies from both the United States and Europe suggest that the incidence of otitis media has increased over the past 2 decades. Lanphear et al[1] have reported a 44% increase in the prevalence of recurrent otitis media in children here in the United States in the period 1981 to 1988, with the greatest increase in infants younger than 1 year. Studies from overseas have also shown an increase in the incidence of otitis media by as much as 70% in Europe.

Although the incidence of otitis media has been increasing overseas, so has the writing of prescriptions for this entity. Antibiotic prescribing rates for otitis media vary from a low of 31% in certain European countries such as The Netherlands, to as high as 98% here in the United States and in Australia.[2] With the literature, including the preceding report, showing that antibiotics are not necessary for every child with otitis media, we have begun to see a slight downward trend in the use antibiotics in our country.

The report abstracted is from The Netherlands, which gives us a glimpse of what is happening in western European countries with respect to the prevalence of otitis media and how physicians deal with it. There, the referral rates from general practitioners for patients with acute otitis media have declined fairly significantly. Also, the incidence rates of acute otitis media seem to have declined as well. This applies, however, only to older children. In younger children, the incidence rates of acute otitis media seem to be actually increasing along with antibiotic prescription rates. This rising antibiotic prescription rate for otitis media in a country that has been very conservative with antibiotic use in the past raises significant concern because it may result in added medical costs as well as antibiotic resistance.

See the Bauchner et al report (Effectiveness of Centers for Disease Control and Prevention recommendations for outcomes of acute otitis media) that shows how effective, or actually not effective, the Centers for Disease Control and Prevention (CDC) recommendations have been for managing acute otitis media. Back in 1999, the CDC released recommendations for the use of specific antibiotic agents for the treatment of acute otitis media. These recommendations were reached through a consensus and were based on data available at that time. In general, these recommendations advocated the use of amoxicillin as first-line therapy for children at low risk for resistant pathogens and high-dose amoxicillin, high-dose amoxicillin/clavulanate, or cefuroxime for children at higher risk. Antibiotic use in the previous 30 days was the principal risk factor for antibiotic-resistant pathogens in the CDC recommendations. Daycare attendance was also cited as a risk factor, but was not incorporated into the decision scheme. What we learn from the CDC report is that despite evidence-based literature, there seems to be very little adherence to the CDC recommendations for treatment of acute otitis media.

The bottom line here is: will we ever learn?

J. A. Stockman III, MD

References

1. Lanphear BP, Byrd RS, Auinger P, Hall CB. Increasing prevalence of recurrent otitis media among children in the United States. *Pediatrics* [serial online]. 1997;99:E1. Available at: http://www.pediatrics.org/cgi/content/full/99/3/e1. Accessed June 5, 2007.
2. Froom J, Culpepper L, Grob P, et al. Diagnosis and antibiotic treatment of acute otitis media: report from international primary care network. *BMJ*. 1990;300: 582-586.

Effectiveness of Centers for Disease Control and Prevention Recommendations for Outcomes of Acute Otitis Media

Bauchner H, for the Boston-Based Pediatric Research Group (Boston Univ)
Pediatrics 117:1009-1017, 2006

Objectives.—To determine whether we could increase adherence to the Centers for Disease Control and Prevention (CDC) recommendations with well-accepted approaches to improving quality of care and adherence to the CDC recommendations resulted in improved outcomes for acute otitis media (AOM).

Methods.—A cluster randomization study was conducted in 12 pediatric practices (6 intervention and 6 control sites). The main outcome measures were adherence to the CDC recommendations (modified to include 2 additional antimicrobial agents) and a subsequent antibiotic prescription for AOM within 30 days after diagnosis.

Results.—Of 3152 patients referred to research assistants, 2584 (82%) were eligible. Of those eligible, 1368 (99%) of 1382 at the intervention sites and 1138 (99%) of 1146 at the control sites consented to participate. Rates of adherence to the CDC recommendations were not significantly higher at the intervention sites than at the control sites, for initial enrollment episodes (78.2% vs 70.6%) or second episodes (62.6% vs 59.9%). After controlling for clustering according to site and covariates, children who were not treated in adherence to the CDC recommendations for both episodes had 1.60 times the odds of a subsequent prescription within 12 days, compared with those treated in adherence at both episodes.

Conclusions.—Despite using evidence-based approaches that are known to influence physician behavior, we were unable to increase adherence to the CDC recommendations for treatment of AOM. However, we did establish that prescription of antimicrobial therapy consistent with the CDC recommendations for a second episode of AOM was associated with improved outcomes, measured as the need for subsequent antibiotic prescription. Because of the selection of resistant otopathogens, adherence to the CDC recommendations is likely more important in subsequent episodes of AOM than in the initial episode.

Tympanostomy Tubes and Development Outcomes at 9 to 11 Years of Age

Paradise JL, Feldman HM, Campbell TF, et al (Univ of Pittsburgh, Pa; Stanford Univ, Calif; Univ of Texas, Dallas; et al)
N Engl J Med 356:248-261, 2007

Background.—Developmental impairments in children have been attributed to persistent middle-ear effusion in their early years of life. Previously, we reported that among children younger than 3 years of age with persistent middle-ear effusion, prompt as compared with delayed insertion of tympanostomy tubes did not result in improved cognitive, language, speech, or psychosocial development at 3, 4, or 6 years of age. However, other important components of development could not be assessed until the children were older.

Methods.—We enrolled 6350 infants soon after birth and evaluated them regularly for middle-ear effusion. Before 3 years of age, 429 children with persistent effusion were randomly assigned to undergo the insertion of tympanostomy tubes either promptly or up to 9 months later if effusion persisted. We assessed literacy, attention, social skills, and academic achievement in 391 of these children at 9 to 11 years of age.

Results.—Mean (±SD) scores on 48 developmental measures in the group of children who were assigned to undergo early insertion of tympanostomy tubes did not differ significantly from the scores in the group that was assigned to undergo delayed insertion. These measures included the Passage Comprehension subtest of the Woodcock Reading Mastery Tests (mean score, 98±12 in the early-treatment group and 99±12 in the delayed-treatment group); the Spelling, Writing Samples, and Calculation subtests of the Woodcock-Johnson III Tests of Achievement (96±13 and 97±16;

104±14 and 105±15; and 99±13 and 99±13, respectively); and inattention ratings on visual and auditory continuous performance tests.

Conclusions.—In otherwise healthy young children who have persistent middle-ear effusion, as defined in our study, prompt insertion of tympanostomy tubes does not improve developmental outcomes up to 9 to 11 years of age.

▶ If there were such a thing as the "article of the year" for 2007, this report would be the Oscar winner. It takes our understanding of a common pediatric problem to a new and significantly higher level.

Many studies in the second half of the last century proposed an association between middle ear infection early in life and subsequent developmental impairments in children. The supposition was that sensorineural hearing loss caused irreversible developmental impairments. The placement of tympanostomy tubes became the second most frequent surgical procedure performed in the United States (after neonatal circumcision) not just to help clear or prevent recurrent infection, but rather to restore normal hearing as a preventive measure to abort the likelihood of developmental delay. In July 1994, what we now call the Agency for Healthcare Research and Quality published a clinical practice guideline that recommended the insertion of tympanostomy tubes when bilateral middle ear effusion had persisted for 4 to 6 months with a hearing threshold of 20 dB or higher in otherwise healthy children 1 to 3 years of age.[1]

The report by Paradise et al helps close the gap between what we know and do not know about the relationship between otitis media and developmental delay. Recognizing the deficiencies of previous retrospective studies, Paradise et al designed a prospective study to answer 3 key questions: (1) is there an association between early otitis media and later impairments of speech, language, and cognitive development? (2) if such an association exists, is it a cause-and-effect relationship? and (3) if developmental impairments result from otitis media, are they reversible? More than 6000 healthy infants in the Pittsburgh area were followed up to answer these questions. They had extensive developmental testing at 3, 4, 6, and 9 to 11 years of age. Four hundred twenty-nine of these children had bilateral middle ear effusion lasting for 90 days or unilateral middle ear effusion lasting for 130 days. These youngsters were assigned to receive tympanostomy tubes promptly or up to 9 months later if the effusion persisted. It was expected that if a causal relationship exists between persistent effusion and developmental impairments, the test scores of the children receiving tympanostomy tubes earlier should have been better than the scores of the children with tubes placed later in life. The bottom line of the study was that at 3, 4, and 6 years of age, no significant differences were found in the test scores for any of the outcomes between children who received tympanostomy tubes early in life and those who received tympanostomy tubes later.

The article by Paradise et al confirms the lack of significant differences between infants with persistent middle ear effusions who receive or do not receive tympanostomy tubes early in life with respect to academic achievement, attention, and social skills. When one puts the data from this report together with information from a report from a national conference sponsored by the National Institutes of Health, which reviewed all the available literature, one can conclude that the effect of otitis media with effusion on speech and language development and academic achievement is "generally very small, accounting for 0% to about 4% of the variance in children's development, after controlling for factors that typically co-vary."[2]

Paradise et al strongly caution that the findings of their study cannot be generalized to children who are not otherwise healthy or have disabling conditions such as sensorineural hearing loss or Down syndrome; to children with longer periods of effusion than those studied; or to children in whom effusion is consistently accompanied by extreme degrees of hearing loss. Such children, however, are seen relatively infrequently in general pediatric practice.

The implications of this study to the general practice of pediatrics are straightforward. Given the consistency of current findings from several studies, it can be concluded that for otherwise healthy children who are younger than 3 years and who have asymptomatic middle ear effusion that is persistent (as defined in the study), prompt insertion of tympanostomy tubes does not improve the developmental outcomes as compared with delayed insertion in children in whom effusion continues unremittingly. Watchful waiting in such circumstances for at least 6 additional months when effusion is bilateral and for at least 9 months when the effusion is unilateral would seem to be the preferred management option. For more on this topic, see the superb editorial by Berman.[3]

J. A. Stockman III, MD

References

1. Otitis Media Guideline Panel, Agency for Healthcare Policy and Research. *Otitis Media With Effusion in Young Children. Clinical Practice Guideline No 12.* Rockville, Md: Dept of Health and Human Services; 1994: AHCPR Publication No 94-0622.
2. Roberts J, Hunter L, Gravel J, et al. Otitis media, hearing loss, and language learning: controversies and current research. *J Dev Behav Pediatr.* 2004;25: 110-122.
3. Berman S. The end of an era in otitis research [editorial]. *N Engl J Med.* 2007;356:300-302.

Post–tympanostomy tube otorrhea: A meta-analysis
Hochman J, Blakley B, Abdoh A, et al (Univ of Manitoba, Winnipeg, Canada)
Otolaryngol Head Neck Surg 135:8-11, 2006

Introduction.—Post–tympanostomy tube otorrhea is the most common complication of tympanostomy tube placement. The incidence of this problem varies from 3.4% to 74%. Trials that study post–tympanostomy tube otorrhea may involve valid randomization "by patient" or "by ear." In an attempt to define "best practice," we conduct a meta-analysis to quantify the benefit of using topical prophylactic antibiotic drops in the postoperative period. We then compare our findings with previous results found in the literature.

Methods.—We selected randomized studies for which antibiotic drops had been used for at least 48 hours after tympanostomy tube insertion. Nine studies, 3 "by ear" and 6 "by patient," met our inclusion criteria. The odds ratio and 95% confidence intervals were calculated for each to conduct the meta-analysis.

Results.—Overall, prophylaxis appears to be effective at reducing the incidence of post–tympanostomy tube otorrhea. The odds ratios for all studies were less than 1.0. However, none of the 3 "by ear" studies and only 3 of the 6 "by patient" studies were statistically significant. The mean odds ratio was 52%, suggesting that prophylaxis may reduce the incidence of post–tympanostomy tube otorrhea by half.

Conclusion.—This meta-analysis suggests that routine post–tympanostomy tube prophylaxis is beneficial, but this finding is dependent on selection criteria used.

▶ This study shows us how little science there is in medicine that relates to certain problems, even ones as common as otorrhea post–tympanostomy tube placement. The question asked in this report is whether using topical prophylactic antibiotic drops in the postoperative period diminishes the prevalence of post–tympanostomy tube otorrhea. The investigators pulled all the literature pertaining to this topic to attempt to answer this question. What they found were 9 studies that suggest some degree of protection derived from the use of topical antibiotics in the prevention of postoperative otorrhea. Unfortunately, only 3 of the studies are actually statistically significant in their findings. In the aggregate, the evidence-based review suggests that the use of prophylactic eardrops reduces the incidence of post–tympanostomy tube otorrhea by about 50%. No study suggests that treated ears fared worse than untreated ears.

One would think that with such a pervasive problem as otorrhea post–tympanostomy tube placement, there would be more than 9 studies appearing in the literature on this topic. Apparently, some things do not turn investigators on, one of them being ooze in the external auditory canal.

J. A. Stockman III, MD

Postpartum splinting of ear deformities
Lindford AJ, Hettiaratchy S, Schonauer F (Queen Victoria Hosp, East Grinstead, England)
BMJ 334:366-368, 2007

Background.—Congenital deformities of the ear are common and are usually corrected surgically in childhood. These deformities are often first noticed by parents or non-specialist health care providers. Splinting of ear deformities in the early neonatal period has been shown to be a safe and effective non-surgical treatment. Three cases that demonstrated how different congenital ear deformities can be successfully treated without surgery were examined.

> *Case 1.*—A male child was born at full term with bilateral con-
> stricted ears. There was no family history of ear deformities. The ap-
> pearance of the rim of the ear in this deformity is tightened, as though
> a purse string has been pulled closed. The ear was splinted for 3 days
> after birth, and the program was continued for 1 month. By 10 days
> the upper pole had expanded, and a good result was seen at 6
> months.
>
> *Case 2.*—A male child was born at full term with a unilateral
> Stahl's ear deformity. This is a helical rim deformity characterized by
> a third crus, flat helix, and malformed scaphoid fossa. Splinting was
> initiated 3 days after birth and continued for 3 weeks. By 10 days the
> correction was already apparent, with disappearance of the third
> crus and a normal helical rim. The good initial result was maintained
> at 6 months.
>
> *Case 3.*—A female child was born at full term with bilateral promi-
> nent ears. This deformity is characterized by excessive height of the
> conchal wall or a wide conchoscaphal angle (>90°). Splinting was
> initiated 3 days after birth and continued for 4 weeks. The ear was
> protuberant initially, with an increased conchoscaphal angle, but af-
> ter splinting the angle was reduced and the ear sat in a more natural
> position.

Conclusions.—Splinting of the ears in the early neonatal period has been advocated as an effective non-surgical treatment that often produces better results than surgery. Many kinds of splints and molding materials have been described. Splinting is a simple, effective, and inexpensive method for treating even the most complex congenital ear deformities.

▶ We pediatricians are often the first to fully examine a newborn baby. All too often when we notice ear deformities, such as those described in this report, we do little or nothing about the deformity; either we are hoping that it will go away or that a later surgical repair will take care of the problem, when, in fact, just a touch of early management will produce a cure of the problem. This statement particularly applies to the constricted ear, the Stahl's ear, and prominent ears. A constricted ear is one in which the rim of the ear looks as if it has been tightened, rather like a purse string that has been pulled closed. A Stahl's ear is a helical rim deformity characterized by a third crus, flat helix, and malformed scaphoid fossa. Prominent or "outstanding" ears we have all seen. This deformity is defined by excessive height of the conchal wall or a wide conchoscaphal angle (>90°). The causes of these deformities are variable. Abnormal development and functioning of the intrinsic and extrinsic muscles of the ear may generate deforming forces. External forces applied to the ears, such as malpositioning of the head in the prenatal and early neonatal period may also contribute. The actual incidence of these deformities is not known, but about 1 in 20 newborns are thought to have prominent ears, though this may be an underestimate. Although some of these deformities do in fact resolve spontaneously, the large proportion does not. In today's society, which puts great emphasis on appearance, the pressure on parents to seek surgical treatment if their child has an ear deformity is quite great. Several surgical techniques are available for each of these deformities, and the results are usually good, but they do involve anesthesia and, at times, the results may be unpredictable.

Splinting of ears in the early neonatal period has been advocated as an effective nonsurgical treatment that often produces better results than later surgery. The best results with splinting, as described in this report are when the splinting is done immediately following birth. Molding of the ears is possible then because of the presence of maternal estrogens, rendering the ear of the neonate soft and malleable. After only a few days of life, the ear of a newborn becomes significantly stiffer and less amenable to molding, which makes splinting more difficult and, in fact, less effective.

Many kinds of splints and molding materials have been described. Splinting is a simple, effective, and cheap way of treating even the most complex congenital ear deformities. Even beyond the immediate neonatal period devices such as the "Auri-Clip" have been successfully used to improve the appearance of prominent ears.

The authors of this report suggest that pediatricians, neonatologists, obstetricians, general practitioners, and midwives become experienced in the detection and initial treatment involving splinting of ear deformities. By assuming responsibility for early management, the delay that is often incurred by referral to otolaryngologists or plastic surgeons is avoided and in many cases obviated. You will have to be the one to decide whether you want to take on the challenge of reshaping a newborn's ear. If so, read this report in detail. The techniques involved look fairly simple.

This report represents a topic that is somewhat of an oddball one, so we will conclude this commentary with an oddball, totally unrelated query: who were the winners of the Ig Nobel Awards back in 2006? Readers of the YEAR BOOK OF PEDIATRICS will be familiar with the Ig Nobel Awards, based on previous questions on this subject. The annual Ig Nobel Awards ceremony is held at Harvard University, where prizes are awarded for science that "makes you laugh, then makes you think." The most recent Ig Nobel prize for medicine went to Francis Fesmire of the University of Tennessee College of Medicine for finding a unique way to terminate intractable hiccups. Dr Fesmire found himself at a loss after many attempts to help a patient who could not stop hiccupping. He eventually decided to attempt to terminate the hiccups by performing a rectal examination (done in the usual manner) and to his and the patient's delight, the patient stopped hiccupping—an event he reported in a journal article entitled: "Termination of intractable hiccups with digital rectal massage."[1]

Two investigators from an agricultural university in The Netherlands won the biology prize for finding that the female malaria mosquito, *Anopheles gambiae* craves equally the smell of stinky feet and Limburger cheese. The investigators' "eureka" moment came when they realized that Limburger cheese is cultured with *Brevibacterium epidermidis*, a bacterium found on human skin. This finding actually has practical implications. By using an organism that emits an odor-alluring scent for mosquitoes, scientists are now building traps that will monitor malaria infestation to aid investigators at mosquito extermination. The Bill and Melinda Gates Foundation awarded these investigators some $8 million to continue their work to reduce the spread of malaria in Africa.

Other Ig Nobel prizes in 2006 included the Peace Prize, which was awarded to Howard Stapleton for inventing a "teenager repellant." The repellant is an electromechanical machine that emits high frequency shrieking that can be heard by teenagers but not by most adults . . . gotta buy one of those. The Literature Prize was awarded to Daniel Oppenheimer of Princeton University for his report "Consequences of erudite vernacular utilized irrespective of necessity: problems with using long words needlessly." Dr. Oppenheimer found that when smart people use big words, they do not sound smarter than others; in fact, they don't seem as smart as those who use simple, clear language.

Finally, the winning prize in ornithology went out to Ivan Schwab, an ophthalmologist, who investigated and explained why woodpeckers do not get headaches.[2] Dr. Schwab found that the North American pileated woodpecker strikes trees at a rate of up to 20 times per second, up to 12,000 times a day, with deceleration forces that in a human would be equivalent to "striking a wall at 16 miles an hour—face first—each time." You will have to look up the reference to see exactly how the average woodpecker is able to survive all this when the average boxer cannot take a simple punch in the head without passing out.

For more on the topic of the Ig Nobel Awards, see a summary of the 2006 events by Lenzer.[3]

J. A. Stockman III, MD

References

1. Fesmire FM. Termination of intractable hiccups with digital rectal massage. *Ann Emerg Med*. 1988;17:872.
2. Schwab IR. Cure for a headache. *Br J Ophthalmol*. 2002;86:843.
3. Lenzer J. The importance of smelly feet and stinky cheese. *BMJ*. 2006;333:771.

Foreign Body Removal From the External Auditory Canal in a Pediatric Emergency Department
Marin JR, Trainor JL (Children's Hosp, Seattle; Children's Mem Hosp, Chicago)
Pediatr Emerg Care 22:630-634, 2006

Objectives.—To describe the experience with external auditory canal foreign body removal in a pediatric emergency department. To identify factors associated with procedural complications and/or failed removal.

Methods.—Retrospective case series of patients treated in the emergency department over a 5-year period. Primary outcomes include success and complication rates. Secondary outcomes include removal rates in the otolaryngology clinic and operating room.

Results.—Physicians in our pediatric emergency department successfully removed 204 (80%) of 254 foreign bodies. In 30 cases (12%), there was a complication. Multiple attempts at removal were associated with failure (relative risk [RR], 6.0; 95% confidence interval [CI], 3.0–12.0) and complications (RR, 3.1; 95% CI, 1.5–6.3). The use of multiple instruments was also associated with failure (RR, 5.4; 95% CI, 2.7–10.8) and complications (RR, 4.0; 95% CI, 2.0–7.6). Of the 244 patients in whom emergency department attempts at removal were made, 26 were successfully removed in otolaryngology clinic, and 14 were removed in the operating room. Foreign bodies present in the canal for more than 24 hours were not at higher risk of failed removal or complications. Patients younger than 4 years also were not at increased risk of having failed removal or complications.

Conclusions.—Physicians in a pediatric emergency department remove most foreign bodies from the external auditory canal successfully with minimal complications and need for operative removal. These data suggest that referral to otolaryngology be considered if more than 1 attempt or instrument is needed for removal.

▶ This is the first report this editor recalls seeing that deals with such a large number of patients presenting with foreign bodies in the ear canal. It illustrates the travails that emergency room physicians may experience when attempting to remove a foreign body. Clearly, the longer a foreign body is lodged in the external canal, the more inflammation that exists and the more difficulty in removing the foreign body. Higher failure rates are seen in small children and with insects in the external canal. Erasers and foam have the same problem. Erasers, popcorn, foam, and bread—in that order—represent those types of foreign bodies that have the highest likelihood of requiring operative removal.

While on the topic of "foreign bodies" in the external ear canal, a patient was recently reported who was thought to have dark impacted wax in his external auditory canal. This could not be removed easily and on further inspection and biopsy the "wax" turned out to be a malignant melanoma.[1]

We close this commentary with a question about dentistry and its history. What is the earliest time recorded in history in which dentistry appears to have been practiced? Welcome to a time so long ago that people without dental insurance still could get their teeth drilled and perhaps filled. The earliest that we know this may have happened is somewhere between 9000 and 7500 years ago, and it appears that flint-wielded specialists performed the work. A total of 11 teeth from 9 adults who lived during that period of time were found to have holes drilled with sharpened flint points. The teeth came from residents of a prehistoric farming village called Mehrgarh in what is now Pakistan. These discoveries appear to represent the earliest known examples of dental work. The teeth involved were molars that would not have been visible, and therefore indicate that the dental alterations were not intended for display or decorations, but more likely were done for therapeutic reasons. A number of the drilled holes were associated with decay, suggesting that the latter was the reason why the teeth were drilled.

Interestingly, no evidence of drilling of teeth was found in teeth from a 6500-year-old cemetery at the same site, suggesting that the practice of dentistry disappeared some time between 7500 to 6500 years ago. The holes that were drilled in the Mehrgarh teeth were relatively small, 1.3 mm to 3.2 mm in diameter with a depth of 0.5 mm to 3.5 mm. Edge smoothing indicates that the drilling was performed on living individuals who continued chewing that further produced dental wear. Some type of filling material may also have been placed in the drilled holes, which would have exposed sensitive tooth areas. Scanning electron microscopy and computerized tomography scanning has identified concentric ridges on the inside walls of the holes in the teeth that were found, clearly indicating that the holes were the products of prehistoric drilling tools. So who practiced such dentistry? It appears that skilled artisans who made beads were more likely than not to have acquired the skills to do this. Bead production did require flint drilling and investigators wielding a flint-type model of prehistoric tools were able to reproduce the drilled holes in molar teeth from a modern human jawbone at the rate of about one hole per minute.

If you want to read more about the first insights into human dentistry, see the summary of this topic by Bower.[2]

J. A. Stockman III, MD

Reference

1. Hannan SA, Parikh A. Malignant melanoma of the external ear canal. *Lancet.* 2006;368:1680.
2. Bower B. Mystery drilling: ancient teeth endured dental procedures. *Sci News.* 2006;169:213.

6 Endocrinology

Clinical Features Affecting Final Adult Height in Patients With Pediatric-Onset Crohn's Disease

Sawczenko A, Ballinger AB, Savage MO, et al (Univ of London)
Pediatrics 118:124-129, 2006

Background.—Growth failure is a recognized complication of pediatric-onset Crohn's disease, but there are few data on final adult height.

Objective.—Our purpose with this work was to determine adult height and the clinical features that influence long-term growth impairment.

Methods.—We retrospectively studied 123 patients with Crohn's disease (65 male and 58 female) who had reached adult height. All of the case subjects were diagnosed before age 16.0 years. Heights were converted to SD scores and univariate analysis performed of factors postulated to influence final height, that is, interval from onset of symptoms to diagnosis, prepubertal onset of symptoms, gender, jejunal disease present at diagnosis, systemic steroid therapy, intestinal surgery, and midparental height SD scores. Significant univariate factors were additional analyzed in regression models.

Results.—Mean height deficit at diagnosis was −0.50 SD scores, which improved to, −0.29 SD scores at final height. Mean final height compared with target height, calculated from parental height, was −2.4 cm (range: −20.0 to 9.0 cm). Nineteen percent of the case subjects achieved a final height >8.0 cm below target height. The length of the interval between symptom onset and diagnosis correlated negatively with height SD scores at diagnosis. Height SD scores at diagnosis were related to final height SD scores, independent of midparental height. The presence of jejunal disease was negatively related to final height.

Conclusions.—Mean final adult height showed a modest deficit compared with target height, but in one fifth of patients, final height was significantly less than target height. Earlier diagnosis and improved treatment of jejunal disease would be likely to improve final height.

▶ One of the hallmarks of Crohn's disease in some, if not most, children is impairment in growth. Short stature and concerns about adult height cause considerable distress to the youngster and certainly to the parents, particularly during adolescence when one's peers seem to be growing quickly, and the child with inflammatory bowel disease may not. Some youngsters seem to be more affected than others in this regard. Those with delayed diagnosis, the presence of jejunal disease at presentation, prepubertal onset of symptoms, male sex, and severity of illness all correlate with short stature. There are some data on the effect of therapy on final height. Systemic steroids, when used to control the inflammatory bowel disease, can significantly, positively affect height. We see in this series that achievement of a relatively favorable final height does occur for the majority of patients, albeit if cared for in a highly specialized center in which maintenance of adequate nutrition is the mantra. The latter includes enteral feeding when necessary.

Exactly why some children have more problems with diminished growth velocity is not entirely clear. Growth velocity has been reported to be abnormally decreased in about one half of Crohn's cases before diagnosis. It has been shown that the interleukin-6 −174 G/C polymorphism determines poor growth at diagnosis, although DNA from the majority of the current patients in this series was not available to confirm this. Clearly delayed growth at presentation underscores the need for earlier diagnosis since delayed growth at presentation is a key risk factor for long-term height reduction. This study also showed that jejunal disease does affect final height. It is clear from the growth perspective that particular attention should be focused on this group of youngsters with Crohn's disease.

Here in the United States, steroids are most often used as the initial treatment for Crohn's disease. Elsewhere, such as in Great Britain, where this report originated, enteral feeding is the favored therapy for inducing remission and has been for more than 20 years because of concerns about potential systemic effects of steroids leading to growth impairment. Elsewhere, steroid use is generally restricted to those who have failed dietary therapy and who may, therefore, have more intractable disease. This does not mean that steroids should not be used, rather that they should be used judiciously.

One other comment, that having to do with the effects of surgery. This series found no effect of intestinal surgery on final height, concurring with previous reports that surgery as an intervention for poor growth is not a wise decision in most instances.

Many pediatricians are using innovative therapies these days for management of idiopathic short stature. One wonders if clinical trials, for example, of recombinant insulin-like growth factor-I would be useful for those with inflammatory bowel disease. To read more about recombinant insulin-like growth factor-I for the treatment of idiopathic short stature, see the report of Rosenbloom.[1] Also, see the Papadimitriou et al report (Early growth acceleration in girls with idiopathic precocious puberty) that discusses early growth acceleration in girls with idiopathic precocious puberty.

J. A. Stockman III, MD

Reference

1. Rosenbloom AL. Is there a role for recombinant insulin-like growth factor-I in the treatment of idiopathic short stature? *Lancet*. 2006;368:612-616.

Early growth acceleration in girls with idiopathic precocious puberty

Papadimitriou A, Beri D, Tsialla A, et al (Penteli Children's Hosp, Athens, Greece; Univ of Athens School of Medicine, Greece)
J Pediatr 149:43-46, 2006

Objective.—To determine the growth pattern of girls with idiopathic precocious puberty (IPP) from birth until diagnosis.

Study Design.—We studied 47 girls with IPP and 35 control girls. In each subject, height and weight were measured at diagnosis, whereas data on height from birth until diagnosis were taken from the personal health book of the patient. Height standard deviation score (HSDS) and body mass index SDS were calculated.

Results.—Mean age (±SD) of the girls with IPP was 7.6 (1.1) years and of control girls was 7.5 (0.9) years. At birth, HSDS of the patients with IPP was −0.01 (0.8); at the age of 2 years, 0.42 (1.2); at the age of 4 years, 0.64 (1.1); and at diagnosis, 1.23 (1.7) ($P < .001$). HSDS of control girls was 0.02 (0.8) at birth, 0.25 (0.8) at 2 years, 0.12 (0.9) at 4 years, and 0.19 (1.1) at assessment ($P > .05$). There was no statistical difference between body mass index SDS of the patients 0.6 (1.1) versus that of control girls 0.5 (1.0).

Conclusions.—The early growth acceleration pattern may be used as an additional clue to the diagnosis of idiopathic precocious puberty (Fig 1).

▶ How we grow up has been the source of many studies for many decades. IPP results from premature reactivation of the hypothalamic–pituitary–gonadal (HPG) axis, not related to intracranial pathology. This axis is actually first activated during infancy, when there is a physiologic postnatal surge of gonadotropins, a phenomenon designated as the "mini-puberty" of infancy.

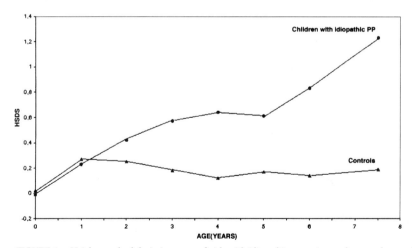

FIGURE 1.—Height standard deviation score of girls with idiopathic precocious puberty and control girls. *HSDS*, Height standard deviation score; *PP*, precocious puberty. (Courtesy of Papadimitriou A, Beri D, Tsialla A, et al. Early growth acceleration in girls with idiopathic precocious puberty. *J Pediatr*. 149:43-46. Copyright 2006 by Elsevier.)

In female infants, the gonadotropin surge is follicle-stimulated hormone (FSH)-predominant and peaks at about 3 to 6 months of life. Thereafter, gonadotropin levels decrease to prepubertal levels because of the increasing sensitivity of the hypothalamus and pituitary to the very low levels of circulating estrogens and because of the development of endogenous mechanisms in the CNS that suppress the human pituitary gonadotropin (HPG) axis. Puberty is initiated when this suppression is released. The mechanisms responsible for the suppression and subsequent activation of the HPG axis involve neuronal input to the hypothalamic gonadotropin-releasing hormone (GnRH) pulse generator. What the primary timing mechanism is that initiates this activation remains unknown. In most developed countries, the cutoff age that determines precocious sexual maturation in girls is 8 years, although this is somewhat lower here in the United States (7 years for white girls and 6 years for black girls).[1]

Most pediatricians have recognized that girls with IPP are unusually tall for their age. Despite this, final height attainment is usually within or less than target height, leading most to suspect that these girls are seen with growth acceleration well before the onset of puberty. This is exactly what this report from Athens documents. The typical growth pattern of a girl with IPP is that of a youngster with average birth length followed by growth acceleration soon after birth, reaching a zenith centile in the first 2 to 4 years of life; she then grows along this centile until she enters puberty, usually between 6 and 8 years, when growth acceleration again resumes. This is a classic growth pattern that may be used as an additional clue to the diagnosis of IPP.

It is important to recognize that there are other causes of early growth acceleration, including in girls born of families with tall stature. Babies born with intrauterine growth restraint may exhibit catch-up growth acceleration in the first few years of life. Also, obese children tend to grow more quickly early in life. One would need to differentiate these circumstances from the girl who is tall simply because she will enter puberty early.

There remains much controversy about how far one should go to evaluate whether precocious puberty is, in fact, idiopathic. This controversy somewhat relates to the debate about the normal age of onset of puberty. The Drug and Therapeutics Committee of the Lawson Wilkins Pediatric Society has stated that the normal age of puberty here in the United States is 7 years in white girls and 6 years in black girls. The Joint Committee has issued the following statement: "In most cases, evaluation of girls with early breast and/or pubic hair development to look for a pathologic etiology of precocious puberty need not be performed for white girls older than 7 years and African-American girls older than 6 years of age." There are opponents elsewhere in the world who suggest that the classic cutoff age of 8 years for breast development or pubic hair development should still be used. An additional controversy is whether every girl with precocious puberty needs neuroimaging. Because there is no consensus whether a healthy 6- to 8-year-old girl with breast development but no central nervous signs or symptoms needs brain imaging, in practice, clinicians have to develop their own criteria for deciding whether to order an MRI. The data from this report would suggest that a longstanding pattern of growth acceleration might be consistent with early onset of puberty and therefore might at the marginal age ranges, if present, dissuade one from doing too much in the way of studies.

When one thinks about it, early growth acceleration leading to early onset of puberty is the other end of the bell-shaped curve of constitutional delay of growth. In the latter circumstance, growth is characterized by growth deceleration in the first 2 to 3 years of life. As a result, the child's height may fall to a nadir centile that is at or below the third centile, depending on parent height. Growth then resumes at a normal rate, and the child grows along this centile until the onset of puberty, which is usually delayed. All of life seems to be a bell-shaped curve, doesn't it?

Before closing this commentary, it seems worthwhile to mention something about the origin of the term "endocrine gland." Gland comes from the French *glande* (it is self-derived from the old English *glandre*). The term has continuously simply meant clusters of anything. Since the 19th century, in medicine, glands have been of two types—with ducts and without ducts. The ductless or endocrine (from the Greek *endon* meaning "inside") pour their secretions directly into the blood, and so affect the whole organism. In 1905, the British physiologist Ernest H. Starling, after consultations with Cambridge classicist, named these secretions "hormones" (from the Greek *hormao*, meaning "to excite").

Thus it is that endocrine glands in part are ductless clusters that pour exciting stuff into one's humors.[2] So much for history.

J. A. Stockman III, MD

References

1. Kaplowitz PB, Oberfield SE. Reexamination of the age limit for defining when puberty is precocious in girls in the United States: implications for evaluation and treatment: drug and therapeutics and executive committees of the Lawson Wilkins Pediatric Endocrine Society. *Pediatrics*. 1999;104:936-941.
2. Sengoopta C. Endocrine glands. *Lancet*. 2005;366:977.

Reproductive outcome in patients treated and not treated for idiopathic early puberty: Long-term results of a randomized trial in adults
Cassio A, Bal MO, Orsini LF, et al (Univ of Bologna, Italy)
J Pediatr 149:532-536, 2006

Objective.—To evaluate the adult reproductive outcome in girls with early puberty who participated in a previous random study.

Study Design.—A total of 22 subjects treated with triptorelin 3.75 mg every 4 weeks (group 1), 18 subjects not treated (group 2), and 22 age-matched normal volunteers (control group) underwent a physical examination, serum hormone level determination, and pelvic ultrasonography.

Results.—The characteristics of menstrual cycles, serum hormone levels, and ultrasound results did not differ significantly among the 3 groups examined. The mean ovarian volume and the uterine volume tended to increase in the subjects of group 2, but the differences were not significant. The percentage of subjects who reported being sexually active at the time of the examination was greater in the 2 groups with previous early puberty than in the controls (76% of cases in group 1, 72% in group 2, and 59% in the control group).

Conclusions.—Neither early puberty nor its treatment seems to significantly affect the normal adult function of the pituitary-gonadal axis.

▶ This report is reassuring. To date, few studies have looked at the long-term outcomes of young ladies who have had early onset of puberty (with or without treatment for this problem). The current results seem to confirm that girls with early puberty exhibit normal menstrual patterns and have the same reproductive capabilities as their peers. Treatment with gonadotropin-releasing hormone analog also does not seem to adversely affect outcomes. If there is one down side to the early onset of puberty, it is the observation in this report that many of these girls became pregnant earlier than their peers. This warrants further investigation to evaluate the psychosocial impact on sexual behavior of early maturation, given that pregnancies were noted as young as 13 to 14 years of age.

Let's leave the subject of early sexual development in girls; see what you would do with the following scenario. A 4-year-old presents to your office for his yearly physical examination. This boy has a normal examination except for the development of gynecomastia. You order a number of laboratory tests including thyroid function studies, follicle-stimulating hormone, luteinizing hormone, testosterone, estriol, dehydroepiandrosterone, 17-alpha-hydroxyprogesterone, and prolactin levels. All of these return normal, including liver function studies. You suspect that this boy somehow has been getting into some exogenous source of estrogen. There appears, however, to be no possibility that he has taken oral contraceptives nor has he had any access to soya products. He is probably too young to be smoking pot, another known cause of gynecomastia in men. What do you think about as other possibilities?

This is a real case. As the youngster's gynecomastia slowly worsened, the boy's mother remembered the lavender oil she had been rubbing on her son's skin. Because this was the only possible source of trouble, she was advised to stop its application. The gynecomastia gradually resolved. This case, along with two others, was recently reported in the *New England Journal of Medicine.*[1] One of the other cases involved a 10-year-old boy who believed that the enlargement of his breasts seemed more prominent in the evening and less so first thing in the morning. On questioning it was determined that the patient was not using drugs, herbal supplements, or herbal lotions, but was applying a styling gel to his hair and scalp every morning and regularly using a shampoo. The labels of both the gel and the shampoo listed *Lavandula angustifolia* (lavender) oil and *Melaleuca alternifolia* (tea tree) oil as ingredients. Reevaluation 9 months after the use of these products was discontinued showed that his physical examination was now in line with his normal male pubertal development. The third patient was a 7-year-old who presented with a 1-month history of gradual onset of gynecomastia with firm, nontender breast tissue that corresponded to Tanner stage 2. His history was positive only for the use of lavender-scented soap and intermittent use of lavender-scented commercial skin lotions. The gynecomastia resolved completely a few months after the use of scented soap and skin lotions was discontinued.

Gynecomastia is quite common in boys. Some 60% will manifest this during puberty, but prepubertal gynecomastia is extremely uncommon. Because there is no known physiologic cause of prepubertal gynecomastia, pathologic causes should be looked for in every case. In most instances, however, prepubertal gynecomastia will finally be labeled idiopathic. It is thought that in such patients, the condition may be caused by exposure to an environmental chemical that disrupts the endocrine system and leads to disproportionate estrogen and androgen pathway signaling, a finding reported in a limited number of adults with gynecomastia.

The most common causes of gynecomastia from exogenous sources are oral contraceptives, marijuana use, and soy products. To these must now be added the repeated topical application of one or more over-the-counter personal care products that contain lavender oil or lavender oil and tea tree oil. It is suspected that these oils may possess endocrine-disrupting activity that causes an imbalance in estrogen and androgen pathway signaling. Lavender oil and tea tree oil are sold over the counter in their "pure form" and are present in an increasing number of commercial products, including shampoos, hair gels, soaps, and body lotions. It is not known whether these oils elicit similar endocrine-disrupting effects in prepubertal girls, adolescent girls and women. Because gynecomastia is not infrequently seen in men, one might suspect that these substances are also a cause of gynecomastia in adult males.

Remember the phenomenon of lavender oil gynecomastia. The next time you see a child with prepubertal gynecomastia, it might save everyone a whole ton of money if you ask about shampoos and creams instead of ordering a lot of laboratory tests.

J. A. Stockman III, MD

Reference

1. Henley DV, Lipson N, Korach KS, Bloch CA. Prepubertal gynecomastia linked to lavender and tea tree oils. *N Engl J Med.* 2007;356:479-485.

Growth and Health in Children With Moderate-to-Severe Cerebral Palsy
Stevenson RD, for the North American Growth in Cerebral Palsy Study (Univ of Virginia, Charlottesville; et al)
Pediatrics 118:1010-1018, 2006

Background.—Children with cerebral palsy frequently grow poorly. The purpose of this study was to describe observed growth patterns and their relationship to health and social participation in a representative sample of children with moderate-severe cerebral palsy.

Methods.—In a 6-site, multicentered, region-based cross-sectional study, multiple sources were used to identify children with moderate or severe cerebral palsy. There were 273 children enrolled, 58% male, 71% white, with

Gross Motor Function Classification System levels III (22%), IV (25%), or V (53%). Anthropometric measures included: weight, knee height, upper arm length, midupper arm muscle area, triceps skinfold, and subscapular skinfold. Intraobserver and interobserver reliability was established. Health care use (days in bed, days in hospital, and visits to doctor or emergency department) and social participation (days missed of school or of usual activities for child and family) over the preceding 4 weeks were measured by questionnaire. Growth curves were developed and z scores calculated for each of the 6 measures. Cluster analysis methodology was then used to create 3 distinct groups of subjects based on average z scores across the 6 measures chosen to provide an overview of growth.

Results.—Gender-specific growth curves with 10th, 25th, 50th, 75th, and 90th percentiles for each of the 6 measurements were created. Cluster analyses identified 3 clusters of subjects based on their average z scores for these measures. The subjects with the best growth had fewest days of health care use and fewest days of social participation missed, and the subjects with the worst growth had the most days of health care use and most days of participation missed.

Conclusions.—Growth patterns in children with cerebral palsy were associated with their overall health and social participation. The role of these cerebral palsy-specific growth curves in clinical decision-making will require further study.

▶ It probably should come as no surprise that children with cerebral palsy have been unequivocally shown to not grow as well as their peers. It should also come as no surprise that a major contributory factor to the rate of fall off in growth is the overall health status of the affected child. Children with moderate-or-severe cerebral palsy who have better health will be larger. Nonetheless, it is clear that even in good health, children affected with cerebral palsy, particularly as they pass their 10th to 12th birthday will be shorter and leaner than their peers. This report is important because it helps sort out what is "normal" in this population, although it is sometimes difficult to tell whether normal short stature and lean body mass might be the result of poor health overall.

J. A. Stockman III, MD

Characteristics at diagnosis of type 1 diabetes in children younger than 6 years

Quinn M, Fleischman A, Rosner B, et al (Children's Hosp Boston; Harvard Univ, Cambridge, Mass)
J Pediatr 148:366-371, 2006

Objective.—To characterize the prodrome, presentation, family history, and biochemical status at diagnosis of type 1 diabetes mellitus (T1D) in children under age 6 years.

Study Design.—This was a retrospective chart review of patients hospitalized at diagnosis with T1D from 1990 to 1999 in a children's hospital.

Results.—A total of 247 children were hospitalized, 44% of whom presented in diabetic ketoacidosis (DKA). When stratified by 2-year age intervals, only total carbon dioxide (tCO_2) was significantly lower in the youngest children ($P = .02$), and the duration of candidiasis was significantly longer in those children presenting in DKA ($P = .004$). Parents were more likely to recognize symptomatic hyperglycemia in children older than 2 years ($P < .0001$). Most parents sought care for their child suspecting that the child had diabetes; the other children were diagnosed when presenting with another concern. Only gender and tCO_2 were significantly correlated with hemoglobin A1c (HbA1c); age-adjusted HbA1c was 0.64% higher in girls compared with boys ($P = .045$), and each 1-mmol/L decrement in tCO_2 increased the age- and gender-adjusted HbA1c by 0.086% ($P < .001$).

Conclusions.—A high proportion of children under age 6 years present critically ill at the diagnosis of T1D. When any of the classic symptoms of diabetes or a yeast infection is present, a serum glucose level should be measured.

▶ Most of us recognize that a young child who presents with diabetes mellitus often does so differently than the older child. The symptoms of T1D in infants and toddlers may be subtle or masquerade as an intercurrent illness. The diagnosis is frequently misinterpreted, ignored, or remarkably delayed, all to the detriment of the youngster. One other difference at a young age is the greater likelihood of the concomitant occurrence of an infectious illness at the time of presentation of diabetes. This report from the Children's Hospital of Boston helps us understand more about the young child (<6 years of age) at the time of presentation with T1D.

The Boston study has some interesting observations. A total of 247 children were evaluated in this report. The finding of comparable HbA1c levels across a 6-year age interval contrasts with previous reports that younger children have a shorter prodrome than older children before diagnosis. It is suggested that younger children do not have a shorter period of inadequate insulin secretion but do have a more severe metabolic decompensation at the time of diagnosis. The data from Boston support this explanation because the investigators found no correlation between age and HbA1c across a 6-year age span, although they did identify an age-related inverse correlation with the degree of acidosis at diagnosis. As one would have predicted, also observed was a very high probability that young children would present with DKA. For young children to present in DKA, they must exhaust the capacity to secrete a minimal amount of insulin, not merely to have sustained exposure to hyperglycemia.

The classic symptoms of diabetes in young children may be subtle and often elude even an experienced family member or clinician. For example, until children can reach the faucet, they must depend on care providers to quench their thirst; only if they can ask for or obtain their own fluids can parents readily recognize the presence of polydipsia. Detecting polyuria in diapered children has become more challenging with the advent of highly absorbent disposable diapers. Furthermore, as parents work outside the home, an increase in urinary frequency may not be noted by a care provider and thus may go unrecognized for days. Once children are verbal and toilet trained, their frequent request to use the bathroom may be more likely to be noted by caregivers, although a more independent child may urinate frequently without informing an adult. Enuresis, the symptom recognized earliest in the course of new-onset T1D in school-age children, is likewise age dependent.

This report reminds us of something we already know, namely, that there is a high proportion of young children presenting with diabetes who have a first-degree family member with T1D, thus suggesting a strong genetic contribution to early-onset disease. Also, like many other investigators, the authors found a male-to-female ratio for children developing early-onset diabetes that ranges from 1.2:1 to 1.5:1.

In most cases, recognition of the classic signs and symptoms of new-onset diabetes in children younger than 6 years will be made by parents. How to properly educate without overalarming large populations of parents about the problem remains a conundrum. Parents should certainly be aware that contact with a physician is important if their child has developed an unexplained yeast infection, particularly in the perineal area. Candidiasis is common in infants, and over-the-counter availability of topical antifungal preparations may leave parents with the false impression that a persistent or recurrent yeast infection need not be brought to the attention of a child's primary care provider. The authors of this report recommend that when a young child presents for evaluation of dehydration, abdominal pain, or fatigue (albeit nonspecific complaints), the presence of a yeast infection should immediately prompt the suggestion that the child might have diabetes, and a serum glucose level should be obtained.

One other tidbit about the initial presentation of diabetes: see what you would do with the following scenario. You are caring for a newly diagnosed diabetic. The presenting blood sugar is 400 mg/dL and the glycosylated hemoglobin level is 17.5%. You begin therapy. The blood sugar promptly responds and the patient is out of trouble. Unfortunately, over the next day or two, the patient complains of blurry vision. The best corrective visual acuity is now 20/80 in both eyes. The intraocular pressure is normal. You refer the patient to an ophthalmologist. The question is, what do you suspect the ophthalmologist will find on careful examination?

The problem being described relates to changes in the lens of the eye following treatment for uncontrolled diabetes. The patient described had a slit-lamp examination, which revealed multiple bilateral, crack-shaped lines transversing the lenses of both eyes. These cracks were located primarily in the central portion of the lens (nucleus), running more or less parallel to the nuclear curvature. In addition, a larger crack continued as a fairly straight band near both ends of the equator, seemingly transversing the nuclear lens fibers tangentially. These cracks had the same optical density as the aqueous in the anterior chamber, suggesting the presence of fluid-filled cavities within the lens. Other ophthalmologic findings were unremarkable. Fundoscopy revealed no signs of diabetic retinopathy. Over a few months, the vision returned to normal and the lens cracks vanished spontaneously.

What is being described here is what, in the eye literature, is called "sugar cracks." The cracks presumably are due to fluid-filled cavities created within the interstitium of the lens. The most likely cause of this is the fact that the lens of the eye becomes somewhat hypertonic during prolonged states of high blood sugar. With correction of the blood sugar, the lens takes some time for its tonicity to correct, causing fluid to enter the lens fracturing it. Fortunately the lens is capable of repairing itself.

To learn more about this interesting problem, see a recent review of the topic in the *New England Journal of Medicine*.

J. A. Stockman III, MD

Reference

1. Tangelder GJ, Dubbelman M, Ringens PJ. Sudden reversible osmotic lens damage ("sugar cracks") after initiation of metformin. *N Engl J Med.* 2005;353:2621-2622.

Age at Onset of Childhood-Onset Type 1 Diabetes and the Development of End-Stage Renal Disease: A nationwide population-based study

Svensson M, for the Swedish Childhood Diabetes Study and the Swedish Registry for Active Treatment of Uraemia (Umeå Univ, Sweden; et al)
Diabetes Care 29:538-542, 2006

Objective.—To analyze the impact of age at onset on the development of end-stage renal disease (ESRD) due to diabetic nephropathy in a nationwide population-based cohort with childhood-onset type 1 diabetes.

Research Design and Methods.—A record linkage between two nationwide registers, the Swedish Childhood Diabetes Registry, including 12,032 cases with childhood-onset diabetes, and the Swedish Registry for Active Treatment of Uraemia was performed. Log-rank test was used to test differences between cumulative risk curves of developing ESRD due to diabetic nephropathy in three different strata of age at onset (0–4, 5–9, and 10–14 years).

Results.—At a maximum follow-up of 27 years, 33 patients had developed ESRD due to diabetic nephropathy and all had a diabetes duration >15 years. In total, 4,414 patients had diabetes duration >15 years, and thus the risk in this cohort to develop ESRD was 33 of 4,414 (0.7%). A significant difference in risk of developing ESRD was found between the youngest (0–4 years) and the two older (5–9 and 10–14 years) age-at-onset strata ($P = 0.03$ and $P = 0.001$, respectively). A significant difference in the risk of developing ESRD was also found between children with prepubertal (0–4 and 5–9 years, $n = 2,424$) and pubertal (10–14 years, $n = 2000$) onset of diabetes ($P = 0.002$). No patient with onset of diabetes before 5 years of age had developed ESRD.

Conclusions.—With a median duration of 21 years in this population-based Swedish cohort with childhood-onset diabetes, <1% of the patients had developed ESRD due to diabetic nephropathy, and a prepubertal onset of diabetes seems to prolong the time to development of ESRD.

▶ A lot is written about type 2 diabetes in adults and children. What we see from this report from Sweden is the ravaging outcome on the kidneys of childhood-onset type 1 diabetics. Poor glucose control is a necessary but not sufficient factor for the development of diabetic nephropathy. Other factors, including perinatal, hormonal, and genetic ones seem to contribute as well. What we see in this report is that children with diabetes are not likely to develop end-stage renal disease on our watch. Nonetheless, what happens on our watch does affect the long-term outcome of the renal problem. In the nationwide population study abstracted, less than 1% of diabetics whose disease duration is more than 15 years (median time to follow of 21 years) develop end stage renal disease. This low prevalence of end-stage renal disease may be due to the relatively short time of follow-up, 15 to 27 years, because the peak incidence of diabetic nephropathy in other studies has been found to occur some 25 to 30 years after the onset of type 1 diabetes. The problem of renal failure comes later in life.

If there is any good news in the report from Sweden, it is that young children who had diabetes develop seem to survive their disease without the development of end-stage renal disease for a longer period. No patient with onset of diabetes before 5 years of age in fact was shown to actually develop end-stage renal disease.

See the Berhe et al report (Feasibility and safety of insulin pump therapy in children aged 2 to 7 years with type 1 diabetes: a retrospective study) that tells us about the feasibility and safety of insulin pump therapy in young children with type 1 diabetes.

J. A. Stockman III, MD

Feasibility and Safety of Insulin Pump Therapy in Children Aged 2 to 7 Years With Type 1 Diabetes: A Retrospective Study

Berhe T, Postellon D, Wilson B, et al (Loyola Univ, Maywood, Ill; DeVos Children's Hosp, Grand Rapids, Mich)
Pediatrics 117:2132-2137, 2006

Background and Objectives.—Although insulin pump therapy has been successful in adults, adolescents and school children, its use has been limited in young children. The purpose of this study was to evaluate the glycemic control, safety and efficacy of continuous subcutaneous insulin infusion via pump in young children (2–7 years old) with type 1 diabetes who were transitioned from twice-a-day insulin injection (neutral protamine Hagedorn/Lente + Humalog/Novalog) to insulin pump therapy. Hemoglobin A1c, BMI, average fasting blood glucose, episodes of severe hypoglycemia, episodes of diabetic ketoacidosis, episodes of lipohypertrophy, blood glucose variability, and number of sick day calls were compared before and after insulin pump therapy.

Methods.—Data were collected retrospectively by chart review over a 2-year period during quarterly diabetes clinic visits from 33 patients who were managed on neutral protamine Hagedorn/Lente + Humalog/Novolog twice-a-day injections for at least 1 year prior to transitioning to insulin pump therapy.

Results.—There was a significant improvement in the average hemoglobin A1c after continuous subcutaneous insulin infusion therapy. The average fasting blood sugar was lower in the continuous subcutaneous insulin infusion group. Severe episodes of hypoglycemia and episodes of lipohypertrophy were significantly higher before insulin pump therapy initiation. There were significantly fewer sick day calls after continuous subcutaneous insulin infusion. Blood sugar variability improved significantly after insulin pump therapy. There was no significant difference in BMI or amount of carbohydrate consumed. None of the patients experienced diabetic ketoacidosis requiring emergency treatment before or after insulin pump therapy.

Conclusions.—Continous subcutaneous insulin infusion therapy in young children with type 1 diabetes is a safe, effective and superior alternative to a twice-a-day insulin regimen.

► This report from the United States and the Nimri et al report (Insulin pump therapy in youth with type 1 diabetes: a retrospective paired study) from Israel have similar findings. Specifically, continuous subcutaneous insulin infusion does in fact improve diabetic control in youngsters with type 1 diabetes.

Insulin pump therapy use has dramatically increased since its introduction in the late 1970s. Although its use in this regard has been most significant in adults, adolescents, and school-age children, it has not been fully extended in its use to preschool-age children, a group that in fact might benefit most from it. This report from Michigan focuses on this age group and studied 33 children aged 2 to 6 years to determine whether insulin pump therapy might improve diabetic control. It was found to do so. These findings are important because preschool-age children with type 1 diabetes are at greatest risk for neurodevelopmental impairment from hypoglycemia and hyperglycemia. The ability to level out control with insulin pump therapy makes this an extremely attractive option for diabetic care in this young age group.

The Nimri et al report (Insulin pump therapy in youth with type 1 diabetes: a retrospective paired study) confirms that continuous insulin infusions work for children even beyond the preschool age. The decrease in hemoglobin HbA1c levels observed was associated with a significant reduction in the rate of severe hypoglycemic events. These findings are important because hypoglycemia has historically been the limiting factor in the implementation of intensive therapy in children and adolescents who have diabetes.

If there is any risk associated with continuous insulin infusions, it is the rapid development of diabetic ketoacidosis secondary to pump or infusion-set failure. Fortunately, the more we learn about the use of subcutaneous insulin infusion pumps, the less frequent such complications tend to be.

J. A. Stockman III, MD

Insulin Pump Therapy in Youth With Type 1 Diabetes: A Retrospective Paired Study

Nimri R, Weintrob N, Benzaquen H, et al (Inst of Endocrinology and Diabetes, Petah Tiqva, Israel; Tel Aviv Univ, Israel)
Pediatrics 117:2126-2131, 2006

Objective.—To compare by age and glycemic control continuous subcutaneous insulin infusion with multiple daily injections in youth with type 1 diabetes.

Methods.—The files of 279 patients who had type 1 diabetes and switched from multiple daily injections to continuous subcutaneous insulin infusion between 1998 and 2003 were reviewed for glycemic control, body mass index standard deviation score, and adverse events. Patients were divided by age as follows: 23 prepubertal (median age: 5.4; range: 1.6–8.6 years), 127 adolescent (median age: 13.7; range 9–17 years), and 129 young adult (median age: 22.8; range: 17–40 years). The data were compared between the 12 months of multiple daily injections that preceded continuous subcutaneous insulin infusion and the period after the start of continuous subcutaneous insulin infusion for the whole cohort and by age group.

Results.—A significant decrease in hemoglobin A1c was demonstrated after the start of continuous subcutaneous insulin infusion use for the entire cohort (-0.51%) and for the prepubertal (-0.48%), adolescent (-0.26%), and young adult (-0.76%) groups. There was a significant interaction between the change in hemoglobin A1c level and hemoglobin A1c value at initiation of pump therapy (-1.7% for patients with hemoglobin A1c $\geq 10\%$; 0.2% for patients with hemoglobin A1c $\leq 7\%$). The rate of severe hypoglycemic episodes decreased significantly in the adolescent group, from 36.5 to 11.1 events per 100 patient-years, and in the young adult group, from 58.1 to 23.3. There was no significant change in the rate of diabetic ketoacidosis between the 2 periods. The young adults showed a significant decrease in body mass index standard deviation scores (-0.08 ± 0.37).

Conclusions.—Continuous subcutaneous insulin infusion improves glycemic control in youth with type 1 diabetes, especially in those with a history of poor glycemic control. This improvement is associated with a decrease in the rate of severe hypoglycemia in the absence of weight gain.

Optimal control of type 1 diabetes mellitus in youth receiving intensive treatment

Springer D, Dziura J, Tamborlane WV, et al (Yale Univ, New Haven, Conn)
J Pediatr 149:227-232, 2006

Objective.—To investigate the impact of factors that might interfere with optimal glycemic control in youth with type 1 diabetes mellitus (T1DM) in the current era of intensive management, including the interplay of race/ethnicity and socioeconomic status (SES) on HbA1c levels.

Study Design.—This study comprised a database review of all patients under age 18 years with T1DM for at least 6 months duration. Sex, age, race/ethnicity, duration of diabetes, mode of insulin administration (pump vs injection), body mass index, SES, and HbA1c level were recorded at each patient's most recent visit between January and September 2003.

Results.—Mean HbA1c level for the 455 patients was 7.6% ± 1.4%; only 31% of patients failed to meet the therapeutic goal of < 8.0%. Multiple linear regression analysis identified female sex (P = .02), older age (P = .001), longer duration of diabetes (P < .001), injection therapy (P < .001), and lower SES (P = .001) as significantly associated with higher HbA1c level. After adjustment for SES, race/ethnicity was not a determinant of HbA1c level.

Conclusions.—Low SES had a greater association with poor metabolic control than did race/ethnicity, which was not associated with differences in HbA1c level after controlling for SES. Most children were able to attain glycemic targets at least as good as the Diabetes Control and Complications Trial recommendations in a large clinical practice.

▶ This report should be read in some detail. It tells us how a well-performing clinic that manages children with diabetes can be successful in an economically diverse community. Many studies have suggested that race and ethnicity are risk factors for poor diabetic control, with African-American and Hispanic youth having higher HbA1c levels than Caucasian children. One possible explanation for this disparity is that predominantly Caucasian and non–Spanish-speaking clinical care provider teams may not be able to provide ethnically and culturally sensitive counseling for minority families. What this report, however, shows is that when differences in SES are controlled for, it is low income, rather than race and ethnicity, that is the important factor associated with higher HbA1c levels in certain racial and ethnic populations.

There is a lot of new information evolving that may mature into better ways to treat diabetic patients, particularly information about stem cells. Research has shown that adult pancreatic beta cells are formed by self-duplication of preexisting cells rather than adult stem cell differentiation. Therefore, it is likely that an individual is born with a certain number of beta cells derived from a small number of progenitors, and those beta cells are the only source of new cells throughout an individual's life. While it may be impossible to coax other cells in the body to become insulin-producing beta cells, scientists have tried to do so in the laboratory. Researchers have been able to induce fibroblast-like cells derived from islets donated postmortem to differentiate into insulin-expressing islet-like cells.[1] Others have manipulated culture conditions to cause differentiation of human fetal liver cells. Still others have shown that bone marrow stem cells are capable of turning into beta cells. These findings are still very preliminary. Researchers have also tried isolating beta cells from human cadavers and cultivating them in the laboratory, but without much sustained success.

The real problem with beta-cell replacement therapy, if it ever comes about, is that even if optimal beta-cell regeneration—by whatever method—is achieved in patients with T1DM, the autoimmune process that caused the condition in the first place must also be addressed. Beta cells may be gunned down, as it were, by the immune system as quickly as they are medically delivered. The unfortunate thing is that researchers remain puzzled about the role of autoimmunity in T1DM. The key issue is whether one can effectively suppress ongoing autoimmune processes.

To read more about how stem cells are being probed as a treatment for T1DM, see the excellent perspective by Hampton.[2]

J. A. Stockman III, MD

References

1. Gershengorn MC, Hardikar AA, Wei C, Geras-Raaka E, Marcus-Samuels B, Raaka BM. Epithelial-to-mesenchymal transition generates proliferative human islet precursor cells. *Science.* 2004;306:2261-2264.
2. Hampton T. Stem cells probed as diabetes treatment. *JAMA.* 2006;296:2785-2786.

International Trial of the Edmonton Protocol for Islet Transplantation
Shapiro AMJ, Ricordi C, Hering BJ, et al (Univ of Alberta, Edmonton, Canada; Univ of Miami, Fla; Univ of Minnesota, Minn; et al)
N Engl J Med 355:1318-1330, 2006

Background.—Islet transplantation offers the potential to improve glycemic control in a subgroup of patients with type 1 diabetes mellitus who are disabled by refractory hypoglycemia. We conducted an international, multicenter trial to explore the feasibility and reproducibility of islet transplantation with the use of a single common protocol (the Edmonton protocol).

Methods.—We enrolled 36 subjects with type 1 diabetes mellitus, who underwent islet transplantation at nine international sites. Islets were prepared from pancreases of deceased donors and were transplanted within 2 hours after purification, without culture. The primary end point was defined as insulin independence with adequate glycemic control 1 year after the final transplantation.

Results.—Of the 36 subjects, 16 (44%) met the primary end point, 10 (28%) had partial function, and 10 (28%) had complete graft loss 1 year after the final transplantation. A total of 21 subjects (58%) attained insulin independence with good glycemic control at any point throughout the trial. Of these subjects, 16 (76%) required insulin again at 2 years; 5 of the 16 subjects who reached the primary end point (31%) remained insulin-independent at 2 years.

Conclusions.—Islet transplantation with the use of the Edmonton protocol can successfully restore long-term endogenous insulin production and glycemic stability in subjects with type 1 diabetes mellitus and unstable control, but insulin independence is usually not sustainable. Persistent islet function even without insulin independence provides both protection from severe hypoglycemia and improved levels of glycated hemoglobin.

▶ Since the first clinical use of insulin more than 80 years ago, injections of insulin have been the mainstay for the treatment of type 1 diabetes mellitus. The report of Shapiro et al changes all that. The report represents a multinational, prospective trial to disseminate the complicated knowledge and techniques required to prepare and transplant human islets and to evaluate the ability to provide a durable cure for a highly selected group of patients with type 1 diabetes. It is absolutely amazing to see how far this field has moved in just a very few short years. Before 2000, the preceding 2 decades' experience with islet cell transplantation achieved only a 1-year rate of allograft survival of less than 2%. It was in 2000 that the group in Canada published a groundbreaking study in which investigators demonstrated that islet cell transplantation could result in what appeared to be a durable diabetes cure, with 1-year graft survival rates of more than 80%.[1] This study launched a new era in islet transplantation with what is now called the "Edmonton protocol."

In the report abstracted, we see the results of a multinational study of islet cell transplantation, a study directed by the Edmonton group. Thirty-six patients were recruited into this study. The study showed how tough it is to achieve a perfect set of outcomes, but nonetheless, the results were very impressive. Multiple islet infusions were required to achieve a adequate transplant. Just 31% of patients received a successful single infusion, 25% received 2 infusions, and 44% received 3 infusions. This shows the difficulty of isolating and engrafting with adequate numbers of islet cells. Of the 36 patients who entered the study, 44% attained the stringent primary endpoint of insulin independence, defined as a HbA1c value of less than 6.5%, a glucose level after an overnight fast not to exceed 140 mg/dL more than 3 times per week, and a 2-hour postprandial glucose level not exceeding 180 mg/dL. In addition, a total of 28% of patients had partial graft function and another 28% experienced complete graft loss. If you shake out the data another way, some 58% of subjects achieved insulin independence at some time during the trial, but 76% had become insulin-dependent again by 2 years after transplantation.

The results of this study from Canada can be seen according to the metaphor of the glass half full or half empty. Without question, the Edmonton protocol results are clearly of magnitude better than previous attempts at islet cell transplantation. The problem that remains is that medium- to long-term cures are not durable. Much more work is needed. As of now, islet cell transplantation remains primarily a research initiative available to a small number of highly selected patients. It may not be long, however, before we have to decide whether the amazing technology should be more broadly disseminated. Outcomes should also be compared to other forms of therapy, such as whole-organ pancreas transplantation, which may significantly better than islet cell transplantation, with a 5-year graft survival rate in the range of 50% to 70%.

To learn more about islet cell transplantation, see the excellent review of this topic by Bromberg and LeRoith.[2] The review reminds us that islet cell transplantation is at a crossroads. It is clear that marginal long-term results, high cost, and the relatively high incidence of major and minor serious adverse effects make it difficult to argue for expansion of islet transplantation to the general population. At the same time, the dramatic discoveries and successful dissemination of information occurring in a relatively short period should encourage all to believe these advances will continue.

J. A. Stockman III, MD

References

1. Shapiro AM, Lakey JR, Ryan EA, et al. Islet transplantation in seven patients with type 1 diabetes mellitus using a glucocorticoid-free immunosuppressive regimen. *N Engl J Med.* 2000;343:230-238.
2. Bromberg JS, LeRoith D. Diabetes cure—is the glass half full? *N Engl J Med.* 2006;355:1372-1374.

The Natural History of Euthyroid Hashimoto's Thyroiditis in Children

Radetti G, for the Study Group for Thyroid Diseases of the Italian Society for Pediatric Endocrinology and Diabetes (SIEDP/ISPED) (Regional Hosp, Bolzano, Italy; et al)

J Pediatr 149:827-832, 2006

Objective.—To study the natural history of Hashimoto's thyroiditis (HT) in children and identify factors predictive of thyroid dysfunction.

Study Design.—We evaluated 160 children (43 males and 117 females, mean age 9.10 ± 3.6 years, with HT and normal (group 0; 105 patients) or slightly elevated (group 1; 55 patients) serum thyroid-stimulating hormone (TSH) concentrations. The patients were assessed at presentation and then followed for at least 5 years if they remained euthyroid or if their TSH did not rise twofold over the upper normal limit.

Results.—At baseline, age, sex, thyroid volume, free thyroxine, free triiodothyronine, thyroid peroxidase antibody (TPOab), and thyroglobulin antibody (TGab) serum concentrations were similar in the 2 groups. During follow-up, 68 patients of group 0 remained euthyroid, and 10 patients moved from group 0 to group 1. In 27 patients, TSH rose twofold above the upper normal limit (group 2), and 9 of these patients developed overt hypothyroidism. Sixteen patients of group 1 ended up in group 0, 16 remained in group 1, and 23 moved to group 2. A comparison of the data of the patients who maintained or improved their thyroid status with those of the patients whose thyroid function deteriorated revealed significantly increased TGab levels and thyroid volume at presentation in the latter group. However, none of these parameters alone or in combination were of any help in predicting the course of the disease in a single patient.

Conclusions.—The presence of goiter and elevated TGab at presentation, together with progressive increase in both TPOab and TSH, may be predictive factors for the future development of hypothyroidism. At 5 years of follow-up, more than 50% of the patients remained or became euthyroid.

▶ This report is significant because it is one of the very first that gives us a reasonably accurate probability of which children will develop hypothyroidism after an episode of HT. HT is turning out to be a fairly common entity in pediatrics. It will develop in 1% to 2% of children. Youngsters with Turner's syndrome, celiac disease, and type 1 diabetes mellitus are at particular risk for getting into trouble with Hashimoto's thyroiditis. To date, little has been known about the natural history of this autoimmune form of thyroiditis or about the prognostic factors for permanent thyroid impairment. It is known that about 50% of affected youngsters will come out of an episode of immune thyroiditis unscathed and will have persistent normal thyroid function. The other half will have some degree of thyroid insufficiency. Growth failure secondary to hypothyroidism may be the presenting sign of a prior episode of HT in many.

As far as the prognosis is concerned, having a goiter and increased levels of TGab at presentation together with an increase over time in TPOab and TSH levels seem to be the most significant predictors for the development of hypothyroidism.

J. A. Stockman III, MD

Combined ultrasound and isotope scanning is more informative in the diagnosis of congenital hypothyroidism than single scanning
Perry RJ, Maroo S, Maclennan AC, et al (Royal Hosp for Sick Children, Glasgow, Scotland)
Arch Dis Child 91:972-976, 2006

Background.—Thyroid imaging is helpful in confirming the diagnosis of congenital hypothyroidism and in establishing the aetiology. Although isotope scanning is the standard method of imaging, ultrasound assessment may be complementary.

Aim.—To determine the strengths and weaknesses of thyroid ultrasound and isotope scanning in neonates with thyroid stimulating hormone (TSH) elevation.

Methods.—Babies from the West of Scotland with raised capillary TSH (>15 mU/l) on neonatal screening between January 1999 and 2004 were recruited. Thyroid dimensions were measured using ultrasonography, and volumes were calculated. Isotope scanning was carried out with a pinhole collimator after an intravenous injection of 99m-technetium pertechnetate.

Results.—40 infants (29 female) underwent scanning at a median of 17 days (range 12 days to 15 months). The final diagnosis was athyreosis (n = 11), ectopia (n = 12), hypoplasia (n = 8; 3 cases of hemi-agenesis), dyshormonogenesis (n = 5), transient hypothyroidism (n = 2), transient hyperthyrotropinaemia (n = 1) and uncertain status with gland in situ (n = 1). 6 infants had discordant scans with no isotope uptake but visualisation of thyroid tissue on ultrasound. This was attributed to TSH suppression from thyroxine (n = 3); maternal blocking antibodies (n = 1); cystic degeneration of the thyroid (n = 1); and possible TSH receptor defect (n = 1).

Conclusions.—Isotope scanning was superior to ultrasound in the detection of ectopic tissue. However, ultrasound detected tissue that was not visualised on isotope scanning, and showed abnormalities of thyroid volume and morphology. We would therefore advocate dual scanning in newborns with TSH elevation as each modality provides different information.

▶ Since the initial description of the thyroid transcription factor Pax8 in 1992, advances have been made in the understanding of both normal thyroid development and the etiology of congenital hypothyroidism. These include the identification of further transcription factors, TTF-1 in 1995 and TTF-2 in 1997, and the description of people with inactivating TSH receptor defects. Infants with congenital hypothyroidism due to a thyroid gland in situ show a greater diagnostic yield in terms of specific etiology. Determining the thyroid site and size by imaging is therefore desirable. Currently, isotope scanning is the gold standard in imaging infants and children with congenital hypothyroidism, and the only reliable method of disclosing an ectopic gland, although it is less helpful in assessing thyroid size and morphology. The rub with isotope scanning is that it is not available in every setting and cannot be performed on sick preterm infants. Alternatively, US may be suitable in certain circumstances, but this technology has not been fully evaluated in infants with congenital hypothyroidism, thus the value of the study performed in Scotland, which compared isotope scanning with US.

So what wins in a head-to-head contest between isotope scanning and US in the detection of ectopic thyroid tissue? It is isotope scanning, which has a sensitivity of 91.7% in picking up ectopic thyroid tissue. Although isotope scanning does turn out to be superior in detecting ectopic thyroid tissue, US bested isotope scanning in some cases. This was in those patients who were receiving thyroid replacement treatment and who presumably had suppression of TSH, which diminished thyroid activity sufficiently to ablate isotope uptake. Also, US scanning can help to identify those neonates with TSH receptor blocking antibody, inactivating TSH receptor defect, or iodine-trapping defect. In other words, there will be circumstances in which ectopic thyroid tissue will not pick up isotope, but might be detectable with US.

The bottom line here is that US scanning can in some situations detect nonfunctioning thyroid tissue not visualized with isotope scanning. It can also show abnormalities in volume and morphology, which are not fully appreciated on 2-dimensional isotope scans. A blood sample for TSH measurement on the day of isotope scanning is recommended in order to accurately interpret the scan results. Also, be aware that if an infant has been exposed to iodine-containing skin cleaning products, iodine may be absorbed and suppress thyroid function as well. That is a pearl we should all remember.

J. A. Stockman III, MD

Adrenal responses to low dose synthetic ACTH (Synacthen) in children receiving high dose inhaled fluticasone

Paton J, Jardine E, McNeill E, et al (Univ of Glasgow, Scotland; Univ of Strathclyde, Glasgow, Scotland)
Arch Dis Child 91:808-813, 2006

Background and Aims.—Clinical adrenal insufficiency has been reported with doses of inhaled fluticasone propionate (FP) >400 μg/day, the maximum dose licensed for use in children with asthma. Following two cases of serious adrenal insufficiency (one fatal) attributed to FP, adrenal function was evaluated in children receiving FP outwith the licensed dose.

Methods.—Children recorded as prescribed FP ≥500 μg/day were invited to attend for assessment. Adrenal function was measured using the low dose Synacthen test (500 ng/1.73 m^2 intravenously) and was categorised as: biochemically normal (peak cortisol response >500 nmol/l); impaired (peak cortisol ≤500 nmol/l); or flat (peak cortisol ≤500 nmol/l with increment of <200 nmol/l and basal morning cortisol <200 nmol/l).

Results.—A total of 422 children had been receiving FP alone or in combination with salmeterol; 202 were not investigated (137 FP within license; 24 FP discontinued); 220 attended and 217 (age 2.6–19.3 years) were successfully tested. Of 194 receiving FP ≥500 μg/day, six had flat responses, 82 impaired responses, 104 were normal, and in 2 the LDST was unsuccessful. Apart from the index child, the other five with flat responses were asymptomatic; a further child with impairment (peak cortisol 296 nmol/l) had encephalopathic symptoms with borderline hypoglycaemia during an intercurrent illness. The six with flat responses and the symptomatic child were all receiving FP doses of ≥1000 μg/day.

Conclusion.—Overall, flat adrenal responses in association with FP occurred in 2.8% of children tested, all receiving ≥1000 μg/day, while impaired responses were seen in 39.6%. Children on above licence FP doses should have adrenal function monitoring as well as a written plan for emergency steroid replacement.

▶ The authors of this report studied the potential problem of adrenal insufficiency resulting from high-dose inhaled steroids as a result of a terrible experience back in 2001 when a 5-year-old girl presented to a Scottish hospital with a day's history of vomiting, impaired consciousness, and visual disturbance. She developed progressive unconsciousness and seizures and died within 9 hours. Postmortem examination showed cerebral edema and small adrenal glands. Four weeks later, her 7-year-old brother was admitted with almost identical symptoms. He had hyponatremia and cerebral edema, but responded to intensive care. After discharge, his initial plasma cortisol level was noted to be inappropriately low. Subsequent adrenal testing showed a severely impaired cortisol response to a low-dose ACTH test. Both siblings had been receiving FP for asthma for several years in doses up to 2000 μg/d. The symptoms that both these children exhibited were clearly due to adrenal insufficiency induced by high-dose inhaled steroids. When a large number of children were more thoroughly evaluated with adrenal testing, flat adrenal responses were seen in about 3% and impaired adrenal responses were seen in almost 40% of those receiving very high-dose inhaled steroids.

There are children with asthma who respond only to very high-dose inhaled steroids, but such children are few and far between. One of the most worrisome features of the reported cases of adrenal failure has been that clinicians sometimes appear to have persevered with increasing doses of what obviously had been unsuccessful treatment, rather than reviewing the situation to ensure that the diagnosis was correct, that unavoidable triggers for asthma had been identified and avoided, that compliance with treatment was satisfactory, and that the use of nonsteroidal medication was being maximized. In managing routine cases of asthma with conventional doses of inhaled steroids, the objective is to abolish or minimize the impact of the disease, knowing that systemic side effects will be minimal. When very high doses of inhaled steroids are contemplated, however, the impact of the disease must be balanced against the known risk posed by this treatment. Such treatment should clearly be reserved for children whose disease is unresponsive to conventional steroid use and severe enough to justify a potentially very dangerous treatment. These cases are indeed unusual and should be under the care of seasoned allergists or pulmonologists. These children should also be regularly tested for the development of adrenal insufficiency. It is not enough to rely on normal growth patterns to exclude the systemic effects of inhaled steroids. A notable feature of the children with adrenal failure has been that many of them are growing normally. There is no option but to perform regular endocrine assessments on children so managed. The best solution, however, would be to avoid using high-dose inhaled steroids in the first place.

For an excellent commentary on very high-dose inhaled steroids, see the excellent review of this topic by Russell.[1] Last, recognize that adrenal insufficiency is an infrequent, but serious cause of hyperkalemia. Recognize, also, the phenomenon known as pseudohyperkalemia. Pseudohyperkalemia can be a cause of major concern and confusion in practice. By definition, pseudohyperkalemia is an elevated laboratory result in which the patient does not have true elevations of serum potassium levels. Things as simple as a difficult venipuncture, severe fist clinching during blood sampling, or shaking of a sample can produce pseudohyperkalemia. Forcibly expressing blood through a needle into a collection tube can hemolyze blood, increasing the potassium concentration. Storage at excessively high temperatures can also cause blood to hemolyze. Cold temperature disables red blood cell membrane ATPase, also leading to higher potassium results, particularly in winter months if samples are left in environments that are chilly.[2]

J. A. Stockman III, MD

References

1. Russell G. Very high dose inhaled steroids: panacea or poison? *Arch Dis Child.* 2006;91:802-804.
2. Smellie WS. Spurious hyperkalemia. *BMJ.* 2007;334:693-695.

Isolated scrotal hair in infancy

Papadimitriou A, Beri D, Nicolaidou P (Penteli Children's Hosp, Athens, Greece; Univ of Athens School of Medicine, Greece)

J Pediatr 148:690-691, 2006

Background.—The development of genital hair in infancy is rare. It is usually manifest as scrotal hair with no other signs of virilization. The development of scrotal hair in an infant is often a source of concern to parents and pediatricians, but there are no data as to the significance of this development. The purpose of the present study was to describe the experience of one group with scrotal hair development in infants and to highlight the benign nature of this event.

Methods.—A retrospective study was conducted of 9 male infants referred to the endocrinology clinic of a Greek children's hospital for development of isolated scrotal hair. Endocrinologic investigation with serum DHEA-S, 17OH progesterone, androstenedione, and testosterone was conducted in 6 of the 9 infants. The infants were followed up at 3-month intervals for at least 6 months after presentation. All of the infants were of Greek origin and born at term after uncomplicated pregnancies with normal birth weight and length. The mothers received no medications, with the exception of vitamins and iron, during gestation, so the infants were not exposed to any hormonal medications.

Results.—The median age of development of scrotal hair was 4.5 months (range, 3-7 months). The median age at presentation was 7 months (range, 4-10 months). On clinical examination, all 9 infants had more than 10 long pigmented hairs on the scrotum, except for 1 infant who had only 5 dark hairs. None of the infants had any pubic hair or exhibited other signs of virilization. The body weight and length of each infant were within normal ranges. Endocrinologic investigations in 6 of the infants showed normal levels of serum testosterone, 17-hydroxyprogesterone, androstenedione, and dehydroepiandrosterone. In all of the patients the scrotal hair receded at a median age of 12 months (range 8-17 months), about 3 to 12 months after its development. Follow up for this report indicated that there were no cases of reappearance of scrotal hair in any of the patients (current age 2-8 years). The parents of 8 of the 9 patients indicated that they had excessive body hair, presumably of an idiopathic nature.

Conclusions.—The development of scrotal hair during infancy in the absence of any other signs of virilization is a benign, self-limited condition.

▶ Needless to say, parents get fairly excited when they see hair on the scrotum of their little infant boy. Indeed, genital hair in infancy is rare and usually it manifests itself as scrotal hair without any other sign of virilization. All too often, these babies are referred to a pediatric endocrinologist for a full and thorough evaluation when in fact, as we see in this report, such an evaluation during infancy is probably rarely needed. In such cases, scrotal hair recedes by an average age of 1 year, suggesting that the whole event was a transient and benign one. This is very different than boys who develop genital hair beyond infancy but well before the age of puberty. The latter circumstance suggests a possible underlying pathologic etiology, such as congential adrenal hypoplasia, adrenal or genital tumor, or true precocious puberty. It may also simply be due to premature adrenarche.

The authors of this report suggest that if scrotal hair is found in the first year of life, one should examine the infant male fairly closely to look for phallic enlargement, which would be consistent with a pathological cause for the problem. They also suggest that it may be worthwhile to measure androgen levels if there is any reason for concern. Otherwise, careful follow up is all that is necessary for what in most cases is a benign and transient condition.

We close this commentary with a gender-related topic posed in the form of a question. How are women doing these days as authors of manuscripts that are published in leading journals? In order to answer this query, one has to look back in time to see the change in authorship of manuscripts in prominent journals in the United States. Such a study was recently undertaken.[1] In carrying out the study, original articles from 6 prominent medical journals— *New England Journal of Medicine*, *Journal of the American Medical Association*, *Annals of Internal Medicine*, *Annals of Surgery*, *Obstetrics and Gynecology*, and *Journal of Pediatrics*—were categorized according to the sex of both the first and the senior (last listed) author. Sex was also determined of the authors of guest editorials in the *New England Journal of Medicine* and the *Journal of the American Medical Association*. Data were collected for the years 1970, 1980, 1990, 2000, and 2004. The study was restricted to authors from United States institutions holding MD degrees. The author's sex was able to be determined for 98.5% of the 7,249 United States authors of original research with MD degrees. Such a sex determination is an amazing feat in itself.

From the period 1970 through 2004, the proportion of first authors who were women increased from 5.9% to 29.3%, and the proportion of senior authors who were women increased from 3.7% to 19.3%. The greatest proportionate rise was seen in *Obstetrics and Gynecology* (from 6.7% of first authors and 6.8% of senior authors to 40.7% of first authors and 28.0% of senior authors) and *Journal of Pediatrics* (from 15% first authors and 4.3% of senior authors to 38.9% of first authors and 38% of senior authors). Unfortunately, the proportion of women as first and senior authors remained low in the *Annals of Surgery* (moving from 2.3% of first authors and 0.7% of senior authors in 1970 to 16.7% of first authors and just 6.7% of senior authors in 2004). In 2004, 11.4% of the authors of guest editorials in the *New England Journal of Medicine* and 18.8% of authors of guest editorials in the *Journal of the American Medical Association* were women.

So is the glass half-full or half-empty when it comes to the "gender gap" in authorship of academic medical literature? Perhaps in a few more years, we won't even have to ask this question.

J. A. Stockman III, MD

Reference

1. Jagsi R, Guancial EA, Worobey CC, et al. The "gender gap" in authorship of academic medical literature—a 35-year prospective. *N Engl J Med*. 2006;355: 281-287.

7 Gastroenterology

Acute Liver Failure in Children: The First 348 Patients in the Pediatric Acute Liver Failure Study Group

Squires RH, Shneider BL, Alonso E, et al (Univ of Pittsburgh, Pa; Mt Sinai Med Ctr; Cincinnati Children's Hosp, Ohio; et al)
J Pediatr 148:652-658, 2006

Objectives.—To determine short-term outcome for children with acute liver failure (ALF) as it relates to cause, clinical status, and patient demographics and to determine prognostic factors.

Study Design.—A prospective, multicenter case study collecting demographic, clinical, laboratory, and short-term outcome data on children from birth to 18 years with ALF. Patients without encephalopathy were included if the prothrombin time and international normalized ratio remained ≥20 seconds and/or 2, respectively, despite vitamin K. Primary outcome measures 3 weeks after study entry were death, death after transplantation, alive with native liver, and alive with transplanted organ.

Results.—The cause of ALF in 348 children included acute acetaminophen toxicity (14%), metabolic disease (10%), autoimmune liver disease (6%), non-acetaminophen drug-related hepatotoxicity (5%), infections (6%), and other diagnosed conditions (10%); 49% were indeterminate. Outcome varied between patient sub-groups; 20% with non-acetaminophen ALF died or underwent liver transplantation and never had clinical encephalopathy.

Conclusions.—Causes of ALF in children differ from in adults. Clinical encephalopathy may not be present in children. The high percentage of indeterminate cases provides an opportunity for investigation.

▶ In early 2006, the American Board of Pediatrics and the American Board of Internal Medicine sought agreement from the American Board of Medical Specialties (ABMS) to offer a certificate of added qualifications in transplantation hepatology. These petitions were approved by the ABMS, and the first examinations in pediatric transplant hepatology have already been administered. The examination process for certification in transplantation hepatology had to be designed in such a way to accommodate the differences in the manifestations of liver failure that occur between children and adults. The examination has a core component that is common to both pediatric and adult diseases and a separate module that is unique to pediatrics. Indeed, the data from the report of Squires et al shows how different children are from adults when it comes to ALF. Acute acetaminophen toxicity is the most identifiable cause of ALF in children 3 years of age and older, but the frequency of ALF in children from such exposure is actually only about half of that seen in adults.

Drug-related hepatotoxicity is relatively common in children, particularly those taking neuroleptic medications, yet acute liver failure from such medications is actually rare. In most instances, the mechanism of injury leading to ALF in such situations is believed to be an idiosyncratic reaction. Nonetheless, children with ALF related to valproic acid should be evaluated for an underlying mitochondrial disorder. In addition, genetic polymorphisms associated with drug detoxification or cytokine expressions may enhance a patient's susceptibility to liver injury.

A few final comments are necessary regarding acute liver failure in children. Hepatic encephalopathy is not an absolute requirement to establish the diagnosis of ALF in children, even though this is the situation in adult medicine. Second, a specific diagnosis for the cause of ALF is found in only about half of all infants and children. Interestingly, an infectious agent as a cause was identified in this report in just 6% of patients. Last, the causes of ALF in children in fact do differ from those seen in adults.

See the Watkins et al report (Aminotransferase elevations in healthy adults receiving 4 grams of acetaminophen daily: a randomized controlled trial) that tells us just how frequently acetaminophen causes elevations in liver enzymes.

J. A. Stockman III, MD

Aminotransferase Elevations in Healthy Adults Receiving 4 Grams of Acetaminophen Daily: A Randomized Controlled Trial

Watkins PB, Kaplowitz N, Slattery JT, et al (Univ of North Carolina, Chapel Hill; Univ of Southern California, Los Angeles; Univ of Washington, Seattle; et al)
JAMA 296:87-93, 2006

Context.—During a clinical trial of a novel hydrocodone/acetaminophen combination, a high incidence of serum alanine aminotransferase (ALT) elevations was observed.

Objective.—To characterize the incidence and magnitude of ALT elevations in healthy participants receiving 4 g of acetaminophen daily, either alone or in combination with selected opioids, as compared with participants treated with placebo.

Design, Setting, and Participants.—A randomized, single-blind, placebo-controlled, 5-treatment, parallel-group, inpatient, diet-controlled (meals provided), longitudinal study of 145 healthy adults in 2 US inpatient clinical pharmacology units.

Intervention.—Each participant received either placebo (n = 39), 1 of 3 acetaminophen/opioid combinations (n = 80), or acetaminophen alone (n = 26). Each active treatment included 4 g of acetaminophen daily, the maximum recommended daily dosage. The intended treatment duration was 14 days.

Main Outcomes.—Serum liver chemistries and trough acetaminophen concentrations measured daily through 8 days, and at 1- or 2-day intervals thereafter.

Results.—None of the 39 participants assigned to placebo had a maximum ALT of more than 3 times the upper limit of normal. In contrast, the incidence of maximum ALT of more than 3 times the upper limits of normal was 31% to 44% in the 4 treatment groups receiving acetaminophen, including those participants treated with acetaminophen alone. Compared with placebo, treatment with acetaminophen was associated with a markedly higher median maximum ALT (ratio of medians, 2.78; 95% confidence interval, 1.47-4.09; *P*<.001). Trough acetaminophen concentrations did not exceed therapeutic limits in any participant and, after active treatment was discontinued, often decreased to undetectable levels before ALT elevations resolved.

Conclusions.—Initiation of recurrent daily intake of 4 g of acetaminophen in healthy adults is associated with ALT elevations and concomitant treatment with opioids does not seem to increase this effect. History of acetaminophen ingestion should be considered in the differential diagnosis of serum aminotransferase elevations, even in the absence of measurable serum acetaminophen concentrations.

▶ The Squires et al report (Acute liver failure in children: the first 348 patients in the pediatric acute liver failure study group) gave us a great deal of information about the causes of acute liver failure in children. The administration of acetaminophen is a common cause of this problem when the latter drug is given in toxic dose range. This report, one done in healthy adults, shows us just how commonly acetaminophen in relatively modest amounts will raise liver aminotransferase levels.

The authors of this report observed an interesting finding a while back. During early clinical development of a novel combination product containing hydrocodone and acetaminophen, they observed a surprisingly high incidence of elevations in serum ALT in participants receiving the combination product at a total daily dose that contained just 4 g of acetaminophen, commonly considered to be the upper limit of recommended acetaminophen dosing in an adult. The study had to be stopped early because of the frequency and magnitude of ALT elevations in the active treatment group versus the placebo group. Because of these findings, the authors decided to undertake the study abstracted, which was designed to investigate hepatotoxicity among participants receiving acetaminophen alone, opioid/acetaminophen combinations, or placebo. In this study, no one receiving placebo showed an elevation of ALT of more than 3 times the upper limit of normal, whereas the incidence of such elevations of ALT was 31% to 44% in the treatment groups solely receiving acetaminophen. The addition of opioids to acetaminophen did not appear to produce higher levels of ALT than were caused by acetaminophen alone.

The association observed between therapeutic dosing of acetaminophen and elevations in ALT has not been reported previously in adults; there are no data comparable to this in children, although it would be reasonable to assume that children are little adults in this regard in terms of being at risk.

The key issue with this new information is whether or not the data can be translated to the situation involving children. What is worrisome, however, is that ALT elevations noted in adults occurred in the absence of plasma concentrations of acetaminophen that would traditionally be considered hepatotoxic. In fact, at the time of the highest ALT elevations observed, acetaminophen concentrations were frequently near or below the limits of assay detection. Therefore, plasma acetaminophen concentrations would be of limited value in determining whether ALT elevations were due to therapeutic doses of acetaminophen. This basically means that if you observe an elevation in ALT (fairly common in pediatric practice), you should ask for a history of acetaminophen exposure. Last, we don't have a clue, either in adults or in children, as to whether elevations of ALT caused by acetaminophen given in therapeutic dosing ranges is of any clinical significance or whether it is a harbinger of problems in a subset of children.

J. A. Stockman III, MD

The "Red Umbilicus": A Diagnostic Sign of Cow's Milk Protein Intolerance

Iacono G, Di Prima L, D'Amico D, et al ("Di Cristina" Hosp, Palermo, Italy; Univ Hosp of Palermo, Italy)
J Pediatr Gastroenterol Nutr 42:531-534, 2006

Introduction.—Red umbilicus is considered to be an infectious disease typical of neonates. In our experience, umbilical erythema could be due to cow's milk protein intolerance (CMPI).

Aims.—To evaluate the frequency and clinical significance of umbilical erythema in a series of consecutive children referred for suspected CMPI.

Patients and Methods.—Seven hundred ninety-six consecutive patients (median age, 18 months) referred for suspected CMPI diagnosis were studied. CMPI diagnosis was based on the disappearance of symptoms on elimination diet and their subsequent reappearance on double-blind placebo-controlled cow's milk challenge.

Results.—CMPI was diagnosed in 384 patients: 120 with respiratory, 75 dermatologic and 198 gastroenterological symptoms. Although some patients showed more than 1 type of symptom, whether gastroenterological, dermatologic or respiratory, they were classified in 1 category only according to the main reason for referral to the outpatients clinic. Umbilical erythema was observed in 36 patients (median age, 10 months): 16 (8%) with gastroenterological symptoms, 9 (7.5%) with recurrent asthma and 11 (15%) with atopic dermatitis. None of the symptomatic controls without CMPI had umbilical erythema. On elimination diet, the erythema disappeared within the second week. On CMPI challenge, it reappeared within 24 hours.

Conclusions.—Umbilical erythema can be a sign of food intolerance and can be a useful diagnostic tool for CMPI.

▶ What a pearl: a red bellybutton equals CMPI (at least in some infants). The data from this study do in fact seem to demonstrate that umbilical and periumbilical erythema can be a sign of food intolerance. The finding was observed in about 9% of children with cow milk protein intolerance. None of the affected children with red bellybuttons showed evidence of bacterial infection as the cause of the problem, which promptly disappeared after the institution of an elimination diet. It also reappeared with food challenge, thus fulfilling Koch's postulate.

The authors of this report did not even attempt to formulate a theory to explain why umbilical erythema may be a presenting sign of food intolerance. Do you have any suggestions?

While on the topic of inflammation, a recent report tells us just how useful a bidet is. Around half a century after bidets first appeared in bathrooms, colorectal surgeons have finally documented their benefit. Several anal conditions, most commonly pruritus ani are now reported to be benefitted by the use of bidet, which is much more successful than a daily shower for such a symptom. There is no substitute for plunging one's bottom into a bidet after evacuating a stool.[1]

Please note that studies of bidets show that only 13% of those in Great Britain and just 6% of those in Germany have a bidet at home, and most bidet owners admit to using them simply to wash their feet or their clothes. There are no data on household bidets here in the United States. There is one in this editor's home, and it alternates occupations as a medical journal receptacle or a repository for potted plants.

J. A. Stockman III, MD

Reference

1. Basso L. In reappraisal of the bidet, nearly half a century later. *Dis Colon Rectum.* 2006;49:1080-1081.

Wireless Video Capsule in Pediatric Patients With Functional Abdominal Pain

Shamir R, Hino B, Hartman C, et al (Meyer Children's Hosp of Haifa, Israel; Rambam Med Ctr, Haifa, Israel)
J Pediatr Gastroenterol Nutr 44:45-50, 2007

Objectives.—Upper endoscopy (esophagogastroduodenoscopy [EGD]) has a limited role, if any, in the evaluation of functional abdominal pain (FAP). Nevertheless, children with intractable FAP are occasionally referred to EGD to rule out intestinal pathology. We evaluated the role of wireless video capsule endoscopy (VCE) in children referred for EGD with a diagnosis of FAP.

Patients and Methods.—Ten children older than 10 years of age were prospectively enrolled. Children were first studied with the PillCam SB (VCE; Given Imaging, Yokneam, Israel) followed by standard EGD within 2 weeks. After the completion of the study, a questionnaire of tolerance and content regarding the 2 procedures was completed by the patients.

Results.—Physical examinations and laboratory tests were within normal limits in all of the patients. Patients swallowed the endoscopic capsules without difficulty. There were no complications. VCE identified gastritis in 4 patients (confirmed by biopsies), whereas EGD detected erosive gastritis in only 1 of the 4 children. EGD detected no duodenal abnormalities. VCE detected Crohn disease in the small intestine and cecum in 1 patient. VCE was ranked by 8 patients as convenient and as a preferable procedure compared with EGD.

Conclusion.—The results of this small cohort suggest that in children with FAP, VCE is more sensitive than EGD for detection of macroscopic gastric and small bowel pathologies.

▶ In August 2001, the Food and Drug Administration (FDA) approved wireless capsule endoscopy as an adjunctive tool for the evaluation of small-intestinal diseases. By July 2003, the FDA had approved it as a first-line modality for the evaluation of all suspected small-bowel disorders. In January 2004, the FDA approved its use for pediatric patients between 10 and 18 years of age. Studies in adults have clearly shown the diagnostic capabilities of capsule endoscopy. Among 100 adults who had undergone some 620 negative diagnostic tests including endogastroduodenoscopy, colonoscopy, small-bowel follow-through radiographs, enteroclysis, enteroscopy, red blood cell scans, Meckel scans, CT scans, and laparoscopy, capsule endoscopy provided a diagnosis in almost half of the cases. The best candidates for capsule endoscopy appear to be patients with active gastrointestinal bleeding.[1]

The first preliminary results of capsule endoscopy in children were reported in 2003 by Mallet et al.[2] A year later, Seidman et al[3] described potential applications of wireless capsule endoscopy among pediatric patients with obscure gastrointestinal bleeding. In a study of 30 patients, 10 to 18 years of age, arteriovenous malformations were found in 75% of capsule studies.[3] In 1 patient, the capsule was retained for 10 days at the site of a small-bowel stenosis but was passed spontaneously after a 4-day course of steroid therapy. Wireless capsule endoscopy was also successful in diagnosing gastrointestinal bleeding related to a jejunal, juvenile, mixed capillary hemangioma–angiomatosis.[4]

In this current report of wireless VCE in pediatric patients with FAP, we see that this form of endoscopy was able to identify an etiology in a small but real subset of patients. The term *recurrent abdominal pain* was coined by the British pediatrician John Apley back in 1958, and we now recognize that it is a real entity. The problem is trying to determine whether a cause for FAP exists. Most youngsters with FAP do not require endoscopy of any sort, but when they do, VCE may just be the way to go in selected cases.

If you are not familiar with capsule endoscopy, it involves the swallowing of a small wireless camera. For young children who are unable to swallow the capsule, a variety of endoscopic techniques have been described for placement of the capsule in the stomach or the duodenum. These include the use of a foreign body "Roth net." Foreign-body grasping forceps or snares may also be useful with "front-loading" of the capsule on the end of a gastroscope. An innovative capsule-delivery device has been patented by US Endoscopy. FDA approval appears to be imminent for the latter, which is specifically designed to deliver and release the capsule into the duodenum for patients with dysphagia, gastroparesis, or anatomical problems. It could also turn out to be very useful in the pediatric age group.

Very little is left in the way of privacy these days, except in hospitals. Now, even there, the inside of our guts are no longer private either. See the Little et al article (Multiple somatic symptoms linked to positive screen for depression in pediatric patients with chronic abdominal pain) that tells us about the relationship between FAP and depression in the pediatric population.

J. A. Stockman III, MD

References

1. Pennazio M, Santucci R, Rondonotti E, et al. Outcome of patients with obscure gastrointestinal bleeding after capsule endoscopy: report of 100 consecutive cases. *Gastroenterology*. 2004;126:643-653.
2. Mallet E, Cron J, Stoller J. Wireless capsule video-endoscopy: preliminary results in children. *Arch Pediatr*. 2003;10:244-245.
3. Seidman EG, Sant'Anna AM, Dirks MH. Potential applications of wireless capsule endoscopy in the pediatric age group. *Gastrointest Endosc Clin N Am*. 2004;14:207-217.
4. Kavin H, Berman J, Martin TL, Feldman A, Forsey-Koukol K. Successful wireless capsule endoscopy for a 2.5-year-old child: obscure gastrointestinal bleeding from mixed, juvenile, capillary hemangioma–angiomatosis of the jejunum. *Pediatrics*. 2006;117:539-543.

Multiple Somatic Symptoms Linked to Positive Screen for Depression in Pediatric Patients With Chronic Abdominal Pain

Little CA, Williams SE, Puzanovova M, et al (Vanderbilt Univ, Nashville, Tenn)
J Pediatr Gastroenterol Nutr 44:58-62, 2007

Objectives.—Abdominal pain is a frequent childhood complaint, comprising 2% to 4% of all reasons for pediatric office visits. Patients referred for evaluation of chronic abdominal pain (CAP) frequently present with comorbid nonspecific somatic symptoms that may complicate the medical evaluation and lead to unnecessary diagnostic tests and procedures. We tested the hypothesis that multiple nongastrointestinal (GI) symptoms in children presenting with CAP is a marker for clinically significant levels of depressive symptoms.

Methods.—Participants were 400 consecutive new patients (ages 8–17 years; 63% female) referred to the pediatric gastroenterology clinic for evaluation of abdominal pain of >3 months' duration. Patients reported how frequently they experienced 7 non-GI symptoms. Patients were screened for depression with the Children's Depression Inventory.

Results.—On the basis of their Children's Depression Inventory scores, 58 (15%) patients had a positive screen for clinically significant depressive symptoms. Patients with a positive versus negative depression screen did not differ by sex, pain duration or laboratory evidence of organic disease. Patient report of ≥3 non-GI symptoms maximized sensitivity (71%) and specificity (75%) in prediction of depression screening results. With each addition of a non-GI symptom, the odds of a positive screen for depression doubled.

Conclusions.—For patients with and without organic disease findings associated with CAP, the presence of ≥3 non-GI symptoms should signal the practitioner to evaluate for depression and may be used as an indicator of the likelihood of depression in the absence of specific inquiry into emotional symptoms.

► Studies have shown that functional abdominal pain comprises the majority of referrals to pediatric gastroenterologists, at least in parts of the country where chronic constipation is still managed by the generalist. The diagnosis of CAP, as defined by the American Academy of Pediatrics, is persistent or intermittent abdominal pain of at least 2 months' duration for which no apparent etiology exists. Many affected with CAP also complain of somatic symptoms that do not involve the GI tract. These symptoms include headaches and fatigue. We see in this article that at least 15% of those with CAP (some call it functional abdominal pain) will also demonstrate evidence of depressive symptoms if the latter are carefully looked for. These symptoms are more often found in patients who, in addition to their abdominal pain, have 3 or more non-GI symptoms.

Unfortunately, this study does not address the potential causal influences in the relationship between abdominal pain, non-GI symptoms, and symptoms of depression. It is entirely possible that depression contributes to the abdominal pain and non-GI symptoms, but at the same time it is also possible that abdominal pain and non-GI symptoms contribute to depression. Either way, affected patients are depressed and need to be managed for their depression. Previous research has shown that psychiatric symptoms and disorders are common in children with chronic or recurrent abdominal pain. The problem is probably more common than suspected because limited time and resources often prohibit primary care providers or consultant gastroenterologists from using mental health assessment tools to conduct psychological assessments in patients with CAP. What is needed is a simple screening test for depression, as is suggested in this study.

J. A. Stockman III, MD

Do Opiates Affect the Clinical Evaluation of Patients With Acute Abdominal Pain?

Ranji SR, Goldman LE, Simel DL, et al (Univ of California, San Francisco; Duke Univ, Durham, NC; Univ of Ottawa, Ont, Canada)
JAMA 296:1764-1774, 2006

Context.—Clinicians have traditionally withheld opiate analgesia from patients with acute abdominal pain until after evaluation by a surgeon, out of concern that analgesia may alter the physical findings and interfere with diagnosis.

Objective.—To determine the impact of opiate analgesics on the rational clinical examination and operative decision for patients with acute abdominal pain.

Data Sources and Study Selection.—MEDLINE (through May 2006), EMBASE, and hand searches of article bibliographies to identify placebo-controlled randomized trials of opiate analgesia reporting changes in the history, physical examination findings, or diagnostic errors (those resulting in "management errors," defined as the performance of unnecessary surgery or failure to perform necessary surgery in a timely fashion).

Data Extraction.—Two authors independently reviewed each study, abstracted data, and classified study quality. A third reviewer independently resolved discrepancies.

Data Synthesis.—Studies both in adults (9 trials) and in children (3 trials) showed trends toward increased risks of altered findings on the abdominal examination due to opiate administration, with risk ratios for changes in the examination of 1.51 (95% confidence interval [CI], 0.85 to 2.69) and 2.11 (95% CI, 0.60 to 7.35), respectively. When the analysis was restricted to the 8 adult and pediatric trials that reported significantly greater analgesia for patients who received opiates compared with those who received placebo, the risk of physical examination changes became significant (risk ratio, 2.13; 95% CI, 1.14 to 3.98). These trials exhibited significant heterogeneity ($I^2 =$ 68.6%; $P = .002$), and only 2 trials distinguished clinically significant changes such as loss of peritoneal signs from all other changes; consequently, we analyzed risk of management errors as a marker for important changes in the physical examination. Opiate administration had no significant association with management errors (+0.3% absolute increase; 95% CI, −4.1% to +4.7%). The 3 pediatric trials showed a nonsignificant absolute decrease in management errors (−0.8%; 95% CI, −8.6% to +6.9%). Across adult and pediatric trials with adequate analgesia, opiate administration was associated with a nonsignificant absolute decrease in the risk of management errors (−0.2%; 95% CI, −4.0% to +3.6%).

Conclusions.—Opiate administration may alter the physical examination findings, but these changes result in no significant increase in management errors. The existing literature does not rule out a small increase in errors, but this error rate reflects a conservative definition in which surgeries labeled as either delayed or unnecessary may have met appropriate standards of care. In published research reports, no patient experienced major morbidity or mortality attributable to opiate administration.

▶ So much has been said about abdominal pain that this editor has little to add except for the fact that some people believe adding fiber to the diet can be of help, not only for constipation, but also for nonspecific abdominal pain. Realize also, that new data suggest that coffee may in fact be a source of fiber. It would seem that a cup of coffee does in fact deliver a significant proportion of one's daily dietary fiber if one partakes of the java. Previously, coffee was not thought to contain any fiber. However, like the cholesterol-lowering substances found in oat bran, fiber in coffee consists of carbohydrates that the body cannot digest, but which dissolve in digestive fluids. Coffee's fiber molecules are small enough to easily pass through most coffee filters. Per unit volume, coffee made using freeze-dried crystals contains 60% more fiber than conventionally filtered coffee. It is suspected that more fiber is extracted from coffee beans by the 200°C process used to make freeze-dried coffee crystals than by the cooler steps used in making typical ground coffee.

The recommended amount of dietary fiber in the United States is about 28 grams per day. Most do not ingest anywhere nearly that amount. The new data suggest that two cups of instant coffee per day might contribute as much as 3.6 grams of fiber, or almost 15% of one's daily requirement.[1]

J. A. Stockman III, MD

Reference

1. Raloff J. Want that fiber regular or decaf? [editorial]. *Sci News.* 2007;171:125.

Treatment of Oesophageal Bile Reflux in Children: The Results of a Prospective Study with Omeprazole

Orel R, Brecelj J, Homan M, et al (Univ Med Centre, Ljubljana, Slovenia; Royal Free Hosp, London)
J Pediatr Gastroenterol Nutr 42:376-383, 2006

Objectives.—Reflux of duodenal juice into the oesophagus has a role in the pathogenesis of both oesophageal and laryngopharyngeal inflammatory and neoplastic lesions. As little is known about effective therapy, we studied the effect of proton pump inhibitor therapy on oesophageal bile reflux in children.

Methods.—Twenty-nine children with moderate to severe erosive oesophagitis and abnormal oesophageal bile reflux were studied before and after treatment with omeprazole 1 mg/kg per day. Outcomes included a clinical symptom score, oesophageal acid and bile reflux (simultaneous 24-hour pH and Bilitec 2000 monitoring), and mucosal healing.

Results.—After 8 weeks of therapy, 17 (59%) of the patients were symptom-free, and 5 (17%) had minimal symptoms. Mucosal healing or reduction to low-grade oesophagitis was achieved in 25 children (86%; $P < 0.0005$). Mean percentages of total, upright, and supine time with oesophageal pH less than 4 were reduced from 17.0%, 16.8%, and 19.2% before treatment, to 2.83%, 3.17%, and 2.07%, respectively, after treatment (all $P < 0.00001$). Similarly, mean percentages of total, upright, and supine time with bile reflux were reduced from 16.96%, 12.67%, and 22.0%, to 2.27%, 1.91%, and 2.23%, respectively ($P < 0.000001$, $P < 0.0001$, and $P < 0.000001$, respectively).

Conclusions.—Omeprazole 1 mg/kg per day is an effective therapy for the majority of children with severe erosive oesophagitis due to abnormal isolated bile reflux or combined acid and bile reflux. It remains unclear how patients with treatment-resistant bile reflux should be managed.

▶ Gastroesophageal reflux disease (GERD) has standard treatments these days that actually do not address the pathophysiologic mechanism underlying the problem. GERD is primarily a motility disorder. Escape of gastric contents into the esophagus occurs as a consequence of a relaxation of the gastroesophageal barrier. This barrier is diminished in the presence of an abnormally functioning lower esophageal sphincter and when there are associated anatomical abnormalities, such as a hiatal hernia. Transient relaxation of the sphincter represents the primary motility dysfunction and leads to acid and nonacid reflux. Although the sphincter is supposed to relax only to allow passage of ingested material and the retrograde escape of swallowed air, transient relaxations can progress to prolonged relaxations without associated swallowing. Once the sphincter has opened, gastric contents will generally follow the rules of physics moving from an area of higher pressure to one of lower pressure, shifting fluid from the stomach to the esophagus. Motility dysfunction associated with GERD includes impaired esophageal peristalsis, delayed gastric emptying, and defective postprandial gastric relaxation.

Despite the fact that GERD is a motility disorder, the standard of care for treatment is to use drugs that have no prokinetic properties, aiming instead at decreasing gastric acid secretion. The reason we use such drugs is pretty clear. They remove symptoms promptly. As importantly, there is little in the way of effective and safe medication that actually improves gastrointestinal motility. The only prokinetic drug that had shown efficacy in the treatment of GERD was cisapride. Given its risk of potentially fatal side effects in cardiac arrhythmias, for all intents and purposes, cisapride remains unavailable for general use. Domperidone had shown some minimal efficacy in the treatment of pediatric GERD but is not available here in the United States. Despite its widespread use in infants and children with GERD, there is no convincing evidence that metoclopramide is effective in treating childhood GERD. Similarly, erythromycin and bethanechol, even though they are prokinetic agents, provide no demonstrative therapeutic benefit in GERD. None of these agents has an effect on transient sphincter relaxation, apparently the reason why they do not work.

It is the failure of our ability to find a good motility agent that we continue on with the use of proton pump inhibitors, such as omeprazole. Unfortunately with these drugs, which change the pH characteristics of the refluxate, regurgitation is minimally affected.

The Tolia et al report (Multicenter, randomized, double-blind study comparing 10, 20 and 40 mg pantoprazole in children (5–11 Years) with symptomatic gastroesophageal reflux disease) tells just how effective omeprazole is for the management of severe erosive esophagitis. This is also true of pantoprazole, which likewise inhibits the final step of gastric acid production. Currently, omeprazole and pantoprazole and other proton pump inhibitors are considered the best therapeutic options for the treatment of acid-related disorders including erosive esophagitis.

To read more about the esophagus as a dysfunctional motility organ, see the excellent commentary on this topic by DiLorenzo.[1] You will learn about a promising new motility agent, baclofen. Baclofen is a gamma-aminobutyric acid receptor agonist, clinically used for the management of spasticity. It inhibits the effects of vagal stimulation on the esophagus. In healthy adults, it has been shown to reduce both acid and nonacid reflux. We now have evidence that it does the same thing in children.[2] Although not a magic bullet, baclofen does seem to target the actual pathophysiologic mechanism underlying GERD although it has some significant side effects that include drowsiness, dizziness, fatigue, and the ability to lower the threshold for seizures. Such side effects will likely preclude its widespread use except in selected circumstances.

J. A. Stockman III, MD

References

1. Di Lorenzo C. Gastroesophageal reflux: not a time to "relax." *J Pediatr.* 2006;149:436-438.
2. Omari TI, Benninga MA, Sansom L, Butler RN, Dent J, Davidson GP. Effect of baclofen on esophagogastric motility and gastroesophageal reflux in children with gastroesophageal reflux disease: a randomized controlled trial. *J Pediatr.* 2006;149:468-474.

Multicenter, Randomized, Double-Blind Study Comparing 10, 20 and 40 mg Pantoprazole in Children (5–11 Years) With Symptomatic Gastro-esophageal Reflux Disease
Tolia V, and Members of the 322 Study Group (Children's Hosp of Michigan, Detroit; Univ of Mississippi, Jackson; Children's Hosp of the King's Daughter, Norfolk, Va; et al)
J Pediatr Gastroenterol Nutr 42:384-391, 2006

Objective.—To evaluate symptom improvement in 53 children (aged 5–11 years) with endoscopically proven gastroesophageal reflux disease (GERD) treated with pantoprazole (10, 20 and 40 mg) using the GERD Assessment of Symptoms in Pediatrics Questionnaire.

Methods.—The GERD Assessment of Symptoms in Pediatrics Questionnaire was used to measure the frequency and severity over the previous 7 days of abdominal/belly pain, chest pain/heartburn, difficulty swallowing, nausea, vomiting/regurgitation, burping/belching, choking when eating and pain after eating. Individual symptom scores were based on the product of the frequency and usual severity of each symptom. The sum of the individual symptom score values made up the composite symptom score (CSS). The primary end point was the change in the mean CSS from baseline to week 8.

Results.—Mean frequency and severity of each symptom significantly decreased (from $P < 0.006$ to $P < 0.001$) over time. Similar significant decreases in CSS at week 8 versus baseline ($P < 0.001$) were seen in all groups. Significant decreases from baseline in CSS were noted from weeks 1 to 8 in the 20-mg ($P < 0.003$) and 40-mg ($P < 0.001$) groups. The 20- and 40-mg doses were significantly ($P < 0.05$) more effective than the 10-mg dose in improving GERD symptoms at week 1. Adverse events were similar among the treatment groups.

Conclusions.—Pantoprazole (20 and 40 mg) is effective in reducing endoscopically proven GERD symptoms in children. Both 20 and 40 mg pantoprazole significantly reduced symptoms as early as 1 week.

Natural History and Symptomatology of *Helicobacter pylori* in Childhood and Factors Determining the Epidemiology of Infection

Özen A, Ertem D, Pehlivanoglu E (Marmara Univ, Istanbul, Turkey)
J Pediatr Gastroenterol Nutr 42:398-404, 2006

Background.—High seroprevalence rates for *Helicobacter pylori* have been reported in developing countries, yet few studies exist determining the pattern of change in the epidemiology of *H. pylori* infection in children. The knowledge of acquisition and loss rates of *H. pylori* and the relevance to the sociodemographic properties and the symptomatology of infection may provide clues for lifestyle changes that might protect children from infection, and also, it may provide rationale for eradication, screening, and protection policies. Our aim was to conduct a prospective study to elucidate the outcome, rate of acquisition, and loss of *H. pylori* infection in a population of healthy children.

Methods.—This study is based on follow-up of 327 healthy Turkish children aged 3 to 12 years. The follow-up was conducted 6 years after the baseline examination. *Helicobacter pylori* status was determined by ^{13}C-urea breath test. Children were investigated for sociodemographic variables and several symptoms.

Results.—Data from 136 (41%) of 327 children were available. The prevalence of infection increased from 52.9% to 56.6%, mainly increasing in children younger than 10 years. The incidence of *H. pylori* infection among previously uninfected children was 14%, and the loss rate of infection among previously infected children was 5.5% during the follow-up. Socioeconomic status, household density, and antibiotic use during last 6 months were inversely related to *H. pylori* prevalence. Children infected with *H. pylori* were complaining more often of headache but not of abdominal pain or dyspepsia.

Conclusions.—In this study, the acquisition rate of *H. pylori* infection was 2.5-fold higher than the loss of infection, and the acquisition mostly occurred before 10 years of age. Data regarding acquisition and loss of *H. pylori* infection are critical for understanding the epidemiology of infection and development of preventive and treatment strategies.

▶ This study on the natural history and symptomatology of *H pylori* in childhood was carried out in Turkey. Nonetheless, there is much to be learned from this report about the problem here in the United States. The data substantiate that the prevalence of *H pylori* infection increases steeply at 4 to 6 years of age. This coincides with the period that many youngsters begin to spend more time in crowded environments such as kindergartens. The data also show that residential crowding seems to be the most important risk factor for *H pylori* infection.

This report also reminds us that *H pylori* can present with manifestations outside the gastrointestinal tract. Iron deficiency anemia, growth retardation, and even migraine headaches have been linked to the presence of *H pylori* infection. Tunca et al[1] reported that *H pylori* was more prevalent among migrainous patients compared with controls, and that patients who were given eradication treatments for *H pylori* seemed to benefit from this treatment.

Most of us do not tend to think about the fact that *H pylori* infection is the most common bacterial infection worldwide, nor do most know how chance favored the prepared mind in the discovery of *H pylori*. Australian pathologist, Robin Warren, lived almost alone with the knowledge of *H pylori* for over 2 years. Until the young Barry Marshall arrived in his office in 1981, the only doctor to take Warren's findings seriously was his wife, Win. The discovery had been made by chance one afternoon in 1979 while Warren was at work on a routine gastric biopsy sample in a pathology laboratory at the Royal Perth Hospital in Australia. On the surface of a sample showing the gross "cobblestone" changes of severe, active chronic gastritis, Warren noticed a bluish line he thought looked "a bit funny." Higher magnification showed that this was composed of numerous small curved bacilli, in a line just below the stomach's protective mucus. Warren remembers the exact date, June 11, 1979, because it was his birthday. Over the next 2 years, working alone and in the disbelief of his colleagues, Warren tried various staining techniques to see whether he could better identify the organisms that he found in the stomachs of patients who were having gastrectomies for ulcers. Photography had been a passion of his since childhood, so it was perhaps not surprising that, finding the usual alternatives for staining unsatisfactory, he should try the Victorian photographer's favorite, silver salts. He found that the tricky Warthin-Starry silver stain picked up the bacterium nicely, differentiating it clearly from surrounding tissue. Going back over the lab's 10-year archive of gastric samples, Warren found the organism present in well over 30% of tissue samples. Given that the bacterium is fragile and decomposes quickly, it is surprising that he found the organisms in as many samples as he did. Still, his colleagues did not believe him.

Dr Barry Marshall entered the picture in 1981. He was a young registrar on a gastroenterology rotation at that time at Royal Perth Hospital. His division chief suggested he become engaged in 1 of 2 research projects: analyze patient records using punched cards to code for sorting by a room-sized computer, or help Dr Robert Warren with his crazy research. Because computers were of no interest to Marshall, he went to see Dr Warren. Indeed, Marshall was the first person to express any interest in what Dr Warren was doing. The two hit it off. Marshall dug into all the patient records of the specimens that Warren had been investigating. He found a pattern of gastritis, ulcers, and cancer. Marshall and Warren wrote 2 research letters to *The Lancet* in 1983 detailing the Warren discovery and their combined work to date. Unfortunately, when the full manuscript was submitted to *The Lancet* within the year, no peer reviewer would recommend it for publication.

Exasperated by their experience in trying to publish their data, Marshall embarked on a self-experiment. He underwent a gastroscopy to document that he did not carry the infection. He then swallowed a beaker full of a fresh culture of the organism that by then he and Warren had been able to grow in the laboratory. His description of his own illness after drinking the brew is somewhat hilarious: from grumbly tummy to uncontrollable vomiting in 8 days. He rapidly became haggard and "cranky," and his breath smelled like a "sewer." Sleep was impossible. When eventually he confessed to his long-suffering wife, Adrienne, what he had done, she insisted he undergo eradication therapy immediately or sleep under a bridge. So after another gastroscopy (confirming active gastritis and the presence of the organism), Marshall took antibiotics, and the symptoms were resolved. This extraordinary episode was the basis of his "Koch's postulates" article, which appeared in the *Medical Journal of Australia* in 1985. In the meantime, *The Lancet* in fact did publish the team's article reporting the culturing of the organism.

Warren and Marshall were jointly awarded the 2005 Nobel Prize for their work. Robin Warren has retired, and Barry Marshall continues to investigate *H pylori* including the possibility of immunization against this bacterium. The manner in which Warren's original discovery was made fully justifies Pasteur's view that chance favors the prepared mind. Warren himself is insistent that his discovery was neither luck, nor brilliant research: it was serendipity, he says. "I found it and described it, under the mucous. I found what I found and I told them what I saw. I was just doing my job."[2]

J. A. Stockman III, MD

References

1. Tunca A, Türkay C, Tekin O, Kargili A, Erbayrak M. Is *Helicobacter pylori* infection a risk factor for migraine? A case-control study. *Acta Neurol Belg.* 2004;104:161-164.
2. Richardson R. Interview. *Lancet.* 2006;368:S46-S47.

Variability of the 13C-Acetate Breath Test for Gastric Emptying of Liquids in Healthy Children

Hauser B, De Schepper J, Caveliers V, et al (Vrije Universiteit Brussels, Belgium; Universita dell'Insubria, Varese, Italy)
J Pediatr Gastroenterol Nutr 42:392-397, 2006

Purpose.—Scintigraphy is considered as the "gold standard" for measuring gastric emptying (GE). The 13C-acetate breath test (13C-ABT) offers an attractive alternative to measure GE of liquids as it is nonradioactive. The aim of this study was to assess the variability of the 13C-ABT for GE of liquids in healthy children using nondispersive infrared spectrometry (NDIRS).

Methods.—The 13C-ABT was repeated at least 2 times in 21 healthy children (6 girls and 15 boys), aged between 6.2 and 16.4 years, 2 to 7 days apart. After an overnight fast, a standardized milk drink, labeled with 50 or 100 mg ^{13}C-acetate according to weight, was administered. Breath samples were taken before feeding, at 5-minute intervals for the first 40 minutes and at 10-minute intervals for the following 140 minutes after feeding. Breath samples were analyzed using NDIRS, and ^{13}C recovery was used to calculate values for gastric half-emptying time ($t_{1/2}$), time of peak ^{13}C exhalation, or gastric lag phase (t_{lag}) and gastric emptying coefficient (GEC). Intraindividual variabilities of the parameters $t_{1/2}$, t_{lag}, and GEC were expressed as coefficient of intrasubject variation (CV).

Results.—The median CV of $t_{1/2}$ was 8.3% (CV range, 1.6%–16.2%; $t_{1/2}$ interindividual range, 65–112 minutes; and $t_{1/2}$ intraindividual range, 4–33 minutes). The median CV of t_{lag} was 16.6% (CV range, 2.0%–26.6%; t_{lag} interindividual range, 31–76 minutes; and t_{lag} intraindividual range, 1–35 minutes). The median CV of GEC was 4.3% (CV range, 0.8%–15.7%; GEC interindividual range, 3.81–4.89; GEC intraindividual range, 0.08–1.31). The CVs of $t_{1/2}$, t_{lag}, and GEC were independent of age, sex, weight, height, and measured values of $t_{1/2}$, t_{lag}, and GEC.

Conclusions.—The ^{13}C-ABT using NDIRS is an easy, noninvasive, and nonradioactive procedure with a large intraindividual variation for measuring GE of liquids in healthy children, but comparable to the variation reported with other techniques.

▶ Most pediatricians do not think about testing for GE. A delay in GE can be the cause of significant symptoms and is found in a variety of pediatric disorders including chronic renal failure, cystic fibrosis, diabetes mellitus type 1, gastroesophageal reflux, and nonulcer dyspepsia. Many techniques are available to evaluate GE: antroduodenal manometry, applied potential tomography, electrogastrography, epigastric impedance, MRI, marker dilution technique, radiologic contrast studies, radioscintigraphy, US, and last, ^{13}C-ABT. The "gold standard" for measuring gastroesophageal emptying has been technetium-99 colloid-based scintigraphy, but this technique is associated with radiation exposure to both patients and hospital personnel. It is therefore largely unsuitable for use in children. On the other hand, a breath test using acetate and octanoic acid as a substrate, labeled with the stable isotope carbon-13, a naturally occurring nonradioactive isotope, is an alternative nonradioactive technique. These breath tests are based on the principle that carbon-labeled carbon dioxide is expired in the air after metabolization of the marker and that the rate of appearance of carbon-labeled carbon dioxide reflects GE.

This article from Italy confirms that the ^{13}C-ABT does represent an easy, noninvasive, and nonradioactive method for detecting abnormalities of GE in otherwise well children. It is as good as "gold" in this regard. It is relatively easy to perform compared with other studies and involves no radiation. Go for it.

J. A. Stockman III, MD

The changing clinical presentation of coeliac disease

Ravikumara M, Tuthill DP, Jenkins HR (Univ Hosp of Wales, Cardiff)
Arch Dis Child 91:969-971, 2006

Background.—There has been a growing recognition that coeliac disease is much more common than previously recognised, and this has coincided with the increasingly widespread use of serological testing.

Aim.—To determine whether the age at presentation and the clinical presentation of coeliac disease have changed with the advent of serological testing.

Methods.—A 21-year review of prospectively recorded data on the mode of presentation of biopsy confirmed coeliac disease in a single regional centre. Presenting features over the past 5 years were compared with those of the previous 16 years. Between 1983 and 1989 (inclusive), no serological testing was undertaken; between 1990 and 1998, antigliadin antibody was used with occasional use of antiendomysial antibody and antireticulin antibody. From 1999 onwards, anti-tissue transglutaminase was used.

Results.—86 patients were diagnosed over the 21-year period: 50 children between 1999 and 2004 compared with 25 children between 1990 and 1998 and 11 children between 1983 and 1989. The median age at presentation has risen over the years. Gastrointestinal manifestations as presenting features have decreased dramatically. In the past 5 years, almost one in four children with coeliac disease was diagnosed by targeted screening.

Conclusion.—This study reports considerable changes in the presentation of coeliac disease—namely, a decreased proportion presenting with gastrointestinal manifestations and a rise in the number of patients without symptoms picked up by targeted screening. Almost one in four children with coeliac disease is now diagnosed by targeted screening. Most children with coeliac disease remain undiagnosed. Paediatricians and primary care physicians should keep the possibility of coeliac disease in mind and have a low threshold for testing, so that the potential long-term problems associated with untreated coeliac disease can be prevented.

▶ Celiac disease was once thought to be rare, with an estimated prevalence of 1 in 2000. This was before the wide availability of antibody screening. The prevalence of celiac disease, based on either cross-sectional or population-based studies in Western populations, is on the order of 0.3% to 2%, with a higher prevalence in at-risk groups. Celiac disease is far more common here in the United States, in Europe, and in North Africa than previously thought, with prevalence rates varying between 1:85 and 1:230. It is probably one of the most underdiagnosed disorders in childhood, with seropositivity in apparently healthy individuals when populations are screened. This is commonly referred to as the silent "celiac iceberg."

The report of Ravikumara et al is important because it shows that gastrointestinal manifestations of celiac disease are now less prominent at diagnosis when detection is made with targeted screening. Only about 1 in 4 patients have any gastrointestinal symptoms when screening for the disorder takes place. Nongastrointestinal manifestations include dermatitis herpetiformis, reduced bone mineral density, dental enamel hypoplasia, short stature, delayed puberty, iron deficiency anemia not responsive to iron supplements, and infertility. Conditions that are associated with celiac disease include type 1 diabetes mellitus, IgA deficiency, Down syndrome, Turner syndrome, and Williams syndrome. First-degree relatives of those with celiac disease are at greater risk as well. Given the broad nature of these nongastrointestinal manifestations, one wonders whether all children should be screened for celiac disease, recognizing, however, the many, many problems associated with mass screening in terms of sensitivity, specificity, positive predictive value, and negative predictive value. Detecting a lot of false positives could drive up health care costs given the relatively common nature of this disorder. High-risk children (defined as above) certainly could be screened, however.

Parents are seeing a lot written about celiac disease these days. If you are thinking about screening a child for the disorder, please be aware of this. If a parent has already started a child on a gluten-free diet, screening tests may be negative. If a child has been started on a gluten-free diet or is eating insufficient amounts of gluten, the child should be referred to a pediatric dietitian and advised to reintroduce gluten into the diet for at least 3 months (preferably longer) with serial serologic testing, and if the index of suspicion is high enough, a small bowel biopsy is in order. It is not usually adequate to return to a normal diet for just 2 to 3 weeks before biopsy. After a period of gluten exclusion, it may take many months for serology to turn positive. Current recommendations suggest that all children with positive serology should have a small bowel biopsy before being started on a gluten-free diet. Children for whom there is a high clinical suspicion—for example, those with growth retardation or chronic diarrhea—should be considered for a small bowel biopsy even if the serology is negative, as celiac disease has been reported in this setting, although rarely, and other enteropathies may be found. If all else fails, human lymphocyte antigen (HLA) typing can be considered in high-risk groups or in children in whom the diagnosis is uncertain. The major predisposing genotypes are HLA-dq2 and HLA-dq8. These are found in at least 98% of patients. Celiac disease is unlikely in those who are not HLA-dq2 or HLA-dq8 positive.

The North American Society for Pediatric Gastroenterology, Hepatology, and Nutrition recommends that celiac disease screening should begin at 3 years of age in asymptomatic, high-risk children who have been on an adequate gluten diet for at least 1 year before testing. There is no consensus on exactly how often screening in such populations should be carried out. The most clear-cut indication for screening is type 1 diabetes. The prevalence of celiac disease in type 1 diabetic children and adults runs about 5%. Also, celiac serologic testing should be a routine part of the initial screening in children with short stature.

If there is a key to making a diagnosis of celiac disease, it is to think of the possibility, particularly in children with nongastrointestinal symptom presentations. Unfortunately, the asymptomatic patient remains a puzzle. Even if these patients are picked up with serologic screening testing, we have no clue what placing individuals on a gluten-free diet will do over the long haul, in terms of benefits.

J. A. Stockman III, MD

Enterobius vermicularis and Colitis in Children

Jardine M, Kokai GK, Dalzell AM (Royal Liverpool Children's NHS Trust, England)
J Pediatr Gastroenterol Nutr 43:610-612, 2006

Objectives.—We observed a cohort of children presenting with rectal bleeding that were identified as having *Enterobius vermicularis* at colonoscopy and questioned the reliability of conventional diagnostic methods of identifying *E. vermicularis.*

Patients and Methods.—The study was retrospective in nature and subjects were investigated by colonoscopy between May 1997 and December 1999. Patients were identified as having *E. vermicularis* infestation by direct visualisation of the adult worms at colonoscopy. Patients were treated with mebendazole and a record of their clinical response documented.

Results.—A total of 180 colonoscopic examinations were performed during the study period. *E. vermicularis* was identified macroscopically in 31 cases (17.2%). The symptom profile of patients with *E. vermicularis* were abdominal pain, 19 of 26 (73%); rectal bleeding, 16 of 26 (62%); chronic diarrhoea, 13 of 26 (50%) and weight loss, 11 of 26 (42%). Ova cysts and parasites were identified in none of the saline swabs analysed in 20 patients. Sellotape testing was performed in only 4 patients and was negative in all. Of the 26 children, 21 (81%) demonstrated histopathological features of nonspecific colitis. There was clinical resolution of symptoms in 19 of 23 patients.

Conclusions.—We suggest that in patients with symptoms suggestive of inflammatory bowel disease, *E. vermicularis* infestation must be excluded as a common cause of nonspecific colitis. We also suggest that diagnostic tests such as saline swabs and Sellotape testing may be lacking in sensitivity.

▶ Whether *E vermicularis* causes serious disease or whether it is merely an annoying "passenger" riding through the gut has generated a lot of debate. Most with this worm are asymptomatic. The chief symptom when present is usually anal itching, which can manifest itself as irritability and insomnia. The most common complication of *E vermicularis* is bacterial infections in broken anal skin.

As this article shows, *E vermicularis* can cause much more than a simple itch. Previous cases of colitis secondary to *E vermicularis* infections have been reported. Patients may present with pain, rectal bleeding, a fever, nausea, vomiting, and increased stool frequency. In all reported cases, symptoms have resolved with antiparasitic therapy alone.

In this article from the United Kingdom, colonoscopy was undertaken in children presenting with rectal bleeding. A total of 180 colonoscopic examinations were performed, and *E vermicularis* was identified macroscopically in 17% of cases. In addition to rectal bleeding, these youngsters had abdominal pain. About half had chronic diarrhea, and a lesser percent experienced weight loss. Treatment of the *E vermicularis* infection led to resolution of symptoms in virtually all.

Infections known to be caused by *E vermicularis* go back almost 100 years in the medical literature. As early as 1919, reports began to appear about this obligate parasite. Humans are the only known natural host. The life cycle of *E vermicularis* is 2 to 4 weeks. Digestive secretions dissolve the egg-releasing larvae in the duodenum. Larvae then mature into adult worms that inhabit and mate in the terminal ilium, caecum, and ascending colon. The female migrates at night to the rectum and lays her eggs in the anal canal. Infection then occurs either by the fecal–oral route or by retroinfection, in which the eggs hatch in the anus and the worms reinfect the colon by migration.

E vermicularis has been demonstrated to be a cause of pinworms of the appendix (mimicking appendicitis). In fact, true appendicitis caused by *E vermicularis* has also been described in circumstances in which the appendix ruptures and the worm is released into the peritoneal cavity. The process can go on to produce granulomata in the liver, spleen, or kidney. Cases of pelvic inflammatory disease caused by *Enterobius* have also been reported.

Please remember that *E vermicularis* can cause more than a bad case of the pinworms. It can mimic colitis. It can cause pelvic inflammatory disease. It can cause peritonitis and other bad things.

J. A. Stockman III, MD

Recommendations for the Care of Individuals With an Inherited Predisposition to Lynch Syndrome: A Systematic Review

Lindor NM, Petersen GM, Hadley DW, et al (Mayo Clinic, Rochester, Minn; NIH, Bethesda, Md; Univ of Utah, Salt Lake City; et al)
JAMA 296:1507-1517, 2006

Context.—About 2% of all colorectal cancer occurs in the context of the autosomal dominantly inherited Lynch syndrome, which is due to mutations in mismatch repair genes. Potential risk-reducing interventions are recommended for individuals known to have these mutations.

Objectives.—To review cancer risks and data on screening efficacy in the context of Lynch syndrome (hereditary nonpolyposis colorectal cancer) and to provide recommendations for clinical management for affected families, based on available evidence and expert opinion.

Data Sources and Study Selection.—A systematic literature search using PubMed and the Cochrane Database of Systematic Reviews, reference list review of retrieved articles, manual searches of relevant articles, and direct communication with other researchers in the field. Search terms included *hereditary non-polyposis colon cancer, Lynch syndrome, microsatellite instability, mismatch repair genes*, and terms related to the biology of Lynch syndrome. Only peer-reviewed, full-text, English-language articles concerning human subjects published between January 1, 1996, and February 2006 were included. The US Preventive Services Task Force's 2-tier system was adapted to describe the quality of evidence and to assign strength to the recommendations for each guideline.

Evidence Synthesis.—The evidence supports colonoscopic surveillance for individuals with Lynch syndrome, although the optimal age at initiation and frequency of examinations is unresolved. Colonoscopy is recommended every 1 to 2 years starting at ages 20 to 25 years (age 30 years for those with *MSH6* mutations), or 10 years younger than the youngest age of the person diagnosed in the family. While fully acknowledging absence of demonstrated efficacy, the following are also recommended annually: endometrial sampling and transvaginal ultrasound of the uterus and ovaries (ages 30-35 years); urinalysis with cytology (ages 25-35 years); history, examination, review of systems, education and genetic counseling regarding Lynch syndrome (age 21 years). Regular colonoscopy was favored for at-risk persons without colorectal neoplasia. For individuals who will undergo surgical resection of a colon cancer, subtotal colectomy is favored. Evidence supports the efficacy of prophylactic hysterectomy and oophorectomy.

Conclusions.—The past 10 years have seen major advances in the understanding of Lynch syndrome. Current recommendations regarding cancer screening and prevention require careful consultation between clinicians, clinical cancer genetic services, and well-informed patients.

▶ This report by Lindor et al, the Balmaña et al report (Prediction of *MLH1* and *MSH2* mutations in Lynch syndrome), and the Chen et al report (Prediction of germline mutations and cancer risk in the Lynch syndrome) deal with a hereditary disorder known as Lynch syndrome, a syndrome we tend not to think too much about in pediatrics. A small but real subset of colorectal cancer occurs in those born with the autosomal dominantly inherited Lynch syndrome. Colorectal cancer is one of the most common malignancies in the United States. Approximately 150,000 individuals are affected each year. If one is going to do well with this form of cancer, early diagnosis is mandatory because long-term survivorship is directly related to the stage at diagnosis: 5-year survival rates are greater than 90% for the rare patient diagnosed with stage I cancer but less than 5% for those who present with metastatic disease.

Needless to say, early diagnosis is essential for the prevention of the morbidity and mortality associated with colorectal surgery. This is the reason why population-based screening for colon polyps and cancer, preferably with colonoscopy in individuals 50 years or older, is recommended. Certain groups, however, are at an even higher risk than the general population. A quarter of all colorectal cancers occur in families containing other members with this malignancy, which suggests a familial basis. Even more striking is the fact that somewhere between 3% and 4% of colorectal cancers occur in families with a clear autosomal dominant pattern of inheritance, the most common of which is Lynch syndrome (ie, hereditary nonpolyposis colorectal cancer). When this syndrome was originally described, the clinical criteria defining it included a history of at least 3 affected family members including 2 generations with at least 1 person diagnosed before 50 years of age. This diagnosis is recognizably restrictive and does not take into account the possibility of later-onset variants of the disease, the implications of extracolonic tumors, or the limitations imposed by small family size. This is the reason why new understandings that have been developed over the last 15 years about Lynch syndrome are so important.

In the early 1990s, the genetic basis for Lynch syndrome was uncovered with the discovery of germline mutations in the mismatch DNA repair genes *MLH1* and *MSH2* (and, subsequently, *MSH6* and, rarely, *PMS2*). These mutations confer a high susceptibility to not only colon and endometrial cancer but also several other cancers including cancers of the ovary, stomach, small bowel, hepatobiliary system, ureteral tract, brain, and other sites. The delineation of these mutations has allowed for genetic testing and counseling of individuals in families with a genetic suspicion of these forms of cancer. Importantly, surveillance for colorectal cancer begins on the pediatrician's watch because it is recommended that such screening begin by age 20 and be carried out at intervals as frequent as every 1 to 2 years. The systematic review by Lindor et al makes such a recommendation. These recommendations should be followed very carefully because the risk of the development of cancer is as high as 70% by 70 years of age, and the mean age of diagnosis of a first cancer is in one's early 40s. Children have also been reported to have been given a diagnosis of these cancers.

In addition to routine colorectal screening with colonoscopy beginning at a young age, surveillance for endometrial cancer is also in order. The average age for development of endometrial cancer in patients with Lynch syndrome is around 50 years, which is more than a decade earlier than the average age of presentation in otherwise nongenetically affected individuals. Fortunately, three quarters of women with Lynch syndrome who develop endometrial cancer present with stage I disease, which is similar to sporadic endometrial cancer. This has a 5-year survival rate of almost 90%. Endometrial cancer screening is not likely to improve on these numbers but can theoretically decrease the amount of treatment needed by detecting cancer at its very earliest stages when surgery alone is curative.

Cancers occurring outside the colorectal area and the uterus account for one third of all malignancies developing in those affected with Lynch syndrome. A regular, yearly complete history and physical examination, a urinalysis with cytologic examination, and the tracking down of every sign and symptom a patient has that cannot be accounted for by some simple explanation are reasonable for the detection of malignancies elsewhere.

J. A. Stockman III, MD

Prediction of *MLH1* and *MSH2* Mutations in Lynch Syndrome

Balmaña J, Stockwell DH, Steyerberg EW, et al (Dana-Farber Cancer Inst, Boston; Harvard Med School, Boston; Myriad Genetic Labs Inc, Salt Lake City, Utah; et al)
JAMA 296:1469-1478, 2006

Context.—Lynch syndrome is caused primarily by mutations in the mismatch repair genes *MLH1* and *MSH2*.

Objectives.—To analyze *MLH1/MSH2* mutation prevalence in a large cohort of patients undergoing genetic testing and to develop a clinical model to predict the likelihood of finding a mutation in at-risk patients.

Design, Setting, and Participants.—Personal and family history were obtained for 1914 unrelated probands who submitted blood samples starting in the year 2000 for full gene sequencing of *MLH1/MSH2*. Genetic analysis was performed using a combination of sequence analysis and Southern blotting. A multivariable model was developed using logistic regression in an initial cohort of 898 individuals and subsequently prospectively validated in 1016 patients. The complex model that we have named PREMM$_{1,2}$ (Prediction of Mutations in *MLH1* and *MSH2*) was developed into a Web-based tool that incorporates personal and family history of cancer and adenomas.

Main Outcome Measure.—Deleterious mutations in *MLH1/MSH2* genes.

Results.—Overall, 14.5% of the probands (130/898) carried a pathogenic mutation (*MLH1*, 6.5%; *MSH2*, 8.0%) in the development cohort and 15.3% (155/1016) in the validation cohort, with 42 (27%) of the latter being large rearrangements. Strong predictors of mutations included proband characteristics (presence of colorectal cancer, especially ≥ 2 separate diagnoses, or endometrial cancer) and family history (especially the number of first-degree relatives with colorectal or endometrial cancer). Age at diagnosis was particularly important for colorectal cancer. The multivariable model discriminated well at external validation, with an area under the receiver operating characteristic curve of 0.80 (95% confidence interval, 0.76-0.84).

Conclusions.—Personal and family history characteristics can accurately predict the outcome of genetic testing in a large population at risk of Lynch syndrome. The PREMM$_{1,2}$ model provides clinicians with an objective, easy-to-use tool to estimate the likelihood of finding mutations in the *MLH1/MSH2* genes and may guide the strategy for molecular evaluation.

▶ This report and the Chen et al report (Prediction of germline mutations and cancer risk in the Lynch syndrome) present 2 new algorithms for predicting the likelihood of carrying a germline mismatch repair gene mutation in Lynch syndrome. The algorithms developed by Balmaña et al use a multivariate logistic regression model to predict carrier status based on a personal and family history of colon and endometrial cancer and other Lynch syndrome cancers. In contrast, in the article by Chen et al, the algorithm involves a detailed parametric model invoking the Bayes rule to estimate the probability that the counselees carry a mutation, given their personal family history of Lynch syndrome malignancies. This model uses more data input, particularly from unaffected relatives of the counselee, than do other predictive models.

Predictive rules to detect Lynch syndrome form very useful tools for clinicians and their patients, as well as for epidemiologists who wish to assess both the magnitude of the nonhereditary polyposis colorectal cancer problem and the potential usefulness of preventative efforts. It should be recognized that because the rules were developed and evaluated with the use of samples primarily composed of white individuals with European ancestry, there is great need to evaluate the performances of these rules when applied to ethnic minorities, as the prevalence and penetrance of Lynch syndrome is poorly understood in nonwhite populations.

It has been more than 40 years since Henry Lynch first described the syndrome that bears his name,[1] and our understanding of the genetics of the syndrome has improved enormously in the interval. As the genome project has matured, it is fairly clear that we pediatricians will be counseling pediatric patients and their families about colorectal cancer and related cancers. It will be up to us to trigger routine colonoscopic screening as affected patients are exiting their teens.

This commentary closes with a question only peripherally related to the GI tract. In the way of "why didn't I think of this" categories, what novel treatment is now being explored to get rid of perianal fistulae? An Israeli team has tested a highly concentrated fibrin glue to treat complex perianal fistulae. The glue, one mixed with antibiotics, is instilled along the fistula tract without the need for a surgical procedure. Of some 60 patients who have undergone the procedure, 53% achieved complete healing of their perianal fistulae, and one-third achieved significant improvement despite incomplete healing. Not a single patient had a problem with incontinence and all resumed normal activity within a day of being "glued." The procedure seems to have avoided the need for surgery in about half or slightly more than half of patients with this problem.[2]

J. A. Stockman III, MD

Reference

1. Lynch HT, Shaw MW, Magnuson CW, Larsen AL, Krush AJ. Hereditary factors in cancer. Study of two large midwestern kindreds. *Arch Intern Med*. 1966;117: 206-212.
2. Zmora O, Neufeld D, Ziv Y, et al. Prospective, multicenter evaluation of highly concentrated fibrin glue in the treatment of complex cryptogenic perianal fistulas. *Dis Colon Rectum*. 2005;48:2167-2172.

Prediction of Germline Mutations and Cancer Risk in the Lynch Syndrome

Chen S, for the Colon Cancer Family Registry (Johns Hopkins, Baltimore, Md; Columbia Univ, New York; Mem Sloan-Kettering Cancer Ctr, New York; et al)
JAMA 296:1479-1487, 2006

Context.—Identifying families at high risk for the Lynch syndrome (ie, hereditary nonpolyposis colorectal cancer) is critical for both genetic counseling and cancer prevention. Current clinical guidelines are effective but limited by applicability and cost.

Objective.—To develop and validate a genetic counseling and risk prediction tool that estimates the probability of carrying a deleterious mutation in mismatch repair genes *MLH1, MSH2,* or *MSH6* and the probability of developing colorectal or endometrial cancer.

Design, Setting, and Patients.—External validation of the MMRpro model was conducted on 279 individuals from 226 clinic-based families in the United States, Canada, and Australia (referred between 1993-2005) by comparing model predictions with results of highly sensitive germline mutation detection techniques. MMRpro models the autosomal dominant inheritance of mismatch repair mutations, with parameters based on meta-analyses of the penetrance and prevalence of mutations and of the predictive values of tumor characteristics. The model's prediction is tailored to each individual's detailed family history information on colorectal and endometrial cancer and to tumor characteristics including microsatellite instability.

Main Outcome Measure.—Ability of MMRpro to correctly predict mutation carrier status, as measured by operating characteristics, calibration, and overall accuracy.

Results.—In the independent validation, MMRpro provided a concordance index of 0.83 (95% confidence interval, 0.78-0.88) and a ratio of observed to predicted cases of 0.94 (95% confidence interval, 0.84-1.05). This results in higher accuracy than existing alternatives and current clinical guidelines.

Conclusions.—MMRpro is a broadly applicable, accurate prediction model that can contribute to current screening and genetic counseling practices in a high-risk population. It is more sensitive and more specific than existing clinical guidelines for identifying individuals who may benefit from MMR germline testing. It is applicable to individuals for whom tumor samples are not available and to individuals in whom germline testing finds no mutation.

▶ Because this editor has little more to say about Lynch syndrome, we will close this series of articles by asking a question having to do with scanning of the abdomen. You are referring a 6-year-old for a CT of the abdomen. The radiologist calls you on the day of the procedure to tell you that the youngster will not drink his barium contrast material. What might you suggest as a suitable substitute, something that the child might very well like?

The answer is that you might suggest a glass of milk, or even better yet, a milkshake. Radiologists looking to replace chalky-tasting barium-based contrast agents used for some computed tomography (CT) imaging need look no further than the dairy case. It appears that whole milk may be an adequate substitute. Researchers from St. Luke's-Roosevelt Hospital in New York City said their preliminary findings from an ongoing study have found that milk achieves similar bowel distention and enhancement as a commonly used barium-based contrast agent, VoLumen. When a CT is used for visualization of the small intestinal wall, it requires a negative oral contrast agent, such as VoLumen. Such an agent allows better visualization of the bowel wall and clearer delineation between the bowel cavity and soft tissue. Using whole milk (not skim or reduced fat milk because the fat content makes a difference), the milk-filled intestinal cavity appears dark while the intestinal wall appears brighter. The investigators studied 62 consecutive patients receiving VoLumen (900 mL 30 minutes before the CT plus 30 mL immediately prior to the test) and 117 consecutive patients receiving milk (400 mL to 600 mL one hour before the test plus 200 mL to 400 mL 20 minutes prior to imaging). The study involved adults. Approximately 42% of the 57 VoLumen patients who subsequently completed a questionnaire experienced abdominal discomfort such as cramps, diarrhea and nausea compared with only 23% of the 117 patients given milk. Of those taking the VoLumen, 40% said they would have preferred milk, and 85% of the milk drinkers said they would select it again. The investigators concluded that milk could very well be an excellent contrast agent for children who tend to balk at drinking barium-based drinks . . . there's a study waiting to be done.

So what about cost? The milk consumed per patient in this study ran about $1.50 while the amount of VoLumen needed was approximately $18.00 per procedure. While this does not sound like a world of difference in terms of dollars and cents, there are some 30 million to 40 million CT scans performed annually here in the United States, about a third of which involve contrast abdominal CTs. This editor's math suggests that utilizing a moo-cow as a source of contrast would save in excess of $100 million per year in healthcare costs.

Obviously, whole cow milk cannot be used in patients who are lactase deficient. Then again, it could be used as a bowel prep in such circumstances. That would make another interesting clinical trial.[1]

J.A. Stockman III, MD

Reference

1. Mitka M. Milk shows potential as CT contrast agent. *JAMA.* 2007;297:353.

Complications of Colonoscopy in an Integrated Health Care Delivery System

Levin TR, Zhao W, Conell C, et al (Kaiser Permanente Med Care Program, Oakland, Calif; Battelle Mem Inst, Seattle; Ctrs for Disease Control and Prevention, Atlanta, Ga)

Ann Intern Med 145:880-886, 2006

Background.—Information about colonoscopy complications, particularly postpolypectomy bleeding, is limited.

Objective.—To quantify the magnitude and severity of colonoscopy complications.

Design.—Retrospective cohort.

Setting.—Kaiser Permanente of Northern California.

Patients.—16 318 members 40 years of age or older undergoing colonoscopy between January 1994 and July 2002.

Measurements.—Electronic records reviewed for serious complications, including hospital admission within 30 days of colonoscopy for colonic perforation, colonic bleeding, diverticulitis, the postpolypectomy syndrome, or other serious illnesses directly related to colonoscopy.

Results.—82 serious complications occurred (5.0 per 1000 colonoscopies [95% CI, 4.0 to 6.2 per 1000 colonoscopies]). Serious complications occurred in 0.8 per 1000 colonoscopies without biopsy or polypectomy and in 7.0 per 1000 colonoscopies with biopsy or polypectomy. Perforations occurred in 0.9 per 1000 colonoscopies (CI, 0.5 to 1.5 per 1000 colonoscopies) (0.6 per 1000 without biopsy or polypectomy and 1.1 per 1000 with biopsy or polypectomy). Postbiopsy or postpolypectomy bleeding occurred in 4.8 per 1000 colonoscopies with biopsy (CI, 3.6 to 6.2 per 1000 colonoscopies). Biopsy or polypectomy was associated with an increased risk for any serious complication (rate ratio, 9.2 [CI, 2.9 to 29.0] vs. colonoscopy without biopsy). Ten deaths (1 attributable to colonoscopy) occurred within 30 days of the colonoscopy.

Limitations.—99.3% (16 204) of colonoscopies were nonscreening examinations. The rate of complications may be lower in a primary screening sample. The small number of observed adverse events limited power to detect risk factors for complications.

Conclusions.—Colonoscopy with biopsy or polypectomy is associated with increased risk for complications. Perforation may also occur during colonoscopies without biopsies.

▶ There really are not any high-quality data available about the complication rates of colonoscopy when carried out in children. The starting point for understanding the "universe" of such complications must come from data in adults, thus the inclusion of this report from the *Annals of Internal Medicine*. The report comes from Kaiser Permanente, Northern California, and looked at some 16,318 colonoscopies. These colonoscopies were being performed because of a family history of colorectal cancer or adenomatous polyp, as a follow-up to a positive screening test (ie, polyp or cancer at sigmoidoscopy, positive results on a fecal occult blood test, or an abnormal barium enema), for surveillance because of a previously detected adenomatous polyp or colorectal cancer, or for primary screening.

What we learn from Kaiser Permanente is that among all patients, the incidence of serious complications of colonoscopy is 5.0 per 1000 procedures, or 1 in 200 examinations. Complications include colonic perforation, the post-polypectomy syndrome, postprocedure bleeding requiring hospitalization, and infrequent other problems such as a flare-up of diverticulitis. The chance of dying as a result of colonoscopy is a risk of 0.6 per 1000 examinations. Some of these deaths are the result of colonoscopy complicating the kinds of diseases that adults have (congestive heart failure, coronary artery disease, etc). The risk of a complication of colonoscopy increases by approximately 9-fold if the colonoscopy involves the performance of a biopsy.

Hopefully, the risk of colonoscopy in children is less than the risk found in this study from Kaiser Permanente. Fortunately, not that many children undergo colonoscopy. It would be helpful, however, for there to be a collaborative reporting of colonoscopy complications in the pediatric age population so we would know more precisely when counseling parents about the pros and cons of this procedure.

J. A. Stockman III, MD

Colonoscopic Withdrawal Times and Adenoma Detection during Screening Colonoscopy

Barclay RL, Vicari JJ, Doughty AS, et al (Rockford Gastroenterology Associates, Ill; Univ of Illinois at Rockford)
N Engl J Med 355:2533-2541, 2006

Background.—Colonoscopy is commonly used to screen for neoplasia. To assess the performance of screening colonoscopy in everyday practice, we conducted a study of the rates of detection of adenomas and the amount of time taken to withdraw the colonoscope among endoscopists in a large community-based practice.

Methods.—During a 15-month period, 12 experienced gastroenterologists performed 7882 colonoscopies, of which 2053 were screening examinations in subjects who had not previously undergone colonoscopy. We recorded the numbers, sizes, and histologic features of the neoplastic lesions detected during screening, as well as the duration of insertion and of withdrawal of the colonoscope during the procedure. We compared rates of detection of neoplastic lesions among gastroenterologists who had mean colonoscopic withdrawal times of less than 6 minutes with the rates of those who had mean withdrawal times of 6 minutes or more. According to experts, 6 minutes is the minimum length of time to allow adequate inspection during instrument withdrawal.

Results.—Neoplastic lesions (mostly adenomatous polyps) were detected in 23.5% of screened subjects. There were large differences among gastroenterologists in the rates of detection of adenomas (range of the mean number of lesions per subject screened, 0.10 to 1.05; range of the percentage of subjects with adenomas, 9.4 to 32.7%) and in their times of withdrawal of the colonoscope from the cecum to the anus (range, 3.1 to 16.8 minutes for procedures during which no polyps were removed). As compared with colonoscopists with mean withdrawal times of less than 6 minutes, those with mean withdrawal times of 6 minutes or more had higher rates of detection of any neoplasia (28.3% vs. 11.8%, P<0.001) and of advanced neoplasia (6.4% vs. 2.6%, P=0.005).

Conclusions.—In this large community-based gastroenterology practice, we observed greater rates of detection of adenomas among endoscopists who had longer mean times for withdrawal of the colonoscope. The effect of variation in withdrawal times on lesion detection and the prevention of colorectal cancer in the context of widespread colonoscopic screening is not known. Ours was a preliminary study, so the generalizability and implications for clinical practice need to be determined by future studies.

▶ When it comes to screening colonoscopy, there has been a dramatic explosion in its use. Obviously, screening colonoscopy is most often done in adults, but some kids do undergo screening colonoscopy. There is good evidence that patients with a normal result on a colonoscopy have a reduced 10-year incidence of colorectal cancer. An important objective of screening colonoscopy is the detection and removal of adenomas, which can prevent many cancers. If, however, colonoscopy is to be a successful screening tool for colorectal cancer, it must be performed with a low rate of missed lesions and complications and by properly trained endoscopists who are committed to continuous quality improvement. Barclay et al report the results of screening colonoscopy within a private practice gastroenterology group. They measured a key outcome—rate of adenoma detection. The authors report an overall rate of adenoma detection of 23.5%, and a rate of 5.2% with advanced adenomas (defined as adenomas with a diameter of at least 10 mm or with villous histologic features, high-grade dysplasia, or invasive cancer). The important contribution of this study is the observation of significant variation among the 12 endoscopists in the rates of detection of adenomas. The variable associated with low rates of detection was a colonoscopic withdrawal time of less than 6 minutes. Longer procedure time does not necessarily mean higher quality; the endoscopist must be able to recognize important pathologic features and have the technical skills to ensure appropriate management. However, the results of this study are intuitive—careful endoscopic examination of the colon should improve the rate of detection of adenomas.

So why is the quality of colonoscopy important, and why is quality a problem? Evidence now shows that colonoscopy, even in the hands of experts, is not performed perfectly every time. Studies have shown that in up to 1% of patients who have had adenomas removed, invasive colorectal cancer develops within 3 years after a baseline colonoscopy during which "all" polyps are removed. This could be due to missed lesions, incomplete removal of adenomas, and new, fast-growing lesions. Missed lesions are certainly part of the equation.

So how can we improve quality? One answer is that it must be built into the tapestry of what we do every day. The rate of detection of adenomas is just one example of practice that cries out for quality improvement initiatives. A task force from the National Colorectal Cancer Roundtable is developing a reporting system for colonoscopy that could be adopted into every clinical practice. The system would capture key quality indicators (including the rate of detection of adenomas) and provide benchmarking information for the endoscopist. If there were transparent data reporting, primary care providers would have needed information to decide where to refer patients for endoscopy. It is time for all endoscopists to routinely measure quality indicators in their practice and strive for continuous quality improvement. It is also time for all of us to do the same thing.

This commentary closes with a "who-dun-it" related to a complication of a bowel prep for a colonoscopy. It is intended to challenge your diagnostic acumen. A 16-year-old with ulcerative colitis and impaired renal function presents to the emergency room with inability to open his jaw and has carpopedal spasm. He also describes skin paraesthesia "like something crawling under my skin." Physical examination shows evidence of tetany. The only significant history in addition to his known ulcerative colitis is that two days before, in anticipation of a followup colonoscopy, he had started a bowel prep with Fleet Phospho-soda. Your diagnosis?

A prerequisite for a good quality colonoscopy is adequate bowel preparation. Various methods are available including the use of the oral sodium phosphate solution (Fleet Phospho-soda), which has become increasingly popular as an alternative to other forms of bowel prep. Its acceptance is largely due to the smaller volume required for ingestion with a recommended dose of 45 ml of sodium phosphate mixed with water, given in two intervals 12 hours a part.[1] It is definitely cheaper than other forms of bowel preparation agents. The rub with phosphate bowel preparations is their associated complication rate. Sodium phosphate bowel preparations can lead to renal failure, particularly in patients who are unable to excrete the acute and excessive phosphate load. The main symptoms relate to hypocalcemia. This results from the raised sodium phosphate concentration. In the patient described, renal failure in association with the phosphate enema was likely to be the cause of the tetany.

If you are not totally familiar with phosphate bowel preparations, sodium phosphate is a hypertonic solution with strong osmotic effects. It acts by retaining fluid in the bowel through osmosis. The product contains 48 g of monobasic sodium phosphate and 18 g of dibasic sodium phosphate per 100 ml. The diluted preparation contains about 34-times the amount of sodium, 2000-times the phosphate, and has more than 30-times the osmolarity of normal plasma. Even in normal people there will be some rise in serum phosphate and a fall in serum calcium after ingestion of sodium phosphate. Fatal hyperphosphatemia has been reported in patients with renal dysfunction. Administration of this product to patients with renal failure has a mortality rate as high as 33%.

If you are one who uses a Fleet's preparation, in addition to its contraindication in patients who have renal failure, there are other vulnerable groups of patients. These include the elderly and debilitated, patients with hepatic and cardiac disease, those with delicate fluid and electrolyte balance and subjects taking drugs that prolong QT interval. The use of sodium phosphate is also contraindicated in children and in patients with gastrointestinal obstruction or megacolon. Anyone taking sodium phosphate should be advised to maintain adequate hydration.

Although sodium phosphate preparations are safe and effective for most patients, all of us who might prescribe sodium phosphate for bowel preparation should be aware of the potential for life threatening complications.[2]

J. A. Stockman III, MD

Reference

1. Fleet Labortories. Phospho-soda E-Z-prep bowel preparation instructions. Available at: http://www.phosphosoda.com. Accessed June 12, 2007.
2. Woo YM, Crail S, Curry G, Geddes CC. A life threatening complication after ingestion of sodium phosphate bowel preparation. *BMJ.* 2006;333:589-590.

Treatment of Faecal Impaction with Polyethelene Glycol Plus Electrolytes (PGE + E) Versus Lactulose as Maintenance Therapy

Candy DCA, Edwards D, Geraint M (Royal West Sussex NHS Trust, England; Norgine Pharmaceuticals Ltd, Harefield, Middlesex, England)
J Pediatr Gastroenterol Nutr 43:65-70, 2006

Objectives.—To assess the efficacy of polyethylene glycol 3350 plus electrolytes (PEG + E; Movicol®) as oral monotherapy in the treatment of faecal impaction in children, and to compare PEG + E with lactulose as maintenance therapy in a randomised trial.

Patients and Methods.—An initial open-label study of PEG + E in the inpatient treatment of faecal impaction (phase 1), followed by a randomised, double-blind comparison between PEG + E and lactulose for maintenance treatment of constipation over a 3-month period (phase 2) in children aged 2 to 11 years with a clinical diagnosis of faecal impaction.

Results.—Disimpaction on PEG + E was achieved in 58 (92%) of 63 of children (89% of 2–4 year olds and 94% of 5–11 year olds) without additional interventions. A maximum dose of 4 sachets (for 2–4 year olds) or 6 sachets (for 5–11 year olds) was required; median time to disimpaction was 6 days (range, 3–7 days). Seven children (23%) reimpacted whilst taking lactulose, whereas no children reimpacted while taking PEG + E ($P = 0.011$). The total incidence rate of adverse events seen was higher in the lactulose group (83%) than in the PEG + E group (64%).

Conclusions.—PEG + E is safe and highly effective in the management of childhood constipation. It allows a single orally administered laxative to be used for disimpaction without recourse to invasive interventions. It is significantly more effective than lactulose as maintenance therapy, both in efficacy in treating constipation and efficacy in preventing the recurrence of faecal impaction.

▶ Impaction of stool frequently presents with soiling, often in a child that has had constipation that was undetected for many months. Chronic constipation is associated with fecal soiling in most cases. The recommended approach to the problem is to empty the constipated bowel and to keep it empty. The rub is that the current means of achieving disimpaction merely add to the distress already affecting the youngster. No one likes repeated enemas and suppositories. Manual evacuation of stool with or without a general anesthetic is equally unpleasant. The latter is associated with a risk of structural injury to the anal sphincter, particularly when the procedure is performed under anesthesia. One possible solution to all these difficulties is the use of polyethylene glycol 3350 (PEG).

PEG is a particularly suitable substance upon which to base an oral laxative because a solution of PEG exhibits a linear dose-response relationship when ingested, retaining water in the bowel to potentially induce an almost unlimited laxative action. This is in contrast to laxatives such as lactulose or senna, which, as prodrugs, need metabolism in the large bowel to produce an active moiety. The ingestion of increasing amounts of agents such as lactulose and senna will saturate the metabolic capability of the colon, and thus the dose-response curve shows a plateau after which raising the dose does not produce any greater effect.

The report abstracted from the United Kingdom was designed to determine whether invasive, unpleasant treatments for fecal impaction could be avoided by the oral administration of PEG + electrolyte solution (PEG + E). The study also looked at whether PEG + E was effective in preventing reimpaction compared with lactulose. The PEG + E was administered orally (dose, 13.8-g powder dissolved in at least 125/ml water per sachet) on a daily regimen until disimpaction was achieved. This regimen used an escalating dose of PEG + E to maximize compliance, with a higher dose given to children in the 5- to 11-year-olds than the 2- to 4-year-olds. Disimpaction was successfully achieved in 92% of the children in an average time of just 6 days. No additional interventions were required. Adverse effects of PEG + E included nausea, vomiting, and abdominal pain, but these were able to be minimized by a reduction in the rate at which the solution was given.

This British report clearly shows that PEG + E is a safe and highly effective, orally administered laxative for the treatment of fecal impaction in children. No additional treatment was required to clear impaction in the children in this study, indicating that the use of invasive treatments had been eliminated or at least substantially reduced for the overwhelming majority of youngsters. The report confirms a previous study on impaction using a PEG-based laxative (Miralax).[1] Treatment with PEG + E can be administered at home in most instances, eliminating any requirement for hospitalization for disimpaction. It also appears that PEG + E can be effectively used as a maintenance therapy in preventing reoccurrences of the problem.

On a totally unrelated gastrointestinal question, have you ever wondered what the origin is of the gas we pass? Three-quarters of flatulence is likely due to bacterial gases, and the pressure in the bubbles created by these gases can be as high as 760 mm Hg. The rest of the gas is from swallowed air. Some bacterial gases are absorbed and eventually exhaled, but the rest have no other way to get out of our bodies but to escape per anum. Scientists believe that flatulence rich in bacterial gases is the price we pay for resorption of water in the large bowel and that little can be done to reduce it.[2]

J. A. Stockman III, MD

References

1. Youssef NN, Peters JM, Henderson W, Shultz-Peters S, Lockhard DK, Di Lorenzo C. Dose of PEG 3350 for the treatment of childhood fecal impaction. *J Pediatr*. 2002;141:410-414.
2. Kurbel S, Kurbel B, Vcev A. Intestinal gases and flatulence: possible causes of occurrence. *Med Hypotheses*. 2006;67:235-239.

Diagnostic Tests in Hirshsprung Disease: A Systematic Review
de Lorijn F, Kremer LCM, Reitsma JB, et al (Emma Children's Hosp, Amsterdam)
J Pediatr Gastroenterol Nutr 42:496-505, 2006

Objective.—We conducted a systematic review to determine and compare the diagnostic accuracy of contrast enema (CE), anorectal manometry (ARM) and rectal suction biopsy (RSB) in infants suspected of Hirschsprung disease.

Design.—This is a systematic review.

Data Sources.—Articles were identified through electronic searches in Medline, EMBASE.com and Cochrane Controlled Trials Register. Searches were limited to articles published after 1966 in PubMed and after 1980 in EMBASE.com.

Study Selection.—Studies were included if infants underwent at least one of the following tests: CE, ARM or RSB, followed by full-thickness biopsy and/or clinical follow-up as the reference standard.

Data Extraction.—Two reviewers independently assessed the methods of data collection, patient selection, blinding and prevention of verification bias and description of the test protocol and reference standard. Data to construct 2 × 2 tables were abstracted for each test.

Results.—Twenty-four studies met our inclusion criteria, but 2 studies were subsequently excluded for statistical analysis because data were missing to construct the 2 × 2 table. RSB (14 studies for a total of 993 patients) was the most accurate test, having both the highest mean sensitivity (93%; 95% confidence interval [CI], 88%–95%) and mean specificity (98%; 95% CI, 95%–99%). Sensitivity and specificity of ARM (9 studies for a total of 400 patients) were similar to those of RSB (91% vs 93%, $P = 0.73$ and 94% vs 98%, $P = 0.08$, respectively). Sensitivity and specificity of CE (12 studies for a total of 425 patients) were significantly lower than those of RSB and

ARM, with mean sensitivity and mean specificity of 70% and 83%, respectively.

Conclusions.—RSB and ARM are the most accurate tests in the diagnostic workup of Hirschsprung disease.

▶ Hirschsprung disease can present in a variety of ways, but most commonly the presentation is that of constipation. Unfortunately, only about 1 in 5000 cases of constipation is caused by Hirschsprung disease. We need to think of the disorder every time we see such a common problem as a child presenting with constipation.

The diagnosis of Hirschsprung disease is not always easy to establish. The report from The Netherlands reminds us that there is some variation in the accuracy of the three most commonly used tests for Hirschsprung disease. The presence of a transitional zone is the critical feature to suspect Hirschsprung disease in a contrast enema test. Anorectal manometry assesses the rectoanal inhibition reflex; failure to elicit this reflex indicates the likelihood of Hirschsprung disease. The third option consists of a rectal suction biopsy, which shows an elevated acetylcholinesterase activity and aganglionosis. These three tests are relatively simple and noninvasive. The gold standard, however, remains a full-thickness biopsy of the rectum and provides the most definitive answer. The classical method for biopsy involves a full-thickness biopsy of rectal mucosa and underlying muscle. However, this requires general anesthesia and the suturing of the biopsy site. Possible complications are perforation, rectal bleeding and infection. Absence of ganglion cells confirms the diagnosis of Hirschsprung disease.

There has been a considerable amount of debate about the most appropriate initial test for diagnosing Hirschsprung disease because everything but a full-thickness biopsy is associated with some degree of false-negative and false-positive test results. This is where the report from The Netherlands helps us. What we learn from this systematic review of diagnostic tests for Hirschsprung disease is that rectal suction biopsy and anorectal manometry are the most accurate noninvasive diagnostic tools for Hirschsprung disease. Rectal suction biopsy will, however, miss about 7% of diagnoses, but the test has almost 100% specificity if positive. The sensitivity and specificity of anorectal manometry runs 91% and 94%, respectively. Basically, this means that if either of these tests is positive, the patient is overwhelmingly likely to have Hirschsprung disease. A negative test does not totally exclude the diagnosis, however.

It can be concluded from this systematic review of the literature that both rectal suction biopsy and anorectal manometry are indeed the most accurate tests in the noninvasive diagnostic workup of patients suspected of having Hirschsprung disease. Anorectal manometry is easy to perform in children older than 1 year. It therefore has been suggested to be the ideal screening tool. However, the equipment to perform this test is expensive, and extensive experience is required to perform the procedure adequately, particularly in children younger than 1 year of age. By comparison, a rectal suction biopsy is a relatively simple, efficient, and, largely, incident-free procedure, although rectal bleeding, perforation, and sepsis have been described as complications.

The contrast enema alone is unlikely to instill confidence in anyone with respect to either making or excluding a diagnosis of Hirschsprung disease. Studies have shown that the sensitivity of this procedure ranges from 80% to 88% and its specificity ranges from a low of 76% to a high of 98% in various series.

See the Garcia et al report (Use of the recto-sigmoid index to diagnose Hirschsprung's disease) that tells us about one more test—the recto-sigmoid index—as a tool to diagnose Hirschsprung disease.

J. A. Stockman III, MD

Use of the Recto-Sigmoid Index to Diagnose Hirschsprung's Disease
Garcia R, Arcement C, Hormaza L, et al (Louisiana State Univ, Baton Rouge)
Clin Pediatr (Phila) 46:59-63, 2007

The recto-sigmoid index on barium enema may aid in the diagnosis of Hirschsprung's disease. However, data on its reliability in different age groups are sparse. The recto-sigmoid index and transitional zone were evaluated blindly in 107 patients with diagnostic rectal suction biopsies. Patients were divided into 3 groups: neonates, infants older than 1 month, and children. The recto-sigmoid index and transitional zone agreed with the histopathologic diagnosis in 79% and 87% of the cases, respectively. Their negative predictive values reached clinical significance in infants and children but not in neonates. Their positive predictive values were not significant in any age group. The recto-sigmoid index identified 4 patients with recto-sigmoid Hirschsprung's disease whose diagnosis was missed by evaluating the transitional zone alone.

▶ In 1975, Pochaczevsky and Leonidas published an innovative article concerning the use of the anterior, posterior, and lateral view of the barium enema to diagnose distal Hirschsprung disease.[1] They calculated a "recto-sigmoid index," the widest diameter of the rectum divided by the widest diameter of the sigmoid colon. Initially, the recto-sigmoid index was used for the diagnosis of Hirschsprung disease in the first few weeks of life. Some suggested that it could also be used in older infants and children to aid in the diagnosis. The intent of the measurement was to refine the ability to identify the transitional zone that, for some, was not clearly visible. In this report, the investigators did not find any significant differences in the reliability of the recto-sigmoid index versus the appearance of a transitional zone in the diagnosis of Hirschsprung disease when performing a barium enema. This, taken together with the de Lorijn et al report (Diagnostic tests in Hirshsprung disease: a systematic review), means that once one performs a barium enema, one will still need to think about doing anorectal manometry or a rectal suction biopsy as the next screening test for the diagnosis of Hirschsprung disease.

For history aficionados in the reading audience, Hirschsprung's disease takes its name from a Danish pediatrician of German extraction, Dr Harald Hirschsprung (1830-1916), who, during a conference of the German Society of Pediatrics in Berlin in March 1886, presented two infants who died of complications of bowel obstruction. Autopsies revealed a marked dilatation and hypertrophy of the large intestine, whereas the rectum seemed to be normal. Hirschsprung considered the condition an inborn disease and named it congenital megacolon. Before this 1886 description, approximately 20 similar cases had been recorded in the medical literature in the period between 1825 and 1886. Hirschsprung himself added an additional 10 more cases before the time of his death on April 11, 1916. The term Hirschsprung's disease, as well as megacolon congenitum, came into widespread use circa 1893. At the beginning of the 20th century, others accurately described the pathological and anatomical findings of the aganglionic bowel. It was not until 1948, however, that theories related to the cause of Hirschsprung disease coordinated with a practical surgical approach to its cure. This was when Swenson published the results of an experimental study on the possibilities of surgical treatment of Hirschsprung's disease and proposed a new concept of its etiology.[2] Swenson's studies conclusively proved that megacolon in Hirschsprung's disease is secondarily related to an obstruction formed by an aganglionic narrow rectosigmoid, which prevents stool propulsion. Swenson's surgery brought, for the first time, a realistic hope that children with Hirschsprung's disease can be successfully cured.

To read more about the historical milestone of Hirschsprung's disease in commemoration of the anniversary of Professor Harald Hirschsprung's death, see the superb review of this topic by Skaba.[3]

J. A. Stockman III, MD

References

1. Pochaczevsky R, Leonidas JC. The "recto-sigmoid index:" a measurement for the early diagnosis of Hirschsprung's disease. *Am J Roentgenol Radium Ther Nucl Med.* 1975;123:770-777.
2. Swenson O, Rheinlander H, Diamond L. Hirschsprung disease: a new concept of the etiology. *N Engl J Med.* 1949;241:551-556.
3. Skaba R. Historic milestones of Hirschsprung disease. *J Pediatr Surg.* 2007;42: 249-251.

A Quantitative Immunochemical Fecal Occult Blood Test for Colorectal Neoplasia

Levi Z, Rozen P, Hazazi R, et al (Beilinson Hosp, Petach Tikva, Israel; Clalit Health Services, Tel Aviv and Bat-Yam, Israel; Tel Aviv Univ, Israel)
Ann Intern Med 146:244-255, 2007

Background.—Guaiac-based fecal occult blood tests (FOBTs) for colorectal cancer screening are not specific for human hemoglobin and have low sensitivity. Automated-development, immunochemical FOBT is quality-controlled, is specific for human hemoglobin, and does not require diet restriction.

Objectives.—To measure the sensitivity and specificity of quantitative immunochemical fecal hemoglobin measurements for detection of cancer and advanced adenoma in patients undergoing colonoscopy, to determine fecal hemoglobin thresholds that give the highest posttest probability for neoplasia, and to determine the number of immunochemical FOBTs needed.

Design.—Prospective, cross-sectional study.

Setting.—Ambulatory endoscopy services of the main health medical organization in Tel Aviv, Israel.

Participants.—1000 consecutive ambulatory patients—some asymptomatic but at increased risk for colorectal neoplasia and some symptomatic—who were undergoing elective colonoscopy and volunteered to prepare immunochemical FOBTs.

Intervention.—The hemoglobin content of 3 bowel movements was measured, and the highest value was compared with colonoscopy findings.

Measurements.—Sensitivity, specificity, predictive values, likelihood ratios, and 95% CIs of fecal hemoglobin measurements for clinically significant neoplasia, their relationship to the amount of fecal hemoglobin measured, and the number of immunochemical FOBTs performed.

Results.—Colonoscopy identified clinically significant neoplasia in 91 patients (cancer in 17 patients and advanced adenomas in 74 patients). Using 3 immunochemical FOBTs and a hemoglobin threshold of 75 ng/mL of buffer, sensitivity and specificity were 94.1% (95% CI, 82.9% to 100.0%) and 87.5% (CI, 85.4% to 89.6%), respectively, for cancer and 67% (CI, 57.4% to 76.7%) and 91.4% (CI, 89.6% to 93.2%), respectively, for any clinically significant neoplasia.

Limitations.—The fecal sampling method is standardized, but the sample size depends on fecal consistency. Some patients were tested while discontinuing aspirin and anticoagulant therapies. Study patients were at increased risk, and results might not apply to average-risk populations.

Conclusions.—Quantitative immunochemical FOBT has good sensitivity and specificity for detection of clinically significant neoplasia. Test performance in screening average-risk populations is not known.

▶ The old-fashioned guaiac-based FOBT may be going the way of the Model T Ford. The guaiac test has fairly low specificity for detecting human haemoglobin, and when used for screening purposes to detect fecal blood, it has fairly low sensitivity. More recently introduced is the office-developed quantitative immunochemical FOBT. The office varieties of these tests are specific for detection of human hemoglobin and have improved test specificity. Laboratory-based, automated immunochemical measurement of fecal human hemoglobin levels eliminates the need for diet restrictions, is specific for human, as opposed to animal, hemoglobin and allows for improved quality control. In addition, the test's sensitivity threshold can be set up or down depending on what a patient's actual risk is otherwise for advanced cancer detection.

The study reported from Israel measured the sensitivity and specificity of quantitative immunochemical fecal hemoglobin levels for the detection of cancer and advanced adenomas in adults who were undergoing colonoscopy to determine the fecal hemoglobin thresholds that would give the highest posttest probability for cancer. While the results of this study have no immediate direct translation to the care of children, it is clear that when studies such as this are done in adults, it is not too long after that we begin to see similar studies in children. In any event, be wary of investing further in companies that make guaiac tests. *Passé* is not a word that investors like to hear. Guaiac-based tests measure the peroxidase activity of hemoglobin. Drawbacks continue to include limited sensitivity and low patient adherence. Another disadvantage is poor specificity resulting in high false-positive rates because guaiac tests react with nonhuman heme in food. One advantage of guaiac tests is that they are cheap. The cost of immunochemical FOBT ranges from $18 to $30.

To close this commentary, here is a little known fact: a rectal examination can actually improve your hearing! Yes, in some instances this may be true, as evidenced by the case of a profoundly deaf, elderly man who was admitted to an emergency room with a history of constipation, a rectal examination did improve hearing. Communication with this individual was somewhat difficult because of his severe lack of hearing. Because of his history of constipation, a digital rectal exam was performed, but at the time of the examination, an unusual "skin tag" was observed. On further examination, the "skin tag" in fact was not anatomical, but a hearing aid firmly wedged between the gentleman's buttocks. The gentleman was as delighted as the ER physician was that his hearing aid had been found since he had been confined to silence for four days upon loss of the device. On rare occasions, rectal examinations can be more useful than one might think at improving one's hearing.[1]

J. A. Stockman III, MD

Reference

1. Mar F. Rectal examinations can improve your hearing. *BMJ.* 2007;334:85.

8 Genitourinary Tract

The 'learning curve' in hypospadias surgery

Horowitz M, Salzhauer E (New York Weill Cornell; SUNY Downstate Med Ctr, Brooklyn, NY)
BJU Internatl 97:593-596, 2006

Objective.—To provide an insight into the 'learning curve' of fellowship-trained paediatric urologists associated with hypospadias repair, as hypospadias surgery is one of the most common yet difficult procedures used by the paediatric urologist.

Patients and Methods.—Prospective data were collected on 231 consecutive hypospadias operations performed by one paediatric urologist (M.H.) over a 5-year period, beginning with his first year after completing his fellowship. All patients were having their first surgery and none had a staged repair. Fistula formation was used as a surrogate for the complication rate, as it is an objective measurable outcome that is easily identified with little interobserver or parental/physician variability. The follow-up included several visits in the 15 months after repair, during which virtually all complications could be identified and addressed.

Results.—The operative results improved throughout the 5 years of observation; there was a statistically significant decline in the fistula rate in each year of observation ($P < 0.001$; Kruskal-Wallis exact test for ranked groups). The absolute reduction in fistula rates between the first 2 and the last 2 years was 12.7% ($P < 0.02$; chi squared).

Conclusions.—The science and surgery of hypospadiology is mostly and correctly delegated to the paediatric urologist. Even in the hands of a fellowship-trained paediatric urologist, a successful repair, as measured by complication rate, statistically improves with time and experience.

▶ In Ladd's article, "Pediatric surgery fellowship compliance to the 80-hour work week," there is information on how compliant pediatric surgical residency training programs are with the Accreditation Council for Graduate Medical Education's requirement that all trainees spend no more than 80 hours a week in hospital. The assumption is that a reduced number of work hours produces improvements in the quality of care delivered as well as in patient safety while, hopefully, not decreasing the surgical training experience significantly, if at all. It is hard to imagine, however, that you can have it both ways. A reduction in work hours does mean a reduction in the number of patient contacts that one has. The article abstracted from the *British Journal of Urology* is an interesting one in that it provides insight into just how good an individual is after a surgical fellowship (this one in the field of pediatric urology). The article looks at the experiences of one very busy pediatric urologist to determine whether, over time, postfellowship improvements occurred in the quality of the surgical care related to hypospadias surgery.

The most commonly reported complication of hypospadias surgery is a urethrocutaneous fistula. If a fistula is going to develop, it almost certainly does so within 12 months of surgery; thus, it is a clear marker of quality surgery. In the article abstracted, fistula rates for the 231 boys who were operated on by this single surgeon declined each year the surgeon was in practice from a maximum incidence of 23% in the first year of practice to 6% in the fifth year. The surgical procedure performed was exactly the same each time. A more careful analysis of the surgical data shows that almost all of the improvement had occurred by the middle of the third year in practice, and a relative plateau is seen thereafter. In terms of actual surgical cases performed, this represents some 80 to 90 hypospadias repairs. Thus, if a pediatric surgical fellow were going to gain all the experience necessary during the 2 years of fellowship training to perform the very best hypospadias repair, the fellow would have to personally perform about 7 dozen of these highly technical procedures. This is not possible. Needless to say, surgeons over time learn "best practices" from their own experiences. The time to implement best practices could be significantly shortened if those in practice worked in collaboratives with other experienced practitioners to learn from one another.

It was in 1951 that Davis wrote, "The repair of hypospadias is no longer dubious, unreliable, or even extremely difficult. If tried and proven methods are scrupulously followed, a good result can be obtained in every case. Anything less than this suggests that the surgeon is not temperamentally fit for this kind of surgery."[1] Temperament aside, with tincture of time and experience in practice, a collaborative practice may, hopefully, prove the half-century old comments of Dr Davis to be true.

This commentary addressing physicians and their experiences in practices closes with two queries. The first question is: if you were to do a study of adults and ask them their preferences for what they think their doctor should wear, what do you think those preferences would be? The answer to this query comes from a report that appeared in the *American Journal of Medicine*.[2] Almost 8 in 10 patients preferred their doctor wear a white coat. Results from a survey of 400 people, mean age 52, showed that 76% favored professional attire with a white coat, followed by surgical scrubs (10.2%), business attire (8.8%), and casual dress (4.7%). It would be interesting to see how these data would look in pediatric practice.

With respect to trustworthiness, where do physicians stand relative to politicians and journalists? A survey to answer this question has not been carried out here in the United States, but was in Great Britain. It seems that 9 out of 10 people on the Isles still trust their physician. When surveyed by the Royal College of Physicians, 92% of patients trusted their doctor. Teachers, professors, and judges were equally trusted. However, politicians and governmental officials came in at just 20%. Journalists were at the bottom with a trustworthiness average of just 19% of people that believed journalists were not lying in their writings.[3]

J. A. Stockman III, MD

Reference

1. Davis DM. Surgical treatment of hypospadias, especially scrotal and perineal. *J Urol.* 1951;65:595-602.
2. Rehman SU, Nietert PJ, Cope DW, Kilpatrick AO. What to wear? Effect of doctor's attire on the trust and confidence of patients. *Am J Med.* 2005;118:1279-1286.
3. Hall, S. Doctors enjoy the greatest public trust. *The Guardian.* November 2, 2006. Available at: http://www.guardian.co.uk/medicine/story/0,,1937019,00.html. Accessed June 6, 2007.

Testicular microlithiasis in patients with Down Syndrome

Vachon L, Fareau GE, Wilson MG, et al (Univ of Southern California, Los Angeles)
J Pediatr 149:233-236, 2006

Objectives.—Testicular microlithiasis (TM) occurs with benign as well as with pathological conditions, such as testicular cancer. Since Down syndrome (DS) may be associated with increased frequency of testicular cancer, we determined the prevalence of TM in DS in patients from a DS clinic and evaluated the prevalence by age group.

Study Design.—We compared results of research scrotal ultrasounds obtained from 1998 to 2001 from 92 Latino patients with DS (ages newborn to 29.7 years) and clinical ultrasounds obtained from 1998 to 2004 from 200 Latino patients without DS (ages newborn to 18.3 years). We also reviewed the medical records.

Results.—The prevalence of TM in DS was 29%, significantly higher than the 7% found in patients without DS ($P < .0001$). Twenty of the 27 patients with DS and TM had no testicular pathology clinically or by history. The TM prevalence in the entire group of patients with and without DS increased with advancing age.

Conclusions.—We found a significantly increased prevalence of TM in DS. The clinical significance of TM needs to be investigated further.

▶ If you are not familiar with TM, this is a fairly uncommon condition in which small calcium concretions develop in the seminiferous tubules. These are readily diagnosed by the US appearance of small hyperechoic foci typically scattered throughout the testis. In the majority of individuals with TM, the condition is benign, but it can be associated with pathologic conditions, such as testicular germ cell tumors, cryptorchidism, delayed testicular descent, testicular torsion, infertility, and hypogonadism. In addition, some individuals with pulmonary alveolar microlithiasis, multiple lentigines, Kliefelter and McCune-Albright syndromes demonstrate TM. The primary interest in TM relates to the clinical concern of the high association of the finding with testicular cancer, which in some series runs as high as 46%. It is controversial whether

TM, when found without tumor, indicates an increased likelihood of later malignant degeneration. So far, follow-up studies of incidentally discovered TM in children are limited and do not suggest a higher-than-expected incidence of later cancer development.

This report from California tells us that TM has an extraordinarily high prevalence in those with DS. Almost 1 in 3 boys with DS will have TM. The clinical significance remains unknown, however. In the California series, 1 patient was found who had a testicular tumor 4 years after TM was identified. Some are considering the development of a registry for patients with TM to determine the natural history of related problems, such as testicular cancer. As of now, it is uncertain whether TM is, in fact, a predisposing factor for cancer, a malignant marker, or a coincidental finding.

One final comment about testicular microlithiasis: there is an extraordinarily high incidence of this in those who are competitive cyclists. It would appear that having one's privates traumatized on bicycle seats does indeed do some damage. It is suspected that this may be 1 of the reasons why there is a decreased sperm count in those engaged in this sporting activity.

J. A. Stockman III, MD

Prevalence of acquired undescended testis in 6-year, 9-year and 13-year-old Dutch schoolboys
Hack WWM, Sijstermans K, van Dijk J, et al (Med Centre Alkmaar, The Netherlands; Institution for Youth Health Care, Alkmaar, The Netherlands)
Arch Dis Child 92:17-20, 2007

Objective.—To investigate the prevalence of acquired undescended testis (UDT) in Dutch schoolboys.

Design and Participants.—As a part of routine school medical examinations, during a 2-year period (2001–3), testis position was determined in 6-year, 9-year and 13-year-old schoolboys. Before the examination, a parent questionnaire was sent inquiring both about the position of the testes and whether the child had been admitted earlier to hospital for orchidopexy. In 6-year and 13-year olds, a physical examination was performed by the school medical officer; in 9-year olds, a school nurse interview was held. Each boy for whom there was any doubt of the scrotal position was referred to the hospital for examination of both testes.

Setting.—Institution for Youth Health Care "Noordkennemerland" and Medical Centre Alkmaar, Alkmaar, the Netherlands.

Results.—Testis position was determined in 2042 boys aged 6, 1038 aged 9 and 353 aged 13. Of these, 47, 53 and 8 boys, respectively, were referred to the hospital and seen for further evaluation. The diagnosis of acquired UDT was made in 25 boys aged 6, 23 aged 9 and four aged 13. In 33 boys, a congenital UDT was diagnosed; 32 (97%) had already been diagnosed and treated at an early age.

Conclusions.—The prevalence of acquired UDT for 6-year, 9-year and 13-year olds was, respectively, 1.2% (25/2042), 2.2% (23/1038) and 1.1%

(4/353). In addition, congenital UDT is treated during the early years of life and, in contrast with popular belief, screening programmes for detecting UDT in the early years are successful.

▶ There are 2 varieties of UDT: one that presents early in life, commonly called congenital UDT, and one that presents a few years later, called acquired or ascending testis. In the second group, it seems that the testis has been positioned properly at an early stage of growth, but subsequently leaves its normal scrotal position to occupy itself within the inguinal area. The latter situation is quite controversial. Some have considered these cases to be mis-diagnoses owing to an error in earlier physical examinations. The cumulative experience of many, however, suggests that acquired UDT is a real phenom-enon, which explains a large proportion of orchidopexies performed after infancy.

If we accept that the ascending or acquired testis is a defined entity, the ob-vious issues are how common it is and how it should be managed. Several ex-tensive clinical trials have tried to evaluate the prevalence of acquired UDT. The current report by Hack et al summarizes a remarkable survey of 3 groups of boys in The Netherlands at the ages of 6, 9, and 13 years. A diagnosis of acquired UDT was made in these age groups, leading to a prevalence of 1.2%, 2.2%, and 1.1%, respectively. These data would suggest that acquired UDT occurs at a higher frequency compared with congenital UDT. The logical ques-tion is whether or not one should treat an acquired UDT. In the Hack study, boys with acquired UDT were followed up through puberty. Two thirds of these boys had spontaneous testicular descent. Nonetheless, Hack et al rec-ommend the use of human chorionic gonadotropin in these patients. Such therapy should be considered debatable, although most everyone would agree that periodic follow-up examinations of children with acquired UDT are mandatory.

You will have to be the judge of whether there is such a thing as acquired UDT, or whether these are testes that should still be grouped in the category of the "retractile" testis. Such testes have been called lots of things including the lazy testicle, the vanishing testicle, the yo-yo testis, and the nomad testis. All too often these testes undergo orchidopexy. All too often, the surgeon about to perform an orchidopexy in such patients finds that once the patient is under anesthesia, the testis suddenly has pulled a magic act and has reappeared in front of his or her eyes. In such cases, unfortunately, a surgeon may very well proceed to "tack down" the normal testis so that it is no longer nomadic.

While on the topic of issues with the genitalia, see how you would deal with the following case scenario. You receive a call from a nurse that is working at your triage after-hours service who has a question. She has never dealt with this problem before. The question is from parents of an 8-year-old that have called saying their son, who had been out swimming that day, is unable to get his swimming trunks off. Something that is part of the bathing suit appears to be caught on his penis. What do you think is going on here? If you read the December 2006 issue of *Pediatric Emergency Care*, you have the answer.[1] In that edition, two boys aged 8 years and one boy aged 9 years all presented with "penile bathing suit mesh entrapment." In each instance, the youngsters felt some pain in their groin or penis while swimming and later could not get their bathing suits off. The parents of all three youngsters who presented over a five-week period had uncovered the fact that the foreskins had somehow become entrapped within the tiny holes of the mesh lining of the swimsuits. The parents of all three boys dutifully trimmed off a square of the mesh around the penis and brought their kidos to an emergency room for examination and treatment. In each case, the ER staff was able to remove the mesh with scissors or a scalpel blade with no untoward outcomes. Previously, only zipper injuries have been recorded involving entrapment of the penis or foreskin. In general, zipper injuries are readily managed by removal of the zipper cutting the median bar and disassembling the two pieces of the zipper. Although a relatively simple procedure, zipper removal can be complicated by the anxiety and pain of a child, sometimes requiring procedural sedation. Fortunately, mesh entrapment is readily diagnosed and quickly treated. One wonders why the parents did not figure this out for themselves. Nonetheless, think of penile bathing suit mesh entrapment as an unusual, but not an impossible complication of swimming, at least in boys.

J. A. Stockman III, MD

Reference

1. Hoppa EC, Wiley JF. Bathing suit mesh entrapment: an unusual case of penile injury. *Pediatr Emerg Care.* 2006;22:813-814.

Male circumcision for HIV prevention in young men in Kisumu, Kenya: a randomised controlled trial

Bailey RC, Moses S, Parker CB, et al (Univ of Illinois at Chicago; Univ of Manitoba, Winnipeg, Canada; NIH, Bethesda, Md; et al)
Lancet 369:643-656, 2007

Background.—Male circumcision could provide substantial protection against acquisition of HIV-1 infection. Our aim was to determine whether male circumcision had a protective effect against HIV infection, and to assess safety and changes in sexual behaviour related to this intervention.

Methods.—We did a randomised controlled trial of 2784 men aged 18–24 years in Kisumu, Kenya. Men were randomly assigned to an intervention group (circumcision; n=1391) or a control group (delayed circumcision, 1393), and assessed by HIV testing, medical examinations, and behavioural interviews during follow-ups at 1, 3, 6, 12, 18, and 24 months. HIV seroincidence was estimated in an intention-to-treat analysis.

Findings.—The trial was stopped early on December 12, 2006, after a third interim analysis reviewed by the data and safety monitoring board. The median length of follow-up was 24 months. Follow-up for HIV status was incomplete for 240 (8.6%) participants. 22 men in the intervention group and 47 in the control group had tested positive for HIV when the study was stopped. The 2-year HIV incidence was 2.1% (95% CI 1.2–3.0) in the circumcision group and 4.2% (3.0–5.4) in the control group (p=0.0065); the relative risk of HIV infection in circumcised men was 0.47 (0.28–0.78), which corresponds to a reduction in the risk of acquiring an HIV infection of 53% (22–72). Adjusting for non-adherence to treatment and excluding four men found to be seropositive at enrollment, the protective effect of circumcision was 60% (32–77). Adverse events related to the intervention (21 events in 1.5% of those circumcised) resolved quickly. No behavioural risk compensation after circumcision was observed.

Interpretation.—Male circumcision significantly reduces the risk of HIV acquisition in young men in Africa. Where appropriate, voluntary, safe, and affordable circumcision services should be integrated with other HIV preventive interventions and provided as expeditiously as possible.

▶ This report and the Gray et al report (Male circumcision for HIV prevention in men in Rakai, Uganda: a randomised trial) provide results from 2 randomized trials showing considerable benefit of male circumcision in reducing HIV incidence in men, confirming findings from at least 1 earlier report on this same topic. The South African trial was done in a periurban setting near Johannesburg, in more than 3000 men, 18 to 24 years old, who were selected at random to receive immediate or later circumcision. The trial had to be stopped after a planned interim analysis showed a significant 60% relative reduction in HIV risk associated with circumcision. The participants were from the general population, and loss to follow-up was low, supporting the generalizability of these findings.

This report from Kenya was also done in men 18 to 24 years old, randomly assigned to circumcision or delayed circumcision. This trial was also stopped after an unscheduled interim analysis when evidence emerged of a significant benefit from circumcision. The HIV incidence rate was high, at 1.1 per 100 person years in the circumcised men and 2.1 per 100 person years in the control group (or 2.1% and 4.2%, respectively, over 2 years). These data represent an estimated 53% to 60% reduction in the relative risk of HIV associated with male circumcision.

Unfortunately male circumcision does not provide 100% protection against HIV infection. Condoms remain the mainstay of HIV prevention. The worst possible outcome from these 2 studies is that the street noise on the reports would lead high-risk men to believe that circumcision is the cure-all in prevention and, thus, can reduce condom use and increase risk taking. It is hoped this will not turn out to be the case.

Governments in Africa are weighing the ethics of mass circumcision to reduce HIV transmission. Is it ethical to circumcise everybody even if many will not benefit from the intervention—for example, people who do not engage in risky sexual behavior or are HIV-positive? Whether circumcised men who are infected with HIV are less likely to transmit the infection to their uninfected partners is not known at this time. A trial studying the male-to-female prevention effect of circumcision is in progress. Another ethical issue is whether mandatory circumcision of infants and young children who cannot consent to this procedure is appropriate. A recent law in South Africa banning circumcision in males younger than 16 years is an example of an effort to protect children from unsafe circumcision.[1]

To read more about male circumcision for the prevention of HIV and other sexually transmitted diseases, see the superb commentary by Flynn et al.[2] It is apparent that male circumcision may act directly to reduce the risk of HIV acquisition by reducing the ability of the virus to attach to and enter cells. The inner mucosal surface of the foreskin contains a higher density of Langerhans cells, a target cell for HIV, than stratified squamous epithelium (which is on the surface of the penis) and is more susceptible to HIV infection in vitro. The foreskin is also more susceptible to trauma, which may increase susceptibility to HIV infection during sexual activity.

All in all, circumcision does appear to have many benefits. Newborn circumcision may be preferable to circumcision at an older age because of its enhanced safety. It should be recognized, however, that since 1999, 16 states have eliminated Medicaid payments for circumcisions that were deemed "not medically necessary."[3] These actions were based, in part, on the American Academy of Pediatrics statement that "potential medical benefits . . . are not sufficient to recommend routine neonatal circumcision."[4] Data now clearly demonstrate the benefit of male circumcision as an intervention for the prevention of several forms of sexually transmitted diseases including HIV and genital cancers. Thus, if parents choose circumcision for their newborn male infant, or if an adolescent decides that circumcision might be appropriate to reduce the risk of sexually transmitted disease, it is a medically rational choice that should be included in government health or private insurance benefits. Clearly, the tide is swinging toward routine circumcision. At the time of the writing of the commentary by Flynn et al, the American Academy of Pediatrics was reviewing its 1999 circumcision policy statement that had been reaffirmed most recently in May of 2005.

One final comment about circumcision and the risk of HIV infection. A recent report has shown that circumcision can actually increase the transmission of HIV in Africa unless it is done in hygienic conditions.[5] Needless to say, circumcision is a bloody procedure, and all appropriate precautions need to be taken during the procedure to prevent the spread of HIV resulting from unsafe techniques.

J. A. Stockman III, MD

References

1. Timberg C. South Africa slow to encourage circumcision to curb HIV. *Washington Post*. July 16, 2006. Available at: http://www.washingtonpost.com/wp-dyn/content/article/2006/07/15/ar2006071501015.html. Accessed February 12, 2007.
2. Flynn P, Havens P, Brady M, et al. Male circumcision for prevention of HIV and other sexually transmitted diseases. *Pediatrics*. 2007;119:821-822.
3. National conference of state legislators. Circumcision and infection. State Health Notes. September 18, 2006. Available at: http://www.ncsl.org/programs/health/s8n/2006/hl475.htm#circumcision. Accessed November 6, 2006.
4. American Academy of Pediatrics, Task Force on Circumcision. Circumcision policy statement. *Pediatrics*. 1999;103:686-693.
5. Moszynski P. Unhygienic circumcisions may increase the risk of HIV in Africa. *BMJ*. 2007;334:498.

Male circumcision for HIV prevention in men in Rakai, Uganda: a random-ised trial
Gray RH, Kigozi G, Serwadda D, et al (Johns Hopkins Univ, Baltimore, Md; Rakai Health Sciences Program, Entebbe, Uganda; Makerere Univ, Kampala, Uganda; et al)
Lancet 369:657-666, 2007

Background.—Ecological and observational studies suggest that male cir-cumcision reduces the risk of HIV acquisition in men. Our aim was to inves-tigate the effect of male circumcision on HIV incidence in men.

Methods.—4996 uncircumcised, HIV-negative men aged 15–49 years who agreed to HIV testing and counselling were enrolled in this randomised trial in rural Rakai district, Uganda. Men were randomly assigned to receive immediate circumcision (n=2474) or circumcision delayed for 24 months (2522). HIV testing, physical examination, and interviews were repeated at 6, 12, and 24 month follow-up visits. The primary outcome was HIV inci-dence. Analyses were done on a modified intention-to-treat basis.

Findings.—Baseline characteristics of the men in the intervention and control groups were much the same at enrollment. Retention rates were much the same in the two groups, with 90–92% of participants retained at all time points. In the modified intention-to-treat analysis, HIV incidence over 24 months was 0.66 cases per 100 person-years in the intervention group and 1.33 cases per 100 person-years in the control group (estimated efficacy of intervention 51%, 95% CI 16–72; p=0.006). The as-treated ef-ficacy was 55% (95% CI 22–75; p=0.002); efficacy from the Kaplan-Meier time-to-HIV-detection as-treated analysis was 60% (30–77; p=0.003). HIV incidence was lower in the intervention group than it was in the control group in all sociodemographic, behavioural, and sexually transmitted dis-ease symptom subgroups. Moderate or severe adverse events occurred in 84 (3.6%) circumcisions; all resolved with treatment. Behaviours were much the same in both groups during follow-up.

Interpretation.—Male circumcision reduced HIV incidence in men with-out behavioural disinhibition. Circumcision can be recommended for HIV prevention in men.

Circumcision Status and Risk of Sexually Transmitted Infection in Young Adult Males: An Analysis of a Longitudinal Birth Cohort
Fergusson DM, Boden JM, Horwood LJ (Christchurch School of Medicine and Health Sciences, New Zealand)
Pediatrics 118:1971-1976, 2006

Objectives.—Previous research suggests that male circumcision may be a protective factor against the acquisition of sexually transmitted infections; however, studies examining this question have produced mixed results. The aim of this study was to examine the association between circumcision status and sexually transmitted infection risk using a longitudinal birth cohort study.

Methods.—Data were gathered as part of the Christchurch Health and Development Study, a 25-year longitudinal study of a birth cohort of New Zealand children. Information was obtained on: (1) the circumcision status of males in the cohort before 15 years old, (2) measures of self-reported sexually transmitted infection from ages 18 to 25 years, and (3) childhood, family, and related covariate factors.

Results.—Being uncircumcised had a statistically significant bivariate association with self-reported sexually transmitted infection. Adjustment for potentially confounding factors, including number of sexual partners and unprotected sex, as well as background and family factors related to circumcision, did not reduce the association between circumcision status and reports of sexually transmitted infection. Estimates of the population-attributable risk suggested that universal neonatal circumcision would have reduced rates of sexually transmitted infection in this cohort by 48.2%.

Conclusions.—These findings suggest that uncircumcised males are at greater risk of acquiring sexually transmitted infection than circumcised males. Male circumcision may reduce the risk of sexually transmitted infection acquisition and transmission by up to one half, suggesting substantial benefits accruing from routine neonatal circumcision.

▶ This report provides important new data that links circumcision status to the risk of acquiring a sexually transmitted disease. The study reports the findings of a 25-year longitudinal study of more than 500 males born in New Zealand. The purpose of the study was to examine the extent to which circumcision status is related to the subsequent risk of contracting a sexually transmitted infection. This study is an important one because of its longitudinal nature over more than two decades, which makes it possible to examine links between circumcision status and the risks of infection over more than a third of the average lifespan. Longitudinal studies are always better than cross-sectional studies, for which information is gathered at a particular point in time. The study also was of great value because it was able to integrate social, family, and individual factors into the analysis of potential linkages between circumcision status and the risk of acquiring a sexually transmitted disease. The conclusions were pretty straightforward: uncircumcised males have a risk of developing a sexually transmitted infection that is 3.19 times greater than that of circumcised males.

The data from this report are in fact consistent with several other reports, including those that have suggested that circumcision lowers the risk of HIV acquisition by 60% or more. Data from the United States suggest that circumcision could reduce rates of sexually transmitted infections in males by about at least one third overall, if not more.[1]

Please note that, if one looks at all of the data available about the benefits of circumcision for reducing the risk of sexually transmitted disease, there will be some variation with regard to the types of infections that are prevented. For example, there have been ongoing debates about the extent to which circumcision may play a protective role in reducing the risk of chlamydia infection.

Most of the data does suggest a lower risk of contracting syphilis and gonorrhea, and the data are also clear about the reduction in the risk of acquiring HIV infection.

Over the past 25 years, there has been growing opposition to the practice of routine neonatal circumcision on the grounds that the procedure has some complication risks and few long-term benefits. This report by Fergusson and colleagues, as well as other studies, suggests that this argument must be more finely balanced than critics of circumcision have implied. Both during infancy and after infancy, those who have been circumcised seem to experience small but consistent benefits in terms of reduced risks of penile infection (during middle childhood), urinary tract infection, and sexually transmitted infection. A carefully designed study needs to be performed to determine whether the risks of performing a circumcision outweigh these later benefits. Math is math, and someone should be able to do the analysis better than what has been done in the past based on these new data from New Zealand.

To read more about circumcision and the risk of sexually transmitted disease, see the superb commentary by Dickerman.[2] Dickerman notes that it is "disturbing" to note that the prevalence of circumcision has declined in the United States from 91% in the 1970s to 83% in the 1980s. By the turn of the millennium it had declined to 79%. In 2004, our colleagues in obstetrics and gynecology stated that, "A consensus is forming that circumcision offers protection against urinary tract infection, penile cancer, cervical cancer, genital ulcer disease and HIV."[3] Dickerman believes that there is now sufficient new information to call for a revised AAP policy statement regarding neonatal circumcision, considering the very significant beneficial effects and the very minor risks associated with the newborn procedure.

J. A. Stockman III, MD

References

1. Diseker RA, Peterman TA, Kamb ML, et al. Circumcision and STD in the United States: cross-sectional and cohort analyses. *Sex Transm Infect.* 2000;76:474-479.
2. Dickerman JD. Circumcision in the time of HIV: when is there enough evidence to revise the American Academy of Pediatrics' policy on circumcision? *Pediatrics.* 2007;119:1006-1007.
3. Alanis MC, Lucidi RS. Neonatal circumcision: a review of the world's oldest and most controversial operation. *Obstet Gynecol Surv.* 2004;59:379-395.

Predictors of Fatality in Postdiarrheal Hemolytic Uremic Syndrome
Oakes RS, Siegler RL, McReynolds MA, et al (Univ of Utah, Salt Lake City)
Pediatrics 117:1656-1662, 2006

Objectives.—Describe the cause of deaths among patients with postdiarrheal hemolytic uremic syndrome (HUS) and identify predictors of death at the time of hospital admission.

Methods.—Case-control study of 17 deaths among patients with HUS identified from the Intermountain HUS Patient Registry (1970–2003) compared against all nonfatal cases.

Results.—Of the 17 total deaths, 15 died during the acute phase of disease. Two died because treatment was withdrawn based on their preexisting conditions, and 1 died because of iatrogenic cardiac tamponade; they were excluded from analysis. Brain involvement was the most common cause of death (8 of 12); congestive heart failure, pulmonary hemorrhage, and hyperkalemia were infrequent causes. Presence of prodromal lethargy, oligoanuria, or seizures and white blood cell count (WBC) >20 × 10^9/L or hematocrit >23% on admission were predictive of death. In multivariate analysis, elevated WBC and elevated hematocrit were independent predictors. The combination of prodromal dehydration, oliguria, and lethargy and admission WBC values >20 × 10^9/L and hematocrit >23% appeared in 7 of the 12 acute-phase deaths.

Conclusions.—Diarrheal HUS patients presenting with oligoanuria, dehydration, WBC >20 × 10^9/L, and hematocrit >23% are at substantial risk for fatal hemolytic uremic syndrome. Such individuals should be referred to pediatric tertiary care centers.

▶ You do not hear much about HUS these days, largely because there has not been much new learned about it. Some 90% of childhood cases of HUS occur after a diarrheal episode that is usually bloody. The predominant cause of this is infection with shigatoxin-producing *Escherichia coli*, particularly, *E coli* 0157:H7. Patients who have HUS develop usually experience the triad of microangiopathic hemolytic anemia, thrombocytopenia, and acute nephropathy. Dialysis has dramatically reduced the mortality of this syndrome from just over 20% before the mid 1970s to less than 5% in the last 15 to 20 years.

The importance of the study from Utah is that a registry of cases now tells us exactly why some children with HUS die. Hemorrhagic CNS stroke and cerebral edema are the most common causes of death, along with colonic necrosis. The predictors of death at the time of admission to hospital include the duration of oliguria and anuria. Curiously, and contraintuitively, a hematocrit >23% seems to be the strongest predictor of a fatal outcome. The authors of this report speculate that in those who are destined to die there is such widespread microvascular disease at the time of presentation that blood actually does not perfuse the microvascular system thus minimizing red blood cell fragmentation and limiting the severity of anemia. It is also possible that the comparatively higher hematocrits might reflect a more fulminant toxic insult in which the full pathophysiology that leads to severe anemia may not have had time to kick in. In any event, woe betides the situation in which the hematocrit has not fallen remarkably.

Worry a great deal about a patient with HUS and really worry about those who have had a prolonged period of oligoanuria before admission along with an elevated white blood cell count (>20 × 10^9/L) and a hematocrit (>23%). It would behoove a care provider to get a patient presenting with such risk factors to a tertiary care center as quickly as possible, assuming that tertiary care center has an excellent track record in the management of children requiring dialysis.

J. A. Stockman III, MD

Chronic prostatitis during puberty

Li Y, Qi L, Wen JG, et al (Central South Univ, PRC China; Zhengzhou Univ, PRC China)

BJU Int 98:818-821, 2006

Objective.—To investigate the features of chronic prostatitis (CP) during puberty and the effects of biofeedback on young males with this disease.

Patients and Methods.—In all, 40 patients were divided into two groups; group 1 included 25 pubertal patients with CP (mean age 16.5 years, sd 1.1) and group 2 was a control group including 15 patients (mean age 16.2 years, SD 1.2) with a normal lower urinary tract. National Institute of Health-Chronic Prostatitis Symptom Index (NIH-CPSI) scores (three parts) were assessed individually in both groups. Expressed prostatic secretions and urine samples after prostate massage from group 1 were cultured to determine whether patients were infected with bacteria, and group 1 was categorized into various NIH types. Each patients in the two groups underwent urodynamics and group 1 were treated with biofeedback.

Results.—In group 1, there were one, three and 21 patients with type II, IIIA and IIIB prostatitis. The incidence of staccato voiding and detrusor-sphincter dyssynergia (DSD), and the maximum urinary flow rate (Q_{max}), postvoid residual urine volume (PVR), maximum detrusor pressure ($Pdet_{max}$) and maximum urethral closure pressure (MUCP) between the groups were significantly different ($P < 0.05$). The total NIH-CPSI scores and all the subdomains between the groups before biofeedback were significantly different ($P < 0.001$). In group 1 the difference in NIH-CPSI scores and Q_{max} before and after biofeedback was significant ($P < 0.05$).

Conclusions.—The main type of CP during puberty is IIIB; the dominating symptom is a voiding disorder. The impact on life and psychological effects are substantial. Pubertal boys with CP have pelvic floor dysfunction and several abnormal urodynamic values, i.e. staccato voiding, DSD, decreasing Q_{max}, and increasing $Pdet_{max}$ and MUCP. The effect of biofeedback strategies for treating pubertal CP is satisfactory.

▶ As common as CP is in young and middle aged men, it is rare in boys before puberty. During puberty, however, as the prostatic gland develops, boys may experience CP. The literature has been bereft of any information about this problem in teens, at least until this report from China appeared. It describes the many features of CP in young pubertal boys. The diagnosis usually follows a symptomatic complex set of voiding symptoms, including frequency, urgency, split stream, and sense of residual urine. Pain and discomfort, particularly testicular, penile, scrotal, and pelvic are frequent. Although there is no worldwide consensus as to the definition of chronic prostatitis, especially in younger men, the symptoms mentioned along with perineal and ejaculatory pain are the clues to the diagnosis. The real and perceived impacts of CP in those affected are substantial. Think of the diagnosis, otherwise the problem is only likely to get worse. Treatment with antibiotics helps as noted in this report, and ancillary therapies, including biofeedback, are often necessary in well-established cases of CP.

On a topic only broadly related to prostatitis, how would you deal with the following? One tends to associate the prevalence of erectile dysfunction with aging. Aging, of course, begins at birth. The question is, just how common is erectile dysfunction in teens and young adults such as college-age men?

A recent report gives us rather starling information about how common erectile dysfunction is in college-age males. An anonymous, self-administered survey was taken of 302 young men at three national universities in Chicago. Erectile dysfunction was defined as "ever having had difficulty getting or keeping an erection." Some 13% of college age males indicated that they had had this problem. Fewer than 3% experiencing the problem had discussed this condition with a medical care provider. Particularly common was erectile dysfunction when defined as "ever lost an erection while putting on a condom." Some 6% of those surveyed reported using Viagra, obtained largely from friends or non-medical sources, including the Internet.[1]

J. A. Stockman III, MD

Reference

1. Musacchio NS, Hartrich M, Garofalo R. Erectile dysfunction and Viagra use: what's up with college-age males? *J Adolesc Health*. 2006;39:452-454.

Single Kidney and Sports Participation: Perception Versus Reality
Grinsell MM, Showalter S, Gordon KA, et al (Univ of Virginia, Charlottesville)
Pediatrics 118:1019-1027, 2006

Objectives.—Physician opinions and practice patterns regarding the participation of children and adolescents with single, normal kidneys in contact/collision sports are widely varied. We hypothesize that limitation of participation from play based only on the presence of a single kidney is not supported by available data. We sought to determine recommendations of pediatric nephrologists regarding the participation of patients with single, normal kidneys in contact/collision sports and review the literature to determine the rate of sports-related kidney injury compared with other organs.

Methods.—Members of the American Society of Pediatric Nephrology were surveyed regarding their recommendations for participation of patients with single, normal kidneys in contact/collision sports. Medical and sports literature databases were searched to determine sports-related kidney, brain, spinal cord, and cardiac injury rates and the sports associated with kidney injury.

Results.—Sixty-two percent of respondents would not allow contact/collision sports participation. Eighty-six percent of respondents barred participation in American football, whereas only 5% barred cycling. Most cited traumatic loss of function as the reason for discouraging participation. The literature search found an incidence of catastrophic sports-related kidney injury of 0.4 per 1 million children per year from all sports. Cycling was the most common cause of sports-related kidney injury causing > 3 times the kidney injuries as football. American football alone accounted for 0.9 to 5.3 fatal brain injuries and 4.9 to 7.3 irreversible spinal cord injuries per 1 million players per year. Commotio cordis causes 2.1 to 9.2 deaths per year.

Conclusions.—Most pediatric nephrologists prohibit contact/collision sports participation by athletes with a single kidney, particularly football. The available evidence suggests that cycling is far more likely to cause kidney injury. In addition, kidney injury from sports is much less common than catastrophic brain, spinal cord, or cardiac injury. Restricting participation of patients with a single, normal kidney from contact/collision sports is unwarranted.

▶ In a report by Accadbled et al (Meniscal tears in children and adolescents: results of operative treatment), the long-term outcome is shown for meniscal tears in children and adolescents. Many of these knee injuries are the consequence of engagement in sporting activity. This article from the University of Virginia provides information about the risks of sports participation for youngsters who have a single kidney. We pediatricians are commonly asked to assess a patient for participation in contact and collision sports. For the purposes of evaluation, a single kidney historically has precluded engagement in such sporting activity. A single kidney is usually defined as a morphologically normal kidney without congenital abnormalities that resides in the usual anatomical site. Such kidneys may be somewhat larger than paired kidneys, but they are otherwise normal. Some controversy exists about whether youngsters with single kidneys can safely participate in contact/collision sports. Before 1994, the American Academy of Pediatrics (AAP) and the American Medical Association identified the presence of a single kidney as a disqualifying condition for participation in contact/collision sports. In addition, the National Kidney Foundation has advised kidney donors to avoid contact sports. Since 1994, however, the AAP has recommended a "qualified yes, pending individual assessment" regarding the participation of athletes with single kidneys in contact/collision sports. Unfortunately, a clear definition of "individual assessment" is not provided by the AAP. No other organization of medical professionals, including the American Urologic Association, American College of Sports Medicine, or the American Pediatric Surgery Association, has position statements regarding sports participation by athletes with a single kidney. Published opinions of medical professionals regarding these patients show little consensus on this issue. The majority of pediatric urologists currently recommend that athletes with a single kidney avoid contact sports. Most members of the American Society for Sports Medicine counsel athletes and families to avoid full sports participation if the athlete has a single kidney.

The authors of this article from the University of Virginia hypothesize that the opinions of physicians regarding the participation of athletes with single kidneys in contact and collision sports may not be supported by available literature. They theorize that the rate of kidney injury in contact/collision sports may, in fact, be lower than the rate of injury of unpaired organs such as the brain, spinal cord, and heart. They reviewed all the available literature to determine the rate of sports-related kidney injury and also surveyed the opinions of members of the American Society of Pediatric Nephrology on this topic.

So what did the Virginia folks find? They observed that pediatric nephrologists, as well as urologists and sports medicine physicians, largely counsel restriction of participation in contact and collision sports for children and adolescents with a solitary kidney. The reasons given were the potential for injury to result in end-stage renal disease or death, an increased risk of injury because of the compensatory hypertrophy of a single kidney, and concern over medicolegal action in case of renal injury. If one looks carefully at the medical literature, however, none of these arguments seem to hold up. Although the loss of a solitary kidney would, indeed, be catastrophic, there appears to be no documentation in the literature that the risk of that event is noteworthy. In fact, the risk of loss of life from injuries to other organs is significantly higher. The literature also does not support the fact that a slightly enlarged solitary kidney is more prone to injury, simply because of its size. With respect to the medicolegal consequences of allowing a child with a single kidney to participate in contact/collision sports, the authors of the article indicate that a full discussion of that topic is outside the scope of the medical literature. It was noted, however, that some athletes have used the legal system to successfully argue that prohibiting sports participation under such circumstances is, in fact, discriminatory.

So what's the punch line here? The conclusions of this article suggest that the current AAP recommendations, even though more liberal than before 1994, may be overprotective. The arguments that the authors use seem to be sound. You have 1 brain, 1 heart, and 1 spinal cord, all of which are more easily catastrophically injured than might be a solitary kidney. That is the basis of the authors' argument. I would suggest, however, that you are born with a fixed number of heartbeats and they should not be wasted on sporting activities. Such a philosophy would protect 100% of brains, hearts, spinal cords, and solitary kidneys. Because this belief is not likely to be accepted, you will have to be the judge, and bear all the consequences, of your decision to allow, or not allow, a patient with a single kidney to participate in contact sports.

To close this commentary, here is a diagnostic challenge for you. See what you would do with the following circumstance. Twenty-four hours after you admit a patient to the hospital, the urine collection bag of this patient turns an intense purple color. Even more curious is the fact that urine in the collecting tube proximal to the bag has stayed its usual yellow color. The question is: what is going on here and what diagnosis have you made for a problem the patient may have?

This turns out to be a real case. The explanation is that the patient had a urinary tract infection. Some bacteria are able to convert a metabolite of tryptophan into a substance that interacts with the plastic of urine collection bags to produce pigments. The pigments are either indirubin or indigo blue. Although quite dramatic, the "purple urine bag syndrome" is actually harmless and is easily curable by treatment of the urinary tract infection.[1]

J. A. Stockman III, MD

Reference

1. Beunk J, Lambert M, Mets T. The purple urine bag syndrome. *Age Ageing.* 2006;35:542.

9 Heart and Blood Vessels

Managed Care Network for the assessment of cardiac problems in children in a district general hospital: a working model
Pushparajah K, Garvie D, Hickey A, et al (Univ Hosp Lewisham, London; Guy's and St Thomas' Hosps Found Trust, London)
Arch Dis Child 91:892-895, 2006

Aim.—To assess a model for cardiology assessments in children with suspected heart disease by a general paediatrician with special expertise in paediatric cardiology (PsePC) in a district general hospital.

Methods.—A new monthly "screening" clinic was established in May 2004 by the PsePC to reduce the burden of new referrals on outreach tertiary paediatric cardiology services. All patients were to have echocardiograms as part of their referral for cardiac assessment. Over a one year period (May 2004–April 2005), through audit, details of referrers, indications for referral, echocardiography assessments, and subsequent management were recorded. This was compared with the pattern of patients seen in the joint paediatric cardiology outreach clinics over a two year period (May 2003–April 2005).

Results.—In the "screening" clinic, there were 75 appointments for 65 patients seen in 12 months. Fifty five of these patients had normal echocardiographic studies. Of the 47 referrals with heart murmurs in asymptomatic children, four had structurally abnormal hearts on echocardiographic assessment. Between May–October 2003 and November 2003–April 2004, the number of new patients with normal echocardiographic studies seen in the paediatric cardiology outreach clinic was 33/106 (31%) and 28/110 (25.4%) respectively. Following the introduction of the "screening" clinic, the number decreased to 21/99 (21%) during May–October 2004, and 10/102 (9.8%) during November 2004–April 2005.

Conclusion.—This model can work effectively in order to identify pathology requiring input of a paediatric cardiologist more appropriately. Paediatricians with specific training in paediatric cardiology are potentially well equipped to provide this basic screening service.

▶ There is a great deal to be learned about health services provided elsewhere in the world. We are not unique here in the United States, with increasing demands being placed upon our pediatric subspecialists. In Great Britain, in recent years, there has been a 50% increase in the demand for pediatric cardiology services, as one example. Some of this is driven by the increase in the number of children being referred for echocardiography, youngsters with asymptomatic murmurs. The number of well-trained pediatric cardiologists in Great Britain is fairly modest. To handle the problem, some general pediatricians have gained special expertise in certain areas of pediatric cardiology, what we call in the United States a general pediatrician with an area of special interest. Specifically, pediatricians in Great Britain are being trained to read echocardiograms of patients referred by general practitioners, largely patients with asymptomatic murmurs.

What we see in this report from London is an interesting hub-and-spoke model of health care delivery in which selected general pediatricians are trained in echocardiography under the regular supervision of a pediatric cardiologist. The training involves a minimum of 200 echocardiograms performed annually under the direct supervision of the cardiologist in monthly joint clinics. In the "screening" clinic, the echocardiogram is read by the generalist pediatrician who has a special interest in echocardiography. A pediatric cardiologist subsequently reviews all the echocardiograms. This allows for an efficient screening referral process to the pediatric cardiologist, when necessary. Of the echocardiograms screened by generalist pediatricians, 91.5% were found to be normal. Of the 8.5% of echocardiograms with abnormal findings, the most common abnormality was pulmonary stenosis, followed by ventricular septal defect and mild aortic stenosis. The model described remarkably reduces the number of referrals to pediatric cardiology centers.

It is hard to say whether the model described will ever catch on here in the United States. While the number of referrals to pediatric subspecialists has increased significantly, the marketplace in terms of supply of pediatric subspecialists is finally beginning to catch up. It is also hard to say whether parents would be satisfied with being seen by a non–fully trained subspecialist, but frankly, many problems seen by subspecialists can, all other things considered, be properly evaluated and managed by a generalist. All other things considered means being adequately reimbursed for those services and having the time to perform those services in a busy generalist practice.

While on the topic of things having to do with the heart, how would you handle the following situation in which you are being asked for some guidance? A teenager in your practice asks for some career advice. He has considered a number of options, but is enchanted with the possibility of becoming a firefighter. He knows all the usual risks associated with such a high-hazard job, but wants to ask about some of the associated remote risks such as an increased probability of illness and death due to cardiovascular disease. How would you answer his questions about his career choice? The most precise answer you could give this teen comes from a recent report about emergency duties and deaths from heart disease among firefighters here in the United States.[1] The story regarding cardiovascular disease in such an occupation as firefighting is not a simple one. It is not surprising that firefighters face an increased risk of illness and death due to cardiovascular disease during periods of intense physical and even psychological stress while at work, but firefighters as a group quintessentially show a "healthy worker effect." By the very nature of their generally high levels of fitness and health (mandated for all entry-level career firefighters and sometimes required for volunteers), they are indeed expected to have a lower risk of death (particularly due to cardiac events) than the general population. And they do—on average, a firefighter's risk of dying from coronary heart disease is about 90% of a peer population. Thus, firefighters overall do not have an excess risk of dying from heart disease, or if they do, the excess risk must be very small.

So does that mean firefighters are off the hook entirely with respect to heart attacks? The answer is no. During actual periods of fire suppression, the odds of death from coronary heart disease rise to somewhere between 10 and 10 times as high for a firefighter compared with firefighters during non-emergency duties. This risk exists not only during periods of fire suppression, but also during the alarm response phase of a call. During periods of actual firefighting, there are other factors that also may amplify this risk of heart attack, including exposure to chemicals (such as carbon monoxide), fine particulate matter, and other cardiac toxins. Thermal and emotional stress obviously play a role. Likewise, although there has been marked improvement in respiratory protection during active fire suppression, firefighters frequently abandon this equipment during overhaul (the period immediately after fire suppression), when exposure to fine particulate matter, which has been shown to increase the risk of sudden myocardial infarction and other toxic chemicals, may be particularly high.

Firefighters (like many police officers) enter the workforce particularly healthy having coming off of the equivalent of "basic training," but they do not necessarily maintain this attribute over time. There is more than ample evidence to suggest that firefighters in particular are not immune to the hazards of overeating and inadequate regular off-the-job exercise. Just look at the menu that firefighters serve themselves in the firehouse. Volunteer firefighters, in particular, often serve with fewer entry and ongoing fitness requirements and serve until older ages, when most cardiac events occur. Seventy percent of cardiac events occur among volunteer firefighters.

Needless to say, you can advise this teenager that if he wishes to maintain a healthy career as a firefighter, he should stay physically active. One wonders whether older firefighters might pop a beta-blocker before buckling up next to the dalmatian when heading out to douse the flames. In other circumstances, beta-blockers do in fact suppress the sudden responses to adrenaline seen in "emergency" situations.

J. A. Stockman III, MD

Reference

1. Kales SN, Soteriades ES, Christophi CA, Christiani DC. Emergency duties and deaths from heart disease among firefighters in the United States. *N Engl J Med.* 2007;356:1207-1215.

How effectively can clinical examination pick up congenital heart disease at birth?
Patton C, Hey E (Wansbeck Hosp, Ashington, Northumberland, England; Newcastle upon Tyne, England)
Arch Dis Child Fetal Neonatal Ed 91:F263-F267, 2006

Aims.—To assess what proportion of all cardiac abnormality can be suspected at birth when all clinical examination before discharge is undertaken by a small stable team of clinicians.

Methods.—A prospective audit of all the 14,572 births in a maternity unit only staffed by nurse practitioners between 1996 and 2003.

Results.—1.2% of all babies born in the unit were found to have a structural defect (as confirmed by echocardiography) within a year of birth. The number not suspected before discharge declined over time, and only 6% were first suspected after discharge in the last four years of this eight year study. Four potentially life threatening conditions initially went unsuspected in 1996–8, but none after that. A policy of referring every term baby with a murmur at 1 day of age that was still present at 7–10 days resulted in 4.2% requiring cardiac referral; 54% of these babies still had a murmur when assessed one to two weeks later, and 33% had a structural defect. Parents said in independent, retrospectively conducted, interviews that they found it confidence building to have any possible heart defect identified early and the cause of any murmur clearly and authoritatively explained.

Conclusions.—Effective screening requires experience and a clear, structured, referral pathway, but can work much better than most previous reports suggest. Whether staff bring a medical or nursing background to the task may well be of less importance.

▶ Congenital heart disease is a major cause of death in infancy and term infants. It accounts for 3% of all infant deaths and 46% of all deaths from congenital malformations. Those surviving beyond infancy have a 96% chance of living into young adulthood and longer. For these reasons, adequate screening for congenital heart disease in the nursery is essential. Routine antenatal screening for congenital heart defects is also important, but most data suggest that at best fewer than 25% of structural lesions are identified by prenatal ultrasound. For these reasons, routine clinical examination of all newborn infants remains mandatory with the expectation that the physical examination is capable of picking up most lesions. In fact, as this report shows, physical examination misses some disease. The question is, however, can we do better?

The majority of congenital heart disease lesions presenting in the immediate newborn period is fairly limited. The vast majority of early deaths, particularly those occurring in the first 2 weeks of life, are due to a handful of conditions. These are the so-called ductal-dependent lesions, namely, coarctation of the aorta, critical aortic stenosis, interrupted aortic arch, hypoplastic left heart syndrome, transposition of the great arteries, pulmonary atresia, and critical pulmonary stenosis. To these must be added obstructed total anomalous pulmonary venous connection. These lesions, although individually rare, do form the large majority of the life-threatening heart conditions in the newborn period. The aim of any screening program for congenital heart disease in a nursery therefore should be to identify these conditions.

Most studies of the value of the newborn physical examination to detect congenital heart disease have shown uniformly poor detection abilities with less than half the infants with heart defects of all types detected in the nursery. In contrast, the study abstracted from Ashington in the north of England shows what can be achieved if a newborn service puts its mind to it. In a hospital in Ashington, a newborn congenital heart disease service was created to be delivered by nurse practitioners with maximum support and training from neonatal consultant pediatricians and a regional pediatric cardiac center. The experience shows an initial learning curve that is a bit long, but ultimately a trained nurse is able to detect more than 90% of congenital heart disease with a specificity >97% in terms of referral accuracy. No infant with a life-threatening condition was missed once a nurse practitioner was fully trained. One key to success here was keeping infants around long enough for some of the clinical manifestations of congenital heart disease to manifest. For example, assessment performed within 6 hours of birth in infants who were set for early discharge clearly was more likely to miss ductal-dependent lesions because in many infants the duct may still be widely patent. Ideally, examinations should be performed on the second or third day of life, which may not be a possibility here in the United States for many infants.

The newborn detection of congenital heart disease requires training, training, training. In many instances the signs and symptoms will not jump out at you. Heart failure, for example, is quite uncommon in the immediate newborn period. Most infants will look quite well at birth. For this reason, surrogate markers of heart disease must be sought including barely detectable levels of cyanosis, murmurs, and poor pulses. Poor pulses have to be carefully looked for. Murmurs, when present, should be able to be detected. Several studies have suggested that pulse oximetry should be a routine part of the physical examination of a newborn. A carefully performed physical examination complimented by pulse oximetry would go a long way in detecting infants with congenital heart disease. Nonetheless, it must be recognized that clinical examination on its own will never be completely 100% sensitive when it comes to malformations of the heart. The ideal would be for all infants to have a screening echocardiogram before discharge. Given the logistics and costs associated with this, this is not a functional reality, at least at this point in time. Thus, it is up to the eyes and ears and fingers of clinicians, both physicians and nurses, to give every infant with congenital heart disease a fighting chance by early detection in the immediate newborn period.

J. A. Stockman III, MD

Racial and Ethnic Disparities in Mortality Following Congenital Heart Surgery

Benavidez OJ, Gauvreau K, Jenkins KJ (Children's Hosp Boston)
Pediatr Cardiol 27:321-328, 2006

Our objective was to assess risk-adjusted racial and ethnic disparities in mortality following congenital heart surgery. We studied 8483 congenital heart surgical cases from the Kids' Inpatient Database 2000. Black sub-analysis was performed using predetermined regional categories. For our Hispanic sub-analyses, we categorized Hispanics into state groups according to a state's predominant Hispanic group: West (Mexican-American), Southeast (Cuban-American), Northeast (Puerto Rican), and Mixed/Heterogeneous. Risk adjustment was performed using the Risk Adjustment for Congenital Heart Surgery method. Multivariate analyses assessed the effect of race/ethnicity and Hispanic state group on mortality and explored the effects of gender, income, insurance type, and region. Black children had a higher risk for death than Whites odds ratio (OR), [1.65; $p = 0.003$]. Hispanics and the Cuban-American state group showed a trend toward a higher death risk (Hispanic: OR, 1.24; $p = 0.16$; Southeast Cuban-American: OR 1.55; $p = 0.08$). Disparities were not influenced by insurance. Among Blacks, disparities were greatest in the Northeast region (OR, 2.25; $p = 0.007$). After adjusting for gender, income, and region, Blacks (OR, 1.76; $p = 0.002$) and Hispanics (OR, 1.34; $p = 0.05$) had a higher death risk. Racial and ethnic disparities in risk-adjusted mortality following congenital heart disease exist for Blacks and Hispanics. These disparities are not due to insurance but are partially explained by gender and region.

▶ The Agency for Healthcare Research and Quality (AHRQ) developed the healthcare cost utilization project Kids Inpatient Database (KID) back in 2000. The database was developed specifically to examine issues pertinent to healthcare delivery in children and consists of a random sample of more than 2.5 million discharges from almost 3000 institutions in 27 states. What we learn from KID with respect to congenital heart surgery outcomes is that when individuals are risk-adjusted for all variables except race and ethnicity, black children will have a significantly higher likelihood of dying when compared with white children. This finding was not explainable by insurance differences. Adjusting for income increases the magnitude of the disparity. Black children disproportionately resided in the south, which tended to have slightly higher risks-adjusted death rates than other regions, but this accounts for only a small portion of the differences in outcomes between black and white children. In fact, disparities are greatest in other regions, especially the northeast, where black children have more than twice the odds of dying than white children. Similar trends are seen for Hispanic children; however, these differences do not reach statistical significance.

The body of literature is now clearly growing that demonstrate worse outcomes for black and Hispanic children undergoing congenital surgery. The findings seem to suggest that differences in outcome may be related to access to optimal cardiovascular care rather than biology.

Racial and ethnic disparities have been reported in other complex pediatric medical care. In a study of pediatric patients at the time of their first dialysis for end-stage renal disease, it was found that black children were less likely to be wait listed for renal transplantation at any given time in follow-up.[1] Similarly, nonwhite children are twice as likely to be admitted to hospital with complications of diabetes mellitus and have longer hospital stays.

So are the differences seen in healthcare outcomes related to biology or to disparate access in healthcare services across races and ethnicities? Given the wide variation in outcomes across the United States, it would seem that biology is not the key factor. You will need to read this report in some detail to get any inkling about what types of remedies would address the disparities found in this report. Thank goodness for KID 2000, which at least provides us with accurate information about the magnitude of the problem.

J. A. Stockman III, MD

Reference

1. Carr W, Zeitel L, Weiss K. Variations in asthma hospitalization and deaths in New York City. *Am J Public Health.* 1992;82:59-65.

Predictors of Spontaneous Closure of Isolated Secundum Atrial Septal Defect in Children: A Longitudinal Study

Hanslik A, Pospisil U, Salzer-Muhar U, et al (Med Univ of Vienna; Univ of Vienna)
Pediatrics 118:1560-1565, 2006

Objectives.—The goals were to assess the frequency of spontaneous closure of isolated secundum atrial septal defect in children and to identify predictors of spontaneous atrial septal defect closure.

Methods.—A retrospective cohort study was performed in a tertiary care pediatric cardiology center. Consecutive patients ($n = 200$) diagnosed as having isolated atrial septal defects (no multiple or fenestrated atrial septal defects, no additional congenital heart disease, and no syndromes) were monitored for >6 months with serial 2-dimensional echocardiography, according to a standardized protocol.

Results.—The median age at diagnosis was 5 months (minimum: 0 months; maximum: 13.9 years). The atrial septal defect diameter at diagnosis was 4 to 5 mm in 40% of cases, 6 to 7 mm in 28% of cases, 8 to 10 mm in 21% of cases, and >10 mm in 11% of cases. The median age at the final follow-up evaluation was 4.5 years (range: 6.8 months to 16.2 years). Thirty-four percent of atrial septal defects showed spontaneous closure, and 28% decreased to a diameter of ≤3 mm. Logistic regression analysis revealed atrial septal defect diameter and age at diagnosis as independent predictors of spontaneous closure or regression to ≤3-mm defect size. Of atrial septal defects with a diameter of 4 to 5 mm at diagnosis, 56% showed spontaneous closure, 30% regressed to a diameter of ≤3 mm, and none required surgical closure. Of atrial septal defects with a diameter of >10 mm at diagnosis, none closed spontaneously, whereas 77% required surgical or device closure. Gender and observation time were not associated with spontaneous atrial septal defect closure or regression to ≤3 mm.

Conclusions.—In the present study population of children with atrial septal defects, 62% showed spontaneous closure (34%) or regression to ≤3 mm (28%). Initial atrial septal defect diameter was the main predictor of spontaneous closure.

▶ You would think by now that we would have nailed down all of the "demographics" of how and when atrial septal defects (ASDs) close. The natural course and frequency of the spontaneous closure of ASDs has been assessed in a number of studies, but the results are in fact quite divergent: closure rates range from 4% to 87%. Most of this variation is explained by differing selections of study populations with respect to ASD sizes or patient ages. Unfortunately, much of the early data about ASD closures was based on diagnosis achieved through cardiac catheterization, which is no longer performed for this purpose, and these early study populations are hardly comparable with those in more recent investigations with echocardiographic diagnosis. This report out of Austria does us a great service by giving us information not only about size at the time of diagnosis but also about the likelihood of closure on the basis of age at diagnosis.

What we learn from this report is that, when an ASD is detected, the average age of diagnosis will be 5 months, and the ASD size will range from 4 mm to in excess of 10 mm. The female-to-male ratio was shown in this report to be 2:1, which was similar to earlier reports. Unlike earlier studies, however, there was a predominance of small- and moderate-sized defects, which is probably best explained by early detection using echocardiography. Needless to say, there was a positive correlation of ASD size with age at diagnosis. This correlation is probably explained by the fact that, in older children, small defects have already closed spontaneously, leaving mainly large defects to be observed. Of all of the ASDs diagnosed, the majority (77%) showed regression over time, and some 34% of ASDs actually showed spontaneous closure. As compared with prior studies, this is a fairly high closure rate. Also, 28% of ASDs showed regression to a residual size of ≤3 mm; this is roughly the size of a normal patent foramen ovale, which, in general, is left alone. However, we all know from recent literature that persistent foramen ovale has been implicated in cryptogenic stroke and decompression sickness. Device closure has been suggested for adults. Needless to say, this report suggests that youngsters who are ultimately found to have the equivalent of a patent foramen ovale should be followed throughout adolescence to see if these findings go away or whether, on the basis of new information, the "defect" should be closed.

This report also suggests that it may be worth waiting for a while before sending a youngster off for an operative closure or asking the invasive cardiologist to close the lesion with a septal device. The median age at spontaneous ASD closure in this series was 4.2 years, and the 75th percentile for closure was 5.8 years. Thus, the optimum timing for elective device closure for young children with 8-mm to 10-mm defects must be considered quite carefully. The results from this report provide evidence that supports current recommendations that elective closure (either surgical or device) for asymptomatic children should not be performed before the age of 5 to 6 years. This suggestion seems to make sense, because the majority of ASDs do seem to respond with spontaneous complete closure or regression to ≤3 mm. Thus, it is up to us to "hold our horses" and to let the tincture of time do its thing in resolving ASDs during the first few years of life.

J. A. Stockman III, MD

Transitional Medicine: Will Emergency Medicine Physicians Be Ready for the Growing Population of Adults With Congenital Heart Disease?
Cross KP, San Tucci KA (Yale-New Haven Children's Hosp, Conn)
Pediatr Emerg Care 22:775-781, 2006

Background.—Currently, approximately 85% of children with significant congenital heart problems survive to adolescence and adulthood. This survival rate represents a dramatic improvement in the medical and surgical care of congenital heart disease (CHD) during the last 35 years. Nevertheless, these patients remain at increased risk for significant cardiac problems long after primary interventions are completed. They are more likely than the general population to seek urgent medical care, often in an emergency department setting. They represent a new and growing population of emergency department patients with a specialized set of problems not traditionally part of the training for emergency medicine (EM) physicians.

Objective.—We investigated the current scope and status of training for EM physicians in the immediate management of CHD patients as they grow to adolescence and adulthood.

Methods.—We conducted 2 cross-sectional surveys to assess the current training environment for 2 specific groups: (1) US general EM (GEM) residency programs, and (2) US and Canadian pediatric EM (PEM) fellowship programs. Surveys were mailed to program directors during the summer of 2005. A total of 198 surveys were sent out: 134 to GEM residency directors and 64 to PEM fellowship directors.

Results.—The response rate overall was 68%, with a 64% response rate from the GEM residency directors and 77% from the PEM fellowship directors. Across all programs, 43% (56/130 respondents) were "unsure" about the existence or location of an adult CHD (ACHD) clinic in their area. When asked to rate the importance of ACHD as a training topic, 40 (85%) of 47 PEM fellowship directors and 62 (74%) of 84 GEM residency directors ranked it as "low priority" or "unnecessary." However, 70 (55%) of 127 respondents were "unsure," "uncomfortable," or "worried" about the ACHD training their trainees receive (PEM, 59%; GEM, 53%). In addition, most program directors (75%) estimated that their trainees care for 5 or fewer ACHD patients annually.

Conclusions.—There seems to be a mismatch between the growing need for ACHD emergency care and the current state of this topic in both GEM residency and PEM fellowship training programs.

▶ There are lots of orphans in this world. The adult with CHD frequently is such an orphan. The incidence of complex and moderate CHD has been estimated at 1.5 and 2.5 per 1000 live births, respectively. This converts to 9000 new cases of CHD annually in the United States. More than 85% of these children will grow up to be adult CHD survivors. As of the year 2000, there were an estimated 420,000 adult survivors of CHD. There are roughly twice as many survivors older than 15 years than there are children living with CHD. This high survival rate is a testimony to the quality of care given by pediatricians, pediatric cardiologists, and pediatric cardiac surgeons as well as other providers.

As youngsters with CHD transition into adulthood, they remain at risk for significant medical problems. They are more likely than the general population to need urgent medical care. Patients with CHD who have had a surgical repair have been shown to be 25 to 100 times more likely to experience sudden death than age-matched controls without CHD.[1] There is a much higher prevalence of arrhythmias, acute congestive heart failure, and infections in this population. What we see in this report is that there seems to be a growing need for training for these disorders in both GEM residency programs and PEM fellowship programs. This problem represents an example of the difficulties with transitional medicine of all types in our current training programs. Patients with cystic fibrosis and regional enteritis experience similar difficulties as they move into adulthood. This problem is only more likely to become worse now that graduates of PEM training programs increasingly enter community emergency department settings and, thus, are further away from the training sites where they had a fair volume of experience in handling these problems.

Clearly, we must do better for our patients with CHD during the transition to adulthood. Cystic fibrosis, childhood cancer, and congenital myopathies are examples of once-fatal pediatric illnesses that today have many adult survivors, often with very unique and special needs. Our internal medicine colleagues are beginning to recognize the necessity for them to gain greater skill in the care of such disorders.

While on the topic of life expectancy, among large developed countries, which has the longest life expectancy at birth and which has the shortest? The following table provides the answer to this query. It is wise to be born in Japan and even wiser not to be a man living in Russia[2]:

Life Expectancy at Birth, by Sex - Selected Countries, 2001

Females	Country	Males
84.9	Japan	78.1
84.6	Hong Kong	78.4
83.0	Switzerland	77.4
82.9	Spain	75.6
82.9	France	75.5
82.8	Italy	76.7
82.4	Australia	77.0
82.2	Canada	77.1
82.1	Sweden	77.6
81.6	Israel	77.1
81.5	Norway	76.2
81.5	Finland	74.6
81.5	Austria	75.6
81.3	Germany	75.6
81.1	Singapore	76.5
81.1	Belgium	74.9
80.9	New Zealand	76.0
80.7	Netherlands	75.8
80.7	Greece	75.4
80.6	England and Wales	76.0
80.3	Portugal	73.5
80.1	Northern Ireland	75.2
80.0	Puerto Rico	71.0
79.9	Costa Rica	75.6
79.8	United States	74.4
79.7	Ireland	74.7
79.3	Denmark	74.7
79.2	Cuba	74.7
78.8	Scotland	73.3
78.7	Chile	72.7
78.5	Czech Republic	72.1
78.3	Poland	70.2
77.7	Slovakia	69.6
76.4	Hungary	68.1
75.4	Bulgaria	68.6
75.0	Romania	67.7
72.3	Russia	59.1

J. A. Stockman III, MD

Reference

1. Silka MJ, Hardy BG, Menashe VD, Morris CD. A population-based prospective evaluation of risk of sudden cardiac death after operation for common congenital heart defects. *J Am Coll Cardiol*. 1998;32:245-251.
2. National Center for Health Statistics. QuickStats: life expectancy at birth, by sex-selected countries 2001. *MMWR* [serial online]. 2006;55:631. Available at: http://www.cdc.gov/mmwr/preview/mmwrhtml/mm5522a6.htm. Accessed June 14, 2007.

Aneurysm Syndromes Caused by Mutations in the TGF-β Receptor

Loeys BL, Schwarze U, Holm T, et al (Johns Hopkins Univ, Baltimore, Md; Kennedy Krieger Inst, Baltimore, Md; Univ of Washington, Seattle; et al)
N Engl J Med 355:788-798, 2006

Background.—The Loeys–Dietz syndrome is a recently described autosomal dominant aortic-aneurysm syndrome with widespread systemic involvement. The disease is characterized by the triad of arterial tortuosity and aneurysms, hypertelorism, and bifid uvula or cleft palate and is caused by heterozygous mutations in the genes encoding transforming growth factor β receptors 1 and 2 (*TGFBR1* and *TGFBR2*, respectively).

Methods.—We undertook the clinical and molecular characterization of 52 affected families. Forty probands presented with typical manifestations of the Loeys–Dietz syndrome. In view of the phenotypic overlap between this syndrome and vascular Ehlers–Danlos syndrome, we screened an additional cohort of 40 patients who had vascular Ehlers–Danlos syndrome without the characteristic type III collagen abnormalities or the craniofacial features of the Loeys–Dietz syndrome.

Results.—We found a mutation in *TGFBR1* or *TGFBR2* in all probands with typical Loeys–Dietz syndrome (type I) and in 12 probands presenting with vascular Ehlers–Danlos syndrome (Loeys–Dietz syndrome type II). The natural history of both types was characterized by aggressive arterial aneurysms (mean age at death, 26.0 years) and a high incidence of pregnancy-related complications (in 6 of 12 women). Patients with Loeys–Dietz syndrome type I, as compared with those with type II, underwent cardiovascular surgery earlier (mean age, 16.9 years vs. 26.9 years) and died earlier (22.6 years vs. 31.8 years). There were 59 vascular surgeries in the cohort, with one death during the procedure. This low rate of intraoperative mortality distinguishes the Loeys–Dietz syndrome from vascular Ehlers–Danlos syndrome.

Conclusions.—Mutations in either *TGFBR1* or *TGFBR2* predispose patients to aggressive and widespread vascular disease. The severity of the clinical presentation is predictive of the outcome. Genotyping of patients presenting with symptoms like those of vascular Ehlers–Danlos syndrome may be used to guide therapy, including the use and timing of prophylactic vascular surgery (Figs 2 and 3).

▶ Most pediatricians are not familiar with the Loeys–Dietz syndrome, but they should be. The syndrome represents one end of a spectrum of genetic disorders associated with problems in connective tissue development, particularly that involving blood vessels. Mutations in the genes encoding transforming growth factor β (TGF-β) receptors 1 and 2 (*TGFBR1* and *TGFBR2*, respectively) have been noted in association with these clinical disorders. On the mild end, the mutations have been found in association with a presentation very similar to that of Marfan's syndrome or with thoracic aortic aneurysm and dissection conditions found within certain families. On the severe end, they are associated with a complex phenotype in which aortic dissection or rupture

A Loeys–Dietz Syndrome Type I

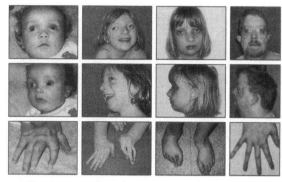

B Loeys–Dietz Syndrome Type II

C Loeys–Dietz Syndrome Type I

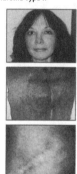

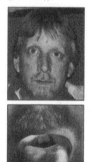

D

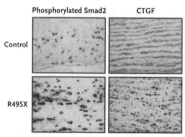

FIGURE 2.—Characteristics of the Loeys–Dietz Syndrome. Panel A shows typical facial characteristics of patients with Loeys–Dietz syndrome type I at different ages: blue sclerae, hypertelorism, proptosis, malar flattening, retrognathia, camptodactyly, and arachnodactyly. Panel B shows the facial characteristics of a patient with Loeys–Dietz syndrome type II. The translucency of the skin is evident, with visible veins and distended scars. Panel C shows a patient who had type I with a nonsense mutation (R495X) in *TGFBR2*, hypertelorism, and bifid uvula. Panel D shows the results of immunostaining of aortic tissue from a patient who was heterozygous for the R495X mutation, revealing increased nuclear accumulation of phosphorylated Smad2 and levels of expression of connective-tissue growth factor (CTGF), both indicative of increased TGF-β signalling, as compared with an age-matched control. (Reprinted by permission from Loeys BL, Schwarze U, Holm T, et al. Aneurysm syndromes caused by mutations in the TGF-β receptor. *N Engl J Med.* 355:788-798. Copyright 2006, Massachusetts Medical Society. All rights reserved.)

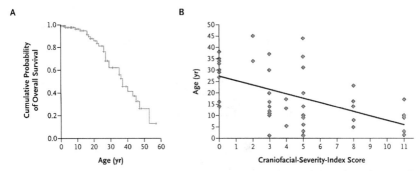

FIGURE 3.—Kaplan–Meier Estimates of Overall Survival (Panel A) and the Relation between the Craniofacial-Severity-Index Score and the Age at the First Major Cardiovascular Event (Surgery, Dissection, or Death) (Panel B) among Patients with the Loeys–Dietz Syndrome. (Reprinted by permission from Loeys BL, Schwarze U, Holm T, et al. Aneurysm syndromes caused by mutations in the TGF-β receptor. *N Engl J Med*. 355:788-798. Copyright 2006, Massachusetts Medical Society. All rights reserved.)

commonly occurs in childhood. This childhood phenotype is characterized by the triad of widely spaced eyes (hypertelorism); a bifid uvula, cleft palate, or both; and generalized arterial tortuosity with widespread vascular aneurysm and dissection. Since this presentation occurs on the watch of pediatricians, it is critical for us to be aware of the phenotype. Previously described in 10 families, the phenotype has been classified as the Loeys–Dietz syndrome (Online Mendelian Inheritance in Man 609192).

What we see in this report is the natural history of families affected with the Loeys–Dietz syndrome. The average survival for the disorder is just 37 years and the mean age of death is even lower at 26.0 years. Thoracic aortic dissection is the leading cause of death (in two-thirds of affected individuals) followed by abdominal aortic dissection (22%) and cerebral bleeding (7%). Children as young as 6 months of age have had these vascular complications. The average age for first vascular surgery, often for ascending aortic aneurysm or dissection, is just 19.8 years.

The three connective tissue disorders that tend to most affect blood vessels in childhood include the Ehlers–Danlos syndrome, Marfan's syndrome, and now the Loeys–Dietz syndrome. While the median survival for those with the Loeys–Dietz syndrome, as seen in this study, is 37 years, it is 48 years among patients with vascular involvement with Ehlers–Danlos syndrome and 70 years among patients with Marfan's syndrome who are properly managed. In the past it is clear that many who have been diagnosed with Marfan's syndrome in fact more properly should have been diagnosed as having Loeys–Dietz syndrome. Testing for the *TGFBR* mutation will distinguish these disorders because such mutations are not found in classic Marfan's syndrome.

The next time you see a youngster who has wide-set eyes and a bifid uvula, look carefully at other family members for the autosomal dominant findings of Loeys–Dietz syndrome. Refer that youngster to a geneticist quickly. Children and their families should be advised of and evaluated for the life-threatening manifestations of the disease that are treatable, including cervical-spine instability, spontaneous or traumatic organ rupture, and catastrophic complications of pregnancy. There is fairly significant wide intrafamilial variation in the clinical presentation of the disorder and thus all family members should be tested for the genetic marker. The exact mechanism by which mutations in the TGF-β receptor caused the multisystem manifestations of the Loeys–Dietz syndrome remains poorly understood, but the gene marker is an excellent tool for determining who is or is not affected. Periodic CT scanning, MRI, and echoes are warranted in subjects bearing the autosomal dominant mutation.

See the Aryan et al report (Aneurysms in children: review of 15 years experience) that tells us about intracranial aneurysms in children, their location, size, presentation, and causation. You will see a table of disorders associated with pediatric intracranial aneurysms. The table should have Loeys–Dietz syndrome added to it.

J. A. Stockman III, MD

Aneurysms in children: Review of 15 years experience
Aryan HE, Giannotta SL, Fukushima T, et al (Univ of California, San Diego)
J Clin Neurosci 13:188-192, 2006

Introduction.—Intracranial aneurysms in children are rare. The location, size, age, and presentation in the young are markedly different from that of adults. The 15-year experience of the senior author in southern California is presented.

Methods.—All paediatric patients treated for cerebral aneurysm over a 15-year period were identified. Intraoperative and postoperative data were collected retrospectively from the medical records. The need for additional surgery as well as the incidence of complications including death, hemiparesis, seizures, memory disturbances, and the need for subsequent cerebrospinal fluid (CSF) diversion were identified.

Results.—Fifty children were identified (54 lesions). Subarachnoid haemorrhage was the most common mode of presentation with the average Hunt–Hess grade being I-II. The locations of the lesions were middle cerebral (10), internal carotid (8), anterior communicating (7), posterior cerebral (6), posterior communicating (5), pericallosal (4), anterior cerebral (3),

---

TABLE 6.—Disorders Associated With Paediatric
Intracranial Aneurysms

Aortic coarctation	Polycystic kidney disease
Fibromuscular dysplasia	Tuberous sclerosis
Arteriovenous malformation	Vascular anomalies
Cardiac myxoma	Cerebral tumours
Ehlers-Danlos syndrome	Marfan syndrome
Irradiation	Moyamoya syndrome
Human immunodeficiency virus	Syphilis
Thalassaemia	Glucose-6-phosphate
Sickle cell anaemia	dehydrogenase deficiency
	Pseudoxanthoma elasticum

(Courtesy of Aryan HE, Giannotta SL, Fukushima T, et al. Aneurysms in children: review of 15 years experience. *J Clin Neurosci.* 13:188-192. Copyright 2006, Elsevier.)

choroidal (3), posterior inferior cerebellar (3), basilar (2), vertebral (2) and frontopolar (1) arteries. Clinical vasospasm was encountered in eight of our patients, but no cases were observed in those younger than nine years. Long-term outcome was excellent in 22 cases, good in 20 and poor in nine, with one death and two patients lost to follow-up.

Conclusion.—Analysis of our data suggested a predilection for the posterior circulation compared to adults, larger size, more complex architecture, and a decreased incidence of clinical vasospasm in the younger age group. This series and a review of the literature suggest that aneurysmal disease in children may be distinct from that of adults (Table 6).

Randomized Trial of Pulsed Corticosteroid Therapy for Primary Treatment of Kawasaki Disease

Newburger JW, for the Pediatric Heart Network Investigators (Harvard Med School, Boston; New England Research Insts, Watertown, Mass; Univ of Toronto; et al)
N Engl J Med 356:663-675, 2007

Background.—Treatment of acute Kawasaki disease with intravenous immune globulin and aspirin reduces the risk of coronary-artery abnormalities and systemic inflammation, but despite intravenous immune globulin therapy, coronary-artery abnormalities develop in some children. Studies have suggested that primary corticosteroid therapy might be beneficial and that adverse events are infrequent with short-term use.

Methods.—We conducted a multicenter, randomized, double-blind, placebo-controlled trial to determine whether the addition of intravenous methylprednisolone to conventional primary therapy for Kawasaki disease reduces the risk of coronary-artery abnormalities. Patients with 10 or fewer days of fever were randomly assigned to receive intravenous methylprednisolone, 30 mg per kilogram of body weight (101 patients), or placebo (98 patients). All patients then received conventional therapy with intravenous immune globulin, 2 g per kilogram, as well as aspirin, 80 to 100 mg per kilogram per day until they were afebrile for 48 hours and 3 to 5 mg per kilogram per day thereafter.

Results.—At week 1 and week 5 after randomization, patients in the two study groups had similar coronary dimensions, expressed as z scores adjusted for body-surface area, absolute dimensions, and changes in dimensions. As compared with patients receiving placebo, patients receiving intravenous methylprednisolone had a somewhat shorter initial period of hospitalization ($P=0.05$) and, at week 1, a lower erythrocyte sedimentation rate ($P=0.02$) and a tendency toward a lower C-reactive protein level ($P=0.07$). However, the two groups had similar numbers of days spent in the hospital, numbers of days of fever, rates of retreatment with intravenous immune globulin, and numbers of adverse events.

Conclusions.—Our data do not provide support for the addition of a single pulsed dose of intravenous methylprednisolone to conventional intravenous immune globulin therapy for the routine primary treatment of children with Kawasaki disease.

▶ You would think by now that we would have figured out the very best way to manage children with Kawasaki disease. At least 2 generations of us have tackled this problem. As pointed out in a commentary by Burns, "How can an illness look like an infectious disease but not have a recoverable agent, look like an immune-mediated vasculitis but not be easily treated with corticosteroids, and look like a benign, self-limited illness but be the leading cause of acquired heart disease in children?"[1]

With respect to the initial management of Kawasaki disease, our Japanese colleagues have suggested that high doses of intravenously administered immune globulin are most effective in relieving patients of symptoms and reducing the risk of coronary artery disease. From these early Japanese experiences with immune globulin, randomized prospective clinical trials here in the United States that took place a quarter of a century ago established that IV immune globulin is, indeed, effective and safe therapy for reducing the rate of coronary artery aneurysms. The mechanism of action of this form of therapy has never been clearly understood, although many theories abound. Aspirin is also administered, usually in high dosages, for its anti-inflammatory effects, and good data exist to support its use as well.

IV immune globulin is not effective in every patient with Kawasaki disease. Failure rates as high as 20% have been described. The findings of Newburger et al suggest that adding corticosteroid therapy to IV immune globulin does not improve the outcome in such children. Why steroids do not work in this form of vasculitis but are the mainstay of therapy for most other vasculitides remains an enigma. Perhaps only when we find out the true etiology of Kawasaki disease will we have a definitive therapy for it. The 4-decade long search for a causative agent has yielded only a long list of ruled-out pathogens. The findings of studies implicating a superantigen in the upregulation of the immune response have not been confirmed. Current evidence suggests the involvement of an oligoclonal antibody response to a conventional antigen.[2]

It is now more than 40 years since the original description of the clinical signs of this illness by the Japanese pediatrician Tomisaku Kawasaki. Hopefully, it will not take another 40 years before we pin down the etiologic agent, if one exists, or understand everything there is to be understood about the pathophysiology of this curious entity.

J. A. Stockman III, MD

References

1. Burns JC. The riddle of Kawasaki disease. *N Engl J Med.* 2007;356:659-661.
2. Rowley AH, Shulman ST, Spike BT, Mask CA, Baker SC. Oligoclonal IgA response in the vascular wall in acute Kawasaki disease. *J Immunol.* 2001;166:1334-1343.

A multicenter prospective randomized trial of corticosteroids in primary therapy for Kawasaki disease: Clinical course and coronary artery outcome

Inoue Y, for the Gunma Kawasaki Disease Study Group (Gunma Univ, Japan; et al)
J Pediatr 149:336-341, 2006

Objective.—To investigate the role of corticosteroids in the initial treatment of Kawasaki disease (KD).

Study Design.—Between September 2000 and March 2005, we randomly assigned 178 KD patients from 12 hospitals to either an intravenous immunoglobulin (IVIG) group (n = 88; 1 g/kg for 2 consecutive days) or an IVIG plus corticosteroid (IVIG+PSL) group (n = 90). The primary endpoint was coronary artery abnormality (CAA) before a 1-month echocardiographic assessment. Secondary endpoints included duration of fever, time to normalization of serum C-reactive protein (CRP), and initial treatment failure requiring additional therapy. Analyses were based on intention to treat.

Results.—Baseline characteristics of groups were similar. Fewer IVIG+PSL patients than IVIG patients had a CAA before 1 month (2.2% vs 11.4%; $P = .017$). The duration of fever was shorter ($P < .001$) and CRP decreased more rapidly in the IVIG+PSL group than in the IVIG group ($P = .001$). Moreover, initial treatment failure was less frequent (5.6% vs 18.2%; $P = .010$) in the IVIG+PSL group. All patients assigned to the IVIG+PSL group completed treatment without major side effects.

Conclusions.—A combination of corticosteroids and IVIG improved clinical course and coronary artery outcome without causing untoward effects in children with acute KD.

▶ It has been some time since we have seen the topic of steroid use for the primary treatment of patients with KD appearing in the literature, and there remains no consensus about the value of steroids for this purpose. The debate about steroid use, of course, is not new at all. In fact, back in the 1960s, Dr Kawasaki did report the use of oral, intravenous, and intramuscular steroids. This report by Inoue and colleagues represents the results of a Japanese multicenter prospective randomized trail of IVIG plus aspirin with or without the addition of corticosteroids (methylprednisolone 2 mg/kg/day). It was concluded that patients treated with the regimen that included steroids had a more rapid fall in CRP levels, a more rapid resolution of fever, and fewer CAAs at 1 month after treatment. Additionally, fewer of the steroid-treated patients had evidence of initial treatment failure requiring additional therapy. Just 8.9% of those treated with a regimen that included steroids required additional therapy for either persistent or recurrent fever as compared with 19.3% of those treated with IVIG plus aspirin alone.

Readers are encouraged to read an editorial that accompanied this report by Dr Jane Burns. Dr Burns points out a number of methodologic issues that should caution us about embracing the use of steroids solely on the basis of this one Japanese report. For example, the study used only about half the amount of IVIG that is used in the United States. In addition, there are many difficulties associated with studying adjuvant therapies for children with acute KD (the problem stemming from the fact that IVIG plus aspirin is so remarkably effective as a treatment). Here in the United States, clinical trials of IVIG and aspirin show only a 3% to 5% rate of the development of coronary artery aneurysms. Dr Burns reminds us of the wisdom of *primum non nocere* and to carefully consider the wisdom of additional primary therapies for a disease that has a 95% satisfactory response rate with what we would now consider traditional treatment.

The Nigrovic et al report (Extreme thrombocytosis predicts Kawasaki disease in infants) tells us that extreme thrombocytosis predicts KD in infants. Specifically, among babies presenting with fever without an identified source and who have a platelet counts in excess of 800,000 cells/mm³, there is a markedly increased probability of KD. Platelet counts that high or higher raise the risk of the infant having KD by a factor of 17.

J. A. Stockman III, MD

Extreme Thrombocytosis Predicts Kawasaki Disease in Infants
Nigrovic LE, Nigrovic PA, Harper MB, et al (Children's Hosp Boston; Brigham and Women's Hosp, Boston)
Clin Pediatr (Phila) 45:446-452, 2006

Infants with Kawasaki disease are at high risk of developing life-threatening coronary complications, yet may elude timely diagnosis because they often lack the full complement of classic clinical features. We retrospectively studied 26,540 children 1 year of age or less who were evaluated at a tertiary care pediatric emergency department in whom a platelet count was performed. Among those infants with fever without a source identified, 8.5% with platelet counts of 800,000 cells/mm³ or greater had Kawasaki disease compared to 0.4% with platelet counts of less than 800,000 cells/mm³ (likelihood ratio for Kawasaki disease was 17 [95% confidence interval, 8-34]). Because many infants present atypically, Kawasaki disease should be considered in all children of 1 year or less with prolonged fever, extreme elevation of the platelet count, and no compelling alternative diagnosis.

Prediction of resistance to intravenous immunoglobulin treatment in patients with Kawasaki disease
Egami K, Muta H, Ishii M, et al (Kurume Univ, Japan; Kitasato Univ, Sagamihara, Japan)
J Pediatr 149:237-240, 2006

Objectives.—The objective of this study was to find the predictors and generate a prediction score of resistance to intravenous immunoglobulin (IVIG) in patients with Kawasaki disease (KD).

Study Design.—Patients diagnosed as having KD were sampled when they received initial high-dose IVIG treatment (2 g/kg dose) within 9 days of illness (n = 320). These patients were divided into 2 groups: the resistance (n = 41) and the responder (n = 279). The following data were obtained and compared between resistance and responder: age, sex, illness days at initial treatment, and laboratory data.

Results.—Multivariate logistic regression analysis identified age, illness days, platelet count, alanine aminotransferase (ALT), and C-reactive protein (CRP) as significant predictors for resistance to IVIG. We generated prediction score assigning 1 point for (1) infants less than 6 months old, (2) before 4 days of illness, (3) platelet count $\leq 30 \times 10^{10}$/L, (4) CRP ≥ 8 mg/dL, as well as 2 points for (5) ALT ≥ 80 IU/L. Using a cut-off point of 3 and more with this prediction score, we could identify the IVIG-resistant group with 78% sensitivity and 76% specificity.

Conclusions.—Resistance to IVIG treatment can be predicted using age, illness days, platelet count, ALT, and CRP. Randomized, multicenter clinical trials are necessary to create a new strategy to treat these high-risk patients.

▶ This is a very useful report. Anyone who has been involved with the care of patients with KD knows that not every child seems to respond well to high-dose IVIG treatment, and those who are resistant to initial IVIG treatment tend to be the ones who are at greatest risk for the development of coronary artery aneurysms somewhere during the course of the disease. Previous studies have suggested that a high neutrophil count, a low hemoglobin, high CRP, a high lactate dehydrogenase (LDH), and a low albumin might be predictors of poor response to IVIG. Unfortunately, studies that have attempted to draw correlations predicting poor outcome have been based on small numbers of patients. Therefore, the reliability of the correlations has proven to be fairly modest. The importance of this report from Japan is that it examined a database that goes back several decades allowing the selection of more than 300 patients who were treated with high-dose IVIG. Resistance to treatment was found in 13% of this population, a sizable number allowing a good analysis of risk factors for poor response.

What we learn from this study is that young age (< 6 months), shorter duration of illness prior to treatment (< 4 days), a normal platelet count (< 300,000×107/L) an elevated aspartate aminotransferase (AST) (> 80IU/L), and an elevated CRP (> 8 mg/dL) are the factors predicting resistance to IVIG. By using a combination of these factors, the authors demonstrated a sensitivity of 61% in picking out patients who would not respond to IVIG (with an 81% specificity).

So what do you do with the information from this report? The authors suggest that patients presenting with adverse risk factors predictive of failure with IVIG might be best treated initially with even higher doses of IVIG, or IVIG plus steroid, or IVIG plus infliximab. These recommendations would require additional studies that would be difficult to perform absent a large collaborative investigation, but the recommendations do seem reasonable given the fact that one has only 1 shot at early management of these patients to prevent the development of coronary artery disease.

See the Singh-Grewal report (A prospective study of the immediate and delayed adverse events following intravenous immunoglobulin infusions) that describes the immediate and delayed adverse effects associated with the administration of IVIG.

J. A. Stockman III, MD

A prospective study of the immediate and delayed adverse events following intravenous immunoglobulin infusions

Singh-Grewal D, Kemp A, Wong M (Children's Hosp of Westmead, Sydney)
Arch Dis Child 91:651-654, 2006

Aim.—To document the incidence of immediate and delayed adverse events (AE) following intravenous immunoglobulin (IVIG) infusion in children.

Methods.—Immediate and delayed adverse events were prospectively recorded for 345 infusions in 58 children receiving IVIG for immunodeficiency (n = 33) or immunomodulation (n = 25). For each infusion adverse events were documented during the infusion and by follow up interview 4–7 days later.

Results.—Immediate adverse events occurred in 10.3% and delayed adverse events in 41.4% of children treated during the study period. Three and a half per cent of the infusions were associated with immediate AE and 20.9% with delayed adverse events. Headache was the most common delayed AE, occurring in 24.1% of patients and 12.8% of infusions.

Conclusions.—Delayed adverse events to IVIG infusions are common in children. They occur more frequently than immediate adverse events and are the cause of significant morbidity. Recognition of the high frequency of delayed adverse events is important in the care of children receiving IVIG therapy.

▶ Anyone who has been involved with the care of children receiving IVIG infusions knows that such infusions are not trouble-free in all instances. IVIG is derived from pooled donor serum and is produced by ethanol fractionation with additional steps taken to remove immunoglobulin aggregates. Preparations are then stabilized using a variety of substances such as human albumin, glycine, polyethylene glycol and sugars such as sucrose, maltose, or glucose. As the result of fractionation and the addition of stabilizers, reactions may occur to either immunoglobulin aggregates or to the stabilizing agents. Steps to remove or minimize immunoglobulin aggregation reduce the immediate adverse events in many children, but do not eliminate them. Adverse events after IVIG infusions are generally classified as immediate (occurring during the infusion) or delayed (occurring after the infusion has ceased). Infusion of IVIG preparations can be associated with fever, flushing, headache, rash, arthralgia, malaise, renal failure, aseptic meningitis, hemolysis, and anaphylaxis. In most instances, these reactions are mild and can be controlled.

The study from Sydney, Australia turns out to be the first to prospectively document the rates of delayed events related to IVIG infusions. Some 21% of infusions are associated with this problem. The frequency of delayed events was 4 times greater per infusion in comparison with the frequency of acute events. Headache is the most consistent delayed transfusion problem, followed by fatigue, abdominal pain, myalgia and nausea, followed then by a sprinkling of other signs and symptoms. Interestingly, no episodes consistent with aseptic meningitis were observed in this series, but absent a lumbar puncture having been performed, it is not clear how many episodes of headache might have been due to this problem. Needless to say, there is nothing worse than a child who has a severe headache develop who has received IVIG for the management of severe thrombocytopenia as part of the treatment for idiopathic thrombocytopenic purpura. Such a problem may result in further study and cost the patient in excess of $1000 for a CT scan for what otherwise is a relatively minor side effect of IVIG.

The adverse reactions to IVIG clearly are more likely to be delayed than acute. These delayed reactions rarely are life threatening, but are a principle cause of lost school time and the need for additional diagnostic studies and therapies.

J. A. Stockman III, MD

Vasospastic Angina in a 13-Year-Old Female Patient Whose Only Symptom Was Toothache

Okajima Y, Hirai A, Higashi M, et al (Chiba Prefectural Togane Hosp, Togane City, Japan; Chiba Children's Hosp, Chiba City, Japan)
Pediatr Cardiol 28:68-71, 2007

Vasospastic angina was confirmed in a 13-year-old female patient at autopsy. The patient's only symptom was recurrent toothache, which began when she was 10 years old. In November 2000, she was evaluated at our medical center; however, all examinations were judged normal. Six months later, she suffered a severe toothache. She went to school the next morning after the symptoms improved. She lost consciousness at school and was given cardiopulmonary resuscitation but could not be revived. At autopsy, her three coronary vessels showed marked intimal hyperplasia, and multiple focal myocardial infarctions were observed in the lateral wall of the left ventricle. The patient's only clinical symptom was toothache and none of the physicians realized that this was caused by angina. Vasospastic angina begins at a young age and is one of the causes of sudden death in adolescents.

▶ This case report relates a sad tale of a 13-year-old girl. It is an important case because it warns us that even children can have heart attacks. The youngster had been having recurrent toothaches, but dental examination showed no abnormalities. A thorough medical examination also showed no abnormalities. She had normal exercise tolerance and electroencephalogram (EEG) and chest radiograph were normal. She was followed up without medication. There was some consideration that her symptoms might be caused by psychological stress. She was evaluated several times in several months and was discharged from care to return only if there was recurrence of her severe toothache. Six months after the final visit, she experienced a severe toothache at night. This subsided and she went to school the following morning. However, she lost consciousness as she was entering her classroom. Cardiopulmonary resuscitation was performed immediately, but she could not be revived. At autopsy, multiple focal myocardial infarctions were found scattered on the lateral side of the left ventricle. It was clear at autopsy that the multifocal myocardial infarction had existed for several months. The coronary blood vessels showed severe intimal hyperplasia, especially in the left circumflex artery, with no evidence of atherosclerotic change or thrombosis. The intimal hyperplasia was considered to be consistent with an entity called vasospastic angina.

Vasospastic angina was first described in 1959 and was initially thought to occur only in older patients. Angina caused by vasospasm is an uncommon finding in the pediatric population, but there have been case reports in children and adolescents. It is fairly likely that the toothache this youngster experienced was referred pain from angina. Referred pain from angina has not been previously reported in the pediatric literature. On the basis of this single case report, we must think about referred pain and its association with angina in the pediatric population. The findings reported in this youngster are not consistent with Kawasaki disease.

On a heart-related subject, many readers of the YEAR BOOK OF PEDIATRICS know this editor's philosophy on exercise: you are born with a fixed number of heartbeats, and they should not be so wasted. Recently an article appeared to support this philosophy, one which demonstrates the value of resting in a chair. What do the data show? The data show resting in a chair for just 16 minutes results in a significant drop in both systolic and diastolic blood pressure in untreated hypertensive patients.[1] This drop is due to a systemic vasodilatation, and 75% of the fall takes place in the first 10 minutes of resting. Measurement of blood pressure in clinics might be more accurate if patients could rest for 10 minutes before seeing the health professional who will be examining them.

J. A. Stockman III, MD

Reference

1. Sala C, Santin E, Rescaldani M, Magrini F. How long shall the patient rest before clinic blood pressure measurement? *Am J Hypertens.* 2006;19:713-717.

Trends in Sudden Cardiovascular Death in Young Competitive Athletes After Implementation of a Preparticipation Screening Program

Corrado D, Basso C, Pavei A, et al (Univ of Padua, Italy; Ctr for Sports Medicine and Physical Activity, Padua, Italy)
JAMA 296:1593-1601, 2006

Context.—A nationwide systematic preparticipation athletic screening was introduced in Italy in 1982. The impact of such a program on prevention of sudden cardiovascular death in the athlete remains to be determined.

Objective.—To analyze trends in incidence rates and cardiovascular causes of sudden death in young competitive athletes in relation to preparticipation screening.

Design, Setting, and Participants.—A population-based study of trends in sudden cardiovascular death in athletic and nonathletic populations aged 12 to 35 years in the Veneto region of Italy between 1979 and 2004. A parallel study examined trends in cardiovascular causes of disqualification from competitive sports in 42,386 athletes undergoing preparticipation screening at the Center for Sports Medicine in Padua (22,312 in the early screening period [1982-1992] and 20,074 in the late screening period [1993-2004]).

Main Outcome Measures.—Incidence trends of total cardiovascular and cause-specific sudden death in screened athletes and unscreened nonathletes of the same age range over a 26-year period.

Results.—During the study period, 55 sudden cardiovascular deaths occurred in screened athletes (1.9 deaths/100,000 person-years) and 265 sudden deaths in unscreened nonathletes (0.79 deaths/100,000 person-years). The annual incidence of sudden cardiovascular death in athletes decreased by 89% (from 3.6/100,000 person-years in 1979-1980 to 0.4/100,000 person-years in 2003-2004; *P* for trend <.001), whereas the incidence of sudden death among the unscreened nonathletic population did not change significantly. The mortality decline started after mandatory screening was implemented and persisted to the late screening period. Compared with the prescreening period (1979-1981), the relative risk of sudden cardiovascular death in athletes was 0.56 in the early screening period (95% CI, 0.29-1.15; *P*=.04) and 0.21 in the late screening period (95% CI, 0.09-0.48; *P*=.001). Most of the reduced mortality was due to fewer cases of sudden death from cardiomyopathies (from 1.50/100,000 person-years in the prescreening period to 0.15/100,000 person-years in the late screening period; *P* for trend =.002). During the study period, 879 athletes (2.0%) were disqualified from competition due to cardiovascular causes at the Center for Sports Medicine: 455 (2.0%) in the early screening period and 424 (2.1%) in the late screening period. The proportion of athletes who were disqualified for cardiomyopathies increased from 20 (4.4%) of 455 in the early screening period to 40 (9.4%) of 424 in the late screening period (*P*=.005).

Conclusions.—The incidence of sudden cardiovascular death in young competitive athletes has substantially declined in the Veneto region of Italy since the introduction of a nationwide systematic screening. Mortality reduction was predominantly due to a lower incidence of sudden death from cardiomyopathies that paralleled the increasing identification of athletes with cardiomyopathies at preparticipation screening.

▶ Exercise-related sudden death in adults is primarily due to coronary artery disease. Events in younger individuals are usually due to a variety of congenital and genetic cardiovascular disorders, including inherited cardiomyopathies and arrhythmias, to anomalies of the coronary arteries, or to acquired cardiomyopathy. Hypertrophic cardiomyopathy accounts for more than one third of fatal cases in the United States, and arrhythmogenic right ventricular cardiomyopathy accounts for approximately one fourth of fatal cases.

Preparticipation cardiac evaluation of athletes is intuitively attractive for identifying athletes at risk. Both the American Heart Association and the Sports Cardiology Study Group of the European Society of Cardiology recommend screening high school and college athletes before athletic participation. Both organizations' guidelines recommend a personal and family history as well as a physical examination. The European guidelines go further and recommend obtaining a routine ECG. Unfortunately, these types of recommendations are largely based on consensus development as few, if any, large studies of screening protocols exist to provide mortality data. This is where the article of Corrado et al becomes helpful. The article clearly supports the cardiovascular screening techniques used in Europe that require ECGs. Italy, for example, has had a national mandated preparticipation screening program for athletes in place since 1982. The study reported in *JAMA* provides incidence data for sudden cardiac deaths in Italian athletes and nonathletes aged 12 to 35 years in the Veneto region of Italy before and during this screening program. The annual incidence of sudden cardiac death in athletes decreased from 3.6 deaths per 100,000 person-years in 1979 and 1980 to just 0.4 deaths per 100,000 person-years in 2003 and 2004, which is an 89% reduction. In terms of actual deaths, this reduction was from 1 death per year per 27,777 athletes to 1 death per year per 250,000 athletes. No change occurred in the incidence of sudden death among nonathletes, which suggests that this reduction was not due to changes in the population death rate. Most of the decrease in death was due to fewer deaths attributable to cardiomyopathies, whereas the number of athletes disqualified because of cardiomyopathies increased. Both the decrease in deaths and increase in disqualifications were primarily due to changes in the frequency of arrhythmogenic right ventricular cardiomyopathy. Of the 42,386 screened athletes, 9% required additional cardiovascular testing, and 2% were ultimately prohibited from athletic participation.

An editorial accompanied the *JAMA* article. This editorial suggested that the results of the Italian study, while provocative, do not definitively prove the value of screening or establish the importance of routine ECGs in the screening process. It was noted that this study was not a controlled comparison of screening versus nonscreening of athletes but rather a population-based observational study. This study did not evaluate the routine use of ECGs compared with more limited screening based on a history and physical examination. The authors attribute their success to the routine use of ECGs, but this component was not examined separately from the start-up of a comprehensive history and physical examination screening back in 1982. Last, the sudden death rate in young athletes in Italy currently is no different than the sudden death rate seen here in the United States, where ECGs are not used routinely. This suggests that the less formal screening process practiced in the United States might be as effective as the more formal Italian program that includes ECGs.

The study of Corrado et al does provide the best evidence to date supporting the preparticipation screening of athletes and also gives some provocative evidence for including ECGs in this process. It does not prove, however, that the latter is necessary. What we need is a large collaborative study to develop a rigorous, comprehensive, regional or national registry to evaluate the preparticipation screening process prospectively to determine how such programs can be ideally designed to reduce sudden death in young athletes. Obviously, such a study would need to be randomized to include ECGs as part of the process. If it turns out that ECGs should be employed, a lot of pediatricians will need to bone up, once again, on interpreting the ECG. Congenital arrhythmias and the ECG findings of myocardial hypertrophy are relatively easy to detect, but you need to know what you are looking for when interpreting the ECG.

This report from *JAMA* should be read by every generalist practitioner. It is full of numbers. If you are really into numbers, also read the *Wall Street Journal* edition published June 20, 2005. You will see a lot of numbers related to secrets of successful living. Today, the average person in the United States lives nearly 78 years. Some people beat the average significantly, however. Numerous studies of rats, monkeys, nuns, British government workers, and centenarians have unlocked many of the secrets of successful aging. People age better if they do not smoke, do not abuse alcohol, maintain a healthy weight, and get regular exercise. One of the biggest culprits in unhealthy aging also receives the least respect from the medical community and that is stress. Increasingly, researchers are viewing stress—how much stress we face in a lifetime, and how well we cope with it—as one of the most significant factors for predicting how well we age.

Consider the following numbers:

- 11 — Number of additional years a 75-year-old man can expect to live
- 13 — Number of additional years a 75 year-old woman can expect to live
- 17 — Number of additional years a 65-year-old man can expect to live
- 30 — Percentage of 80- to 102-year-old women still having sex
- 40 — Waistline measurement, in inches, at which risk for heart attack increases exponentially
- 63 — Percentage of 80- to 102-year-old men still having sex
- 78 — Average age of death in the United States overall
- 85 to 94 — Fastest growing age group in the United States[1]

J. A. Stockman III, MD

Reference

1. Parker-Pope T. The secrets of successful aging. *Wall Street Journal.* June 20, 2005.

One-Month Therapy with Simvastatin Restores Endothelial Function in Hypercholesterolemic Children and Adolescents

Ferreira WP, Bertolami MC, Santos SN, et al (Instituto Dante Pazzanese de Cardiologia, São Paulo, Brazil; Rua Napoleão de Barros, São Paulo, Brazil; Rua Comendador Gabriel Calfat, São Paulo, Brazil)
Pediatr Cardiol 28:8-13, 2007

Simvastatin has been shown to restore endothelial function in children with familial hypercolesterolemia after 28 weeks of treatment. The aim of this study was to evaluate 1-month simvastatin treatment effect on endothelial function in hypercholesterolemic children and adolescents. Eighteen hypercholesterolemic patients (HC group) and 18 healthy controls, aged 6–18 years, were studied with medical history, physical examination, full lipid profile, serum apolipoprotein B (apo B), fibrinogen, hepatic transaminases, and creatine kinase concentrations. Flow-mediated dilatation (FMD) was performed by high-resolution ultrasound of the brachial artery. The HC group received simvastatin 10 mg/day for 1 month. Arterial diameter was measured by two experienced sonographers who were unaware of subjects' conditions. At baseline, FMD was impaired in the HC group (mean, 5.27 ± 4.67%) compared to controls (mean, 15.05 ± 5.97%) (p < 0.001). After treatment, we observed a significant reduction in total cholesterol (TC) (29%), low-density lipoprotein cholesterol (LDL-C); (37%), apo B concentrations (36%) and FMD restoration (mean, 12.94 ± 7.66%), with an absolute increase of 7.66 ± 8.58 ($p = 0.001$). These results show that children and adolescents with hypercholesterolemia present endothelial dysfunction, and simvastatin, in addition to significantly reducing TC, LDL-C, and apo B concentrations, restores endothelial function with 1-month treatment.

▶ Statins are amazing drugs. They are HMG coenzyme A reductase inhibitors that have been shown not only to lower cholesterol levels, but also to improve endothelial function in adults with hypercholesterolemia. Several studies reporting the use of statins in children have been undertaken, but few have assessed its effect on endothelial function. It can be seen in this report that 6 months of statin use in youngsters with hypercholesterolemia will improve endothelial function in those who have some initial impairment. Arterial endothelial function was studied by examination of brachial artery responses to endothelium-dependent stimuli. This is done by taking 2-dimensional scans of the brachial artery with US measuring flow velocity by means of a pulse Doppler signal.

Before this report, no study had shown restoration of endothelial function in children and adolescents with only 1 month of statin therapy. This observation is important because it shows real and early benefits on the atherogenic process by the use of such drugs. Exactly how statins so quickly improve endothelial function remains speculative. A simple lowering of serum cholesterol levels is not the likely sole reason for the improvement. There may also be up-regulation of nitric oxide synthetase, which has a significant positive effect on arterial blood flow.

If there is any message worth taking home from this report, it is that the benefits of statin use in children and adolescents with hypercholesterolemia kick in quite early, perhaps sufficiently early in the phase of the development of atherosclerosis to make it reversible. The Im et al article (Association between brachial-ankle pulse wave velocity and cardiovascular risk factors in healthy adolescents) shows just how powerful brachial (and ankle) pulse wave velocity is as a cardiovascular risk factor in otherwise healthy appearing adolescents.

While on the topic of high cholesterol and statins, how would you deal with the following situation? A teen in your practice has a hyperlipidemia. This patient's mother has been giving her red yeast rice as a home therapy for the problem. The patient is also receiving a statin. The problem is that the teen now has developed severe and diffuse myalgias. Laboratory studies show markedly elevated serum levels of the muscle enzyme creatine kinase. Should you stop the statin?

There are a number of side effects of statin therapy. All of us recognize that myalgias can develop in patients on statins and elevated levels of muscle enzymes may also occur. In such circumstances, statins should be withdrawn. That is the exact circumstance of a woman who was recently reported that was taking simvastatin for hyperlipidemia. When her statins had to be discontinued, the patient decided to begin taking the over-the-counter herbal preparation red yeast rice (rice that has been fermented by the red yeast *Monascus purpureus*). Red rice is a dietary supplement that contains 3-hydroxy-3-methylglutaryl coenzyme A reductase inhibitors, commonly used for the self-treatment of hyperlipidemia. Within 3 months of starting red yeast rice, the woman again developed severe diffuse myalgias, and laboratory studies showed markedly elevated serum creatine kinase levels. The red yeast rice was withdrawn and the patient's symptoms resolved.[1]

If you are not familiar with red yeast rice, it has been used as a food preservative in medicine in China since the year 800. The main antihyperlipidemic ingredients in red yeast rice are its 3-hyrdoxy-methylglutaryl coenzyme A reductase inhibitors. Data are clear. Compared with placebo, red yeast rice substantially decreases total cholesterol, low-density lipoprotein, and triglyceride levels. Unfortunately, myopathy is a well-known complication of such inhibitors because these inhibitors are the key ingredients of some statins such as lovastatin.

Thus it is that any 3-hydroxy-3-methylglutaryl coenzyme A reductase inhibitor, red yeast rice included, can cause a myopathy. It does not take a prescription drug to cause the problem. Given the widespread use of over-the-counter herbal preparations, we should all be aware of this important potential adverse reaction.

J. A. Stockman III, MD

Reference

1. Mueller PS. Symptomatic myopathy due to red yeast rice. *Ann Intern Med.* 2006;145:474-475.

Association between Brachial-Ankle Pulse Wave Velocity and Cardiovascular Risk Factors in Healthy Adolescents

Im J-A, Lee J-W, Shim J-Y, et al (MizMedi Hosp, Seoul, Korea; Yonsei Univ, Seoul, Korea)
J Pediatr 150:247-251, 2007

Objective.—To investigate the associations between cardiovascular risk factors and arterial stiffness, measured as brachial-ankle pulse wave velocity (baPWV), in healthy adolescents.

Study Design.—In this cross-sectional study, 178 male and 84 female adolescents, aged 12 to 18 years, were recruited. Total homocysteine levels, serum lipid profiles, high-sensitivity C-reactive protein (hs-CRP) levels, fasting glucose levels, fasting insulin levels, and baPWV were measured.

Results.—baPWV was significantly higher in male adolescents than in female adolescents. In both sex groups, baPWV was positively correlated with body mass index (BMI), waist circumference, waist-hip ratio, systolic and diastolic blood pressures, fasting insulin levels, homeostatic model assessment of insulin resistance, triglyceride levels, hs-CRP levels, and total homocysteine levels. In male adolescents, age, total cholesterol level, low-density lipoprotein cholesterol levels, and white blood cell counts were positively correlated with baPWV, and, in female adolescents, high-density lipoprotein cholesterol levels were negatively correlated with baPWV. In multivariate analysis, sex, mean blood pressure, BMI, and total homocysteine levels were found to be independent factors associated with baPWV.

Conclusion.—Blood pressure, BMI, sex, and total homocysteine levels were independently associated with arterial stiffness, measured as baPWV, in healthy adolescents, suggesting that these risk factors may be associated with an increased risk of atherosclerosis in adolescents.

▶ The Ferreira et al study (One-month therapy with simvastatin restores endothelial function in hypercholesterolemic children and adolescents) reported how effective statins were on improving endothelial function in patients with hypercholesterolemia. The study used brachial pulse wave velocity as measured by Doppler flow study, a barometer of vascular impairment. In recent years, several noninvasive techniques have been developed to measure vascular properties, and these have been used to predict later-onset cardiovascular morbidity and mortality rates. Measures of blood vessel wall stiffness, distensibility, and compliance have been used for such purposes. We see in this report by Im et al analysis of pressure waveforms, vessel diameter changes in response to pressure changes, and measurement of pulse wave velocity as markers of vascular endothelial compromise. Arterial pulse wave analysis is performed by what is known as application tonometry, which requires a transfer function to derive central aortic waveforms. The derivation and validation procedures used require intra-arterial catheter measurements excluding this particular technology for most children. Arterial distensibility is the change in vessel size in response to pressure change. In a sense, it is the reciprocal of arterial stiffness, estimating blood vessel elastic properties. The vessel diameters are measured with US scanning. Studies in adults have shown impairments of blood vessel function in patients with high blood pressure, diabetes, and dyslipidemia. These measures can also predict future adverse cardiovascular outcomes. What studies have been performed in children (few in number) using this technique have shown data roughly paralleling the adult results.

Im et al report their findings of baPWV and the correlations with known risk factors for cardiovascular disease, all done in a population of healthy Korean adolescents. Wave velocity studies are now done routinely, using automated devices. The technique is completely noninvasive. Studies in adults by researchers using the technology are now plentiful and have been performed in patients with many chronic diseases known to increase cardiovascular pathology. Studies in children have been fairly limited but have included youngsters with diabetes mellitus, neurofibromatosis, obstructive airway disease, Kawasaki disease, polyarteritis nodosa, and coarctation of the aorta after surgical repair. Im et al found abnormalities of baPWV in children with a variety of cardiovascular risk factors, including high BMI, high waist circumference, elevated waist-hip ratio, systolic and diastolic blood pressure elevations as well as in youngsters with abnormal levels of insulin, triglycerides, CRP, and homocysteine.

More and more you will be reading about noninvasive markers for vascular disease. Chances are, in the not-widely-distant future, these automated devices will be used as part of routine primary care for the detection of atherosclerosis in high-risk teens. It is not necessary to be a pediatric cardiologist to know how to interpret the results of such testing, assuming the procedure has been competently performed by well-trained technicians.

In terms of prevention of coronary artery disease, you might consider drinking 1 cup of tea per day. There is some evidence that drinking tea does have cardiovascular benefits. At the same time, adding milk to a cup of tea may destroy these benefits, as indicated in a study published this past year.[1] The German researchers who performed this study found that catechins found in tea do in fact help dilate blood vessels, but caseins in milk essentially eliminate this benefit.

In addition, many claims have been made about the potential benefits of green tea. Research in humans has been inconsistent, possibly because the studies undertaken thus far have been too small to find a modest effect. The largest study so far reports that drinking several cups of green tea a day is associated with a reduced risk of death and a reduced risk of cardiovascular death in particular, stroke being the most notable. This study involved over 400,000 Japanese adults.[2] The same study also found no evidence that green tea can help prevent cancer deaths. In the Japanese study, most of the participants drank at least one small cup of green tea a day. This translates to about just over 3 ounces daily. The strongest association between green tea and cardiovascular mortality was found in women, particularly for those drinking three or more cups a day. In men, the associations related to reduced mortality were significant only for those who drank five or more cups a day, and the actual benefit was somewhat smaller.

Green tea contains polyphenols, which scavenge free radicals among other things. Thus, a link with good cardiovascular help is certainly biologically plausible. If only the polyphenols came in tablet form so we did not have to look at the icky stuff.

J. A. Stockman III, MD

References

1. Black tea is better than white [editorial]. *BMJ*. 2007;334:60.
2. Kuriyama S, Shimazu T, Ohmori K, et al. Green tea consumption and mortality due to cardiovascular disease, cancer, and all causes in Japan: the Ohsaki study. *JAMA*. 2006;296:1255-1265.

Inhibition of Microsomal Triglyceride Transfer Protein in Familial Hypercholesterolemia

Cuchel M, Bloedon LT, Szapary PO, et al (Univ of Pennsylvania; St Joseph Univ, Beirut, Lebanon; Jikei Univ, Tokyo; et al)
N Engl J Med 356:148-156, 2007

Background.—Patients with homozygous familial hypercholesterolemia have markedly elevated cholesterol levels, which respond poorly to drug therapy, and a very high risk of premature cardiovascular disease. Inhibition of the microsomal triglyceride transfer protein may be effective in reducing cholesterol levels in these patients.

Methods.—We conducted a dose-escalation study to examine the safety, tolerability, and effects on lipid levels of BMS-201038, an inhibitor of the microsomal triglyceride transfer protein, in six patients with homozygous familial hypercholesterolemia. All lipid-lowering therapies were suspended 4 weeks before treatment. The patients received BMS-201038 at four different doses (0.03, 0.1, 0.3, and 1.0 mg per kilogram of body weight per day), each for 4 weeks, and returned for a final visit after a 4-week drug washout period. Analysis of lipid levels, safety laboratory analyses, and magnetic resonance imaging of the liver for fat content were performed throughout the study.

Results.—All patients tolerated titration to the highest dose, 1.0 mg per kilogram per day. Treatment at this dose decreased low-density lipoprotein (LDL) cholesterol levels by 50.9% and apolipoprotein B levels by 55.6% from baseline (P<0.001 for both comparisons). Kinetic studies showed a marked reduction in the production of apolipoprotein B. The most serious adverse events were elevation of liver aminotransferase levels and accumulation of hepatic fat, which at the highest dose ranged from less than 10% to more than 40%.

Conclusions.—Inhibition of the microsomal triglyceride transfer protein by BMS-201038 resulted in the reduction of LDL cholesterol levels in patients with homozygous familial hypercholesterolemia, owing to reduced production of apolipoprotein B. However, the therapy was associated with elevated liver aminotransferase levels and hepatic fat accumulation.

▶ Currently, there are no truly effective therapies for the management of homozygous familial hypercholesterolemia. This hereditary disorder is caused by loss-of-function mutations in both alleles of the LDL receptor gene. Children and young adults with the disease have plasma cholesterol levels of more than 500 mg/dL (12.9 mmol/L); if untreated, affected individuals have cardiovascular disease before the age of 20 and generally do not survive past 30 years of age. Affected individuals have a poor response to conventional drug therapy with statins, which generally lower LDL cholesterol levels through upregulation of the hepatic LDL receptor. The current standard of care for these patients is LDL apheresis. This procedure will transiently reduce LDL cholesterol levels by about half and may delay the onset of atherosclerosis, but apheresis must be repeated frequently, usually every 1 to 2 weeks. Compliance obviously is a major problem with this management technique. Thus, new therapies have been badly needed for patients with homozygous familial hypercholesterolemia as well as for other patients with severe refractory hypercholesterolemia who are candidates for LDL apheresis.

The "pie in the sky" therapy for homozygous familial hypercholesterolemia would be an agent that would reduce LDL production. The microsomal triglyceride transfer protein is responsible for transferring triglycerides onto apolipoprotein B within the liver in the assembly of very low density lipoprotein (VLDL), the precursor to LDL. In the absence of functional microsomal triglyceride transfer protein, as in the rare recessive genetic disorder abetalipoproteinemia, the liver cannot secrete VLDL, leading to the absence of all lipoproteins containing apolipoprotein B in the plasma. Thus, the pharmacologic inhibition of microsomal triglyceride transfer protein might be a strategy for reducing LDL production and plasma LDL cholesterol levels.

This study from the University of Pennsylvania evaluated the cholesterol-lowering efficacy of the microsomal triglyceride transfer protein inhibitor BMS-201038 in the management of patients with homozygous familial hypercholesterolemia. The study also examined the mechanism of cholesterol reduction, the tolerability of the inhibitor, and its effects on hepatic fat. The results of the investigations are a good news/bad news story. The microsomal triglyceride transfer protein inhibitor was highly effective in reducing plasma LDL cholesterol levels, with a reduction of more than 50% at the highest dose. The mechanism of this reduction in LDL cholesterol was documented to be due to a markedly reduced rate of production of LDL apolipoprotein B. One side effect was predictable, that of loose stools at high-dose inhibitor administration. Because the microsomal triglyceride transfer protein is expressed in the intestine and is required for chylomicron assembly and secretion, inhibition of the protein would be expected to cause steatorrhea. For this reason, study patients were informed that they should have a diet containing less than 10% of energy from fat.

The real problem, however, with the use of transfer inhibitors is the accumulation of fat in the liver. In this study, there was substantial variability in the amount of fat accumulated in the liver, but fat indeed was accumulated. In 5 of

6 patients, when the transfer inhibitor was stopped, hepatic fat accumulation returned to normal. The clinical significance of hepatic fat accumulation and the probability of its evolution to fibrotic liver disease are speculative, but worrisome.

Thus, all in all, microsomal triglyceride transfer protein inhibitor BMS-201038 is effective in reducing the levels of atherogenic apolipoprotein B–containing lipoproteins by reducing their production in patients with homozygous familial hypercholesteremia. In concept, such inhibition may be the way to go in patients who are not likely to live much past 30 years of age. Before such therapies are recommended, however, studies on outcomes of liver function will be needed to see whether the cure turns out to be worse than the disease.

This commentary closes with a few remarks about dog walking and how it may be good for your cardiovascular health. In United States households, there are about 65 million dogs. A large percentage of these dogs are taken for walks on more than one occasion daily. Investigators from the CDC have analyzed data from 1,280 individuals who say they take their dog out regularly to go potty. The data show that 80% of the dog walkers take at least one 10-minute walk daily, 59% took two or more daily 10-minute walks, and 42% walked their dogs at least 30 minutes.[1] The current recommendation for physical exercise here in the United States is that adults should accumulate 30 minutes or more of moderate intensity physical activity on most or all days of the week. Moderate intensity could very well be a brisk walk taken with a larger dog that prompts one to walk at a fairly intense pace. Indeed, a study has shown that the average dog owner will walk approximately 300 minutes per week, more than twice the number of minutes walked per week for non-dog owners.[2]

If you believe that dog walking improves your health may be a bunch of whoowie, recognize that statisticians have analyzed all published data to date and report that 9% of human coronary disease could be prevented if dog owners walked their dogs for at least 150 minutes per week.[3] Dogs that are put on diets that include extra walking have owners that simultaneously lose about 5% of their body weight during the period of canine obesity reduction.[4]

While on the topic of dog walking, what constitutes one of the single largest sources of refuge going into landfills these days? It turns out that China's Year of the Dog (2006) and President Bush's plan for alternative fuel services have proudly come together in San Francisco. The city is planning to turn the waste of its 120,000 dogs into usable energy. A study in San Francisco has shown that nearly 4% of the refuge collected from homes comes from pet waste, a percentage virtually identical to the waste generated by disposable diapers. The traditional means of collecting such waste results in doggy dung mummified in plastic baggies in landfills. It is the latter that the city of San Francisco is attacking by developing recyclable doggie poo bags. In fact, Norcal Waste is trying out special collection carts and biodegradable bags at Duboce Park, a popular dog-walking park in San Francisco. Along with food leftovers, the dog waste will go into a methane digester, where bacteria will feed on the combination and emit methane to be used as natural gas.

Cat lovers take heart. Norcal is extending its dung-to-methane project to other pets and collecting cat dung from private homes. No one would want Muffin left out.[5]

J. A. Stockman III, MD

References

1. Ham SA, Epping J. Dog walking and physical activity in the United States. *Prev Chronic Dis.* 2006;3:A47.
2. Brown SG, Rhodes RE. Relationships among dog ownership and leisure-time walking in Western Canadian adults. *Am J Prev Med.* 2006;30:131-136.
3. Bauman AE, Russell SJ, Furber SE, Dobson AJ. The epidemiology of dog walking: an unmet need for human and canine health. *Med J Aust.* 2001;175:632-634.
4. Voelker R. Studies suggest dog walking a good strategy for fostering fitness. *JAMA.* 2006;296:643.
5. Dung into methane: the year of the dog; recycling in San Francisco takes a dirty step forward [editorial]. *The Economist.* March 4, 2006.

Risk of Aborted Cardiac Arrest or Sudden Cardiac Death During Adolescence in the Long-QT Syndrome

Hobbs JB, Peterson DR, Moss AJ, et al (Univ of Rochester, NY; Mayo Clinic, Rochester, Minn; Bikur Cholim Hosp, Jerusalem; et al)
JAMA 296:1249-1254, 2006

Context.—Analysis of predictors of cardiac events in hereditary long-QT syndrome (LQTS) has primarily considered syncope as the predominant end point. Risk factors specific for aborted cardiac arrest and sudden cardiac death have not been investigated.

Objective.—To identify risk factors associated with aborted cardiac arrest and sudden cardiac death during adolescence in patients with clinically suspected LQTS.

Design, Setting, and Participants.—The study involved 2772 participants from the International Long QT Syndrome Registry who were alive at age 10 years and were followed up during adolescence until age 20 years. The registry enrollment began in 1979 at 5 cardiology centers in the United States and Europe.

Main Outcome Measures.—Aborted cardiac arrest or LQTS-related sudden cardiac death; follow-up ended on February 15, 2005.

Results.—There were 81 patients who experienced aborted cardiac arrest and 45 who had sudden cardiac death; 9 of the 81 patients who had an aborted cardiac arrest event experienced subsequent sudden cardiac death. Significant independent predictors of aborted cardiac arrest or sudden cardiac death during adolescence included recent syncope, QTc interval, and sex. Compared with those with no syncopal events in the last 10 years, patients with 1 or 2 or more episodes of syncope 2 to 10 years ago (but none in the last 2 years) had an adjusted hazard ratio (HR) of 2.7; (95% confidence interval [CI], 1.3-5.7; *P*<.01) and an adjusted HR of 5.8 (95% CI, 3.6-9.4; *P*<.001), respectively, for life-threatening events; those with 1 syncopal episodes in the last 2 years had an adjusted HR of 11.7 (95% CI, 7.0-19.5; *P*<.001) and those with 2 or more syncopal episodes in the last 2 years had an adjusted HR of 18.1 (95% CI, 10.4-31.2; *P*<.001). Irrespective of events occurring more than 2 years ago, QTc of 530 ms or longer was associated with increased risk (adjusted HR, 2.3; 95% CI, 1.6-3.3; *P*<.001) compared with those having a shorter QTc. Males between the ages of 10 and 12 years had higher risk than females (HR, 4.0; 95% CI, 1.8-9.2; *P* = .001), but there was no significant risk difference between males and females between the ages of 13 and 20 years. Among individuals with syncope in the past 2 years, β-blocker therapy was associated with a 64% reduced risk (HR, 0.36; 95% CI, 0.18-0.72; *P*<.01).

Conclusions.—In LQTS, the timing and frequency of syncope, QTc prolongation, and sex were predictive of risk for aborted cardiac arrest and sudden cardiac death during adolescence. Among patients with recent syncope, β-blocker treatment was associated with reduced risk.

▶ Congenital LQTS is a rare cardiac disorder. Affected persons present with prolongation of the QT interval corrected for heart rate (QTc). Patients are at increased risk for syncope and sudden death because of life-threatening ventricular arrhythmias. In most cases, inheritance of the LQTS is autosomal dominant, but can be recessive, with or without associated deafness. The genetic causes of the LQTS have been well characterized. Mutations in the potassium-channel genes *KCNQ1* and *KCNH2* cause the most frequent forms of the LQTSs) (types 1 and 2 respectively).

In this report from the University of Rochester, the authors report about risk factors for sudden death in adolescents who have the LQTS. Using the large LQTS cohort derived from the International Long QT Syndrome Registry, the effects of various clinical factors and therapeutic interventions on the risk of aborted cardiac arrest and sudden cardiac death during the high-risk adolescent period were evaluated. This registry turns out to be the largest LQTS study to date and is the first to identify risk factors specific for aborted cardiac arrest and sudden cardiac death in the high-risk adolescent period. It appears that the timing and frequency of recent syncope, the degree of QT interval prolongation, and sex are independent predictors of life-threatening events in adolescents with the LQTS. Assessment of these 3 factors during a routine office visit can be used to stratify the risk of a patient. β-blockers reduce the overall risk in everyone by about 64%. Despite β-blocker therapy, those in the very high-risk category, on average, experience a 1% per year life-threatening event between the ages of 10 and 20 years. Boys are much more likely than girls to experience such an event before they are 15 years old, but girls have a higher risk thereafter. For whatever reason, boys eventually experience a shortening of the QT interval during adolescence, and girls do not. This suggests that androgens somehow achieve this shortening, and estrogens appear to decrease potassium-channel density in the myocardium. An unusual finding in this report was the observation of no correlation between the QT interval syndrome genotype of a patient and the risk of a life-threatening event. All in all, the importance of this study is based on the fact that 3 identifiable risk factors for estimating the probability of life-threatening events were identified: timing and frequency of recent syncope, the duration of the QT interval, and sex (increased risk in boys before age 15 and increased risk in girls after the age of 15).

Shortly after this report appeared, another showed up in the literature telling us that more girls than boys are affected with QT interval syndrome on the basis of the fact that classic mendelian-inheritance ratios expected for an autosomal dominant trait are not observed among the offspring of female carriers of the LQTS type 1 allele or among mothers and fathers carrying an allele for the LQTS type 2. This results in about 68% of LQTS individuals affected with types 1 and 2 being female. The etiology of this predilection is based on something known as "transmission distortion," which has been previously reported in invertebrates as well as in mammals. The actual mechanism of transmission distortion is very complicated, well beyond this editor's ability to explain. Read up on the article by Imboden to learn more about this for yourselves.[1]

Let's close this commentary with two questions. The first is: what is turning out to be the real problem with mobile phones in hospitals? Most of us are familiar with the "bans" on the use of mobile phones within the hospital setting. Such bans were put into place because of concerns with interference with sensitive medical equipment. Indeed, a study by the Medical Devices Agency reported that mobile phones could interfere with 4% of medical devices at a distance of 1 meter.[2] In general, however, the interference observed was merely an irritation and ultimately harmless to patients—for example, alarms might be theoretically triggered and ECG recordings may need to be repeated. Effects on pacemakers, such as disruption to the atrial sensing circuitry or ventricular inhibition may occur, but in reality this only happens when a patient holds their phone directly against his or her chest rather than to his or her ear, and the effect stops immediately once the phone is removed. Thus, caution regarding the proximity of mobile phones to medical equipment is warranted, but concerns about patient safety alone do not justify zealously enforced no-phone areas, which frequently lead to more arguments between staff, patients, and visitors than they do good to patients. On the other hand, beeping, ringing, and singing phones are an absolute nuisance and the tendency of patients to ask their care providers to wait a minute or two while they finish their conversation on their cell phone is irritating at best, and poor care at worst. In reality, this is no different than when as a medical student, I was asked to wait a minute or two while an adult female patient finished watching *General Hospital* on her hospital room TV. What really is of concern, however, these days are the HIPPA violations inherently possible with allowing camera cell phones inside of hospitals. The use of camera phones can easily compromise patient confidentiality, an issue that has not been carefully evaluated.[3]

Last, should police vehicles be equipped with automated defibrillators? The answer here is yes, especially if the police are equipped with taser stun guns. Recently, an adolescent was described who developed ventricular fibrillation following the use of a stun gun. This adolescent was subdued with a taser stun gun and subsequently collapsed. Paramedics quickly arrived at the scene who began to perform cardiopulmonary resuscitation within two minutes of the collapse. After four shocks and the administration of epinephrine, atropine, and lidocaine, a perfusing cardiac rhythm was restored. The adolescent made a nearly complete recovery and was discharged from the hospital after several days.[4] Deaths have been reported after discharges from taser stun guns, although no definite causative link between death and the use of a stun gun has been made. The case of this teen who arrested following stunning, however, seems to be proof positive that these things kill by inducing ventricular fibrillation. This case of ventricular fibrillation after a discharge from a stun gun suggests that the availability of automated external defibrillators to law enforcement personnel carrying stun guns should be considered.

J. A. Stockman III, MD

References

1. Imboden M, Swan H, Denjoy I, et al. Female predominance and transmission distortion in the long-QT syndrome. *N Engl J Med.* 2006;355:2744-2751.
2. Department of Health, Social Services and Public Safety. *MDA device bulletin DB 9702.* London: DHSSPS; 1997.
3. Derbyshire SWG, Burgess A. Use of mobile phones in hospitals. *BMJ.* 2006;333:767-768.
4. Kim PJ, Franklin WH. Ventricular fibrillation after stun-gun discharge. *N Engl J Med.* 2005;353:958-959.

10 Infectious Diseases and Immunology

Nonmedical Exemptions to School Immunization Requirements: Secular Trends and Association of State Policies With Pertussis Incidence
Omer SB, Pan WKY, Halsey NA, et al (Johns Hopkins Bloomberg School of Public Health, Baltimore, Md; Ctrs for Disease Control and Prevention, Atlanta, Ga; Univ of Florida, Gainesville; et al)
JAMA 296:1757-1763, 2006

Context.—School immunization requirements have played a major role in controlling vaccine-preventable diseases in the United States. Most states offer nonmedical exemptions to school requirements (religious or personal belief). Exemptors are at increased risk of acquiring and transmitting disease. The role of exemption policies may be especially important for pertussis, which is endemic in the United States.

Objective.—To determine if (1) the rates of nonmedical exemptions differ and have been increasing in states that offer only religious vs personal belief exemptions; (2) the rates of nonmedical exemptions differ and have been increasing in states that have easy vs medium and easy vs difficult processes for obtaining exemptions; and (3) pertussis incidence is associated with policies of granting personal belief exemptions, ease of obtaining exemptions, and acceptance of parental signature as sufficient proof of compliance with school immunization requirements.

Design, Setting, and Participants.—We analyzed 1991 through 2004 state-level rates of nonmedical exemptions at school entry and 1986 through 2004 pertussis incidence data for individuals aged 18 years or younger.

Main Outcome Measures.—State-level exemption rates and pertussis incidence.

Results.—From 2001 through 2004, states that permitted personal belief exemptions had higher nonmedical exemption rates than states that offered only religious exemptions, and states that easily granted exemptions had higher nonmedical exemption rates in 2002 through 2003 compared with states with medium and difficult exemption processes. The mean exemption rate increased an average of 6% per year, from 0.99% in 1991 to 2.54% in 2004, among states that offered personal belief exemptions. In states that easily granted exemptions, the rate increased 5% per year, from 1.26% in

1991 to 2.51% in 2004. No statistically significant change was seen in states that offered only religious exemptions or that had medium and difficult exemption processes. In multivariate analyses adjusting for demographics, easier granting of exemptions (incidence rate ratio = 1.53; 95% confidence interval, 1.10-2.14) and availability of personal belief exemptions (incidence rate ratio = 1.48; 95% confidence interval, 1.03-2.13) were associated with increased pertussis incidence.

Conclusions.—Permitting personal belief exemptions and easily granting exemptions are associated with higher and increasing nonmedical US exemption rates. State policies granting personal belief exemptions and states that easily grant exemptions are associated with increased pertussis incidence. States should examine their exemption policies to ensure control of pertussis and other vaccine-preventable diseases.

▶ The number of children who are opted out of immunization by their parents varies fairly extensively by state. Some states make exemptions widely available to parents either by offering a personal belief exemption or by making the exemption option easy to obtain. All states and the District of Columbia require children entering school to provide documentation that they have met the state vaccine requirements. As of 2006, all states permitted medical exemptions to school and day care immunization requirements: 48 states allowed religious exemptions, and 19 states had provision for personal belief exemptions. Personal belief exemptions include religious, philosophical, or any other unspecified nonmedical exemption. Two states (Arkansas and Texas) added personal belief exemptions during the 2003 and 2004 school years.

Some states make exemptions widely available to parents either by offering a personal belief exemption rather than a religious exemption or by easing permission for exemptions. For example, California offers a personal belief exemption whereby the parent simply signs a prewritten statement on the school immunization form. This personal belief exemption is available to anyone, regardless of the nature of their beliefs (religious or philosophical), and it is easier to claim this exemption than to complete the school immunization form that requires the healthcare clinician to obtain the child's medical record and transcribe the dates of vaccine administration. Other states, such as Maryland, call their exemption religious, but they also make it extremely easy for parents to take the exemption option. The Maryland school immunization form states, "Because of my bona fide religious beliefs and practices, I object to any immunizations being given to my child." As in California, parental signature to this Maryland statement provides for an exemption without any other administrative requirement, and some Maryland parents are likely to use this exemption even though their reasons for not vaccinating are not religiously grounded. Some states that offer either religious or personal belief exemptions have administrative requirements, such as requiring a signature from a local health department official, annual renewal, notarization, or a personally written letter from the parents explaining the reasons for vaccine refusal.

The study described in the abstract attempts to determine whether the rates of nonmedical exemptions differ among states and whether the findings correlate with how easy it is to obtain an exemption to the immunization requirements. It is clear that states that permit personal belief exemptions have a higher nonmedical exemption rate than states that only offer religious exemptions, and states that easily grant exemptions have higher exemption rates as compared with states with medium and difficult processes for granting objections. The Centers for Disease Control and Prevention databases clearly show that the availability of personal belief exemptions and easily obtained exemptions are associated with increased pertussis infection incidence rates. Children with nonmedical exemptions are at increased risk for disease, and they also increase the community risk of disease transmission. From 1985 though 1992, exempted children in all states were 35 times more likely to contract measles than nonexempt children. In Colorado, exempted children were observed to be 22 times more likely to have had measles and 5.9 times more likely to have had pertussis than vaccinated children.

This study also reported one other interesting finding: nonmedical exemptions tend to be geographically clustered, thus providing the critical mass of susceptible children to disease transmission while also increasing individual and community risks. For example, exemption rates of 15% to 18% are found in Ashland, Oregon, and Vashon, Washington. Such social clustering of exemptions increases the risk of disease outbreaks, as was recently exemplified in an Indiana measles outbreak.[1]

There are many reasons why parents opt out of immunizations. The success of immunizations has paradoxically shifted many parents' concerns from the risks of vaccine-preventable diseases to the risks of vaccine-adverse events. Safety concerns about vaccines have increased markedly given the publicity associated with these events. Most studies to date show that vaccine safety concerns are the primary reasons that parents claim nonmedical exemptions. This was the principal reason why parents in Indiana opted out, and, thus, their kids got measles. The report described in the abstract also produces one other interesting finding, which is that the majority of parents are selective about their exemptions. Only about 25% of children with nonmedical exemptions receive no vaccines at all; the remainder of the children are vaccinated to varying degrees, depending on their parents' beliefs and concerns about a specific vaccine's safety.

One final comment about nonmedical exemptions to school immunization requirements: some children do not attend school and are instead homeschooled. Most states do not collect or report exemption rates among homeschooled children. This loophole in data collection tends to affect certain communities more than others. Overall, it is clear that states must balance parent autonomy with the tremendous public health benefit that vaccines afford when considering the types of exemptions allowed. Just how much latitude should be allowed with these exemptions does vary tremendously. The easiest state in which to get an exemption is likely to be Vermont, and it is clear that Vermonters exercise their option to opt out of vaccines at a far, far higher rate than do the citizens of other states. At the same time, Vermont trails only Minnesota in being among the healthiest states in the United States (see the UnitedHealthcare Foundation Website for detailed data, http://www.unitedhealthfoundation.org/ahr2006/findings.html).

J. A. Stockman III, MD

Reference

1. Parker AA, Staggs W, Dayan GH, et al. Implications of a 2005 measles outbreak in Indiana for sustained elimination of measles in the United States. *N Engl J Med.* 2006;355:447-455.

Safety of reduced-antigen-content tetanus–diphtheria–acellular pertussis vaccine in adolescents as a sixth consecutive dose of acellular pertussis-containing vaccine
Zepp F, Knuf M, Habermehl P, et al (Johannes Gutenberg Univ, Mainz, Germany; GlaxoSmithKline Biologicals, King of Prussia, Pa)
J Pediatr 149:603-610, 2006

Objective.—The safety of a booster dose of a reduced–antigen–content tetanus-diphtheria-acellular pertussis (Tdap) vaccine was evaluated in adolescents previously vaccinated with five doses of acellular pertussis–containing vaccine.

Study Design.—Adolescents (n = 319) previously vaccinated with either 5 doses of diphtheria–tetanus–acellular pertussis (DTaP) (n = 193) or 4 doses of DTaP plus another acellular pertussis-containing vaccine received one dose each of Tdap and hepatitis A vaccine in a double-blinded, randomized, crossover trial. Rates of adverse events (AEs) after vaccination with Tdap versus hepatitis A and rates of local AEs among adolescents vaccinated with Tdap (sixth acellular pertussis-containing vaccine dose) versus rates in these same individuals after vaccination with their fifth DTaP dose were assessed.

Results.—After Tdap, pain (63.6%), redness (51.7%), and swelling (41.4%) were the most frequently reported AEs. Large injection site swelling (swelling > 100 mm, arm circumference increase > 50 mm or diffuse swelling interfering with daily activities) occurred in three adolescents and resolved without sequelae. After the sixth dose of acellular pertussis-containing vaccine, adolescents reported more pain and less redness and swelling compared with incidences of these AEs reported when these same individuals received their fifth DTaP dose.

Conclusions.—These results suggest that Tdap is well tolerated as a sixth consecutive dose of acellular pertussis-containing vaccine.

▶ Adults with uncertain histories of a complete primary vaccination series with diphtheria and tetanus toxoid-containing vaccines should begin or complete a primary vaccination series. A primary vaccination series for adults is 3 doses; administer the first two doses at least 4 weeks apart and the third dose 6 to 12 months after the second. Administer a booster dose to adults who have completed a primary series and if the last vaccination was received more than 10 years previously. The same rules apply to adolescents with an uncertain history of a complete primary vaccination. Tdap or tetanus and diphtheria (Td) vaccine may be used; Tdap should replace a single dose of Td for adults under 65 years of age who have not previously received a dose of Tdap (either in a primary series, as a booster, or for wound management). Only one of the two Tdap products (Adacel) is licensed for use in adults.

Injection-site reactions tend to increase with increasing numbers of doses of acellular pertussis vaccine, with rates after the fourth dose exceeding those of the first three doses. Rates of injection-site erythema and swelling over 2 cm can exceed 50% after the fifth consecutive dose of acellular pertussis vaccine. The cause of these injection-site reactions has not been determined but may be related, in part, to preexisting antibody levels against one or more of the antigens, as well as to cell-mediated immunity. With regards to the fifth consecutive dose of an acellular pertussis-containing vaccine and preadolescents and adolescents, although this dose is generally well tolerated despite erythema and swelling, there have been concerns that a sixth consecutive dose might not be tolerated. In a number of pre-licensure studies, Tdap was tolerated well by adolescents and adults with the nature and rate of adverse events associated with immunization not substantially different from those associated with the licensed and widely used Td vaccine. There is some concern that the rates of adverse events in the pre-licensure studies of Tdap underestimate the rates that would be seen in adolescents who received acellular pertussis vaccine for all of their previous doses.

Although it will be several years before the general adolescent population routinely receives their sixth consecutive dose of acellular pertussis vaccine, the study by Zepp et al provides some reassurance that this dose will be well tolerated and will not adversely affect the pertussis immunization strategy. These first reassuring safety data on six consecutive doses of acellular pertussis vaccine are indeed timely, given the recent recommendations for universal adolescent pertussis immunization and early indications on the effectiveness of this strategy in decreasing rates of pertussis in adolescents. It will be interesting to see what the effect of the adolescent and adult immunization programs is on the incidence of pertussis among vulnerable newborns. It will also be important to study the safety and effectiveness of Tdap during pregnancy and its effects on the newborn.

For more on the topic of recommendations for an adolescent dose of tetanus and diphtheria toxoids and acellular pertussis vaccine, see the excellent editorial by Halperin.[1] Last, if you were to name the most significant medical advance since 1840, what would you say? Interestingly, 11,300 readers of the *British Medical Journal* were queried on this question by being provided with a list of 15 major milestones in medical advances occurring since 1840. The most votes went to the "sanitary revolution" as being the most important medical milestone since 1840. The work of the 19th century lawyer, Edwin Chadwick, who pioneered the introduction of piped water to people's homes and sewers rinsed by water, attracted 15.8% of the votes, while antibiotics took 15%, and anesthesia 14%. The next two most popular responses were the introduction of vaccines, with 12%, and the discovery of the structure of DNA at 9%. Of those voting, almost a third of the voters were physicians while a fifth were members of the general public and 1 in 7 were students. Another tenth were academic researchers. Almost two-fifths of the voters were from the United Kingdom and a fifth were from the United States.[2]

Please note that the true original champion of sanitation was John Snow, who showed that cholera was spread by water. Later, Edwin Chadwick did come up with the idea of sewage disposal and the piping of water into homes.

J. A. Stockman III, MD

References

1. Halperin SA. Recommendations for an adolescent dose of tetanus and diphtheria toxoids and acellular pertussis vaccine: reassurance for the future. *J Pediatr.* 2006;149:589-591.
2. Ferriman A. *BMJ* readers choose the "sanitary revolution" as greatest medical advance since 1840. *BMJ.* 2007;334:111.

Ultrasound Examination of Extensive Limb Swelling Reactions After Diphtheria-Tetanus-Acellular Pertussis or Reduced-Antigen Content Diphtheria-Tetanus-Acellular Pertussis Immunization in Preschool-Aged Children

Marshall HS, Gold MS, Gent R, et al (Women's and Children's Hosp, North Adelaide, Australia; Univ of Adelaide, Australia)
Pediatrics 118:1501-1509, 2006

Objective.—The aim of this study was to determine the site, extent, and resolution of tissue involvement when extensive limb swelling occurred in the injected limb for children who received diphtheria-tetanus-acellular pertussis or reduced-antigen content diphtheria-tetanus-acellular pertussis vaccine at 4 to 6 years of age.

Methods.—Children who had experienced an injection site reaction at 18 months of age were assigned randomly to receive an intramuscular injection of either reduced-antigen content diphtheria-tetanus-acellular pertussis vaccine or diphtheria-tetanus-acellular pertussis vaccine between 4 and 6 years of age. Children who developed extensive limb swelling were recruited for assessment by clinical examination; ultrasound studies of the affected and opposite (control) arms were performed 24 to 48 hours after immunization and 48 to 96 hours later.

Results.—Twelve children with extensive limb swelling were enrolled in the study. Ultrasound examinations demonstrated swelling of both the subcutaneous and muscle layers of the vaccinated arm. Ultrasound assessment showed that the swelling exceeded the clinical measurements of skin redness and swelling. Subcutaneous and muscle tissues expanded to 281% and 111% of the tissue thicknesses of the control arm, respectively. Repeat ultrasound examinations after 48 to 96 hours showed considerable resolution of muscle swelling, compared with subcutaneous tissue swelling. There was no significant difference in the extent of swelling detected between children who received diphtheria-tetanus-acellular pertussis vaccine and those who received reduced-antigen content diphtheria-tetanus-acellular pertussis vaccine.

Conclusion.—Extensive limb swelling reactions after diphtheria-tetanus-acellular pertussis or reduced-antigen content booster immunizations involved swelling of subcutaneous and muscle tissues with swelling and duration more marked in subcutaneous tissue.

▶ Sometimes you pick up a report and say to yourself, "Why didn't I do this study myself?" This is one such report. Ultrasonography is easily used and ideal for examining subcutaneous tissue and muscle layers. One wonders why some smart investigator had not previously used ultrasound to examine the anatomical changes underlying limb swelling following immunization in children. The latter is exactly what these investigators did.

Ultrasonography has been used to measure the thickness of subcutaneous and muscle layers and to determine the appropriate needle length for intramuscular injections. It has not been used for formal assessment of injection site reactions after diphtheria-tetanus-acellular pertussis or reduced-antigen content diphtheria-tetanus-acellular pertussis immunization. Without question, extensive limb swelling reactions after booster doses of acellular pertussis combination vaccines have been alarming to parents and to providers as well. If the reaction is not recognized as an immunization reaction, sometimes diagnoses are given of infective cellulitis, resulting in inappropriate treatment with antibiotics. The importance of the study is that it shows that extensive limb swelling reactions are largely attributable to marked edema in both the subcutaneous and muscle tissue spaces, with fluid accumulation being greater in the subcutaneous tissue space. It is interesting that there is significant subcutaneous edema given that vaccines are administered via the intramuscular route. Swelling in the muscle tissue is generally not as extensive and seems to resolve more rapidly than swelling in subcutaneous tissue. This is likely due to the better supply of blood to muscle than to subcutaneous tissue. Even when there is massive swelling, there is no evidence of associated joint effusion. The findings are highly suggestive of angioedema rather than an inflammatory cellulitis.

The authors of this report should be thanked for a great service in revealing the anatomical basis of swelling post immunization. Although this was not looked at in the study, the data from this report could guide clinicians in using ultrasound to differentiate between an immunization reaction and cellulitis. There are differences between the two that are visible on ultrasound should it be necessary to make a specific diagnosis. Last, one key finding from this report is that when the fifth dose of acellular pertussis vaccine is given, the incidence of reactions causing tissue redness greater than the size of an Oreo cookie is just 25%. One more use for the Oreo cookie, a reference for immunization reaction size.

Finally, just what evidence exists to tell us what the best size is for selecting a needle for vaccination of infants? Specifically, does a long (25mm) needle work better than a shorter needle? What gauge needle is ideal? We finally have detailed information on this topic from Great Britain. Investigators have actually assessed the immunogenicity of vaccines for infants along with the incidence of reactions to vaccination based on the use of needles of varying lengths and gauges. The diphtheria, tetanus, whole cell pertussis and *Hae-*

mophilus influenzae type B vaccine and a serogroup C meningococcal glycoconjugate vaccine were studied administering them using a wide, long needle, a narrow, short needle, or a narrow, long needle. Eighteen general practices were able to be recruited to carry out this task using healthy infants who were being vaccinated at 2, 3, and 4 months of age with a followup to 5 months of age. So what do the data show? The incidence of any local reaction after each immunization dose in the United Kingdom schedule for infants age 2, 3, and 4 months was significantly reduced when a wide, long (25mm) needle was used rather than a narrow, short (16mm) needle. The weight of the evidence clearly favored the wide, long needle in achieving comparable, if not superior, immunogenicity in relation to a narrow, short needle while at the same time remarkably reducing reactions.

Thus it is that needle length is associated with reduced reactions to immunizations. In addition, some authors have suggested that a narrower gauge needle might produce an injection jet under pressure, causing increased trauma at local reaction rates, but little difference was observed in this study between needle gauges.[1]

So why does a longer needle works better? Several trials of vaccines in adults and adolescents have shown that intramuscular delivery minimizes adverse reactions. A longer needle is more likely to achieve deposit of the vaccine into the muscle. Intramuscular delivery is particularly recommended for vaccines containing aluminum adjuvant, as inadvertent subcutaneous administration may increase irritation or lead to lumps at the injection site. Injection with a 16mm needle inserted at 90° has been shown not to reach the muscle in a significant number of infants at four months of age. Compared with subcutaneous tissue, muscle has an even abundant blood supply, one of the reasons why seroconversion rates also appear to be higher.

J. A. Stockman III, MD

Reference

1. Diggle L, Deeks JJ, Pollard AJ. Effect of needle size on immunogenicity and reactogenicity of vaccines in infants: randomized controlled trial. *BMJ.* 2006;333:571.

Prevention of Antigenically Drifted Influenza by Inactivated and Live Attenuated Vaccines

Ohmit SE, Victor JC, Rotthoff JR, et al (Univ of Michigan, Ann Arbor)
N Engl J Med 355:2513-2522, 2006

Background.—The efficacy of influenza vaccines may decline during years when the circulating viruses have antigenically drifted from those included in the vaccine.

Methods.—We carried out a randomized, double-blind, placebo-controlled trial of inactivated and live attenuated influenza vaccines in healthy adults during the 2004–2005 influenza season and estimated both absolute and relative efficacies.

Results.—A total of 1247 persons were vaccinated between October and December 2004. Influenza activity in Michigan began in January 2005 with the circulation of an antigenically drifted type A (H3N2) virus, the A/California/07/2004-like strain, and of type B viruses from two lineages. The absolute efficacy of the inactivated vaccine against both types of virus was 77% (95% confidence interval [CI], 37 to 92) as measured by isolating the virus in cell culture, 75% (95% CI, 42 to 90) as measured by either isolating the virus in cell culture or identifying it through real-time polymerase chain reaction, and 67% (95% CI, 16 to 87) as measured by either isolating the virus or observing a rise in the serum antibody titer. The absolute efficacies of the live attenuated vaccine were 57% (95% CI, −3 to 82), 48% (95% CI, −7 to 74), and 30% (95% CI, −57 to 67), respectively. The difference in efficacy between the two vaccines appeared to be related mainly to reduced protection of the live attenuated vaccine against type B viruses.

Conclusions.—In the 2004–2005 season, in which most circulating viruses were dissimilar to those included in the vaccine, the inactivated vaccine was efficacious in preventing laboratory-confirmed symptomatic illnesses from influenza in healthy adults. The live attenuated vaccine also prevented influenza illnesses but was less efficacious.

▶ The report of Ohmit et al provides a comprehensive, direct assessment of the inactivated influenza vaccine and the live attenuated influenza vaccine. Earlier studies reported similar efficacies for the inactivated and live attenuated vaccine formulations, but this randomized, double-blind, placebo-controlled trial involving individuals over a wide age range, from healthy adults to teenagers, is the most comprehensive study to date comparing the two very different vaccines. The most important finding is that the inactivated and live attenuated vaccines appear to have roughly similar efficacies against culture-confirmed influenza A infections (74%). The inactivated vaccine was superior to the live vaccine against culture-confirmed type B influenza infections, at 80% versus 40%, which leads to an overall higher efficacy of the inactivated vaccine against influenza A and B infections combined.

If one takes all existing data comparing the two vaccines, one can say that they are roughly comparable in their protection against influenza A in healthy adults. The annual development of influenza vaccines is an exemplary model of public-private cooperation. The World Health Organization coordinates global influenza-virus surveillance, so that appropriate vaccine candidates can be identified by the World Health Organization and national authorities, and vaccines can be reformulated each year. Vaccine viruses must be selected every year, because genetic mutations arise continuously in influenza viruses—a process termed *drift* that results in the emergence of immunologically distinct variant viruses. Several regulatory and production steps must then be completed to ensure safe, effective, and adequate vaccine supplies before the vaccine is administered each influenza season. The process must be repeated each year, which imposes severe time restrictions on all groups involved with the production and supply of the vaccine.

While on the topic of agents that cause pneumonia, see how you would address the following situation. The mother of one of your patients recently came down with pneumonia related to an unusual organism, *Legionella longbeachae*. Is there anything about the environment in the home that might also put the offspring of this woman at some risk for the same infection? What questions might you ask of the mother about her hobbies? The next time you are potting out plants, or are around someone who is, beware. A case-controlled study from South Australia identified *Legionella longbeachae*, which is found in commercial potting mixes, as a cause of infection. Recent use of a potting mix, in association with poor handwashing and exposure to hanging flower pots that drip seem to be the risk factors for the development of infection with this particular organism. Inhalation and ingestion are the likely modes of transmission.[1]

J. A. Stockman III, MD

Reference

1. O'Connor BA, Carman J, Eckert K, Tucker G, Givney R, Cameron S. Does using potting mix make you sick? Results from a *Legionella longbeachae* case-control study in South Australia. *Epidemiol Infect*. 2007;135:34-39.

Effectiveness of School-Based Influenza Vaccination

King JC Jr, Stoddard JJ, Gaglani MJ, et al (Univ of Maryland, Baltimore; MedImmune, Gaithersburg, Md; Texas A&M Univ, Temple; et al)
N Engl J Med 355:2523-2532, 2006

Background.—Vaccination of children in school is one strategy to reduce the spread of influenza in households and communities.

Methods.—We identified 11 demographically similar clusters of elementary schools in four states, consisting of one school we assigned to participate in a vaccination program (intervention school) and one or two schools that did not participate (control schools). During a predicted week of peak influenza activity in each state, all households with children in intervention and control schools were surveyed regarding demographic characteristics, influenza vaccination, and outcomes of influenza-like illness during the previous 7 days.

Results.—In all, 47% of students in intervention schools received live attenuated influenza vaccine. As compared with control-school households, intervention-school households had significantly fewer influenza-like symptoms and outcomes during the recall week. Paradoxically, intervention-school households (both children and adults) had higher rates of hospitalization per 100 persons than did control-school households. However, there was no difference in the overall hospitalization rates for children or adults in households with vaccinated children, as compared with those with unvaccinated children, regardless of study-group assignment. Rates of school absenteeism for any cause (based on school records) were not significantly different between intervention and control schools.

Conclusions.—Most outcomes related to influenza-like illness were significantly lower in intervention-school households than in control-school households.

▶ This report gives us information on whether the vaccination of children 5 years or older with a live attenuated influenza vaccine reduces the spread of influenza to households and the community through "herd effect" (the indirect protection from influenza at the community level). Herd immunity is an attractive concept, particularly if it could extend protection to highly vulnerable groups—especially very young persons and older adults—who often do not have an adequate protective immune response to immunization. Apart from health-care workers, for whom vaccination is recommended largely to avoid transmitting the infection to patients, influenza vaccine is currently administered mostly to prevent individuals from having severe complications from influenza—not, as is sometimes believed, to "control" the spread of an influenza epidemic throughout communities. The planned use of influenza vaccination to induce herd immunity would mark a considerable departure from or an addition to current approaches in most countries. Although this use could theoretically provide substantial benefits, very convincing evidence that vaccination can induce substantial levels of community protection through herd immunity will be required before such an approach is embraced widely.

In the study abstracted, the investigators offered the vaccine to children attending several intervention schools, but not to children attending control schools. Using questionnaires provided to all households, the researchers assessed clinical outcomes and outcomes related to the use of health care and medications among children and household members. Additionally, work and school absences were assessed. Overall, there were significant but relatively modest reductions in the number of symptoms of respiratory illness and visits to physicians in the intervention-school households as compared with the control-school households. Absenteeism from elementary and high school, but not middle school, was also reduced in the intervention-school households, as was the number of paid workdays missed.

So what do we learn? The findings suggest but do not conclusively prove that vaccination of children reduces the spread of influenza within households and to other student populations. Although not definitive, the study does provide supporting information for recommendations for influenza vaccination as a measure for more widespread control of infection beyond those who are immunized. By the way, if there was any one positive, albeit unintended learning from the events surrounding September 11, 2001, it was the effects on the spread of certain diseases. If an epidemic of avian influenza becomes likely, restricting airline travel might slow the spread of the disease and buy time for preventative measures. In a study published on September 12, 2006, in the online journal *PLoS Medicine*,[1] investigators found that prior to 2001, mortality peaked around the 17th of February. In the 2001 to 2002 flu season, just after the September attacks, the peak did not occur until a month later and was much less dramatic. Most of us recall that many elected not to travel by air after 9/11, a phenomenon that lasted for some months.

J. A. Stockman III, MD

Reference

1. Brownstein JS, Wolfe, CJ, Mandl KD. Empirical evidence for the effect of airline travel on inter-regional influenza spread in the United States. *PLoS Med* [serial online]. 2006;3:e401. Available at: http://medicine.plosjournals.org/perlserv/ ?request=get-document&doi=10.1371/journal.pmed.0030401. Accessed June 25, 2007.

Comparison of the Efficacy and Safety of Live Attenuated Cold-Adapted Influenza Vaccine, Trivalent, With Trivalent Inactivated Influenza Virus Vaccine in Children and Adolescents With Asthma

Fleming DM, for the CAIV-T Asthma Study Group (Northfield Health Centre, Birmingham, England; et al)
Pediatr Infect Dis J 25:860-869, 2006

Background.—Despite their potential for increased morbidity, 75% to 90% of asthmatic children do not receive influenza vaccination. Live attenuated influenza vaccine (LAIV), a cold-adapted, temperature-sensitive, trivalent influenza vaccine, is approved for prevention of influenza in healthy children 5 to 19 years of age. LAIV has been studied in only a small number of children with asthma.

Methods.—Children 6 to 17 years of age, with a clinical diagnosis of asthma, received a single dose of either intranasal CAIV-T (an investigational refrigerator-stable formulation of LAIV; n = 1114) or injectable trivalent inactivated influenza vaccine (TIV; n = 1115) in this randomized, open-label study during the 2002–2003 influenza season. Participants were followed up for culture-confirmed influenza illness, respiratory outcome, and safety.

Results.—The incidence of community-acquired culture-confirmed influenza illness was 4.1% (CAIV-T) versus 6.2% (TIV), demonstrating a significantly greater relative efficacy of CAIV-T versus TIV of 34.7% (90% confidence interval [CI] 9.4%–53.2%; 95% CI = 3.9%–56.0%). There were no significant differences between treatment groups in the incidence of asthma exacerbations, mean peak expiratory flow rate findings, asthma symptom scores, or nighttime awakening scores. The incidence of runny nose/nasal congestion was higher for CAIV-T (66.2%) than TIV (52.5%) recipients. Approximately 70% of TIV recipients reported injection site reactions.

Conclusions.—CAIV-T was well tolerated in children and adolescents with asthma. There was no evidence of a significant increase in adverse pulmonary outcomes for CAIV-T compared with TIV. CAIV-T had a significantly greater relative efficacy of 35% compared with TIV in this high-risk population.

▶ In the King et al report (Effectiveness of school-based influenza vaccination), the safety of the trivalent inactivated influenza vaccine on children aged 6 to 23 months is discussed. This vaccine is the only vaccine currently approved for use in high-risk children and adolescents. Few trials have specifically evaluated the efficacy of the influenza vaccine in children with asthma. Previous studies have suggested that the efficacy rates of the vaccine run about 67% for influenza A and about 44% for influenza B. This report studies the effectiveness of FluMist, a live attenuated, cold-adapted, and temperature-sensitive trivalent influenza vaccine currently approved for the prevention of influenza in healthy children aged 5 to 19 years. The study looks at children with asthma, comparing the safety and efficacy of a single dose of this vaccine with the injectable trivalent inactivated influenza vaccine.

So, is the live intranasal vaccination as efficacious and safe as an injectable inactivated vaccine in asthmatic children? The answer appears to be *yes* on both counts. Overall, both vaccines appear to be safe and well tolerated. Protection levels run about the same. There was no evidence of significant increases in adverse pulmonary events for the cold-adapted live virus vaccine. A slight nod to the latter is given for its greater relative effectiveness of 35% compared with the injectable vaccine.

J. A. Stockman III, MD

Superior Relative Efficacy of Live Attenuated Influenza Vaccine Compared With Inactivated Influenza Vaccine in Young Children With Recurrent Respiratory Tract Infections

Ashkenazi S, for the CAIV-T Study Group (Schneider Children's Med Ctr, Petah-Tikva, Israel; et al)
Pediatr Infect Dis J 25:870-879, 2006

Background.—Young children have a high incidence of influenza and influenza-related complications. This study compared the efficacy and safety of cold-adapted influenza vaccine, trivalent (CAIV-T) with trivalent inactivated influenza vaccine (TIV) in young children with a history of recurrent respiratory tract infections (RTIs).

Methods.—Children 6 to 71 months of age were randomized to receive 2 doses of CAIV-T (n = 1101) or TIV (n = 1086), 35 ± 7 days apart before the start of the 2002–2003 influenza season and were followed up for culture-confirmed influenza, effectiveness outcomes, reactogenicity, and adverse events.

Results.—Overall, 52.7% (95% confidence interval [CI] = 21.6%–72.2%) fewer cases of influenza caused by virus strains antigenically similar to vaccine were observed in CAIV-T than in TIV recipients. Greater relative efficacy for CAIV-T was observed for the antigenically similar A/H1N1 (100.0%; 95% CI = 42.3%–100.0%) and B (68.0%; 95% CI = 37.3%–84.8%) strains but not for the antigenically similar A/H3N2 strains (−97.1%; 95% CI = −540.2% to 31.5%). Relative to TIV, CAIV-T reduced the number of RTI-related healthcare provider visits by 8.9% (90% CI = 1.5%–15.8%) and missed days of school, kindergarten, or day care by 16.2% (90% CI = 10.4%–21.6%). Rhinitis and rhinorrhea, otitis media, and decreased appetite were the only events that were reported more frequently in CAIV-T subjects. There was no difference between groups in the incidence of wheezing after vaccination.

Conclusions.—CAIV-T was well tolerated in these children with RTIs and demonstrated superior relative efficacy compared with TIV in preventing influenza illness.

▶ Fleming et al (Comparison of the efficacy and safety of live attenuated cold-adapted influenza vaccine, trivalent, with trivalent inactivated influenza virus vaccine in children and adolescents with asthma) looked at the efficacy of a live attenuated influenza vaccine compared with the inactivated influenza vaccine in asthmatic children. The live attenuated influenza vaccine (FluMist) has been shown to reduce the rate of culture-confirmed influenza by 94% and to reduce episodes of febrile otitis media by about 30% compared with placebo. There are few data reporting the safety of the live attenuated inactivated vaccine in children with asthma or wheezing, and only one study has reported an increased risk of asthma in young children after the use of this vaccine. The study by Fleming et al showed no adverse effects in asthmatic children.

This report looks at children with recurrent respiratory infections, many of whom have a history of wheezing illness. Such a population might be expected to benefit significantly from a more effective vaccine against influenza, but also might be particularly susceptible to wheezing associated with the use of such a vaccine. This report, however, showed no evidence of a difference in the incidence of wheezing after vaccination with either type of vaccine. Thus cold inactivated live influenza vaccine is indeed well tolerated in children with a history of recurrent respiratory tract infections and has slightly greater efficacy in the prevention of influenza in comparison with the inactivated vaccine.

J. A. Stockman III, MD

Safety of Trivalent Inactivated Influenza Vaccine in Children 6 to 23 Months Old

Hambidge SJ, for the Vaccine Safety Datalink Team (Kaiser Permanente Colorado, Denver; et al)
JAMA 296:1990-1997, 2006

Context.—Beginning with the winter season of 2004-2005, influenza vaccination has been recommended for all children 6 to 23 months old in the United States. However, its safety in young children has not been adequately studied in large populations.

Objective.—To screen for medically attended events in the clinic, emergency department, or hospital after administration of trivalent inactivated influenza vaccine in children 6 to 23 months old.

Design, Setting, and Participants.—Retrospective cohort using self-control analysis, with chart review of significant medically attended events at 8 managed care organizations in the United States that comprise the Vaccine Safety Datalink. Participants were all children in the Vaccine Safety Datalink cohort 6 to 23 months old who received trivalent inactivated influenza vaccine between January 1, 1991, and May 31, 2003 (45,356 children with 69,359 vaccinations).

Main Outcome Measure.—Any medically attended event significantly associated with trivalent inactivated influenza vaccine in risk windows 0 to 3 days, 1 to 14 days (primary analysis), 1 to 42 days, or 15 to 42 days after vaccination, compared with 2 control periods, one before vaccination and the second after the risk window. All individual *ICD-9* codes as well as predefined aggregate codes were examined.

Results.—Before chart review, only 1 diagnosis, gastritis/duodenitis, was more likely to occur in the 14 days after trivalent inactivated influenza vaccine (matched odds ratio [OR], 5.50; 95% confidence interval [CI], 1.22-24.81 for control period 1, and matched OR, 4.33; 95% CI, 1.23-15.21 for control period 2). Thirteen medically attended events were less likely to occur after trivalent inactivated influenza vaccine, including acute upper respiratory tract infection, asthma, bronchiolitis, and otitis media. After chart review, gastritis/duodenitis was not significantly associated with trivalent inactivated influenza vaccine (matched OR, 4.00; 95% CI, 0.85-18.84 for control period 1; matched OR, 3.34; 95% CI, 0.92-12.11 for control period 2).

Conclusions.—In the largest population-based study to date of the safety of trivalent inactivated influenza vaccine in young children, there were very few medically attended events, none of which were serious, significantly associated with the vaccine. This study provides additional evidence supporting the safety of universally immunizing all children 6 to 23 months old with influenza vaccine.

▶ The trivalent inactivated influenza vaccine has been around for decades to prevent influenza infection. The vaccine currently in use in the United States has been available since 1981, with annual modifications to reflect the predominant three strains of circulating influenza virus. Until recently, its use in children was recommended only for individuals with known chronic medical conditions, such as asthma, that would put them at higher risk from influenza infection. Based on increasing evidence of high morbidity from influenza infection in young children, the Advisory Committee on Immunization Practices of the Centers for Disease Control and Prevention (CDC) has recommended use of trivalent inactivated influenza vaccine in all children 6 to 23 months old, including healthy children with no chronic medical conditions, beginning in the winter season of 2004-2005. By the end of January 2005, about half of all children in this age group in the United States had received trivalent inactivated influenza vaccine.

The influenza vaccine has an excellent record of safety, although there have been documented rare complications from some annual formulations of the vaccine. A population-based study of the safety of trivalent inactivated influenza vaccine in children 0 to 18 years of age found very few medically plausible associations, none of them serious.[1] Studies related to vaccine safety in the youngest of children, however, have been based on relatively modest numbers of immunized children. The report abstracted describes a large population-based study of almost 70,000 vaccinations and evaluates the safety of trivalent inactivated vaccine in very young children. Given the large number of outcomes assessed, there is solid evidence that very few adverse reaction are associated with the vaccine, thereby providing overall assurance that the vaccine is safe for use in this young age group. The only positive association was with an increased risk of gastritis/duodenitis in the 14-day period after vaccination. Noninfectious gastroenteritis was slightly increased during this period. Almost all cases were of acute vomiting, diarrhea, or both in otherwise healthy children. This finding was not unexpected and may be due to chance alone.

Notably, this report also found an unexpected consequence of receiving the influenza vaccine. This was a lower incidence of asthma diagnoses after trivalent inactivated vaccine administration. Although a lower risk of asthma in the 14 days after trivalent inactivated vaccine administration is unlikely to represent protection from infection with influenza virus, it may represent a reduction of asthma exacerbations triggered by other types of upper respiratory tract infections. It is also possible that since children were vaccinated during a visit to a doctor, they may have had some adjustment in their asthma medications. The study also found a lower risk of atopic dermatitis after influenza vaccination in young children. The influenza vaccine does not appear to be associated with an increased risk of febrile seizures unless given with the measles, mumps, and rubella vaccine.

This report from the CDC, the largest safety studies of trivalent inactivated influenza vaccine in children age 6 to 23 months, adds to prior evidence that influenza vaccine is safe for use in infants and young children.

J. A. Stockman III, MD

Reference

1. France EK, Glanz JM, Xu S, et al. Safety of the trivalent inactivated influenza vaccine among children: a population-based study. *Arch Pediatr Adolesc Med.* 2004;158:1031-1036.

Influenza-Related Hospitalizations in Children Younger Than Three Years of Age

Rojo JC, Ruiz-Contreras J, Fernández MB, et al (Hosp Universitario 12 de Octubre, Madrid)
Pediatr Infect Dis J 25:596-601, 2006

Background.—To determine the rates of influenza-related hospitalization and to know the clinical manifestations and underlying diseases in children younger than 3 years who are hospitalized with influenza.

Methods.—Retrospective, descriptive study (1996–2003), performed in a tertiary teaching hospital in Madrid. Data of hospitalized children, younger than 3 years, with influenza virus isolation from nasal aspirates were collected. Rates of hospitalization for every year were calculated.

Results.—Overall, 146 children hospitalized with influenza were identified: 117 had community-acquired influenza as the only disease, 18 had community-acquired influenza and were coinfected with other pathogens, and 11 had nosocomial infection. Rates of influenza hospitalization for years 1996, 1997, 1998, 1999, 2000, 2001, 2002, and 2003 were 0.42, 0.11, 1.46, 1.54, 0.53, 0.25, 0.19, and 0.82, respectively, per 1000 children younger than 3 years of age. Children ≤1 year of age accounted for almost two thirds of admissions.

Bronchitis/bronchiolitis (42 children), pneumonia (11 children), fever without source (36 children), and suspected sepsis (9 children) accounted for almost 90% of all hospitalizations in children with community-acquired influenza.

Forty-seven patients (40%) had underlying diseases, mainly chronic pulmonary disease and congenital heart disease. Ten patients (8.5%) with community-acquired influenza A and underlying conditions were admitted to the intensive care unit.

Conclusions.—Influenza is an important cause of hospitalization in young children. The use of influenza vaccine in high-risk children could prevent hospitalizations and cases of influenza-related diseases.

▶ Here in the United States, yearly influenza vaccination for toddlers aged between 6 months and 2 years is recommended. This recommendation is driven by high rates of hospitalization among young children with influenza. What we see from this report from Spain is that we are not unique here in the United States. It would appear that worldwide, pulmonary symptoms such as bronchitis/bronchiolitis, pneumonia, and also fever without a source and suspected sepsis are the presentations most commonly seen for children who are being hospitalized with what turns out to be influenza.

Obviously hospitalized children with influenza are just the tip of the iceberg according to an active surveillance network operating here in the United States.[1] For every 1000 children younger than 5 years of age, the influenza network recorded 95 visits to outpatient clinics and 27 visits to emergency departments during the 2003-2004 influenza season alone. That is a burden of illness in the outpatient setting that is between 10 and 250 times greater than the burden of hospitalizations for influenza in the same states. In this study, during active surveillance, nurses tested all children younger than 5 years presenting to selected hospitals, clinics, and emergency departments with respiratory tract symptoms or a fever. Of those tested as outpatients, 16% had laboratory-confirmed influenza. The most common symptoms were fever (95%), cough (96%), and runny nose (96%). Pediatricians and other care providers recognized influenza as the source of the infection in only a minority of children— 28% of inpatients and just 17% of outpatients. Very few patients got any kind of antiviral treatment.

Failure to recognize influenza, particularly in toddlers, truly represents a missed opportunity since early treatment can help prevent complications and control spread to other contacts. What we need is a rapid test for influenza to help all of us during flu season to decide who should get antiviral therapy and who would not benefit from it. As we see in this report, somewhere between 1 in 6 and 1 in 7 children presenting with respiratory tract symptoms and fever during flu season will in fact have influenza, a statistic we should all remember.

headache (ARR, 11.3%; 95% CI, 6.50%-16.2%). The combined results from 4 studies of 717 patients showed a nonsignificant decrease in headache in patients who were mobilized after LP (ARR, 2.9%; 95% CI, −3.4 to 9.3%). Four studies on the accuracy of biochemical analysis of CSF in patients with suspected meningitis met inclusion criteria. A CSF–blood glucose ratio of 0.4 or less (likelihood ratio [LR], 18; 95% CI, 12-27]), CSF white blood cell count of 500/μL or higher (LR, 15; 95% CI, 10-22), and CSF lactate level of 31.53 mg/dL or more (≥3.5 mmol/L; LR, 21; 95% CI, 14-32) accurately diagnosed bacterial meningitis.

Conclusions.—These data suggest that small-gauge, atraumatic needles may decrease the risk of headache after diagnostic LP. Reinsertion of the stylet before needle removal should occur and patients do not require bed rest after the procedure. Future research should focus on evaluating interventions to optimize the success of a diagnostic LP and to enhance training in procedural skills.

▶ It is hard to believe that a report such as this would be appearing in the medical literature, since it has been a century and a half since the first descriptions of an LP appeared. In 1891, Quincke[1] first reported having performed an LP for the purposes of examining the CSF. The authors of this report present a fictitious 70-year-old woman who presents to the emergency department with a 3-day history of fever, confusion, and lethargy along with a stiff neck on physical examination. An LP is performed, and then a number of questions arise not only about the performance of the LP, but also the analysis of the results. This fictitious case was used as an example to review the medical literature in a systematic way to update us about how to correctly perform an LP and to analyze data from the findings. The information provided is of direct relevance to the practice of pediatrics. It is suggested that every practitioner read this report, because it is a bit too lengthy to summarize in any detail. The abstract summarizes the key findings.

What is most interesting about this report is the flurry of letters to the editor that quickly followed its publication. Many of the letters took issue with some of the recommendations in the report or in an instructional video on lumbar puncture by Ellenby and colleagues[2] that appeared, also in 2006, in the electronic version of *The New England Journal of Medicine*. The instructional video suggested that as the spinal needle is incrementally advanced, the stylet should be withdrawn periodically to check for CSF and then reinserted until the needle enters the subarachnoid space. While this is how most perform an LP, a letter to the editor suggested this may not be the best method.[3] It is suggested that the main purpose of the stylet is to prevent the formation of an epidermal tumor by avoiding the introduction of a skin plug into the subarachnoid space. Thus, the stylet is of little use after the needle has been advanced beyond the skin. Early removal of the stylet, once it is past the subcutaneous tissue, and needle advancement without the stylet in place allow for better observation of the CSF flow when the subarachnoid space is entered. This technique, it is proposed, may prevent "traumatic taps" by avoiding the inadvertent advancement of the needle beyond the subarachnoid space. In fact, early removal of the stylet has been shown to improve the rate of success of LP in

Methods.—We analyzed blood-contaminated CSF specimens collected from 1-month to 18-year-old children presenting to an urban academic pediatric emergency department between 1993 and 2003. Predictions of leukocytes (total) and neutrophils in CSF were derived from a standard rule and from an alternative rule based on a regression between neutrophils in peripheral blood and CSF. The match between observed and predicted cell counts was estimated by the coefficient of determination (R^2). The value of corrected over uncorrected cells for diagnosing bacterial meningitis was evaluated by comparing the areas under respective receiver operator characteristic curves (AUC).

Results.—At an R^2 of 0.11, predicted leukocytes matched observed leukocytes poorly for 682 CSF specimens that met study criteria. The percent of neutrophils in CSF predicted by the regression 7% + (0.5 × percent of neutrophils in peripheral blood) also fit observed neutrophils only modestly (R^2 0.27). For diagnosing bacterial meningitis, there was no difference between AUC values for corrected and uncorrected leukocytes and percent of neutrophils.

Conclusion.—In blood-contaminated CSF, there is poor to modest correlation between observed and predicted counts of leukocytes and of neutrophils. Adjusted blood counts in CSF have no advantage over uncorrected counts for predicting bacterial meningitis.

▶ The authors of this report are to be congratulated on their perseverance in carrying out this retrospective study that examined whether the formula used to correct the number of leukocytes in the CSF of a child who has experienced a "bloody tap" is of any value in comparison with simply looking at the uncorrected white blood cell count. They examined the results of CSF studies obtained between January 1993 and July 2003, which yielded some 16,280 CSF specimens. They carefully weeded out children who ultimately were documented to have an infectious reason for obtaining the CSF. Also weeded out were specimens obtained from children who had neurologic signs and symptoms. Basically, they ended up with a pool of specimens from otherwise "normal" children. To retrospectively capture CSF specimens that were normal except for blood contamination (defined as a CSF erythrocyte count >500 cells/mL), they applied the following criteria. They excluded children who were given a diagnosis of traumatic head injury, neurologic disease, neurosurgical disease, underlying medical surgical disease, sepsis, meningitis (viral or bacterial), and encephalitis, as well as those with CSF from which a viral or bacterial pathogen was isolated. Predictions of the total leukocyte count expected in blood-contaminated CSF were made in accordance with a previously published rule that predicts the total leukocyte count in blood-contaminated CSF by adjusting the concentration of erythrocytes in the CSF by a factor of 0.002. This conversion is based on the 1:500 ratio of leukocytes to erythrocytes typically found in peripheral blood. Most of us refer to this as the 1:500 rule, which in other studies seems to have a similar utility in comparison with the more complicated rule that adjusts the number of leukocytes based on the actual number of erythrocytes, ratio-wise, in comparison with the counts in a peripheral blood complete blood cell count.

What we see in this report is that when a bloody tap occurs, there is a very poor correlation between the CSF white blood cell count and the predicted number of white blood cells that would be expected as the result of simply performing a bloody tap. The authors concluded that the standard 1:500 rule for adjusting leukocytes in blood-contaminated CSF is a poor match for observed leukocytes in normal CSF. Even when attempting to use the "more precise" and complicated formula that adjusts CSF leukocytes based on the leukocyte-to-erythrocyte ratio in the peripheral blood, the authors found only a modest improvement in the match. The bottom line, as these authors suggest, is that there seems to be no advantage to adjusting leukocytes and neutrophils in blood-contaminated CSF, and the authors recommend support for the utilization of unadjusted leukocytes evaluated against published norms in CSF to lower the risk of missed bacterial meningitis among children with ambiguous findings in blood-contaminated CSF.

J. A. Stockman III, MD

Quick identification of febrile neonates with low risk for serious bacterial infection: an observational study

Marom R, Sakran W, Antonelli J, et al (Rappaport School of Medicine, Haifa, Israel; HaEmek Med Ctr, Afula, Israel; Poria Med Ctr, Tiberias, Israel)
Arch Dis Child Fetal Neonatal Ed 92:F15-F18, 2007

Objective.—To examine the possible usefulness of simple and quick criteria for identifying febrile neonates with low risk for serious bacterial infection (SBI).

Design.—All febrile neonates who were admitted between August 1998 and August 2003 to the Pediatric Emergency Department, HaEmek Medical Center, Afula, Israel, and to the Poriya Hospital, Tiberias, Israel, were included in the study. The recommended evaluation of each neonate included details of medical history and a complete physical examination, including blood culture, erythrocyte sedimentation rate (ESR), white cell count (WBC), and analysis and culture of urine and cerebrospinal fluid. Other tests were carried out as necessary. Patients who met all the following criteria were considered to have low risk for SBI: (1) unremarkable medical history; (2) good appearance; (3) no focal physical signs of infection; (4) ESR <30 mm at the end of the first hour; (5) WBC 5000–15 000/mm^3; (6) a normal urine analysis by the dipstick method.

Results.—Complete data were available for 386 neonates. SBI was documented in 108 (28%) neonates, of whom 14% had a urinary tract infection, 9.3% had acute otitis media, 2.3% had pneumonia, 1.3% had cellulitis, 0.5% had bacterial meningitis and 0.5% had bacterial gastroenteritis. The overall incidence of SBI was 1 in 166 (0.6%) neonates who fulfilled the criteria compared with 107 in 220 (48.6%) in the neonates who did not fulfil the criteria (p<0.001). The negative predictive value for SBI of the combination of the low-risk criteria was 99.4% (95% confidence interval 99.35% to 99.45%).

Conclusions.—Fulfillment of the criteria for low risk might be a reliable and useful tool for excluding SBI in febrile neonates.

▶ One more article on fever in the neonate—are you sick of it yet? What have Marom et al shown that is new information? We see that there is an extremely low rate of severe bacterial infection in neonates who fulfill low-risk criteria for this problem (actual infection rate of just 0.6%). Low risk here means a previously healthy, well-appearing neonate with no focal signs of infection, a low ESR, a WBC count of 5000 to 15,000/mm^3, and a normal urinalysis. These data build on the work of Dagan et al,[1] who considered infants younger than 3 months to be at low risk for severe bacterial infection if they had been previously well, had no signs of ear, soft tissue, or skeletal infection, had a WBC count of 5000 to 15,000/mm^3, had a band cell count of less than 1500/mm^3, and had a normal urinalysis. In the latter group of infants, some did switch into the high-risk group, leading to the admonishment that conservative management for fever of undetermined origin in an otherwise well-looking infant is feasible if meticulous follow-up is provided and adequate laboratory studies are performed and are normal.

So what is your management of the febrile neonate who fulfills low-risk criteria? These infants will still be admitted to the hospital. The issue is whether they will be admitted for observation only without treatment as was done in this study. Folks with more confidence will allow close follow-up to be done as an outpatient. For more on the topic of the "drive-thru" management of fever in the neonate, see the excellent commentary by Rudd.[2]

J. A. Stockman III, MD

References

1. Dagan R, Powell K, Hall C, Menegus MA. Identification of infants unlikely to have serious bacterial infection although hospitalized for suspected sepsis. *J Pediatr.* 1985;107:855-860.
2. Rudd P. Is there a place for "drive-thru" management of neonatal fever? Not yet! *Arch Dis Child.* 2007;92:F2-F3.

Drotrecogin alfa (activated) in children with severe sepsis: a multicentre phase III randomised controlled trial
Nadel S, for the REsearching severe Sepsis and Organ dysfunction in children: a gLobal perspectiVE (RESOLVE) study group (St Mary's Hosp and Imperial College, London; et al)
Lancet 369:836-843, 2007

Background.—Drotrecogin alfa (activated) (DrotAA) is used for the treatment of adults with severe sepsis who have a high risk of dying. A phase 1b open-label study has indicated that the pharmacokinetics and pharmacodynamics of DrotAA are similar in children and adults. We initiated the RESOLVE (REsearching severe Sepsis and Organ dysfunction in children:

a gLobal perspectiVE) trial to investigate the efficacy and safety of the drug in children.

Methods.—Children aged between 38 weeks' corrected gestational age and 17 years with sepsis-induced cardiovascular and respiratory failure were randomly assigned to receive placebo or DrotAA (24 µg/kg/h) for 96 h. We used a prospectively defined, novel primary endpoint of Composite Time to Complete Organ Failure Resolution (CTCOFR) score. Secondary endpoints were 28-day mortality, major amputations, and safety. Analysis was by intention-to-treat.

Findings.—477 patients were enrolled; 237 received placebo, and 240 DrotAA. Our results showed no significant difference between groups in CTCOFR score (p=0.72) or in 28-day mortality (placebo 17.5%; DrotAA, 17.2%; p=0.93). Although there was no difference in overall serious bleeding events during the 28-day study period (placebo 6.8%; DrotAA 6.7%; p=0.97), there were numerically more instances of CNS bleeding in the DrotAA group (11 [4.6%], *vs* 5 [2.1%] in placebo, p=0.13), particularly in children younger than 60 days. For CTCOFR score days 1–14, correlation coefficient was −0.016 (95% CI −0.106 to 0.74); relative risk for 28-day mortality was 1.06 (95% CI 0.66 to 1.46) for DrotAA compared with placebo.

Interpretation.—Although we did not record any efficacy of DrotAA in children with severe sepsis, serious bleeding events were similar between groups and the overall safety profile acceptable, except in children younger than 60 days. However, we gained important insights into clinical and laboratory characteristics of childhood severe sepsis, and have identified issues that need to be addressed in future trials in critically ill children.

▶ This report summarizes the much-anticipated results of the RESOLVE trial. This trial assessed DrotAA (recombinant human activated protein C) in children with sepsis. In this double-blind placebo-controlled international trial, the investigators randomly assigned children with severe sepsis to a 4-day course of DrotAA or placebo (the latter in the form of IV saline). The primary end point was a composite score for resolution of organ failure; secondary end points were all-cause mortality up to 28 days after treatment and safety. The overall results turned out to be quite unexpected and profoundly disappointing: no efficacy signal was detectable from any of the end points, and the survival grafts looked much the same for both treatments.

Intensivists and experts in infectious diseases have been holding on to the belief that new antisepsis agents would improve outcomes in children affected with bloodstream infections. Children with sepsis are an ideal population to study the efficacy of these new antisepsis agents because they usually have no underlying comorbidities. However, they also tend to do much better than adults, which makes studies of antisepsis agents more difficult since large numbers of children have to be studied.

RESOLVE had some interesting findings. First, patients with sepsis who had the most severe coagulation abnormalities were the ones who actually benefitted the most from DrotAA. Second, it became apparent during the study that intracranial bleeding was more common with DrotAA than with placebo. If there is anything to be learned from this report, it is that future trials of this agent, and probably other anticoagulants, should avoid treatment in the neonatal period. Also, the possible role of so-called first-patient effects needs consideration because of the excess mortality rate noted for the initial patients who were enrolled in the placebo-controlled trials of DrotAA. To say this differently, there is a small but real period of learning at the start of trials such as this. When one looks carefully at the data, after the enrollment of the first patient at every site, the number of deaths did not differ between treated and placebo-managed patients.

If one is not familiar with DrotAA, it is a recombinant form of human activated protein C intended to diminish the complications of the coagulopathy so frequently seen in children affected with sepsis. The RESOLVE study is the only placebo-controlled study of this agent in children, and although the results of the trial are disappointing, the report does contain some interesting information in the sense that it is now known exactly what the serious bleeding rate is in severe sepsis. This rate averages about 7% over 28 days. Despite not demonstrating a positive effect, RESOLVE has documented the natural history of severe sepsis and paves the way for future randomized placebo-controlled trials in the field of pediatric critical care medicine. Similar trials are underway in adults using other recombinant products, and sure as shooting we will hear more about this in children as well.

While on the topic of sepsis, see if you can reach a diagnosis with the following case. On October 31, 2004, heavy rains caused an adjacent stream to overflow its banks and flood the campus of the University of Hawaii. A professor at the university waded into his flooded laboratory in sandals to help clean up the mess. He developed blisters in the process. Eight days later, he became ill with fever, chills, and vomiting. The fever subsided over a four-day period, but he also developed other symptoms including tremor, poor balance, and visual flashes of light. A week after the onset of illness, he was seriously ill and was hospitalized. During the same time period, a male graduate student, age 27 years, who worked with the professor, also became ill with fever, chills, vomiting, diarrhea, and headaches. Your diagnosis?

Walking around in murky water can be injurious to your health. Those exposed to fresh water or mud contaminated by the urine of animals infected with the spirochete *Leptospira interrogans* can develop systemic illness if the leptospires enter the body through broken skin or mucus membranes. Indeed, leptospirosis is considered to be the most common zoonosis worldwide and is endemic in tropical environments such as Hawaii, where the mean annual incidence of leptospirosis is 1.29 per 100,000 population. The infection, however, can also occur in milder climates, either as the result of local exposure or in travelers returning from the tropics. It has even been reported in homeless people living on the streets in Baltimore. Natural disasters such as floods and hurricanes increase the risk for human exposure to leptospires through contact with contaminated water or mud.

Initial symptoms of leptospirosis resemble those of any influenza-illness, with fever as the most common sign. A thorough exposure history is essential to diagnosis. Although many infected persons recover spontaneously, somewhere between 5% and 10% of cases progress to a more serious and potentially fatal second stage of illness that affects internal organ systems. Rapid treatment is necessary.

Interestingly, there is very little information regarding any leptospirosis outbreak associated with the flooding in New Orleans. Maybe it was simply missed. To learn more about the epidemiology, clinical findings, diagnosis, treatment and prevention, and reporting of leptospirosis, see the thorough review of this topic in *MMWR*.[1]. The punch line is that medical attention should be sought promptly by any person who has the onset of a febrile illness within one month of participating in the cleanup of a flood-affected area.

J. A. Stockman III, MD

Reference

1. Park SY, Effler PV, Nakata M, et al. Brief report: leptospirosis after flooding of a university campus—Hawaii, 2004. *MMWR*. 2006;55:125-127.

The Effect of Changing From Whole-Cell to Acellular Pertussis Vaccine on the Epidemiology of Hospitalized Children With Pertussis in Canada
Bettinger JA, Halperin SA, De Serres G, et al (Univ of British Columbia, Vancouver, Canada; Dalhousie Univ, Halifax, Canada; Quebec Inst of Public Health; et al)
Pediatr Infect Dis J 26:31-35, 2007

Background.—Between July 1997 and April 1998, universal childhood immunization programs in Canada changed from using a whole-cell pertussis to a 5-component acellular pertussis-containing vaccine. To assess effects on pertussis epidemiology of this nationwide change, we analyzed hospitalizations during 1991–2004 using the Canadian Immunization Monitoring Program, Active (IMPACT) pertussis database.

Methods.—IMPACT is an active surveillance network based in 12 pediatric tertiary-care hospitals across Canada. Characteristics of hospitalized cases of pertussis were compared by type of vaccine received or by birth date (if immunization records were unavailable or the child was unvaccinated). Age-stratified incidence rates were calculated by year and vaccine type.

Results.—Two thousand ninety-six cases of pertussis were admitted to IMPACT centers, 1174 during the whole-cell vaccine program (WCV-P) and 842 during the acellular vaccine program (ACV-P). Pertussis incidence among children <5 years old decreased significantly during the ACV-P, causing an increase in the residual proportion of cases either too young to be immunized (<2 months old: ACV-P 39% versus WCV-P 26.1%; $P < 0.0001$) or too young for a second dose (2–3 months old: 42.9% versus 34.2%, respectively; $P < 0.0001$). A significantly smaller proportion of cases (ACV-P 15.1% versus WCV-P 27.3%) occurred in infants who were old enough (4–11 months of age) to have received 2 or 3 doses of vaccine.

Conclusions.—With ACV-P, pertussis hospitalizations in children 4–59 months old decreased in frequency, consistent with improved vaccine effectiveness, but remained prominent among very young infants. Improved control strategies are needed to reduce infections among infants too young for pertussis vaccination.

▶ This report is from Canada, where a major resurgence of pertussis occurred throughout the country in the early 1990s. Several studies implicated poor efficacy of the whole-cell pertussis vaccine as the reason for the unexpected rise in cases. As all of us know, the whole-cell pertussis vaccine first became available in 1943 and has been the prime source of pertussis vaccination until the introduction in the late 1990s of the acellular pertussis–containing vaccine. The latter produced fewer injection site and systemic adverse events in children, and the acellular vaccine has proven to be safer for use in older children and adults. The report abstracted is the first population-based analysis using the Canadian Immunization Monitoring Program to show the impact of the switch to the acellular vaccine in Canada. The change from whole-cell to acellular vaccine has been associated with the rapid decline in the overall incidence of pertussis in that nation. Unfortunately, the acellular vaccine appears to have had little influence on the incidence of infection in infants younger than 3 months, a group that still accounts for a high proportion of pertussis-related hospital admissions. Despite improvement in vaccine effectiveness, transmission to susceptible infants continues because of ongoing transmission in incompletely immunized children, those left vulnerable despite vaccination, and adolescents and adults without immunity who have remained unvaccinated with the acellular vaccine. The challenge now is to develop effective strategies to protect infants too young to be immunized. The recent Canadian recommendations for one dose of acellular pertussis vaccine during adolescence or adulthood may help to achieve this objective.

The issues reported in Canada are not that very different from what we are seeing here in the United States. Unprotected infants are being infected by adults with pertussis. In the November 2, 2006 issue of the *Boston Globe*, there was a report of an outbreak of whooping cough affecting 1 patient and 15 staff members at Boston Children's Hospital. At Dartmouth-Hitchcock Medical Center in Lebanon, New Hampshire, more than 4500 hospital employees were given acellular pertussis vaccine in response to cases of pertussis among health care workers in the spring of 2006. In Texas in 2005, more than 2000 cases of pertussis were reported. Nine patients died, 8 of them infants. In 2003, more than 1900 cases of pertussis were reported in Wisconsin, predominantly among adolescents and adults. In New York State in 1998 and 1999, more than 600 cases of pertussis were confirmed by a single private laboratory.[1]

Have we lost our long-standing control of whooping cough? During the past 2 decades, there has been a slow, steady resurgence of pertussis, though rates have not approached the levels of the prevaccine era. The shift in the 1990s from whole-cell vaccines to less reactogenic acellular vaccines here in the United States was associated with significantly reduced rates of vaccine-associated adverse events, but the incidence of pertussis here has continued to increase. The problem relates to the existence of a susceptible cohort of adults who received the less effective whole-cell pertussis vaccine years ago. Recently, in Canada, the United States, and elsewhere, programs of universal immunization of adolescents with acellular pertussis vaccine have been implemented to address this changing epidemiology. After administration of whole-cell pertussis vaccine, immunity against pertussis begins to diminish after 3 to 5 years. There is no demonstrable protection by 10 to 12 years. The duration of protection after administration of acellular vaccine is not yet established, but immunity begins to decline after 4 or 5 years, suggesting that a 10-year dose interval will be appropriate with these vaccines.

Some have suggested that we are not seeing a significant rise in the true prevalence of pertussis, merely a better laboratory recognition of the infection with improved techniques that allow documentation of the infection (polymerase chain reaction methodologies). The return of pertussis cannot be dismissed as the effect of increased laboratory testing, however. Large outbreaks of clinically typical pertussis in adolescents and adults, documented by both culture and polymerase chain reaction, have occurred and would not have been missed previously. In view of the clear burden of pertussis in older age groups, more attention should be paid to following the recommendations of the Advisory Committee on Immunization Practices that all adolescents and adults be given a dose of acellular pertussis vaccine combined with diphtheria and tetanus toxoid (Tdap). Given the demonstrated safety and efficacy of such a vaccine in clinical trials involving adolescents and adults, and early evidence of the effectiveness of adolescent-vaccination programs, broader use of the vaccine may prevent pertussis disease and circumvent the difficulties of establishing its diagnosis. At the same time, we must undertake more epidemiologic studies involving careful laboratory testing if we are to evaluate accurately the burden of pertussis among adults and monitor the effectiveness of our vaccine strategies.

J. A. Stockman III, MD

Reference

1. Halperin SA. The control of pertussis—2007 and beyond. *N Engl J Med*. 2007;356:110-113.

Whooping cough in school age children with persistent cough: prospective cohort study in primary care
Harnden A, Grant C, Harrison T, et al (Univ of Oxford, England; Univ of Auckland, New Zealand)
BMJ 333:174-177, 2006

Objective.—To estimate the proportion of school age children with a persistent cough who have evidence of a recent *Bordetella pertussis* infection.
Design.—Prospective cohort study (October 2001 to March 2005).
Setting.—General practices in Oxfordshire, England.
Participants.—172 children aged 5-16 years who presented to their general practitioner with a cough lasting 14 days or more who consented to have a blood test.

Main Outcome Measures.—Serological evidence of a recent *Bordetella pertussis* infection; symptoms at presentation; duration and severity of cough; sleep disturbance (parents and child).

Results.—64 (37.2%, 95% confidence interval 30.0% to 44.4%) children had serological evidence of a recent *Bordetella pertussis* infection; 55 (85.9%) of these children had been fully immunised. At presentation, children with whooping cough were more likely than others to have whooping (odds ratio 2.85, 95% confidence interval 1.39 to 5.82), vomiting (4.35, 2.04 to 9.25), and sputum production (2.39, 1.14 to 5.02). Children with whooping cough were also more likely to still be coughing two months after the start of their illness (85% *v* 48%; P = 0.001), continue to have more than five coughing episodes a day (P = 0.049), and cause sleep disturbance for their parents (P = 0.003).

Conclusions.—For school age children presenting to primary care with a cough lasting two weeks or more, a diagnosis of whooping cough should be considered even if the child has been immunised. Making a secure diagnosis of whooping cough may prevent inappropriate investigations and treatment.

▶ This report on whooping cough is an eye-opener. Most of us do not tend to think about pertussis in older children who present with an ongoing cough as their main symptom if that youngster had been previously immunized. The data from this report are truly a wake-up call in this regard. The report found that nearly 40% of children age 5 to 16 years presenting in the United Kingdom in general medical practice who had a cough lasting 14 days or more demonstrated serologic evidence of recent pertussis infection. You will have to be the judge of whether this study applies to other countries. Do the findings represent a "flow" in a cycle of pertussis incidence that will "ebb" on its own? Is the problem that is being seen in England a reflection of an outbreak of pertussis in adults who infect youngsters with waning immunity? Lots of questions.

Children who have been immunized against pertussis, will frequently not have the classic clinical features of this disease should they develop it. Persistent cough may be the only hallmark of infection. Thinking about the possibility of *Bordetella pertussis* and then confirming the diagnosis may very well obviate the need for x-ray examination or the use of other therapeutic interventions that would otherwise not be needed in a case of resolving pertussis.

Far and away, Vermont leads the rest of the country by having the highest reported incidence of pertussis. Vermont is followed by Massachusetts, Idaho, New Hampshire, and Wisconsin. These 5 states have more pertussis, on average, than one might suspect, and the most likely reason for this is the unusual ease with which parents can exempt out of immunizations for their children. The lowest incidence of pertussis is found in Mississippi, followed by the District of Columbia, Louisiana, Florida, New Jersey, and Georgia. The latter states either do not permit personal exemptions or make them difficult to obtain.[1]

J. A. Stockman III, MD

Reference

1. Omer SB, Pan WK, Halsey NA, et al. Nonmedical exemptions to school immunization requirements: secular trends and association of state policies with pertussis incidence. *JAMA*. 2006;296:1757-1763.

Tuberculosis in Adolescents: A French Retrospective Study of 52 Cases

do Pontual L, Balu L, Ovetchkine P, et al (Jean Verdier Teaching Hosp, Bondy, France; Sainte-Justine Hosp, Montréal, Québec; Avicenne Teaching Hosp, Bobigny, France)

Pediatr Infect Dis J 25:930-932, 2006

Background.—The only available data about tuberculosis (TB) among adolescents date back to the 1980s, although the incidence of tuberculosis has been increasing in this age group.

Methods.—Medical records were reviewed for all adolescents aged 12 to 18 years hospitalized with the diagnosis of TB in Avicenne/Jean Verdier Teaching hospital (Seine-Saint-Denis, suburb of Paris) between September 2000 and December 2004.

Results.—Of the 52 patients identified, 52% were female. Median age at diagnosis was 15 years (range, 12–18 years). The proportion of adolescents known to be born abroad was 90%. Diagnoses resulted from the examination of a sick child in 79% of cases, a case contact investigation of an adult suspected of having TB in 19% and routine tuberculin skin test in 2%. Twenty-seven of 52 patients (52%) had isolated pulmonary disease. Sixteen patients (31%) had pulmonary and extrapulmonary TB and 8 cases (17%) had exclusively extrapulmonary disease. The site of extrapulmonary TB included pleural (n = 8), meningitis (n = 4), lymph node (n = 4), peritoneal (n = 5), osteoarticular (n = 3) and genitourinary (n = 1). TB was confirmed by the isolation of *Mycobacterium tuberculosis* from sputum (n = 21), gastric aspirate (n = 8), bone (n = 1) or cerebrospinal fluid (n = 2). No case had a relapse or recurrence of disease in median 3.2 years of follow up.

Conclusions.—Our results indicate that demographic and clinical characteristics of adolescents with TB differed from adults and children. A specific approach to the prevention and treatment of TB in adolescents is absolutely necessary.

▶ This report underscores the differences in the clinical manifestations of tuberculosis in adolescents. The most common clinical presentation of tuberculosis in adults is pulmonary. Among adolescents in this report, 31% had pulmonary and extrapulmonary tuberculosis and 17% had exclusively extrapulmonary disease. Adolescents seem to be more likely to have cavitary disease compared with young children. Diagnosing tuberculosis is more difficult in children because of nonspecificity of symptoms and difficulty in confirming the diagnosis microbiologically. Adolescents are more symptomatic. More than half of the adolescents in this series had respiratory signs. The adolescent at highest risk for the development of tuberculosis was one coming from families with recent immigration from endemic countries, exposure to tuberculosis-positive adults, and those with HIV infection.

You may have been hearing a lot recently about interferon-gamma release assays for the diagnosis of tuberculosis in children. Advances in molecular biology and genomics have led to an alternative to the tuberculin skin test for the diagnosis of infection with *Mycobacterium tuberculosis*. Two new in vitro assays have been developed that measure interferon-gamma (IFN) released by sensitized T-cells after stimulation by *M tuberculosis* antigens. The Centers for Disease Control and Prevention has published updated guidelines for the use of these assays. The CDC recommends that the assays be used in all circumstances in which the tuberculin skin test is used, including contact investigations, evaluation of immigrants, and serial testing of healthcare workers. Although the CDC guidelines acknowledge that there are few data regarding the performance of IFN-release assays in children and adolescents, the guidelines clearly imply that such assays can be used for children. Without question, the INF release assays show great promise for improving the diagnosis of tuberculosis infection. Nonetheless, a recent commentary appearing in the *Pediatric Infectious Disease Journal* strongly cautions that there is too little information about these assays in children to recommend their universal use.[1]

J. A. Stockman III, MD

Reference

1. Starke JR. Interferon-gamma release assays for diagnosis of tuberculosis infection in children. *Pediatr Infect Dis J*. 2006;25:941-942.

Microscopic-Observation Drug-Susceptibility Assay for the Diagnosis of TB

Moore DA, Evans CA, Gilman RH, et al (Imperial College London; Asociación Benéfica PRISMA, San Miguel, Peru; Universidad Peruana Cayetano Heredia, San Martín de Porras, Peru; et al)
N Engl J Med 355:1539-1550, 2006

Background.—New diagnostic tools are urgently needed to interrupt the transmission of tuberculosis and multidrug-resistant tuberculosis. Rapid, sensitive detection of tuberculosis and multidrug-resistant tuberculosis in sputum has been demonstrated in proof-of-principle studies of the microscopic-observation drug-susceptibility (MODS) assay, in which broth cultures are examined microscopically to detect characteristic growth.

Methods.—In an operational setting in Peru, we investigated the performance of the MODS assay for culture and drug-susceptibility testing in three target groups: unselected patients with suspected tuberculosis, prescreened patients at high risk for tuberculosis or multidrug-resistant tuberculosis, and unselected hospitalized patients infected with the human immunodeficiency virus. We compared the MODS assay head-to-head with two reference methods: automated mycobacterial culture and culture on Lowenstein-Jensen medium with the proportion method.

Results.—Of 3760 sputum samples, 401 (10.7%) yielded cultures positive for *Mycobacterium tuberculosis*. Sensitivity of detection was 97.8% for MODS culture, 89.0% for automated mycobacterial culture, and 84.0% for Lowenstein-Jensen culture (P<0.001); the median time to culture positivity was 7 days, 13 days, and 26 days, respectively (P<0.001), and the median time to the results of susceptibility tests was 7 days, 22 days, and 68 days, respectively. The incremental benefit of a second MODS culture was minimal, particularly in patients at high risk for tuberculosis or multidrug-resistant tuberculosis. Agreement between MODS and the reference standard for susceptibility was 100% for rifampin, 97% for isoniazid, 99% for rifampin and isoniazid (combined results for multidrug resistance), 95% for ethambutol, and 92% for streptomycin (kappa values, 1.0, 0.89, 0.93, 0.71, and 0.72, respectively).

Conclusions.—A single MODS culture of a sputum sample offers more rapid and sensitive detection of tuberculosis and multidrug-resistant tuberculosis than the existing gold-standard methods used.

▶ Tuberculosis has reemerged with a vengeance. This vengeance has been expressed in 2 ways. One is the association between tuberculosis and the epidemic of HIV infection and AIDS. Also, there is the growing prevalence of drug resistance. Unfortunately, with respect to the latter, in many parts of the world there are no good tests available for drug resistance. Suspicion of drug resistance occurs only when there is a clinical suspicion of the problem on the basis of failure to respond to the usual combination of antituberculous drugs. Patients with multidrug-resistant tuberculosis will have progression of disease or may die while receiving ineffective treatment.

The studies of Moore et al attempt to address the problem of multi-resistant tuberculosis by evaluating a method called microscopic-observation drug-susceptibility (MODS) assay, considered to be an inexpensive tool for the bacteriologic diagnosis of tuberculosis and the detection of drug resistance. This technique was originally described back in 2000 and is based on direct inoculation of the selective 7H9 liquid culture medium in 24-well plates with a sputum specimen subjected to the digestion-decontamination procedure using a mixture of two reagents, *N*-acetyl-L-cysteine and sodium hydroxide. This mixture digests sputum, a requirement for the subsequent concentration of the mycobacteria by centrifugation. The sodium hydroxide allows decontamination, which is required to kill microbes that otherwise would interfere with the isolation of a pure mycobacterial culture. Concentration by centrifugation is the final step in the procedure. Detection of the typical cord formation ("microcolonies") of *M tuberculosis* in the wells on microscopic examination constitutes the basis of diagnosis. Growth (or lack thereof) in drug-containing wells, as compared with growth in drug-free wells, is the basis for reporting the results as "susceptible" or "resistant" to medication. The turnaround time for this assay is short: an average of just 7 days for the detection of growth on culture and testing for drug susceptibility.

This report of Moore et al provides support for an affordable, rapid method of culture-based diagnosis and detection of drug resistance, particularly in countries with limited resources. The major difficulty in the implementation of the

MODS assay or any other new cultivation method is that of biosafety, which is not fully addressed in this report. The methodologies used in the study require concentration of specimens in a centrifuge, which raises this issue of biosafety. Biosafety concerns can only be properly addressed in well-organized tuberculosis laboratories using mandatory implementation of biosafety level 3 standards.

The establishment of microbiology laboratories in countries with a high prevalence of tuberculosis and growing rates of drug-resistant tuberculosis should become one of the urgent priorities in the global fight against tuberculosis epidemics, especially in countries with limited financial resources. The MODS technique may well move this process forward.

For more on the topic, see the excellent commentary by Iseman and Heifets.[1] Last, while on the topic of antibiotic resistance and the need for developing new antibiotics, why may a mushroom a day be better than an apple a day at keeping the doctor away, and what does this have to do with Platensimycin? Platensimycin is a new class of antibiotic produced naturally by the mushroom bacterium *Streptomyces platensi*. The latter bacteria, which grows on mushrooms may be effective against a wide variety of multi-resistant super bugs, including multi-drug resistant *Staphylococcus aureus*. Researchers are now isolating a purified form of the compound from a mixture of the two distinct chemical types found in the bacteria that inhabit mushrooms.[2]

J. A. Stockman III, MD

References

1. Iseman MD, Heifets LB. Rapid detection of tuberculosis and drug-resistant tuberculosis. *N Engl J Med.* 2006;355:1606-1608.
2. Nicolaou KC, Li A, Edmonds DJ. Total synthesis of platensimycin. *Angew Chem Int Ed Engl.* 2006;45:7086-7090.

Sporadic *Campylobacter* Infection in Infants: A Population-Based Surveillance Case-Control Study

Fullerton KE, Ingram LA, Jones TF, et al (Ctrs for Disease Control and Prevention, Atlanta, Ga; Atlanta Research and Education Found, Decatur, Ga; Tennessee Dept of Health, Nashville; et al)
Pediatr Infect Dis J 26:19-24, 2007

Background.—*Campylobacter* is an important cause of foodborne illness in infants (younger than 1 year of age), but little is known about the sources of infection in this age group.

Methods.—Eight sites in the Foodborne Diseases Active Surveillance Network (FoodNet) participated in a 24-month population-based case-control study conducted in 2002–2004. Cases were infants with laboratory-confirmed *Campylobacter* infection ascertained through active laboratory surveillance, and controls were infants in the community.

Results.—We enrolled 123 cases and 928 controls. Infants 0–6 months of age with *Campylobacter* infection were less likely to be breast-fed than controls [odds ratio (OR); 0.2; 95% confidence interval (CI), 0.1–0.6]. Risk factors for infants 0–6 months of age included drinking well water (OR 4.4; CI, 1.4–14) and riding in a shopping cart next to meat or poultry (OR 4.0; CI, 1.2–13.0). Risk factors for infants 7–11 months of age included visiting or living on a farm (OR 6.2; CI, 2.2–17), having a pet with diarrhea in the home (OR 7.6; CI, 2.1–28) and eating fruits and vegetables prepared in the home (OR 2.5, CI 1.2–4.9). *Campylobacter* infection was associated with travel outside the United States at all ages (OR 19.3; CI, 4.5–82.1).

Conclusions.—Several unique protective and risk factors were identified among infants, and these risk factors vary by age, suggesting that prevention measures be targeted accordingly. Breast-feeding was protective for the youngest infants and should continue to be encouraged.

▶ It has been just about 30 years since *Campylobacter* infection was recognized as one of the most common causes of bacterial diarrhea in humans. Despite this several-decades-long experience with this infection, there has been relatively little written about it in young infants, thus the value of this report. Most cases of *Campylobacter* infection occur sporadically, rather than as part of a recognized outbreak. *Campylobacter* outbreaks have been caused by ingestion of untreated water, raw milk, chicken, and cross-contaminated foods. Sporadic *Campylobacter* infections have been associated with similar exposures as well as contact with pets, particularly those with diarrhea, and exposure to the farm environment, particularly through farm work or animal husbandry. Infants represent a unique population whose sources of *Campylobacter* are likely to differ from those of the older age group. Postulated sources of *Campylobacter* infection in infants include exposure to pet chickens, puppies in the house, and untreated drinking water. Breastfeeding is generally protective against diarrhea in infants and maybe protective against *Campylobacter* infection.

In this, the largest case-controlled study to look at potential sources of laboratory-confirmed *Campylobacter* infection in infants, we see that drinking well water, eating fruits or vegetables prepared in the home, having a pet in the home with diarrhea, and visiting or living on a farm are predictive of *Campylobacter* as a cause of a bacterial diarrheal illness. Breastfeeding is indeed protective, as noted again in this report. If there was a novel finding in this study, it was that infants with *Campylobacter* infection are more likely than well infants to have ridden in a shopping cart next to meat or poultry in a food store. *Campylobacter* infection was also associated with international travel, a finding also seen in the broader age population.

If there is a punch line to this report, it is that breastfeeding remains best for the first 12 months of life (the American Academy of Pediatrics' recommendation). Second, when on a trek to your local Piggly Wiggly, leave your infant at home with a care provider. Simply riding in a shopping cart may put that baby at risk for *Campylobacter* infection either by directly touching contaminated meat or poultry packages or by contact with objects that have, including the shopping cart itself. Fruits and vegetables per se are not a risk factor except when they become cross-contaminated on countertops that have been exposed to risky meats.

J. A. Stockman III, MD

The New Pentavalent Rotavirus Vaccine Composed of Bovine (Strain WC3) -Human Rotavirus Reassortants
Clark HF, Offit PA, Plotkin SA, et al (Univ of Pennsylvania, Philadelphia; Merck Research Labs, West Point, Pa)
Pediatr Infect Dis J 25:577-583, 2006

Background.—Infantile gastroenteritis caused by human rotaviruses is a prevalent disease throughout the world, causing dehydration and hospitalization in all countries. In developing countries, it is associated with a high mortality. A licensed vaccine against rotavirus was withdrawn because of a causal association with intussusception. A new vaccine has been developed and is a candidate for licensure.

Methods.—To recount the early development and recent demonstration of the safety and efficacy of the new vaccine. A bovine rotavirus attenuated for humans was isolated and reassorted with human rotaviruses of serotypes G1-4 and P1 to create a pentavalent vaccine. Multiple placebo-controlled clinical trials, including one involving approximately 70,000 infants, were conducted in multiple developed countries.

Results.—The pentavalent vaccine was well tolerated by infants less than 8 months of age, and the incidence of intussusception was similar among vaccine and placebo recipients. More than 90% of infants had a significant rise in serum antirotavirus IgA titer after 3 doses. Efficacy of 95% against severe disease causing hospitalization or emergency care was demonstrated, and pentavalent vaccine prevented 74% of all rotavirus disease.

Conclusions.—If widely used, pentavalent vaccine would control rotavirus disease in the United States and other developed countries and could also have a major effect in developing countries.

▶ This is just one of the reports that appeared in 2006 describing a new pentavalent rotavirus vaccine. All of us remember that back in 1998, the US Food and Drug Administration (FDA) licensed a quadrivalent rotavirus vaccine. Unfortunately, these products contained live viruses that multiplied in the gastrointestinal tract and retained the ability to cause fever and diarrhea in some infants. More important, suspicions engendered before licensure concerning an association of the vaccine with intussusception were confirmed postlicensure by case clusters shortly after the vaccine was introduced. The rotavirus vaccine then was withdrawn from use in 1999. Despite these problems, the vaccine proved to be highly effective in preventing serious rotavirus disease and was moderately effective in preventing all symptomatic infections. Despite a mortality rate resulting from natural infection of 1 in 200 in developing countries and the high effectiveness of this vaccine, once the drug was withdrawn in the United States, even underdeveloped countries withdrew the drug. Thus we reentered a period of time where rotavirus diarrhea continued to kill more than half a million children a year throughout the world.

Unfortunately, after the withdrawal of the rotavirus vaccine in 1999, several laboratories continued to work on rotavirus vaccines, most notably in Philadelphia at the Wistar Institute and the Children's Hospital, and at Cincinnati Children's Hospital. Human rotavirus contains several proteins that elicit protective responses, but the 2 most important are the vp7 protein variable for G serotypes and the vp4 protein variable for P serotypes, each of which elicit neutralizing antibodies. The Cincinnati group collaborated with GlaxoSmithKline on the development of a human rotavirus of serotypes G1 and P1a that had been attenuated by tissue culture passage. This vaccine has shown excellent safety and efficacy and was quickly licensed in Mexico, Brazil, and other countries under the name Rotarix. In Philadelphia, Clark et al isolated a bovine rotavirus and in collaboration with Merck a pentavalent mixture of human-bovine reassortants was developed and it is this vaccine that has been licensed by the FDA in the United States under the name of RotaTeq. The article abstracted recounts the many steps in the development of the latter vaccine. It is worth noting that the project in Philadelphia resulting in this vaccine started back in 1985 and 20 years passed before the finished product was finally submitted to the FDA for licensure.

The RedBook Committee has recommended universal vaccination of infants with the currently available rotavirus vaccines. If vaccine acceptance is high, we are likely to see the virtual disappearance of rotavirus disease here in the United States. An editorial, which accompanied the report of Clark et al, suggests that the safety and efficacy of the 2 new rotavirus vaccines has been proven to the limit of human ability.[1] The effect of licensure here in the United States continues to encourage developing countries to reduce their mortality from infantile gastroenteritis with the use of rotavirus vaccines, hopefully sold at much reduced prices.

If you want to read much more about rotavirus vaccines and rotavirus infection itself, see the superb review of this topic by Glass et al.[2]

J. A. Stockman III, MD

References

1. Plotkin SA. New rotavirus vaccines. *Pediatr Infect Dis J*. 2006;25:575-576.
2. Glass RI, Parashar UD, Bresee JS, et al. Rotavirus vaccines: current prospects and future challenges. *Lancet*. 2006;368:323-332.

Diarrhea- and Rotavirus-Associated Hospitalizations Among Children Less Than 5 Years of Age: United States, 1997 and 2000
Malek MA, Curns AT, Holman RC, et al (Ctrs for Disease Control and Prevention, Atlanta, Ga; US Dept of Health and Human Services, Rockville, Md)
Pediatrics 117:1887-1892, 2006

Objective.—A new rotavirus vaccine may be licensed in the United States in early 2006. Estimates of the burden of severe rotavirus disease, particularly hospitalizations, will help evaluate the potential benefits of a national rotavirus immunization program.

Design.—The Kids' Inpatient Database, a robust sample of 10% of the uncomplicated births and 80% of other pediatric discharges was used to estimate the number and rate of diarrhea- and rotavirus-associated hospitalizations among US children <5 years of age in 1997 and 2000.

Results.—In 1997 and 2000, diarrhea was coded in 13% of all childhood hospitalizations, for an estimated cumulative incidence of 1 diarrhea hospitalization per 23 to 27 children by age 5. Most diarrhea-associated hospitalizations (62%) were coded as unspecified etiology, and 35% as viral. Rotavirus was the most common pathogen recorded for 18% and 19% of diarrhea-associated hospitalizations in 1997 and 2000, respectively. Diarrhea-associated hospitalizations coded as unspecified or viral exhibited a marked winter peak similar to that of hospitalizations coded as rotavirus, suggesting that the rotavirus-specific code captures a fraction of all rotavirus hospitalizations (Figs 1 and 2). Using indirect methods, we estimated that rotavirus was associated with 51,142–60,155 and 46,839–56,820 hospitalizations in 1997 and 2000, respectively. By these estimates, rotavirus is associated with 4% to 5% of all childhood hospitalizations, and 1 in 67 to 1 in 85 children will be hospitalized with rotavirus by 5 years of age.

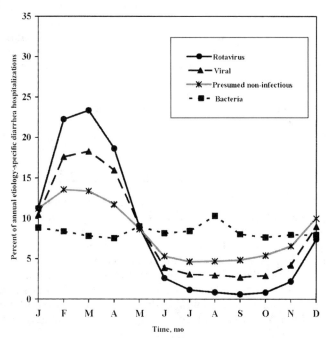

FIGURE 1.—Monthly diarrhea-associated hospitalizations according to etiology: 2000, KID. Monthly percent indicates the proportion of all hospitalizations attributable to a specific etiology that occurred during each month. (Reproduced by permission of *Pediatrics* courtesy of Malek MA, Curns AT, Holman RC, et al. Diarrhea- and rotavirus-associated hospitalizations among children less than 5 years of age: United States, 1997 and 2000. *Pediatrics.* 2006;117:1887-1892.)

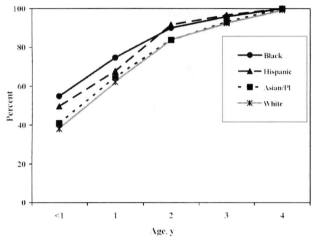

FIGURE 2.—Proportion of diarrhea-associated hospitalizations according to race/ethnicity and age. Other races are not included. (Reproduced by permission of *Pediatrics* courtsy of Malek MA, Curns AT, Holman RC, et al. Diarrhea- and rotavirus-associated hospitalizations among children less than 5 years of age: United States, 1997 and 2000. *Pediatrics*. 2006;117:1887-1892.)

Conclusions.—Diarrhea is an important cause of hospitalization in US children, and rotavirus is the most important etiology. Disease burden estimates have remained stable during the past decade. An effective rotavirus vaccine will likely reduce substantially the burden of severe rotavirus disease, estimated to account for 4% to 5% of all hospitalizations and ~30% of hospitalizations for watery diarrhea among children <5 years of age.

Hospitalizations Associated With Rotavirus Gastroenteritis in the United States, 1993–2002

Charles MD, Holman RC, Curns AT, et al (Ctrs for Disease Control and Prevention, Atlanta, Ga)
Pediatr Infect Dis J 25:489-493, 2006

Background.—In the United States, rotavirus gastroenteritis remains a common disease of children that results in many hospitalizations, clinic visits and medical costs. It is a common cause of morbidity and is associated with a high economic burden in developing countries. Prevention of hospitalizations is the primary target of rotavirus vaccines.

Methods.—To update estimates of rotavirus hospitalization rates in the United States, we conducted a retrospective analysis of 10 years of national hospitalization data associated with gastroenteritis and used both direct and indirect methods to estimate the percentage of cases associated with rotavirus gastroenteritis.

Results.—During 1993–2002, an average of 18% of all hospitalizations with gastroenteritis among children <5 years old were associated with rotavirus infection as determined by the rotavirus-specific International Classification of Diseases, 9th revision, Clinical Modification code. The annual proportion of rotavirus-associated hospitalizations increased from 15% in 1993–1995 to 21% in 2000–2002. Hospitalizations associated with rotavirus and those associated with nonspecific gastroenteritis had a marked winter-time seasonality and similar age distribution, which peaked among children between 3 and 24 months old. Using indirect estimation methods, 58,000 to 70,000 rotavirus-associated hospitalizations were estimated to occur each year in the United States.

Conclusions.—Rotavirus gastroenteritis remains an important cause of hospitalizations in the United States, and the rate has not declined from 1993 through 2002.

▶ This report and the Malek et al report (Diarrhea- and rotavirus-associated hospitalizations among children less than 5 years of age: United States, 1997 and 2000) clearly show that in absence of an effective rotavirus vaccine, rotavirus is still with us. Rotavirus illness is estimated to cause as many as 55,000 hospitalizations and 40 deaths annually here in the United States. As we see in these reports and others, a key characteristic in the epidemiology of rotavirus is its distinct seasonal pattern. In the continental United States, the rotavirus season begins in the southwest in the late autumn and progresses to the northeast by spring. This winter seasonal trend has been described with data from laboratory surveillance and hospital discharges. In recent years, the rotavirus season has begun a bit later (in January rather than in November or December). Interestingly, a report has shown that neither the use of the rotavirus vaccine back in the late 1990s nor the effects of the El Niño and La Niña phenomenon seem to have had evident impacts on the seasonality or distribution of rotavirus infection here in the United States.[1]

Rotavirus infection is nothing to sneeze at. Absent vaccination, the 5500 annual hospitalizations that result from this infection are the tip of the iceberg of the 2.7 million episodes of actual infection. Globally, more than 600,000 children die annually, again a tip of an iceberg of over 100 million infections. Worldwide, it can be expected that 1 of 200 children born in underdeveloped countries will die of this infection.

Last, while on the topic of loose stools, what do calves and human babies share in common when it comes to diarrhea? It is that both humans and calves share *Escherichia coli* enterotoxin-related diarrhea and oral rehydration solutions. Veterinary oral rehydration solutions virtually mimic solutions used by the World Health Organization in its formulations. Veterinary oral rehydration solutions actually take the World Health Organization formulations one step further by producing three varieties of such solutions: type 1 solution corrects dehydration, hypovolemia, and acidosis; type 2 solutions have the properties of type 1 solutions, but avoid the energy deficits imposed by their low glucose content (2%), which is optimal for sodium absorption, but inadequate for metabolism; and type 3 solution, which exploits the ability of glutamine to sustain villus structure and enterocyte function, and renal function, and can be helpful in conditions where reduced food intake imperils villus architecture. Calves are not little cows in the sense that they are pre-ruminants, with GI tracts virtually identical to humans. Calves are functionally simple-stomached until they are weaned onto solid food, well beyond the age at which oral rehydration is usually needed. Indeed, calves have been studied in a laboratory to measure directly the parameters that matter in acute diarrhea including hypovolemia acidosis and prerenal failure.

If you think that oral rehydration solutions are an invention of the last half-century, you would be wrong. Oral rehydration for acute diarrhea was first suggested in remarkable clinical research conducted by W. B. O'Shaughnessy and reported in *The Lancet* in 1831. This report appeared within months of the arrival of a terrifying new disease from Asia—cholera. Sadly, O'Shaughnessy's wisdom was not appreciated until the 1970s, with the arrival of the World Health Organization's oral rehydration solution, the latter often described as the greatest life-saving advance of the 20th century. It converted cholera from a mostly fatal disease in the absence of intravenous rehydration, into one routinely and simply treated orally.[2]

J. A. Stockman III, MD

References

1. Turcios RM, Curns AT, Holman RC, et al. Temporal and geographic trends of rotavirus activity in the United States, 1997-2004. *Pediatr Infect Dis J.* 2006;25:451-454.
2. Michell B. Why shouldn't children benefit from oral rehydration solutions for calves? *BMJ.* 2005;331:1267.

Prolonged Norovirus Shedding in Infant ≤6 Months of Age With Gastroenteritis

Murata T, Katsushima N, Mizuta K, et al (Yamagata Prefectural Inst of Public Health, Japan; Katsushima Pediatric Clinic, Yamagata, Japan; Yamagata Univ, Japan)
Pediatr Infect Dis J 26:46-59, 2007

Background.—Noroviruses (NV) are one of the leading causes of gastroenteritis in young children; however, the duration of NV shedding in young children is not well known.

Methods.—Fecal specimens were collected from children with acute gastroenteritis at a pediatric clinic during the period from November to December 2002 and tested for NV by reverse transcription-polymerase chain reaction.

Results.—Of 71 children infected with NV, 60 (84.5%) were less than 3 years old. Among children aged <2 years and those aged 2 to 5 years, the duration of illness was longer (7 days versus 3.5 days, $P = 0.0069$), the maximum number of stools in a 24-hour period was greater (7 versus 3, $P = 0.0078$) and a 20-point severity score was higher (11 versus 8, $P = 0.0031$) in patients aged <2 years than in patients aged 2 to 5 years. Among the 23 children whose follow-up specimens were obtained, the median duration of NV shedding was 16 days (range, 5–47 days). Virus shedding for more than 2 weeks after onset was observed in 75% (6 of 8), 71.4% (5 of 7) and 25% (2 of 8) of children aged <1 year, 1 year and 2 to 3 years, respectively. Three infants aged ≤6 months continued to excrete NV for an extremely long period (more than 42, 44 and 47 days from onset) after recovery.

Conclusion.—Long-term virus shedding after the disappearance of clinical symptoms was observed. Caution should be exercised when handling the excrement of infants and young children infected with NV.

▶ Before this report appeared, most of us had thought that those infected with Norovirus (NV) recovered from the illness fairly rapidly and promptly cleared their GI tract of the virus. Indeed, NV gastroenteritis, however unpleasant, is usually mild and self-limiting compared with Rotavirus gastroenteritis. Transmission occurs largely by the fecal–oral route. The incubation period generally ranges from just 1 to 2 days, and the duration of illness averages only about 1 to 3 days. Studies on the shedding of the virus in the stool have been previously done in adults, and those studies have suggested that excretion of the virus occurs for up to 2 weeks. As we see in this report from Japan, however, virus shedding for more than 2 weeks after the onset of illness is observed in three-quarters of pediatric patients; in the three infants aged <65 months, NV was excreted for 6 or more weeks after recovery. What we do not know is whether young children and infants are infectious for long periods after the disappearance of their symptoms, a period during which viral shedding is still occurring. Peak viral shedding occurs about 3 days after the onset of illness. Most studies have shown that siblings who become infected usually do so within 2 days from the onset of the index patient becoming symptomatic.

It will likely be a while before we know whether the prolonged period of viral shedding post NV infection in a baby is likely to produce a risk to those around the infant. If nothing else, careful handling of a baby's doo-doo seems reasonable, particularly if there are others around who might be at unusual risk for complications of an episode of gastroenteritis.

For a superb review of acute gastroenteritis in children and its causes and treatment, see the review of this topic by Elliott.[1]

J. A. Stockman III, MD

Reference

1. Elliott EJ. Acute gastroenteritis in children. *BMJ*. 2007;334:35-40.

Acute Human Parvovirus B-19 Infection in Hospitalized Children: A Serologic and Molecular Survey

Miron D, Luder A, Horovitz Y, et al (HaEmek Med Ctr, Afula, Israel; Technion, Haifa, Israel; Sieff Hosp, Safed, Israel; et al)
Pediatr Infect Dis J 25:898-901, 2006

Background.—The extent and clinical manifestations of acute human parvovirus B19 (B19) infection were assessed in previously healthy hospitalized children admitted with clinical syndromes potentially associated with the virus.

Patients and Methods.—The study was prospective and was conducted between October 2002 and August 2004 in the pediatric departments of 3 hospitals in Israel. The survey included previously healthy children who were hospitalized with 1 or more of the following acute diseases: acute nonallergic exanthema, fever for τ1 week, aplastic anemia or pancytopenia, acute nonbacterial arthropathy, immune thrombocytopenic purpura (ITP), Henoch-Schönlein purpura (HSP) and aseptic meningitis. A control group of children with a proven, non-B19 infection was also studied. Serum samples obtained from each child on admission were tested for B19 DNA by real-time PCR and B19 IgM by ELISA. Acute B19 infection was defined by the following criteria: positive serum B19-DNA and/or B19 IgM, negative serum B19 IgG, and no other proven infection.

Results.—Overall, 167 children were included in the study. The mean age was 5.5 ± 4.6 years (range, 0.5–17), males and females equally divided. Acute B19 infection was demonstrated in 12.6% (n = 21) of the children. Both tests were performed in 19 children and were positive in 10 (53%). In 7 and 2 children, only B19-DNA or B19 IgM, respectively, was positive. Acute B19 infection was documented in 27% (10/39) of children who presented with a variety of acute exanthema diseases; 9% (5/57) of children with acute arthropathy (all 5 had transient synovitis); 10% (2/21) of children with fever τ1 week, both presented as mononucleosis syndrome; and in 44% (4/9) of children with transient pancytopenia or aplastic anemia. No acute B19 infection was demonstrated in 15 children with ITP, 9 with HSP, and 6 with aseptic meningitis and among 70 children in the control group. By logistic regression analysis, manifestations significantly associated with acute B19 infection were exanthema (OR 2.9; 95% CI = 1.1–7.5), anemia (OR 6.35; 95% CI = 2.2–18.2) and leucopenia (OR 4.14; 95% CI = 1.2–14.2).

Conclusions.—Acute B19 infection was documented among 12.6% of children hospitalized with clinical syndrome potentially associated with the virus. Clinical and laboratory features associated with acute B19 infection were exanthema, anemia and leucopenia. Determination of both serum B19-DNA and serum B19 IgM should be performed for the accurate diagnosis of acute B19 infection.

▶ This appears to be the first study to assess acute parvovirus B19 infection in hospitalized immunocompetent children. Symptomatic parvovirus B19 infection has been associated in previously healthy children with various exanthematous diseases, acute nonbacterial arthropathies, acute hematological manifestations including transient erythroblastopenia of childhood (TEC), pancytopenia, mononucleosis-like syndrome, Henoch-Schönlein purpura (HSP), immune thrombocytopenic purpura (ITP), aseptic meningitis, and prolonged fever. What we see in this report is that acute parvovirus B19 infection is not infrequent in a hospital setting, having been documented in 12.6% of children admitted with clinical syndromes associated with this pathogen. No cases of ITP, HSP, or aseptic meningitis, however, were associated with parvovirus B19.

The present study shows acute parvovirus B-19 infection to be present in about 15% of hospitalized children presenting with acute exanthema, transient synovitis, transient aplastic anemia, transient pancytopenia, and mononucleosis. The determination of both serum parvovirus B19-DNA and serum parvovirus B19 IgM is best undertaken for the accurate diagnosis of acute parvovirus B19 infection.

J. A. Stockman III, MD

Breastfeeding Plus Infant Zidovudine Prophylaxis for 6 Months vs Formula Feeding Plus Infant Zidovudine for 1 Month to Reduce Mother-to-Child HIV Transmission in Botswana: A Randomized Trial: The Mashi Study

Essex M, for the Mashi Study Team (Harvard School of Public Health, Boston; et al)
JAMA 296:794-805, 2006

Context.—Postnatal transmission of human immunodeficiency virus-1 (HIV) via breastfeeding reverses gains achieved by perinatal antiretroviral interventions.

Objective.—To compare the efficacy and safety of 2 infant feeding strategies for the prevention of postnatal mother-to-child HIV transmission.

Design, Setting, and Patients.—A 2×2 factorial randomized clinical trial with peripartum (single-dose nevirapine vs placebo) and postpartum infant feeding (formula vs breastfeeding with infant zidovudine prophylaxis) interventions. In Botswana between March 27, 2001, and October 29, 2003, 1200 HIV-positive pregnant women were randomized from 4 district hospitals. Infants were evaluated at birth, monthly until age 7 months, at age 9 months, then every third month through age 18 months.

Intervention.—All of the mothers received zidovudine 300 mg orally twice daily from 34 weeks' gestation and during labor. Mothers and infants were randomized to receive single-dose nevirapine or placebo. Infants were randomized to 6 months of breastfeeding plus prophylactic infant zidovudine (breastfed plus zidovudine), or formula feeding plus 1 month of infant zidovudine (formula fed).

Main Outcome Measures.—Primary efficacy (HIV infection by age 7 months and HIV-free survival by age 18 months) and safety (occurrence of infant adverse events by 7 months of age) end points were evaluated in 1179 infants.

Results.—The 7-month HIV infection rates were 5.6% (32 infants in the formula-fed group) vs 9.0% (51 infants in the breastfed plus zidovudine group) ($P = .04$; 95% confidence interval for difference, -6.4% to -0.4%). Cumulative mortality or HIV infection rates at 18 months were 80 infants (13.9%, formula fed) vs 86 infants (15.1% breastfed plus zidovudine) ($P = .60$; 95% confidence interval for difference, -5.3% to 2.9%). Cumulative infant mortality at 7 months was significantly higher for the formula-fed group than for the breastfed plus zidovudine group (9.3% vs 4.9%; $P =$

.003), but this difference diminished beyond month 7 such that the time-to-mortality distributions through age 18 months were not significantly different ($P = .21$).

Conclusions.—Breastfeeding with zidovudine prophylaxis was not as effective as formula feeding in preventing postnatal HIV transmission, but was associated with a lower mortality rate at 7 months. Both strategies had comparable HIV-free survival at 18 months. These results demonstrate the risk of formula feeding to infants in sub-Saharan Africa, and the need for studies of alternative strategies.

▶ This report and the Kuhn et al report (HIV-specific secretory IgA in breast milk of HIV-positive mothers is not associated with protection against HIV transmission among breast-fed infants) tell us about the benefits and the adverse consequences of breastfeeding in relation to protection against HIV transmission to infants. In the study in Botswana, it is clear that breastfeeding with zidovudine prophylaxis is not as effective as formula feeding in preventing postnatal HIV transmission, but is associated with a lower mortality rate at 7 months of age. What is going on here is pretty straightforward. Although avoidance of breastfeeding can minimize the risk of HIV transmission through breast milk, excess morbidity and mortality have been associated with the use of infant formula, particularly where access to clean water is limited. In much of the world, cost and stigma also limit the use of formula feeding. There have been no previous trials, however, of infant zidovudine prophylaxis throughout the breastfeeding period in infants of HIV-infected mothers.

In the aggregate, one cannot recommend the use of extended infant zidovudine prophylaxis for the prevention of breastfeeding-related mother-to-child HIV transmission based on the results of the Botswana study, given the significant number of infant HIV infections that occurred after 1 month of age in the breastfed plus zidovudine group compared with the formula-fed group. If there are lessons to be learned from this report, it is that both formula feeding and breastfeeding with prophylactic infant zidovudine will give similar results of HIV-free survival at 18 months. Unfortunately, formula feeding has a higher risk of early mortality, but breastfeeding with zidovudine prophylaxis has a higher risk of HIV transmission.

This is the first study to compare formula feeding to breastfeeding with extended antiretroviral prophylaxis, and reveals relatively high morbidity and mortality rates associated with formula feeding among infants of HIV-infected mothers, but at the same time, the study did not lend definitive support to the use of infant zidovudine prophylaxis to prevent breastfeeding-related mother-to-child HIV transmission.

The Kuhn et al report shows that HIV-specific secretory IgA in breast milk cannot be expected to be a protective factor against HIV transmission among breastfed infants. There are no surprises in this report.

J. A. Stockman III, MD

HIV-specific secretory IgA in breast milk of HIV-positive mothers is not associated with protection against HIV transmission among breast-fed infants

Kuhn L, Trabattoni D, Kankasa C, et al (Columbia Univ, New York; Univ of Milano, Italy; Univ of Zambia, Lusaka; et al)
J Pediatr 149:611-616, 2006

Objectives.—To test whether secretory immunoglobulin A (sIgA) to human immunodeficiency virus (HIV) antigens in breast milk of HIV-positive women is associated with protection against HIV transmission among breast-fed infants.

Study Design.—Nested, case-control design in which HIV-specific sIgA was measured in breast milk collected from 90 HIV-positive women enrolled in a study in Lusaka, Zambia. Milk samples were selected to include 26 HIV-positive mothers with infected infants (transmitters) and 64 mothers with uninfected infants (nontransmitters).

Results.—HIV-specific sIgA was detected more often in breast milk of transmitting mothers (76.9%) than in breast milk of nontransmitting mothers (46.9%, $P = .009$). There were no significant associations between HIV-specific sIgA in breast milk and other maternal factors, including HIV RNA quantities in breast milk, CD4 count, and plasma RNA quantities.

Conclusions.—HIV-specific sIgA in breast milk does not appear to be a protective factor against HIV transmission among breast-fed infants.

▶ Secretory immunoglobulin A (sIgA) is the predominant immunoglobulin in breast milk and is known to be associated with passive immunity to a number of different pathogens among breast-fed infants. Breast milk will potentially transmit human immunodeficiency virus (HIV) infection to a newborn. A number of studies have quantified this risk and have shown that about 16% of HIV-infected mothers who breast feed will infect their babies as a direct consequence. It has been estimated that the risk of consuming one liter of breast milk from an infected mother may be similar to that of HIV transmission during an episode of unprotected heterosexual sex.[1] Despite this, in parts of the world where infant mortality exceeds 40 per 1000, the survival benefit of breastfeeding statistically exceeds the mortality attributable to breast milk–associated HIV transmission.

One of the interesting mysteries about the association between breast-feeding and HIV transmission is why the majority of babies do not become infected when breastfed from an HIV-infected woman. The report abstracted examines some of the protective aspects of breast milk feeding by looking at the potential role of HIV-specific IgA in human milk from HIV-infected mothers. The authors had hoped that the provision of maternal IgA in the milk of infected mothers might act as a form of passive immunization in protecting against HIV acquisition. Unfortunately, there was no association found between the content of breast milk IgA and protection. In fact, IgA was more common in the milk of transmitting mothers compared with nontransmitting controls. It very well could be that IgA levels in breast milk reflect higher local HIV replication in a heavily infected mother.

Thus it is, and unfortunate it is, that IgA antibodies in the milk of an HIV-infected mother will not protect her child from acquiring HIV if she continues to breastfeed. Wherever possible, breastfeeding should be discouraged except under the circumstances described above.

J. A. Stockman III, MD

Reference

1. Richardson BA, John-Stewart GC, Hughes JP, et al. Breast-milk infectivity in human immunodeficiency virus type 1-infected mothers. *J Infect Dis.* 2003;187:736-740.

Mother-to-child transmission of HIV-1 infection during exclusive breast-feeding in the first 6 months of life: an intervention cohort study
Coovadia HM, Rollins NC, Bland RM, et al (Univ of KwaZulu-Natal, South Africa; Univ College London; Univ of Oxford, England)
Lancet 369:1107-1116, 2007

Background.—Exclusive breastfeeding, though better than other forms of infant feeding and associated with improved child survival, is uncommon. We assessed the HIV-1 transmission risks and survival associated with exclusive breastfeeding and other types of infant feeding.

Methods.—2722 HIV-infected and uninfected pregnant women attending antenatal clinics in KwaZulu Natal, South Africa (seven rural, one semiurban, and one urban), were enrolled into a non-randomised intervention cohort study. Infant feeding data were obtained every week from mothers, and blood samples from infants were taken monthly at clinics to establish HIV infection status. Kaplan-Meier analyses conditional on exclusive breastfeeding were used to estimate transmission risks at 6 weeks and 22 weeks of age, and Cox's proportional hazard was used to quantify associations with maternal and infant factors.

Findings.—1132 of 1372 (83%) infants born to HIV-infected mothers initiated exclusive breastfeeding from birth. Of 1276 infants with complete feeding data, median duration of cumulative exclusive breastfeeding was 159 days (first quartile [Q1] to third quartile [Q3], 122–174 days). 14.1% (95% CI 12.0–16.4) of exclusively breastfed infants were infected with HIV-1 by age 6 weeks and 19.5% (17.0–22.4) by 6 months; risk was significantly associated with maternal CD4-cell counts below 200 cells per μL (adjusted hazard ratio [HR] 3.79; 2.35–6.12) and birthweight less than 2500 g (1.81, 1.07–3.06). Kaplan-Meier estimated risk of acquisition of infection at 6 months of age was 4.04% (2.29–5.76). Breastfed infants who also received solids were significantly more likely to acquire infection than were exclusively breastfed children (HR 10.87, 1.51–78.00, p=0.018), as were infants who at 12 weeks received both breastmilk and formula milk (1.82, 0.98–3.36, p=0.057). Cumulative 3-month mortality in exclusively breastfed infants was 6.1% (4.74–7.92) versus 15.1% (7.63–28.73) in infants given replacement feeds (HR 2.06, 1.00–4.27, p=0.051).

Interpretation.—The association between mixed breastfeeding and increased HIV transmission risk, together with evidence that exclusive breastfeeding can be successfully supported in HIV-infected women, warrant revision of the present UNICEF, WHO, and UNAIDS infant feeding guidelines.

▶ Unfortunately, breastfeeding remains an important cause of acquisition of HIV infection in infants. At the same time, promotion of breastfeeding has been ranked as the most cost-effective intervention for childhood survival and has been said to be capable of preventing anywhere from 13% to 15% of child deaths in low-income countries.[1] Thus, breastfeeding presents a terrible dilemma for patients and policy makers in areas with a high prevalence of HIV infection. It has been estimated that more than 300,000 children are infected with HIV through breastfeeding each year throughout the world. To weigh the pros and cons of breastfeeding, we need to have good data, but such research is fraught with significant difficulties. The report of Coovadia et al helps us in this regard. It represents a meticulous prospective investigation carried out in South Africa and provides crucial confirmatory evidence that when HIV-positive mothers breastfeed exclusively, their babies have a relatively low risk of infection with HIV. This risk is lower than that in babies who receive other food or liquids in addition to breast milk before they are 6 months old. Mixed feeding before or after 14 weeks nearly doubles the transmission risk, and the addition of solid foods increases the risk about 11-fold. The study also reports that the mortality rate by 3 months after birth for replacement-fed babies is more than double that of those who are exclusively breastfed. This result adds to the accumulation of new evidence on the hazards of formula feeding. Early estimates that the risk of postnatal transmission of HIV infection is between 10% and 20% did not distinguish between exclusive and mixed breastfeeding. In 1998, the first report that exclusive breastfeeding might reduce the risk came from a vitamin A trial in South Africa.[2]

You are probably wondering why exclusive breastfeeding would result in a lower risk of HIV transmission than mixed breastfeeding/formula-feeding. Exclusive breastfeeding ordinarily protects the integrity of the intestinal mucosa, which therefore presents a more effective barrier to HIV. Exclusive breastfeeding is also associated with fewer health problems than is mixed feeding, including subclinical mastitis and breast abscess, which, in turn, are associated with increased breast milk viral load. The effect that small departures from exclusive breastfeeding have on the risk of HIV transmission is uncertain, although predominant breastfeeding (the introduction of nonmilk fluids) may also be associated with reduced transmission. Why is the addition of solids especially hazardous? The authors of this report suggest that perhaps large and complex proteins found in solid foods precipitate greater damage than do modified cow milk proteins to gastrointestinal mucosa, allowing easy viral entry between cells. It is also possible that solid food feeding regulates gut receptors differently, thereby increasing the likelihood of virus adherence and infection. If you believe these theories are a bunch of hooey, see the elegant review of this topic by Smith and Kuhn.[3]

Please do not misinterpret the conclusions of this report to mean that in areas of the world where nutrition is not as much of a problem, one should exclusively breastfeed if HIV-positive. That is not true. In such parts of the world, exposure to the HIV virus from any source should be avoided, and, thus, breastfeeding should be avoided in toto. In those parts of the world, however, where things are more marginal, babies are probably better off being exclusively breastfed if they are likely to receive mixed feedings. See the reports by Bailey et al (Male circumcision for HIV prevention in young men in Kisumu, Kenya: a randomised controlled trial) and Gray et al (Male circumcision for HIV prevention in men in Rakai, Uganda: a randomised trial) regarding male circumcision for the prevention of HIV infection.

J. A. Stockman III, MD

References

1. Jones G, Steketee RW, Black RE, et al. How many child deaths can be prevented this year? *Lancet.* 2003;362:65-71.
2. Coutsoudis A, Pillay K, Spooner E, Kuhn L, Coovadia HM. Influence of infant-feeding patterns on early mother-to-child transmission of HIV-1 in Durban, South Africa: a prospective cohort study. South African vitamin A study group. *Lancet.* 1999;354:471-476.
3. Smith MM, Kuhn L. Exclusive breastfeeding: Does it have the potential to reduce breast-feeding transmission of HIV-1? *Nutr Rev.* 2000;58:333-340.

Response to Antiretroviral Therapy after a Single, Peripartum Dose of Nevirapine

Lockman S, Shapiro RL, Smeaton LM, et al (Brigham and Women's Hosp, Boston; Harvard School of Public Health, Boston; Beth Israel Deaconess Med Ctr, Boston; et al)
N Engl J Med 356:135-147, 2007

Background.—A single dose of nevirapine during labor reduces perinatal transmission of human immunodeficiency virus type 1 (HIV-1) but often leads to viral nevirapine resistance mutations in mothers and infants.

Methods.—We studied the response to nevirapine-based antiretroviral treatment among women and infants who had previously been randomly assigned to a single, peripartum dose of nevirapine or placebo in a trial in Botswana involving the prevention of the transmission of HIV-1 from mother to child. All women were treated with antenatal zidovudine. The primary end point for mothers and infants was virologic failure by the 6-month visit after initiation of antiretroviral treatment, estimated within groups by the Kaplan–Meier method.

Results.—Of 218 women who started antiretroviral treatment, 112 had received a single dose of nevirapine and 106 had received placebo. By the 6-month visit after the initiation of antiretroviral treatment, 5.0% of the women who had received placebo had virologic failure, as compared with 18.4% of those who had received a single dose of nevirapine (P=0.002). Among 60 women starting antiretroviral treatment within 6 months after receiving placebo or a single dose of nevirapine, no women in the placebo group and 41.7% in the nevirapine group had virologic failure (P<0.001). In contrast, virologic failure rates did not differ significantly between the placebo group and the nevirapine group among 158 women starting antiretroviral treatment 6 months or more post partum (7.8% and 12.0%, respectively; P=0.39). Thirty infants also began antiretroviral treatment (15 in the placebo group and 15 in the nevirapine group). Virologic failure by the 6-month visit occurred in significantly more infants who had received a single dose of nevirapine than in infants who had received placebo (P<0.001). Maternal and infant findings did not change qualitatively by 12 and 24 months after the initiation of antiretroviral treatment.

Conclusions.—Women who received a single dose of nevirapine to prevent perinatal transmission of HIV-1 had higher rates of virologic failure with subsequent nevirapine-based antiretroviral therapy than did women without previous exposure to nevirapine. However, this applied only when nevirapine-based antiretroviral therapy was initiated within 6 months after receipt of a single, peripartum dose of nevirapine.

▶ Data clearly show that nevirapine administered as one dose to the mother and one to the newborn reduces the mother-to-child transmission of HIV-1 by 41% to 47%. Well over 875,000 women and infants have received a single dose of nevirapine. Single-dose nevirapine is the cornerstone of the regimen recommended by the World Health Organization to prevent mother-to-child transmission among women without access to antiretroviral treatment and among those not meeting treatment criteria. However, nevirapine resistance is detected in 20% to 69% of women and 33% to 87% of infants after exposure to a single peripartum dose of nevirapine (less frequently among HIV-infected infants who had also received a short course of zidovudine prophylaxis). This report from the Harvard School of Public Health examines the consequences of giving nevirapine during labor with respect to the subsequent development of resistance to this agent. It was noted that women who had received a single dose of nevirapine did in fact develop significantly higher rates of virologic failure with subsequent nevirapine-based antiretroviral treatment than did women who had received a placebo. This apparently deleterious effect of a single dose of nevirapine during late pregnancy was largely concentrated in women who initiated antiretroviral treatment within 6 months of receiving the single dose of nevirapine. The study did not find that a single dose of nevirapine compromised the efficacy of subsequent nevirapine-based antiretroviral treatment in women who started antiretroviral treatment 6 months or more after delivery. Among HIV-infected infants, a single dose of nevirapine (one each to mother and infant) as compared with placebo was also associated with significantly higher rates of virologic failure in response to subsequent nevirapine-based antiretroviral treatment.

So what does all this mean? It means a lot for the mother. The study from Boston shows that women who start nevirapine-based antiretroviral treatment 6 months or more after receiving a single dose of nevirapine during pregnancy have high rates of virologic suppression similar to those women who are not exposed to nevirapine, and that nevirapine-based treatment may therefore be considered for such women. Because it may not be safe to delay the initiation of antiretroviral treatment for 6 months or more postpartum, initiation of non–nevirapine-based regimens should be considered for women starting antiretroviral treatment within 6 months after receiving a single dose of nevirapine. Furthermore, exposure to a single dose of nevirapine followed by nevirapine-based antiretroviral therapy is also associated with high rates of virologic failure in the small groups of infants who were studied.

It is clear that every effort should be made to provide antepartum combination antiretroviral treatment to women who qualify for antiretroviral treatment for their own health, because these are the women at highest risk for AIDS-related complications or death, for transmitting HIV to their infants, and for the development of nevirapine resistance after a single dose of nevirapine. However, single-dose nevirapine (with or without additional antiretroviral agents) remains an important component of the global strategy for the prevention of mother-to-child transmission of HIV-1 in women who do not yet qualify for antiretroviral treatment and for areas of the world where treatment is not available. Thus, while there are risks associated with pregnancy prophylaxis, these risks are worth taking for the potential benefit of such prophylaxis.

J. A. Stockman III, MD

Multiple Needle-Stick Injuries With Risk of Human Immunodeficiency Virus Exposure in a Primary School

Thomas HL, Liebeschuetz S, Shingadia D, et al (North East and Central London Health Protection Unit; Queen Mary Univ, London)
Pediatr Infect Dis J 25:933-936, 2006

Background.—Occupational needlestick injuries are generally handled according to established guidelines. Usually the source of the contaminating blood is known, and it can be readily established whether blood-borne viruses (BBV), such as human immunodeficiency virus (HIV), are present. Seroconversion rates for HIV after a needlestick injury are 0.2% to 0.5%, with prophylaxis reducing the rate by about 80%. Cases of community needlestick injuries are more complex. These cases are complicated by less experience, usually limited or no knowledge about the source of and risk from the needles, and a lack of data concerning the efficacy of postexposure prophylaxis in a community setting. An incident occurred in which there were multiple needlesticks in children in a primary school setting.

> *Case Report.*—A young child took about 20 lancets used for diabetic testing to school. The lancets were scattered in a play area, picked up and used to stab several children, then collected by adults, two of whom sustained superficial scratches. More than 24 hours later, the local health protection unit was informed of the incident.
>
> The lancets had been sealed and unused when they were brought to the school, but several children were stabbed with the same ones, so BBVs could have been transmitted. It could not be determined

which children had shared lancets or how often each lancet was used. The extent and depth of the injuries the 21 children sustained were also difficult to ascertain. While information was being gathered, a clinic was set up and offered tetanus boosting as needed, vaccination for hepatitis B, and baseline blood storage for those who were involved. Medical histories were obtained from parents, general practitioners, the local hepatitis B registry, and acute hospital sources to determine if the transmission of BBVs was likely. Within 48 hours, one child was identified as HIV-positive, not on an antiretroviral treatment, and having an HIV-1 viral load of 5,250,000 copies/mL. Individual counseling and HIV postexposure prophylaxis (PEP) was offered to all 20 exposed children. Parents were informed of the exposure and the risk of infection, which was crudely estimated as 1 in 1000. They were also given information concerning potential side effects. All opted to begin PEP and received the drugs and counseling within 72 hours of the exposure. A team dispensed the remainder of the drugs at the school 4 days after the incident. The team remained available for discussion of concerns or issues. Direct monitoring of each child's compliance was not done in view of the low risk of infection.

Results.—Of the 20 children potentially exposed to HIV, hepatitis B virus, and hepatitis C virus, 19 were tested 3 months later, with none showing seroconversion.

Conclusions.—This community needlestick incident illustrates the logistic issues that can arise. Staff must be trained in universal precautions and mechanisms for reporting incidents. The risk of exposure to BBVs must be determined. Confidentiality must be maintained. Difficulties were encountered obtaining details from the young children, gathering medical histories, and quickly setting up the risk assessment and counseling clinic. Managing the incident within 4 days required a strong partnership between health authorities, primary care practitioners, the local hospital, and the school.

▶ This is a fascinating little case report that is highly instructive about how we need to gather our wits when confronted with novel circumstances. Back in 2004, a young child in England took about 20 lancets for diabetic use into a primary school. These lancets became scattered in an outdoor play area. Several children aged 5 to 10 years found and played with the lancets, picking them up, stabbing themselves and/or others, and then discarding the lancets on the ground. Twenty-one children sustained needlestick injuries. Two adults were also scratched while gathering the lancets but sustained only superficial injury. Immediately after the incident, some of the children washed their injuries with soap and water. The local Health Protection Unit, which deals with the public health management of communicable diseases, was informed of the incident the following day, more than 24 hours later. An initial assessment of the likelihood of exposure to blood-borne viruses was conducted based on local estimates of the prevalence of HIV, hepatitis B, and hepatitis C. While more detailed information was gathered, a clinic was set up in a local pediatric unit to offer tetanus boosting (if required), hepatitis B vaccination, and baseline blood storage to those involved in the incident. Within 48 hours after the incident, information became available that one of the children involved in the incident was HIV-positive, was not on antiretroviral treatment, and had an HIV-1 viral load of 5,250,000 copies/mL. Based on this one fact, it was decided to offer individual counseling and HIV postexposure prophylaxis in the form of triple therapy to all 20 children who had sustained needlestick injuries potentially contaminated with HIV-infected blood. The parents of all 20 children did opt to start the prophylaxis. No child on follow-up seroconverted to HIV, hepatitis B, or hepatitis C.

This incident illustrates a number of logistic issues that can occur when dealing with a community needlestick incident involving young children. The first was that there was a delay of more than 24 hours before the relevant health protection unit was informed of the incident by the education authorities. This appears to have been caused by a lack of awareness of the potential for blood-borne viral transmission and the importance of acting quickly to reduce any potential risk. In Great Britain, there is no requirement for an educational establishment to be informed whether a child is infected with a blood-borne virus, and this may have contributed to the delay. Second, it was difficult to assess the risk of exposure to blood-borne viruses in the incident. It was necessary to cross-check the list of children involved in the incident with clinical databases and relevant clinicians to identify the one child who was HIV-positive. Only then was it possible to ascertain whether any of the other children were at risk for having been stabbed with the same needle as the index case. Third, it was necessary to protect the confidentiality of the child who was HIV-positive while offering risk reduction measures to those who had been potentially exposed. Some parents did request information about the source of the HIV risk, but were satisfied that it could not be given when the importance of medical confidentiality for all those involved was explained in detail.

This incident clearly demonstrates the complex logistic difficulties, including eliciting details of exposure from young children, obtaining medical histories from a variety of sources, and setting up a risk assessment and counseling clinic at short notice. Nonetheless, all was able to be accomplished within a 3-day period—not a minor feat.

To close this commentary, here is a simple question that adds to our understanding about why some people are more susceptible than others to the bite of a mosquito. Is it true that people with malaria attract more mosquitoes? It turns out that the malaria-causing protozoan, *Plasmodium falciparum*, may facilitate its own spread by making people more alluring to mosquitoes. After a mosquito bites is victim, protozoa migrate from the wound to the liver. There, the organisms produce offspring that attack red blood cells. When another mosquito bites the infected person, the parasites, now in a form called gametocytes, complete their life cycle in the insect. To see whether carrying the transmissible gametocytes might affect a person's attractiveness to mosquitoes, investigators in Paris devised a simple test in an area of Kenya with endemic malaria. These researchers arranged three tents so that each tent was connected to a central compartment. Then, they had one child enter each tent.

In each of 12 rounds of this test, one child was a carrier of gametocytes; one was infected but carried no *P. falciparum* in its transmissible stage of life, and one child was uninfected. After releasing 100 hungry but malaria-free mosquitos into the central compartment, the researchers counted how many insects got caught in traps on their way toward the children. The mosquitoes were not permitted to reach the children. It was found that roughly twice as many mosquitoes were attracted to the gametocyte-carrying children as to the other two groups. After treating all the children with an antimalarial drug, the experiment was repeated two weeks later. This time, it was found that mosquitos were attracted equally to the children in each of the three different tents.

Thus it is that mosquitos do have a dietary preference. They prefer to munch on those who are already infected. Your guess is as good as anyone as to whether or not infected children give off an aroma of their gametocytes.[1]

J. A. Stockman III, MD

Reference

1. Brownlee C. People with malaria attract more mosquitoes. *Sci News.* 2005; 168:157-158.

11 Miscellaneous

Pediatric surgery fellowship compliance to the 80-hour work week
Ladd AP (Indiana Univ School of Medicine, Indianapolis)
J Pediatr Surg 41:687-692, 2006

Objective.—The goal of this study was to determine the compliance of pediatric surgery fellowships with Accreditation Council for Graduate Medical Education (ACGME) duty hour restrictions while confronting a reduced resident workforce.

Materials and Methods.—An evaluation of training programs was performed by surveying pediatric surgery fellows on aspects of work hours, ACGME guideline compliance, operative case volume, employment of physician extenders, and didactic education.

Results.—A 74% survey response rate was achieved. Of the respondents, 95% felt fully aware of ACGME guidelines. Although 95% of programs had mechanisms for compliance in place, only 45% of fellows felt compliant. Median work hours were 80 to 90 hours per week. Although subordinate residents were felt to obtain better compliance (>86%), only 69% of fellows perceived greater service commitment as a result. No impact on volume of operative cases was perceived. Of the programs, 89% employed physician extenders and 55% used additional fellows, but no overall effect on fellow work hours was evident. Fellows did not identify an improvement in the quality of clinical fellowships with guideline implementation.

Conclusions.—A minority of fellows comply with ACGME guidelines. Vigilance of duty hour tracking correlates to better compliance. A shift of patient care to fellows is perceived. Use of support personnel did not significantly aid compliance.

▶ It was back in 1984 that the catalyst for change in resident work hours occurred. This was when a young woman was admitted to a hospital in New York City with a fever and suspected polypharmacy. The young lady died under the care of residents who had been on duty for over a day and a half. She expired without being seen by a staff attending. Her death triggered a sea change in our thinking about how we change residents' work hours. The State of New York promptly passed laws that did not allow residents to be on duty for more than 80 hours a week. Although it took the better part of a decade, all residents now in training in the United States may not work in excess of 80 hours a week, and other restrictions are placed on how many consecutive hours a resident may be in the hospital. The requirements of the ACGME apply to all residencies, including initial ("categorical") residencies as well as specialty and subspecialty residencies (fellowships). The article from Indianapolis gives us an insight into how pediatric surgical fellows comply with the 80-hour work week regulations. Much can be learned from this article. What we learn is that while virtually all pediatric surgical fellowship training programs are aware of the regulations regarding a ceiling on work hours, the median work hours range from 80 to 90 hours per week, and only 45% of fellows say that they are in full compliance with the regulations. Clearly, a minority of fellowships comply with the ACGME guidelines.

The reduction in resident work hours when introduced did not come without controversy. Many believed that continuity of care would be lost in the search for improved quality of patient care. What we have learned in pediatrics is that a transition to a reduced number of work hours can be accomplished without an apparent reduction in the educational experience of residents. Obviously, this means focusing on quality learning and minimizing wasted time during training. Hospitals have learned to hire physician extenders and hospitalists to pick up the slack. By comparison in the European Union, currently, work hours for those in training may not exceed 50 hours a week. By the end of this decade, there will even be further reductions.

Articles that appear in the *Journal of Pediatric Surgery* sometimes are followed by an active and lively discussion by a panel of individuals. The discussion posted after the publication of this article included a comment by Dr Michael Singh, a pediatric surgeon in the United Kingdom. He noted that, in Britain, the 50-hour work week limitation has produced more than a 30% loss in training opportunities compared with the previous 90-hour work week. A surgical trainee's life there, however, is significantly improved. The downside is that, in Great Britain, a system of continuous monitoring of training hours has been put into place. Residents have to account for every single hour they spend "on the clock." This accounting includes rest breaks every 4 hours, every telephone call that is taken, and even each coffee break, lunch break, and patient encounter times. It is a disciplinary offense if a trainee fails to submit the required documentation. If surgical residents continue to participate in a surgical procedure when they have exceeded the 50-hour work week requirement and if a complication results from the operation, the residents may not be covered by their hospital's medical/legal insurance.

Obviously, a rational middle ground has to be found in the search for quality as far as resident work hours are concerned. Exceptions to the current work limitations can be made if a serious reason to make exceptions exists, but these should be exercised infrequently and only for very, very good reasons. Also, let's hope that the "pond" that separates us from the European Union slows down any transatlantic migration of even shorter work hours until we have learned the most that we can from what we are currently doing with our present programs.

We all know what sleep deprivation does to those who are on call. Exactly what does sleep deprivation do to an intern's likelihood of sustaining a needlestick injury?

Interns (PGY-1) here in the United States are more likely to get needlestick or scalpel injuries during extended shifts. They are also more likely to be injured at night. Some 2737 interns reported their experiences with a percutaneous injury in a web-based survey undertaken for a period of one year. For the one-year period, there were 0.029 injuries per intern per month. Compared with a normal day, the odds of injury went up by 60% during the day after a busy night on call (1.31/1000 opportunities versus 0.76/1000 opportunities, respectively; odds ratio 1.61; 95% confidence interval, 1.46 to 1.78), and more than doubled at night (1.48/1000 opportunities versus 0.70/1000 opportunities; odds ratio 2.04; 1.98 to 2.11). Daytime injuries during long shifts occurred after an average of 29 hours at work. Surgery, pathology, and obstetrics were the riskiest residency programs observed. These findings are consistent with previous research showing that doctors who are deprived of sleep are more likely to crash their car, make more mistakes during simulated driving, and perform tasks about as well as someone with a blood-alcohol concentration of 40 mg to 50 mg/100 ml.[1]

Finally, while on the topic of physician work issues, recognize that the United States "imports" many physicians from overseas for further training. One of the countries from which such physicians come is Pakistan. What has been the impact of emigration for the purposes of training to that nation? In Pakistan, students who are accepted into medical school are congratulated—only half jokingly—on three counts: that they will become doctors; that they will become certified by a Member Board of the American Board of Medical Specialties; and that they will soon be living in the United States. Pakistan has contributed approximately 10,000 international medical school graduates (IMGs) to the United States, even though it faces a continuing shortage of physicians. Take the case of Aga Khan University Medical College in Karachi. By 2004, it had produced 1100 graduates, 900 of whom had gone on to graduate training in the United States—despite the fact that doing so costs up to $20,000 (a fortune for most Pakistanis) and means leaving the comforts of one's home and culture. The United States represents an overpowering lure for international medical school graduates: a rigorous system of graduate medical education, a merit-based structure of professional rewards, and a culture of academic nurturing, and, of course, material rewards. In Pakistan, an intern earns approximately $150 per month (the same salary as an unskilled, illiterate worker), whereas a United States intern earns enough to afford to live independently—and expect a better quality of life after residency. Information from Pakistani medical institutions indicates that only about 300 of the 10,000 United States-trained Pakistani physicians have ultimately repatriated back home. Why did this minority choose to return? The Aga Khan's experience is instructive: the majority of the medical school's 40 or so alumni who have repatriated back from the United States have joined its faculty. The motives for returning include aging parents and family ties, a desire to raise children in a familiar culture, and an emotional need to be home.

For 25 years the number of students admitted to United States allopathic medical schools has remained relatively constant, while the number of post-graduate physicians we import has steadily increased. Without ever enunciating a strategy of dependance on the world, we have created a huge United

States market for physicians educated elsewhere, inadvertently destabilizing the medical systems of countries that are battling poverty and epidemic disease. Perhaps soccer players will always migrate to elite leagues of the world, but if doctors and nurses stayed closer to home, lives would be better served and saved.

J. A. Stockman III, MD

Reference

1. Ayas NT, Barger LK, Cade BE, et al. Extended work duration and the risk of self-reported percutaneous injuries in interns. *JAMA*. 2006;296:1055-1062.

Googling for a diagnosis—use of Google as a diagnostic aid: internet based study

Tang H, Ng JHK (Princess Alexandra Hosp, Brisbane, Australia)
BMJ 333:1143-1145, 2006

Objective.—To determine how often searching with Google (the most popular search engine on the world wide web) leads doctors to the correct diagnosis.

Design.—Internet based study using Google to search for diagnoses; researchers were blind to the correct diagnoses.

Setting.—One year's (2005) diagnostic cases published in the case records of the *New England Journal of Medicine*.

Cases.—26 cases from the *New England Journal of Medicine*; management cases were excluded.

Main Outcome Measure.—Percentage of correct diagnoses from Google searches (compared with the diagnoses as published in the *New England Journal of Medicine*).

Results.—Google searches revealed the correct diagnosis in 15 (58%, 95% confidence interval 38% to 77%) cases.

Conclusion.—As internet access becomes more readily available in outpatient clinics and hospital wards, the web is rapidly becoming an important clinical tool for doctors. The use of web based searching may help doctors to diagnose difficult cases.

▶ Are you feeling tired with a headache, some diarrhea, and a stiff neck and don't know why? Well then, just Google your symptoms; you'll get a pretty good differential diagnosis and, quite possibly, the correct diagnosis. There are thousands of computer systems targeted at medical diagnosis that have been developed during the past half century, but most have had relatively little impact on day-to-day clinical practice. Most are proprietary and have a fairly complex interface. It turns out that a simple Google search just may solve diagnostic problems that mystify the best of practitioners. But is this really true?

The conclusion that Google is a reasonable substitute for a diagnostician is misleading in several ways. First, the Google searches reported in the study described in the abstract were not simple. Although the search only required typing a few words together and clicking a button, the investigators used extensive knowledge and experience to choose the search terms effectively. Second, Google did not actually solve the diagnostic problems. It returned a set of documents that were ranked according to their relation to the search items using metrics that are essentially based on counting the occurrence of word stems. The ability to infer a diagnosis from the returned documents depends on the skill of the doctors. Third, the implication that diagnostic problems can be ordered on a linear scale of difficulty against which human and machine performance can be compared is unwarranted. Nonetheless, the study does show that, in a certain class of diagnostic challenges, experts may gain an advantage by including a Web search in their deliberations.

The last 15 years have shown the extraordinary effect of the Web on clinical medicine. As great as this impact has been, however, the future holds even greater benefits for Web use. Current Web technologies are merely a stepping stone to a more powerful infrastructure: the semantic Web. This new version of the Web aims to create a universal medium for information exchange by putting documents with computer-processable meaning onto the World Wide Web. The semantic Web can overcome current limitations and offer much stronger support for tasks such as medical diagnosis. The development of the semantic Web is already underway. Web-enabled processes using new technologies will be important resources for clinical medicine in the next decade or so. In the meantime, no clinician diagnosing patients should feel insecure about the findings reported by Tang and Ng. However, their study should encourage us to think about strategies for maximizing the benefits of the evolving semantic Web in daily clinical practice.

You can tell a lot about a country and its interest in health issues by the nature of Google searches performed within that country's borders. In fact, a site known as Google Trends tracks such Google searches and reports which nations conduct the most Internet searches on particular items, offering up much in the way of cultural insights on medically-related interests. If one looks at Google Trends, one finds that Pakistanis seem to be most interested in the topics of bird flu and penis enlargement, whereas Indians want information about condoms and metatarsal injuries. South Africans concentrate on malaria and AIDS, and Singaporeans want to know about body odor and slimming. In Ireland, depression and facial hair top the bill, while in England, the most frequently searched items concern chips and chicken tikka masala. Presumably, in Great Britain the Google Trend search was done shortly after an *Emeril Live* airing in that country.[1]

J. A. Stockman III, MD

Reference

1. Minerva. Google searches and health [editorial]. *BMJ.* 2006;332:1282.

Measurement Accuracy of Fever by Tympanic and Axillary Thermometry
Devrim i, Kara A, Ceyhan M, et al (Hacettepe Univ, Ankara, Turkey)
Pediatr Emerg Care 23:16-19, 2007

As the basic sciences develop, temperature measurement methods and devices were improved. For hundreds of years both in clinics and home, mercury-in-glass thermometer was the standard of human temperature measurements. In this study, we aimed to compare tympanic infrared thermometers with the conventional temperature option, mercury-in-glass thermometer, which is historical standard in the clinical conditions.

Methods.—A total of 102 randomly selected pediatric patients who admitted to our hospital were enrolled, and simultaneous temperature measurements were performed via axilla and external auditory canal with 3 different techniques. For external auditory recordings, infrared tympanic First Temp Genius for clinical use and Microlife IR 1DA1 for home usage were used. Classic mercury-in-glass thermometers were used for axillary recording. For each method, 886 measurements were performed.

Results.—The mean results of the axillary mercury-in-glass thermometers, infrared tympanic First Temp Genius, and Microlife IR 1DA1 were 36.8 ± 0.7, 37.5 ± 0.9, 36.9 ± 0.8, respectively. The Bland-Altman plot of differences suggests that 95% of the infrared tympanic clinical use thermometer readings were within the limits of agreement, which is +0.27 and −1.75°C range of mercury-in-glass thermometer. The Bland-Altman plot of differences suggests that 95% of the tympanic home-use thermometer readings were within the limits of agreement, which is +0.98 and −1.27°C range of mercury-in-glass thermometer. In our group, 15% of the patients were misdiagnosed as febrile with home-use tympanic thermometer, whereas this percentage was 4% with clinical tympanic thermometer. Also, 5% and 31% of febrile patients were misdiagnosed as afebrile with clinical tympanic and home-use tympanic thermometer, if axillary mercury-in-glass thermometer recording defines fever.

Discussion.—Our results showed that there is a significant difference in each recording with different thermometers, and this variance was present in both higher and lower readings. We recommend that home-use infrared tympanic thermometer could be used for screening but must not be considered as a tool to decide patients follow-up.

▶ Have you ever wondered what the origins are of the thermometer? To be sure, physicians have recognized the importance of fever since antiquity. Before the rise and fall of body temperature could be used as a window into pathological processes, a reliable means to measure it was needed. Most historians credit Galileo with inventing the first thermometer. This was a crude water thermometer invented about 1595. Duke Ferdinand II of Tuscany experimented with an alcohol-based thermometer during the late 1620s. Newton developed a linseed oil thermometer around 1700. However, it was not until Fahrenheit unveiled his mercury-based thermometer in 1714 that a reliable method of temperature taking was found. These are but a few of the prominent scientific minds who worked on this critical device.[1]

Infrared tympanic thermometers have been in use for some time and have documented benefits including speed, easy usage, and noninvasiveness. Because the blood supply of the tympanic membrane comes from the carotid artery, the temperature of the tympanum is virtually the same as that of the body temperature control center, the hypothalamus. Although it was considered to reflect the core temperature accurately due to this anatomic location, the tympanic thermometer may give higher temperature readings than the oral thermometer, and also some investigators suggested a high degree of variance when compared with the oral thermometer. The varying results of early studies have therefore led to some questions about the actual precision of tympanic thermometers. On the other hand, axillary measurements with mercury-in-glass thermometers have been used for many decades and have the advantages of cheapness, availability, and wide usage in every condition. Unfortunately, mercury-in-glass thermometers also have some disadvantages, including the need to wait for at least 5 minutes for a measurement, the problem of cross-infection when moving from patient to patient, and breakage risks.

In this report, we see a comparison between tympanic and axillary measurements, the latter done with a mercury-in-glass thermometer. The overall difference between the axillary temperature measured with a mercury-in-glass thermometer and the temperature measured with an infrared tympanic thermometer was 0.75°C. The tympanic measurement, as expected, was higher. Fever did not readily change the spread in measured temperature between these 2 sites.

So what is the punch line here? There is no punch line. Believe what you want to believe in terms of what you like and in terms of implications to your practice. The study suggests that tympanic thermometers are useful as a screening tool, but should not be relied on when decisions have to be made about serious illnesses associated with fever.

A closing question related to temperature measurement is posed to you. Just how fast does the temperature inside a closed car rise on a sunny day? We should all be aware of the harm potentially done to children (and pets) by being left in a car on a sunny day, no matter what the time of the year. A study has examined this. This study recorded temperatures in a car over the course of an hour on 16 sunny days. The study found that, regardless of the outside temperature, the rate of temperature rise inside the car did not change. The average rise was 3.2°F (1.7°C) per five-minute interval, with 80% of the rise happening during the first 30 minutes. The average total rise turns out to be 40°F (22.2°C). Leaving a car window opened slightly does not slow the rate of rise in temperature.[2]

J. A. Stockman III, MD

References

1. Estes JW. Quantitative observations of fever and its treatment before the advent of short clinical thermometers. *Med Hist.* 1991;35:189-216.

2. McLaren C, Null J, Quinn J. Heat stress from enclosed vehicles: moderate ambient temperatures cause significant temperature rise in enclosed vehicles. *Pediatrics*. 2005;116:e109-e112.

Can sutures get wet? Prospective randomised controlled trial of wound management in general practice

Heal C, Buettner P, Raasch B, et al (James Cook Univ, Queensland, Australia)
BMJ 332:1053-1054, 2006

Objective.—To compare standard management of keeping wounds dry and covered with allowing wounds to be uncovered and wet in the first 48 hours after minor skin excision.

Design.—Prospective, randomised controlled, multicentre trial testing for equivalence of infection rates.

Setting.—Primary care in regional centre, Queensland, Australia.

Participants.—857 patients randomised to either keep their wound dry and covered (n = 442) or remove the dressing and wet the wound (n = 415).

Results.—The incidence of infection in the intervention group (8.4%) was not inferior to the incidence in the control group (8.9%) (P < 0.05). The one sided 95% confidence interval for the difference of infection rates was infinity to 0.028.

Conclusion.—These results indicate that wounds can be uncovered and allowed to get wet in the first 48 hours after minor skin excision without increasing the incidence of infection.

▶ This tidy little report is not likely to produce a sea of change in the way we practice medicine, but it is still quite instructive. The report shows that minor surgical skin excisions need not be covered, nor must they be kept dry. More than 800 patients were looked at and there was little difference in the incidence of infection whether a sutured area was covered and kept dry or left open and permitted to become wet.

Please note that one person's minor surgery may not be another's minor surgery, and this report does little to tell us exactly what the definition of the latter is. Also, the report did not include any young children. We all know that youngsters like to get down and dirty, so I for one will continue to encourage a coverup and admonish the dressing be kept dry, at least for a few days post suturing. Older kids and teens, however, may be a different story.

J. A. Stockman III, MD

Reference

1. Davis K. Uninsured in America: problems and possible solutions. *BMJ*. 2007; 334:346-348.

Car Seat or Car Bed for Very Low Birth Weight Infants at Discharge Home
Salhab WA, Khattak A, Tyson JE, et al (Univ of Texas, Dallas; Univ of Texas, Houston; Parkland Health and Hosp System, Dallas)
J Pediatr 150:224-228, 2007

Objective.—To compare the incidence of apnea, bradycardia, or desaturation in a car seat with that in a car bed for preterm very low birth weight ($\leq$1500 g) infants.

Study Design.—Infants were studied for 120 minutes in a car seat and in a car bed. Apnea (> 20 seconds), bradycardia (heart rate <80/min for >5 seconds), desaturation (SpO$_2$ <88% for > 10 seconds), and absent nasal flow were monitored.

Results.—We assessed 151 infants (median birth weight, 1120 g [range, 437 to 3105]; median birth gestational age, 29 weeks [24 to 34]) in both devices. Twenty-three infants (15%) had $\geq$ 1 event in the car seat compared with 29 (19%) in the car bed (P = .4). Time to first event was similar in the car seat and car bed (mean, 54 to 55 minutes). In logistic regression analyses, bronchopulmonary dysplasia was a significant predictor for a car seat event and a lower gestational age at birth was a risk factor for a car bed event.

Conclusions.—We found no evidence that an event is less likely in a car bed than in a car seat. Whichever device is used, very low birth weight infants require observation during travel.

▶ Kudos to the authors of this report and the Kinane et al report (Comparison of respiratory physiologic features when infants are placed in car safety seats or car beds). It was almost 20 years ago that the American Academy of Pediatrics recommended that all newborn infants discharged from hospital be transported in infant car safety seats. The rub was that as many as one third of premature babies placed in such car seats were shown to have episodes of apnea, desaturation, and/or bradycardia. Studies in the mid-1990s suggested that a car seat could be adapted to accommodate very small babies, and, based on these studies, the American Academy of Pediatrics recommended in 1996 that each preterm infant be monitored in a car safety seat before hospital discharge and that babies with documented desaturation, apnea, and/or bradycardia should travel in a supine or prone position in a car bed.[1,2] The recommendation, although it was not based on any true science, seemed to be intuitively correct on the theory that apneic episodes, desaturation, and bradycardia would be less likely in a car bed balancing the risk of these problems against the lesser safety of car bed use. What the reports from Salhab et al and Kinane et al show is that no mode of transportation in an automobile is truly safe. Specifically, infant car beds are no safe haven in comparison with an infant car safety seat for the premature baby. Data from both of these studies document that science wins out over intuition any day of the week.

It is important for readers to gain some perspective on the challenge of car safety seats by reading the commentary of Dr James Greenberg that accompanied the report of Salhab et al.[3] Dr Greenberg acknowledges that automobile travel is a fact of life these days, but that infants born prematurely are not anatomically designed to ride in cars for extended periods without some risk. Parents need to know that they must limit the duration of automobile travel when toting premature babies around. A 100-mile trip to see grandma on a holiday should be discouraged or, alternatively, interrupted frequently for stops. Better yet, buy grandma a plane ticket and have her come to visit. If babies must travel for an extended time, it would be good for an adult to sit alongside to keep a careful eye on how things are going.

J. A. Stockman III, MD

References

1. American Academy of Pediatrics Committee on Injury and Poison Prevention and Committee on Fetus and Newborn. Safe transportation of premature and low birth weight infants. *Pediatrics*. 1996;97:758-760.
2. Bull M, Agran P, Laraque D, et al. American Academy of Pediatrics. Committee on Injury and Poison Prevention. Transporting children with special healthcare needs. *Pediatrics*. 1999;104:988-992.
3. Greenberg JM. The challenge of car safety seats. *J Pediatr.* 2007;150:215-216.

Comparison of Respiratory Physiologic Features When Infants Are Placed in Car Safety Seats or Car Beds

Kinane TB, Murphy J, Bass JL, et al (Harvard Med School; Newton-Wellesley Hosp, Boston; Boston Univ School of Medicine)
Pediatrics 118:522-527, 2006

Objective.—The objective of this study was to compare the respiratory physiologic features of healthy term infants placed in either a car bed or a car safety seat.

Methods.—Within the first 1 week of life, 67 healthy term infants were recruited and assigned randomly to be monitored in either a car bed (33 infants) or a car safety seat (34 infants). Physiologic data, including oxygen saturation and frequency and type of apnea, were obtained and analyzed in a blinded manner.

Results.—The groups spent similar amounts of time in the devices (car bed: 71.6 minutes; car seat: 74.2 minutes). The mean oxygen saturation values were not different between the groups (car bed: 97.1%; car seat: 97.3%). The percentages of time with oxygen saturation of <95% were also similar for the 2 groups (car bed: 11.8[corrected]%; car seat: 18.2[corrected]%). In both groups, a number of infants spent high percentages of study time with oxygen saturation of <95%. The 6 infants with the most time at this level were all in the car safety seat group (54%–63% of study time). Values for the 6 infants in the car bed group with the most time at this level were lower (20%–42%). This difference in the duration of oxygen saturation of <95% was not statistically significant. The mean end-tidal carbon dioxide levels and the numbers of episodes of apnea were similar for the 2 groups.

Conclusions.—The respiratory physiologic features of infants in the 2 car safety devices were observed to be similar. Of note, substantial periods of time with oxygen saturation of <95% were surprisingly common in both groups.

Cost-Outcome Analysis of Booster Seats for Auto Occupants Aged 4 to 7 Years

Miller TR, Zaloshnja E, Hendrie D (Pacific Inst for Research and Evaluation, Calverton, Md; Univ of Western Australia, Crawley)
Pediatrics 118:1994-1998, 2006

Objectives.—The purpose of this work was to analyze the societal return on investment in booster seats and in laws requiring their use in the United States. Booster seats reduce crash-related injury. Their use is mandatory for vehicle occupants aged 4 to 7 years in most of the United States. This study estimates the injury cost savings attributable to booster seat use.

Methods.—Seat cost came from pricing on the Web and at retailers. Costs of passing and enforcing a legal mandate were estimated as a percentage of the costs of seat use. Injury risk when belted absent a seat was computed from national probability samples of crashes in the last years before booster seats entered into general use (1993–1999). Published estimates were used of the percentage of reduction in injuries achieved with booster seats, the mix of diagnoses reduced, and injury cost by diagnosis. The computations used a 3% discount rate. We studied the net cost per quality-adjusted life year saved, benefit-cost ratio, and net savings per seat.

Results.—A booster seat costs $30 plus $167 for maintenance and time spent on installation and use. This investment saves $1854 per seat, a return on investment of 9.4 to 1. Even lower bound estimates in sensitivity analysis indicated that society would benefit from the use of booster seats. Seat laws offer a return of 8.6 to 1.

Conclusions.—Belt-positioning booster seats offer a sound return on investment. Booster seat use laws should be passed, publicized, and enforced nationwide.

▶ As of mid 2006, 36 states and the District of Columbia had mandated the use of booster seats or other appropriate restraint devices for children who have outgrown their forward-facing child safety seats but who are still too small to use an adult safety belt system correctly. These laws are based on good science. For example, Durbin and colleagues provide good evidence of the effectiveness of booster seats in highway crashes.[1] The odds of serious injury are almost 60% lower for crash-involved children between the ages of 4 and 7 years who are using booster seats and lap/shoulder belts as compared with those using lap/shoulder belts only. This effectiveness did not vary by seating position. In the study described in the abstract, a cost-outcome analysis of booster seat use is provided. The study analyzes the cost, benefits, and quality-adjusted life year savings associated with booster seats from a societal perspective. Few things in life produce such returns as the investment in a booster seat. If the seat costs an average of $30 plus $167 for maintenance and time spent on installation and use, the investment will produce returns of $1854 per seat, for an outstanding 9.4 to 1 return. Warren Buffet, in his best years, never produced such returns.

If your state does not have a booster seat requirement, make copies of this report, and mail them to your legislators. You do not even need to call; the data speak for themselves.

J. A. Stockman III, MD

Reference

1. Durbin DR, Elliott MR, Winston FK. Belt-positioning booster seats and reduction in risk of injury among children in vehicle crashes. *JAMA.* 2003;289:2835-2840.

Odds of Critical Injuries in Unrestrained Pediatric Victims of Motor Vehicle Collision

Chan L, Reilly KM, Telfer J (Univ of Arizona, Tucson)
Pediatr Emerg Care 22:626-628, 2006

Objectives.—To compare morbidity and mortality between pediatric victims of motor vehicle collisions (MVC) who were unrestrained to those restrained and to describe compliance with child restraint usage in our population.

Materials and Methods.—A retrospective consecutive chart review study was performed on MVC victims 14 years old and younger who presented to our academic, level 1 trauma emergency department in 2003. Each patient's emergency department and hospital course was reviewed and data were collected. Odds ratios (ORs) were calculated for unrestrained children with respect to restrained children for fractures; intraabdominal injuries, intrathoracic injuries, intracranial injuries, admission, surgery, blood transfusion, intubation; and deaths. Hospital charges and length of hospital stay were compared between those unrestrained and restrained. Percentage of children unrestrained was determined.

Results.—Of 336 patients, 81 (24%) were unrestrained. Mean hospital stay for unrestrained children was longer, 1.94 days (95% confidence interval [CI] 0.75–3.12) versus 0.098 days (95% CI 0.02–0.21). Unrestrained victims had higher mean charges, $14,754 (95% CI $7676–$21,831) versus $1996 (95% CI $1207–$2786). Admissions (OR = 14.48, 95% CI 5.91–38.63), fractures (OR = 5.85, 95% CI 2.13–16.89), intraabdominal injuries (OR = 20.16, 95% CI 2.36–930.68), and intrathoracic injuries (OR = 13.09, 95% CI 1.26–647.05) were all more likely in unrestrained patients. No restrained child had intracranial injury, whereas 9/81 (11.11%) of unrestrained did. Odds were higher in unrestrained for surgery [OR = 13.09, 95% CI 3.30–74.33] and transfusion [OR = 27.61, 95% CI 3.56–229.85]. Ten out of 81 (12.35%) of unrestrained children required intubation versus none for restrained. The only 2 mortalities were unrestrained patients.

Conclusion.—Critical injuries and cost of care are higher in unrestrained than restrained children. Improved compliance with child safety restraint in

southern Arizona should decrease childhood morbidity and mortality from MVCs.

▶ By way of historical background, the world's first automobile fatality apparently took place in the Irish midlands in 1869. Mary Ward fell from a steam carriage that had been designed and built for her by her cousin. She died after being crushed by its heavy iron wheels. Mary Ward had enjoyed a multitude of achievements before her untimely and unfortunate premature death at the age of 42. She had been a celebrated microscopist, artist, astronomer, and naturalist.[1]

Read the report of Chan et al in some detail. You will see that about a quarter of a million children sustain injuries in MVCs each year here in the United States. The total annual cost of motor-vehicle-occupant–related death and injury exceeds $25.8 billion for children who are 14 years old and younger. This makes motor vehicle collision the leading cause of death in this overall age group. Most of these injuries are the result of being unrestrained. Also, although 4- to 8-year-old children should be placed in booster seats, many parents mistakenly believe that it is safe to use only a seatbelt after their child reaches the age of 4 years. Clearly there is room for improvement in terms of compliance with child safety restraints in our population. Ongoing educational and stronger legislative efforts are indeed necessary to maintain and maximize child safety restraint use.

Before leaving the topic of motor vehicle accidents, I would like you to consider the idea of traveling in the Middle East. Please recognize that there is a fairly wide variation in the number of road traffic deaths depending on where you are in that part of the world. The World Health Organization estimates that, by 2020, road traffic injuries will be the third leading cause of disability-adjusted years of life lost worldwide. Five countries in the Middle East have among the highest road traffic death rates in the world: in 2000, the United Arab Emirates, Oman, Saudi Arabia, Qatar, and Kuwait all had more than 18 deaths per 100,000 population. By comparison, Israel had just 8 deaths per 100,000 population. The highest death rate in the Middle East is in the United Arab Emirates, with 29 deaths per 100,000 people. Interestingly, in the Middle East, the higher motor vehicle death rates tend to be in the most affluent countries, presumably because of the ability to afford cars and to travel at high speed on quality roads.[2]

Last, on a related topic, what does the *Journal of Trauma* have to say about the TV show *Cops*? Investigators have done a study of *Cops*, a popular TV reality show in the United States. The premise of the show is that cameras follow police around as they perform their duties. *Cops*, however, could do a lot more for injury prevention. A careful review of *Cops'* episodes shows that police frequently do not use their safety belts and do so even more infrequently during low-speed chase scenes. Overall, the use of seat belts by police officers was pitifully low .[3]

Wouldn't you just love to make a citizen's arrest?

J. A. Stockman III, MD

References

1. Minerva. Mary Ward [editorial]. *BMJ.* 2005;330:1516.
2. Christensen-Rand E, Hyder AA, Baker T. Road deaths in the Middle East: call for action. *BMJ.* 2006;333:860.
3. Cowan JA, Jones B, Ho H. Safety belt use by law enforcement officers on reality television: a missed opportunity for injury prevention? *J Trauma.* 2006;61:1001-1004.

School Bus–Related Injuries Among Children and Teenagers in the United States, 2001-2003

McGeehan J, Annest JL, Vajani M, et al (Columbus Children's Research Inst, Ohio; Ctrs for Disease Control and Prevention, Atlanta, Ga; Indiana Univ, Indianapolis; et al)
Pediatrics 118:1978-1984, 2006

Objective.—The purpose of this work was to describe the epidemiology of nonfatal school bus–related injuries among children and teenagers aged ≤19 years in the United States.

Design/Methods.—Nationally representative data from the National Electronic Injury Surveillance System All-Injury Program operated by the US Consumer Product Safety Commission were analyzed. Case subjects included all of the patients in the National Electronic Injury Surveillance System All-Injury Program database who were treated in a hospital emergency department for a nonfatal school bus–related injury from 2001 to 2003.

Results.—There were an estimated 51 100 school bus–related injuries treated in US emergency departments from 2001 to 2003, for a national estimate of 17 000 injuries (rate: 21.0 per 100 000 population) annually. Ninety-seven percent of children were treated and released from the hospital. Children 10 to 14 years of age accounted for the greatest proportion of injuries (43.0%; rate: 34.7) compared with all other age groups. Motor vehicle crashes accounted for 42.3% of all injuries, followed by injuries that occurred as the child was boarding/alighting/approaching the bus (23.8%). Head injuries accounted for more than half (52.1%) of all injuries among children <10 years of age, whereas lower extremity injuries predominated among children 10 to 19 years of age (25.5%). Strains and sprains accounted for the highest percentage of all injuries, followed by contusions and abrasions (28.3%) and lacerations (14.9%). More than three quarters (77.7%) of lacerations were to the head.

Conclusions.—This is the first study to describe nonfatal school bus–related injuries to US children and teenagers treated in US hospital emergency departments using a national sample. This study identified a much greater annual number of school bus–related injuries to children than reported previously.

▶ The pros and cons (as few as they are) of requiring seatbelts on school buses represent a complex set of issues, but one that is important to debate.

Each year in the United States, 23.5 million children travel more than 4 billion miles on almost half a million school buses. The National Highway Safety Transportation Administration sets the standards for school bus travel. A current standard requires school buses with a gross weight rating of >10,000 lb to provide lap belts at all seating positions. School buses under 10,000 lb gross vehicle weight rating are said to provide passive protection to passengers in the form of "compartmentalization." Compartmentalization requires that buses have closely spaced seats and high padded seat backs. Annually, there are about 800 fatalities of school-aged children because of motor vehicle crashes during normal school travel hours. Only about 2% of these fatalities are attributable to school-bus–related crashes, including both passenger- and pedestrian-related fatalities. By comparison, an estimated 152,000 children are injured in motor vehicle crashes during school travel hours, of which 4% are school-bus–related, including school bus passengers and pedestrians. The National Highway Traffic Safety Administration estimates that there are 8500 total school-bus–related injuries per year, of which 86% are minor, 10% are moderate, and 4% are severe. Fatal school-bus–related events tend to occur outside of the bus (pedestrians, bicyclists, or occupants of other vehicles), whereas nonfatal injuries frequently occur to passengers riding in the school bus.

This report is the first to provide national estimates of the numbers of children and teenagers with nonfatal school-bus–related injuries who are treated in United States emergency departments. The number of school-bus–related injuries in this study greatly exceeded those published in previous reports, most likely because this analysis included children who were injured in school buses regardless of the nature of the trip or hours traveled. The data show more than three times the previously reported frequency of school-bus–related injuries. The report looked at injuries occurring at all times of the day throughout the entire year rather than just the "traditional" school year. We see that children between 10 and 14 years old have the highest rate of school-bus–related injuries that are treated in emergency departments. This may simply be because this age group is more independent than younger children, and parents may not feel the need to transport these youngsters by car. In addition, children 16 years old and older may drive to school themselves or hitch a ride with friends.

The data from this report seem to suggest that a significant percentage of injuries on school buses would have been prevented by the use of seatbelts. The National Highway Transportation and Safety Administration crash testing has shown that school bus passengers are better protected from head injury with a lap/shoulder belt as compared with car compartmentalization and lap belts only. Theoretically, a lap/shoulder restraint system would provide protection for crash-related injuries in school buses that is similar to that seen in other motor vehicles. On the basis of these findings and others, the American Academy of Pediatrics recommends that seatbelts be installed on all newly purchased school buses. The Academy also recommends that there be supervision on buses to keep children seated, to ensure the use of seatbelts (when available), and to ensure safe behavior while riding the bus. The presence of a second adult on a school bus might also prevent driver distraction by providing a monitor to supervise passengers, thus allowing the driver to do his or her job, which is focusing on the road. Given the fact that the data from this report suggest a much higher problem with school-bus–related injury than previously observed, the Academy's recommendations really do need to be enforced. It is expensive to retrofit existing buses, but schools should consider this, where feasible. Here in North Carolina, we have no requirement for seatbelts on school buses, although this past year saw the passage of legislation requiring back seat passengers in automobiles to be belted in. We are ever so gradually doing the right thing.

J. A. Stockman III, MD

Sudden infant death syndrome: Risk factors for infants found face down differ from other SIDS cases
Thompson J, for the New Zealand Cot Death Study Group (Univ of Auckland, New Zealand; et al)
J Pediatr 149:630-633, 2006

Objective.—To test the hypothesis that infants with sudden infant death syndrome (SIDS) found face down (FD) would have SIDS risk factors different from those found in other positions (non–face-down position, NFD).

Study Design.—We used the New Zealand Cot Death Study data, a 3-year, nationwide (1987 to 1990), case-control study. Odds ratios (univariate and multivariate) for FD (n = 154) and NFD SIDS (n = 239) were estimated separately, and statistical differences between the two groups were assessed.

Results.—Of 12 risk factors for SIDS, there were 8 with a statistically significant difference between FD and NFD infants. After adjustment for the potential confounders, younger infant age, Maori ethnicity, low birth weight, prone sleep position, use of a sheepskin, and pillow use were all associated with a greater risk of SIDS in the FD than the NFD group. Sleeping during the nighttime, maternal smoking, and bed-sharing were associated with a risk of SIDS only in the NFD group. Pacifier use was associated with a decreased risk for SIDS only in the NFD group, whereas being found with the head covered was associated with a decreased risk for SIDS for the FD group.

Conclusions.—Infants with SIDS in the FD position appear to be a distinct subgroup of SIDS. These differences in risk factors provide clues to mechanisms of death in both SIDS subtypes.

▶ This report is from New Zealand, where investigators have evaluated infants found in the face-down position who die of SIDS and compare these babies with the non–face-down SIDS infants. It does appear that risk factors for SIDS differ significantly between infants found dead face down and those found dead in other positions. The increased risk of SIDS with the use of pillows and sheepskins is seen only with face-down SIDS. These are items of bedding likely to be placed beneath an infant's head and hence likely to be beneath the infant's face when they turn to the face-down position. Both of these bedding items have been shown to be conducive to rebreathing and/or asphyxial death in infant physiological studies.

The report from New Zealand also found that low birth weight infants were at greater risk for face-down SIDS than for non–face-down infants. Infants with low birth weight related to prematurity have a developmental delay in head turning. Effectiveness of motor skills involved in head turning appear to be an important factor contributing to the risk of being face down, and one would expect that preterm and low birth weight infants would have a delay in acquisition of this protective behavior compared with term infants. In addition, the infant's face is an important part of the body for elimination of heat, and heat lost during respiration is also important in thermal regulation. Infants in the face-down position are less able to eliminate body heat, because they are rebreathing fully humidified, warm air and also have increased insulation covering the face. This report also shows that the non–face-down SIDS baby is more likely to die in the morning (6:00 AM to noon) in contrast to face-down deaths, which occur at night.

Bed sharing was also examined as a risk factor relative to baby positioning. Bed sharing proved to be a risk factor only in the non–face-down group. This was substantial even after controlling for potential confounders, including maternal smoking. Nearly all epidemiological studies of SIDS indicate that maternal smoking continues to be a major risk factor. Mechanisms underlying this risk are unclear, but effects on arousal threshold or hypoxia tolerance have been suggested. There was no increased risk of smoking in the face-down group in this study.

The findings from this study add further support for asphyxial rebreathing of expired air as the primary cause of death in face-down SIDS. The data are consistent also with the three-factor risk theory for SIDS mentioned in the Paterson et al article (Multiple serotonergic brainstem abnormalities in sudden infant death syndrome) dealing with serotonin.

J. A. Stockman III, MD

Multiple Serotonergic Brainstem Abnormalities in Sudden Infant Death Syndrome

Paterson DS, Trachtenberg FL, Thompson EG, et al (Harvard Med School; New England Research Insts, Watertown, Mass; Rady Children's Hosp, San Diego, Calif; et al)
JAMA 296:2124-2132, 2006

Context.—The serotonergic (5-hydroxytryptamine [5-HT]) neurons in the medulla oblongata project extensively to autonomic and respiratory nuclei in the brainstem and spinal cord and help regulate homeostatic function. Previously, abnormalities in 5-HT receptor binding in the medullae of infants dying from sudden infant death syndrome (SIDS) were identified, suggesting that medullary 5-HT dysfunction may be responsible for a subset of SIDS cases.

Objective.—To investigate cellular defects associated with altered 5-HT receptor binding in the 5-HT pathways of the medulla in SIDS cases.

Design, Setting, and Participants.—Frozen medullae from infants dying from SIDS (cases) or from causes other than SIDS (controls) were obtained from the San Diego Medical Examiner's office between 1997 and 2005. Markers of 5-HT function were compared between SIDS cases and controls, adjusted for postconceptional age and postmortem interval. The number of samples available for each analysis ranged from 16 to 31 for SIDS cases and 6 to 10 for controls. An exploratory analysis of the correlation between markers and 6 recognized risk factors for SIDS was performed.

Main Outcome Measures.—5-HT neuron count and density, 5-HT_{1A} receptor binding density, and 5-HT transporter (5-HTT) binding density in the medullary 5-HT system; correlation between these markers and 6 recognized risk factors for SIDS.

Results.—Compared with controls, SIDS cases had a significantly higher 5-HT neuron count (mean [SD], 148.04 [51.96] vs 72.56 [52.36] cells, respectively; $P<.001$) and 5-HT neuron density ($P<.001$), as well as a significantly lower density of 5-HT_{1A} receptor binding sites ($P\leq.01$ for all 9 nuclei) in regions of the medulla involved in homeostatic function. The ratio of 5-HTT binding density to 5-HT neuron count in the medulla was significantly lower in SIDS cases compared with controls (mean [SD], 0.70 [0.33] vs 1.93 [1.25] fmol/mg, respectively; $P = .001$). Male SIDS cases had significantly lower 5-HT_{1A} binding density in the raphé obscurus compared with female cases (mean [SD], 16.2 [2.0] vs 29.6 [16.5] fmol/mg, respectively; $P = .04$) or with male and female controls combined (mean [SD], 53.9 [19.8] fmol/mg; $P = .005$). No association was found between 5-HT neuron count or density, 5-HT_{1A} receptor binding density, or 5-HTT receptor binding density and other risk factors.

Conclusions.—Medullary 5-HT pathology in SIDS is more extensive than previously delineated, potentially including abnormal 5-HT neuron firing, synthesis, release, and clearance. This study also provides preliminary neurochemical evidence that may help explain the increased vulnerability of boys to SIDS.

▶ Despite intensive research, the causes of SIDS remain unknown. Moreover, controversies abound about the role of certain practices, such as bed sharing or the use of pacifiers, in SIDS, in part because of the lack of understanding of the basic and biological mechanisms of SIDS. The authors of the study abstracted have proposed a triple risk model, which suggests that sudden infant death results when three factors impinge on the infant simultaneously: (1) an underlying vulnerability, (2) an exogenous stressor (eg, prone sleep position, bed sharing), and (3) the critical development period (ie, the first 6 months of postnatal life when the infant is at greatest risk for SIDS). Paterson and colleagues now report that SIDS cases have a significantly higher number and density of 5-hydroxytryptamine (5-HT) neurons and have a significantly lower density of 5-HT receptor binding sites in regions of the medulla involved in homeostatic function compared with controls. The density of 5-HT transporter binding relative to the number of 5-HT neurons in the medulla is significantly lower in SIDS cases compared with controls. Paterson et al also demonstrate that male infants who succumb to SIDS have lower 5-HT receptor binding density in the raphé obscurus compared with female infants. This evidence strongly supports extensive abnormalities in the 5-HT neuropathology of the medulla in SIDS and begins to address the sex disparity in SIDS incidence, something that has been long known. Recognizing that 5-HT influences a broad range of physiological systems, including respiratory, cardiovascular, and thermoregulatory systems, and the sleep-wake cycle, Paterson et al extend the literature in support of the underlying hypothesis that SIDS is the result of 5-HT–mediated dysregulation of the autonomic nervous system.

Although the neuropathological studies in SIDS are providing remarkable insight into the underlying mechanisms in the 5-HT pathways, identification of the definitive causes for SIDS will necessitate an expanded network of scientists and families working together toward this shared goal. Medical examiners need to join forces in providing autopsy specimens for neuropathology researchers. We do know that the risk of SIDS is about three times more common in African-American babies and that these babies are underrepresented in such studies as the report of Paterson et al. Clinicians and researchers can gently inform parents who have lost an infant to SIDS about autopsy and the opportunity for their lost infant to contribute to the further understanding of SIDS. With more than 2000 babies dying from SIDS in the United States annually, there is no time to lose in determining if serotonin is indeed the key factor in the pathophysiology of the disorder.

It should be noted that 65% of the babies reported by Paterson et al were found in the prone position. The Thompson et al report (Sudden infant death syndrome: risk factors for infants found face down differ from other SIDS cases) tells us a little more about the risk factors associated with SIDS for infants found face down.

J. A. Stockman III, MD

Sleep Environment, Positional, Lifestyle, and Demographic Characteristics Associated with Bed Sharing in Sudden Infant Death Syndrome Cases: A Population-Based Study

Ostfeld BM, Perl H, Esposito L, et al (Univ of Medicine and Dentistry of New Jersey, New Brunswick; Hackensack Univ, NJ; New Jersey Dept of Health and Senior Services, Trenton)
Pediatrics 118:2051-2059, 2006

Background.—In 2005, the American Academy of Pediatrics Task Force on Sudden Infant Death Syndrome recommended that infants not bed share during sleep.

Objective.—Our goal was to characterize the profile of risk factors associated with bed sharing in sudden infant death syndrome cases.

Design/Methods.—We conducted a population-based retrospective review of sudden infant death syndrome cases in New Jersey (1996–2000) dichotomized by bed-sharing status and compared demographic, lifestyle, bedding-environment, and sleep-position status.

Results.—Bed-sharing status was reported in 239 of 251 cases, with sharing in 39%. Bed-sharing cases had a higher percentage of bedding risks (44.1% vs 24.7%), exposure to bedding risks in infants discovered prone (57.1% vs 28.2%), and lateral sleep placement (28.9% vs 17.8%). The prone position was more common for bed-sharing and non–bed-sharing cases at placement (45.8% and 51.1%, respectively) and discovery (59.0% and 64.4%, respectively). In multivariable logistic-regression analyses, black race, mother <19 years, gravida >2, and maternal smoking were associated with bed sharing. There was a trend toward less breastfeeding in bed-sharing cases (22% vs 35%). In bed-sharing cases, those breastfed were younger than those who were not and somewhat more exposed to bedding risks (64.7% vs 45.1%) but less likely to be placed prone (11.8% vs 52.9%) or have maternal smoking (33% vs 66%).

Conclusions.—Bed-sharing cases were more likely to have had bedding-environment and sleep-position risks and higher ratios of demographic and lifestyle risk factors. Bed-sharing subjects who breastfed had a risk profile distinct from those who were not breastfed cases. Risk and situational profiles can be used to identify families in greater need of early guidance and to prepare educational content to promote safe sleep.

▶ For some time now, the American Academy of Pediatrics (AAP) Task Force on Sudden Infant Death Syndrome has wrestled with the conundrum of the benefits of bed sharing on breastfeeding juxtaposed to the risks of sudden infant death syndrome. In its policy statement on breastfeeding, the AAP Section on Breastfeeding has recommended exclusive breastfeeding in the first 6 months of life. It also recognizes that bed sharing is facilitative of breastfeeding. In weighing the pros and cons, however, the AAP policy statement indicates that bed sharing is hazardous, and it recommends that although infants may be taken into the parental bed to support breastfeeding, parents should place their babies on a proximal sleep surface, such as a crib, for sleep.

This report by Ostfeld and colleagues sheds light on the relationship between sudden infant death syndrome and bed sharing, providing new information about the linkages. The investigators have found that bed sharing defines a group within our population with a higher proportion of risk factors for sudden infant death syndrome. Specifically, bed-sharing infants are more likely to have bedding characteristics that have been associated with a higher risk of sudden infant death syndrome. With bed sharing, a higher proportion of infants are placed to sleep laterally in an unstable sleep position. The greatest risk associated with bed sharing is seen with adolescent mothers, African-American mothers, mothers with two or more other children, and mothers who smoke.

No one will argue that bed sharing facilitates breast feeding, but it also facilitates sudden infant death syndrome. One can still breastfeed while not bed sharing, although it is sometimes difficult for mothers to stay awake during breastfeeding, and that is the conundrum. Read this report in detail. It teaches us a lot about the problem.

One closing comment seems appropriate regarding the sudden infant death syndrome. Bed sharing does appear to be one of the greatest risk factors for this problem. Bed sharing seems to be more prevalent among the poor in our society. Recent data tell us the extent of poverty here in the United States when looked at through the lens of who is and who is not insured. Approximately 16% of the population of the United States receive no health coverage in the form of Medicare, Medicaid, voluntary employer-based private insurance, or individual insurance. The number of uninsured has increased from 40 million in 2000 to nearly 47 million in 2005. Nearly all the growth in the uninsured is among people aged 18 to 64, most of whom are working. The average family premium for an employer-based coverage now runs almost $12,000 per year. The Institute of Medicine estimates that 18,000 lives are lost annually as a consequence of gaps in insurance coverage. It calculates the annual cost of achieving full coverage at 34 billion to 69 billion, which is less than the loss in economic productivity from existing coverage (65 billion to 130 billion annually).

As of 2004, the following states had more than 23% of people aged 18 to 64 without insurance: Alaska, California, Montana, New Mexico, Texas, Oklahoma, Arkansas, Louisiana, Florida, and West Virginia. The following states had the lowest percentage of uninsured (less than 14%): Minnesota and Iowa.[1]

J. A. Stockman III, MD

Reference

1. Davis K. Uninsured in America: problems and possible solutions. *BMJ*. 2007; 334:346-348.

Child Maltreatment in the United States: Prevalence, Risk Factors, and Adolescent Health Consequences

Hussey JM, Chang JJ, Kotch JB (Univ of North Carolina, Chapel Hill)
Pediatrics 118:933-942, 2006

Objectives.—The purpose of this study was to estimate the prevalence of child maltreatment in the United States and examine its relationship to sociodemographic factors and major adolescent health risks.

Methods.—The National Longitudinal Study of Adolescent Health is a prospective cohort study following a national sample of adolescents into adulthood. The wave III interview, completed by 15 197 young adults in 2001–2002 (77.4% response rate), included retrospective measures of child maltreatment. We used these measures to estimate the prevalence of self-reported supervision neglect, physical neglect, physical assault, and contact sexual abuse during childhood. Next, we investigated the relationship between sociodemographic characteristics and maltreatment. Finally, we examined the association between child maltreatment and adolescent self-rated health; overweight status; depression; cigarette, alcohol, marijuana, and inhalant use; and violent behavior.

Results.—Having been left home alone as a child, indicating possible supervision neglect, was most prevalent (reported by 41.5% of respondents),

TABLE 1.—Prevalence of Self-Reported Child Maltreatment

Variable	Supervision Neglect (N=10056)[a]			Physical Neglect (N=10324)[a]			Physical Assault (N=10262)[a]			Contact Sexual Abuse (N=10406)[a]		
	No.	%[b]	95% CI	No.	%	95% CI	No.	%	95% CI	No.	%	95% CI
Any report	4184	41.5	(39.9-43.1)	1205	11.8	(10.7-12.9)	3013	28.4	(26.9-29.9)	479	4.5	(3.9-5.2)
Frequency												
1 time	1276	13.1	(12.1-14.1)	471	4.7	(4.1-5.3)	838	8.3	(7.5-9.0)	233	2.4	(1.9-2.9)
2 times	942	9.3	(8.6-10.0)	217	2.1	(1.7-2.5)	649	5.9	(5.3-6.5)	76	0.5	(0.4-0.7)
≥3 times	1966	19.1	(18.0-20.3)	517	5.0	(4.4-5.6)	1526	14.2	(13.2-15.2)	170	1.6	(1.3-1.9)

Because of rounding, frequency percentages may not sum to overall percentage. CI indicates confidence interval.

[a] Total unweighted nonmissing observations.

[b] All percentages and 95% CIs are weighted and provide nationally representative estimates for the target population.

(Reproduced by permission of *Pediatrics* courtesy of Hussey JM, Chang JJ, Kotch JB. Child maltreatment in the United States: prevalence, risk factors, and adolescent health consequences. *Pediatrics* 2006;118:933-942.)

followed by physical assault (28.4%), physical neglect (11.8%), and contact sexual abuse (4.5%). Each sociodemographic characteristic was associated with ≥1 type of maltreatment, and race/ethnicity was associated with all 4. Each type of maltreatment was associated with no fewer than 8 of the 10 adolescent health risks examined.

Conclusions.—Self-reported childhood maltreatment was common. The likelihood of maltreatment varied across many sociodemographic characteristics. Each type of maltreatment was associated with multiple adolescent health risks (Table 1).

▶ In early 2006, the American Board of Pediatrics agreed to create a certificate of special qualifications in the area of child abuse and neglect. This report tells us that such certification comes none too soon given the prevalence of childhood maltreatment. Conservative estimates have placed the number of children that are victimized in our country by maltreatment each year at close to 1 million, and the annual number of child deaths caused by abuse or neglect at nearly 1500. Although we spend a lot on child welfare services (in excess of $20 billion annually), little is done at the governmental level to deal with the problem of childhood maltreatment in terms of prevention.

The abstracted report is critically important when it comes to our understanding of childhood maltreatment. Despite many decades of sustained research on child abuse and neglect, we continue to have voids in our understanding of which children are at greatest risks, what the long-term health consequences are of child neglect and maltreatment, and exactly what the prevalence of these problems may be. Recognizing the problem, the National Research Council Panel on Research on Child Abuse and Neglect has called for including child maltreatment questions on future national surveys as a new strategy for improving the quality of evidence on child abuse and neglect. Indeed, the National Longitudinal Study of Adolescent Health responded to this call by including maltreatment measures in its third wave of interviews, collected from nationally representative samples of more than 15,000 young adults. It is from the latter database that the information reported in the abstract is derived. The data show that somewhere between 1% and 2% of United States children are maltreated annually. This translates into huge numbers of children who have been abused. If anything, these data indicate a lower prevalence than may actually exist in our community because other studies have suggested that the prevalence of child abuse may be as much as twice as great. Either way, the problem is highly prevalent and pervasive.

The most common problem of child maltreatment is current supervision neglect on the part of a care provider (constituting just over 40% of all identified child maltreatment situations). Actual physical neglect occurs at a prevalence of about 12%. Among abused children, physical assault constitutes somewhere between 15% and 20% of all abuse cases. Lastly, some 4.5% of abused individuals have reported sexual abuse by a parent or adult caregiver before the sixth grade.

The information provided by the National Longitudinal Study of Adolescent Health and the understandings derived from the study with respect to child abuse and neglect have important implications for us pediatricians and for residents in training. A recent study shows how badly we train our prodigy (residents in training) when it comes to child abuse and neglect.[1] Although most residency training programs do provide didactics on physical and sexual abuse, only about half include domestic violence. On the other hand, just 41% of programs require mandatory clinical rotations in child abuse and neglect. Some 57% offer elective rotations, and 25% of residencies offer no rotations at all. Only 12% of residents exiting training feel that they are very well prepared to deal with issues related to child abuse and neglect as they arise. Almost half of all residents indicate that they want more training and teaching sessions, a neat trick given the competition for time in an 80-hour workweek.

J. A. Stockman III, MD

Reference

1. Narayan AP, Socolar RR, St Claire K. Pediatric residency training in child abuse and neglect in the United States. *Pediatrics.* 2006;117:2215-2221.

Redefining the Community Pediatric Hospitalist: The Combined Pediatric ED/Inpatient Unit

Krugman SD, Suggs A, Photowala HY, et al (Franklin Square Hosp Ctr, Baltimore, Md; MedStar Research Inst, Hyattsville, Md)
Pediatr Emerg Care 23:33-37, 2007

Background.—The use of pediatric hospitalists in community hospitals has increased over the past decade in response to the desire to provide high-quality pediatric care. Many hospitals are challenged to create financially independent and productive programs.

Objective.—To evaluate an alternative approach to traditional community hospital pediatric care of having pediatricians work in a combined pediatric Emergency Department (PED)/inpatient unit.

Design/Methods.—Franklin Square Hospital Center converted its pediatric hospitalist program from a traditional inpatient with partial Emergency Department (ED) coverage program to one that covers a combined PED/inpatient unit. Outcome categories were compared between the year before opening, 2003, to the year after, 2004. Measures included total part B billing, overall patient satisfaction scores for the PED and inpatient unit from the Press Ganey patient satisfaction survey, perception of wait times and time to admission, and risk-adjusted inpatient length of stay (ALOS).

Results.—Part B billings from the 5.5 Full Time Equivalent (FTE) pediatric hospitalists increased 82% from increased 61% from 2003 to 2004, from $1,631,583 in 2003 to $2,967,715 in 2004 as a result of increased volume of ED patients seen by pediatricians. The mean inpatient satisfaction score did not significantly change, 75.7 in 2003 and 79.0 in 2004 ($P = 0.432$), but the mean PED score significantly increased from 75.8 to 83.4 ($P = 0.0001$). Mean scores of the efficiency measures on the survey increased for PED patients, with the mean score for wait time to treatment increasing from 62.0 to 75.3 ($P < 0.0001$). Total throughput time through the ED improved significantly as well from 143 minutes to 122 minutes ($P = 0.0003$). Risk-adjusted length of stay performance did not change; for calendar year 2003, the mean monthly ALOS was 1.883 (95% range 1.503, 2.263), compared with a 2004 mean monthly ALOS of 1.869 (95% range 1.523, 2.216).

Conclusions.—Implementation of a combined PED/inpatient unit was associated with increased billing by hospitalists, increased satisfaction scores of ED patients, and decreased ED throughput times. Pediatric hospitalist programs that want to improve financial and patient outcomes in a community setting could consider adopting the combined unit approach.

▶ This report reminds us that community hospitals struggle to maintain high-quality, cost-effective pediatric care, and that the majority of hospitalized children wind up in community hospitals rather than in highly specialized children's hospitals. Community hospitals have increasingly used pediatric hospitalists for these youngsters. For cost containment reasons, there is often only one hospitalist on duty at any time. Imagine the scene in which the pediatric hospitalist is working up an inpatient, but has also been called to the ED to evaluate an ill child and just receives a call to evaluate a tachypneic baby in the nursery. Part of the problem may be solved by implementing the model described here, where the Franklin Square Hospital Center combined the PED and inpatient service into one unit.

Franklin Square Hospital Center is a 335-bed community hospital in eastern Baltimore County, Maryland. In 1999, the institution began a hospitalist program utilizing 5.5 FTEs, allowing 24/7 hospital-wide coverage by a general pediatrician. In 1999, the inpatient pediatric service housed 15 acute care beds, and the single ED had 55,000 visits of which 15,000 involved children. A single inpatient service attending rounded on the inpatients in the morning (this was either a hospitalist or other general pediatrician) and signed out to the hospitalist at noon, who would cover the inpatients but be physically present in the ED most of the time from 1 PM to 1 AM. A pediatrician was available to the ED to consult 24 hours a day. From 1999 to 2003, the inpatient census declined from an average of 7 inpatients per day to 3.5 inpatients a day, limiting hospitalist and inpatient nursing staffing productivity. The reasons for the declining census included a decrease in the average length of stay to approximately 2.0 days and the opening of a new hospital north of Baltimore, which resulted in a loss of 125 admissions annually. These changes precipitated a decision to consolidate all pediatric patient care onto one unit, resulting in a physically combined pediatric inpatient unit and PED. Overall, the unit housed 12 to 16 PED beds and 3 to 6 inpatient beds all on one rectangular-shaped floor.

So what happened as a result of combining the PED and inpatient services into one? Billings went up for the 5 hospitalists by some 60%. Patient satisfaction scores stayed the same for the inpatients but significantly increased for patients being seen on the emergency side of the ledger. Efficiency scores went up, which probably explained the improvement in the patient satisfaction scores for the ED.

You will have to decide whether it makes sense to have such small numbers of pediatric patients in-house in a community hospital. This report does not give any quality indicators for measurements of quality other than patient satisfaction and efficiency, and therefore, we do not have a clue as to whether these children were receiving the best of care. At the same time, we have no reason to think they were not. If a hospital must have an inpatient service of such small size for kids, this study does provide some novel insights about how inpatient and emergency services might be combined to make overall care more efficient.

Many here in the United States complain about being tossed out of the hospital after very abbreviated stays. Length of stay here is an important cost driver. If you lived in Burundi, however, what is one surefire way of being able to stay in the hospital, almost as long as you like? In Burundi, patients are detained in the hospital for having unpaid bills. Hundreds have been detained in Burundi's hospitals, sometimes for months, because they cannot afford their medical bills, says a report from Human Rights Watch. Many are women who unexpectedly needed cesarean sections.[1]

The Burundian situation seems a bit counterproductive, doesn't it?

J. A. Stockman III, MD

Reference

1. Kippenberg J. A high price to pay: detention of poor patients in Burundian hospitals. *Human Rights Watch*. 2006;18. Available at:http://hrw.org/reports/2006/burundi0906/. Accessed June 26, 2007.

A non-invasive test for prenatal diagnosis based on fetal DNA present in maternal blood: a preliminary study

Dhallan R, Guo X, Emche S, et al (Ravgen Inc, Columbia, Md; York Hosp/WellSpan Health, Pa; Lancaster Gen Women and Babies Hosp, Pa; et al)
Lancet 369:474-481, 2007

Background.—Use of free fetal DNA to diagnose fetal chromosomal abnormalities has been hindered by the inability to distinguish fetal DNA from maternal DNA. Our aim was to establish whether single nucleotide polymorphisms (SNPs) can be used to distinguish fetal DNA from maternal DNA—and to determine the number of fetal chromosomes—in maternal blood samples.

Methods.—Formaldehyde-treated blood samples from 60 pregnant women and the stated biological fathers were analysed. Maternal plasma fractions were quantified at multiple SNPs, and the ratio of the unique fetal allele signal to the combined maternal and fetal allele signal calculated. The mean ratios of SNPs on chromosomes 13 and 21 were compared to test for potential fetal chromosomal abnormalities.

Findings.—The mean proportion of free fetal DNA was 34.0% (median 32.5%, range 17.0–93.8). We identified three samples with significant differences in the fetal DNA ratios for chromosome 13 and chromosome 21, indicative of trisomy 21; the remaining 57 samples were deemed to be normal. Amniocentesis or newborn reports from the clinical sites confirmed that the copy number of fetal chromosomes 13 and 21 was established correctly for 58 of the 60 samples, identifying 56 of the 57 normal samples, and two of the three trisomy 21 samples. Of the incorrectly identified samples, one was a false negative and one was a false positive. The sensitivity and positive predictive value were both 66.7% (95% CI 12.5–98.2) and the specificity and negative predictive values were both 98.2% (89.4–99.9).

Interpretation.—The copy number of chromosomes of interest can be directly established from maternal plasma. Such a non-invasive prenatal test could provide a useful complement to currently used screening tests.

▶ Another report telling us about the ability to detect free fetal DNA in maternal blood samples and the utility of such testing for prenatal diagnosis. Analysis of fetal cells and free fetal DNA in the maternal circulation provides an alternative to existing prenatal tests. Invasive diagnostic tests such as amniocentesis and chorionic villus sampling are becoming increasingly passé. The use of free fetal DNA in maternal blood has been reported in the diagnosis of achondroplasia and myotonic dystrophy, to determine fetal sex, and in fetal rhesus D genotyping. However, 2 major issues have restricted the clinical use of the analysis of free fetal DNA. First, little free DNA exists in the maternal circulation: initial studies have reported a mean of only 3.4% free fetal DNA in the late first trimester to mid-second trimester. Second, in a heterogeneous mixture of maternal and fetal DNA, it is difficult to distinguish fetal chromosomes of clinical interest—for example, chromosomes 13, 18, and 21—from maternal chromosomes. The authors of this report have previously reported that careful sample processing and the addition of formaldehyde increases the proportion of free fetal DNA recovered from the maternal circulation to as high as 25%. Having increased the proportion of free DNA, the remaining challenge that these authors studied was how to determine the copy number of fetal chromosomes in a heterogeneous mixture of maternal and fetal DNA. Using new technology, these investigators were able to detect and quantify fetal DNA in maternal plasma and were able to determine the copy number of fetal chromosomes of most interest, specifically chromosomes 13 and 21.

With the techniques described, prenatal diagnosis with virtually no risk to a mother and fetus is possible for many of the genetic disorders that previously required invasive techniques like amniocentesis or chorionic villus sampling. Obviously, not every laboratory will be able to reproduce these findings, at least not for some time, but it is clear that, in the not widely distant future, all it will take is a bit of blood from a mother to learn a lot about her unborn baby.

J. A. Stockman III, MD

An Intervention to Decrease Catheter-Related Bloodstream Infections in the ICU

Pronovost P, Needham D, Berenholtz S, et al (Johns Hopkins Univ, Baltimore, Md; Univ of Michigan, Ann Arbor; William Beaumont Hosp, Royal Oak, Mich; et al)

N Engl J Med 355:2725-2732, 2006

Background.—Catheter-related bloodstream infections occurring in the intensive care unit (ICU) are common, costly, and potentially lethal.

Methods.—We conducted a collaborative cohort study predominantly in ICUs in Michigan. An evidence-based intervention was used to reduce the incidence of catheter-related bloodstream infections. Multilevel Poisson regression modeling was used to compare infection rates before, during, and up to 18 months after implementation of the study intervention. Rates of infection per 1000 catheter-days were measured at 3-month intervals, according to the guidelines of the National Nosocomial Infections Surveillance System.

Results.—A total of 108 ICUs agreed to participate in the study, and 103 reported data. The analysis included 1981 ICU-months of data and 375,757 catheter-days. The median rate of catheter-related bloodstream infection per 1000 catheter-days decreased from 2.7 infections at baseline to 0 at 3 months after implementation of the study intervention (P≤0.002), and the mean rate per 1000 catheter-days decreased from 7.7 at baseline to 1.4 at 16 to 18 months of follow-up (P<0.002). The regression model showed a significant decrease in infection rates from baseline, with incidence-rate ratios continuously decreasing from 0.62 (95% confidence interval [CI], 0.47 to 0.81) at 0 to 3 months after implementation of the intervention to 0.34 (95% CI, 0.23 to 0.50) at 16 to 18 months.

Conclusions.—An evidence-based intervention resulted in a large and sustained reduction (up to 66%) in rates of catheter-related bloodstream infection that was maintained throughout the 18-month study period.

▶ This study was conducted in adults. The reason I chose to include it is because a virtually identical collaborative has been formed to reduce catheter-related bloodstream infections in pediatric ICUs. This collaborative is being coordinated by the National Association of Children's Hospitals and Related Institutions. It is being funded, in part, by the American Board of Pediatrics Foundation as an initiative to demonstrate how subspecialists in pediatrics can improve systems of care while fulfilling requirements for maintenance of certification.

Overall, in the United States, some 36 million are admitted to acute care hospitals. About 1 in 10 of these hospitalizations involves an admission to a critical care unit. When one looks at pediatric patients, the proportion of admissions to critical care units is even higher. In such units, central venous catheters are commonly placed and, regrettably, many of these become infected. Not only is this costly in terms of an increase in the length of stay but also significant morbidity and some mortality are associated with IV line infections in ICUs and elsewhere. If one looks at all 6000 acute care hospitals and their associated ICUs in the United States, it is estimated that approximately 17,000 deaths are directly related to catheter-associated infections each year. This is out of approximately 18 million ICU days and 9.7 million catheter-days in ICUs.

With this background, Pronovost et al describe a remarkable intervention cohort study involving 103 ICUs in 67 hospitals with more than 375,000 catheter-days of observation. For adult ICUs, the Centers for Disease Control and Prevention (CDC) has very specific recommendations for minimizing the risk of catheter-related infections. In the study by Pronovost et al, 5 of the CDC's category IA recommendations were championed by local team leaders at the ICUs, and during the 18 months after implementation of the study intervention, the mean rate of catheter-related bloodstream infections fell from 7.7 to 1.4 per 1000 catheter-days, which was a 66% reduction.

As of this writing, it is still too early to accurately report the conclusive findings of the pediatric collaborative related to bloodstream infections in ICUs. During the first 3 months of initiation of the collaborative in late 2006 and early 2007, the initial fall in the incidence of bloodstream infections was brisk, approaching 50%. The intent is to learn best practices from those ICUs that are at the best end of the bell-shaped curve of less catheter-related infections and to spread the knowledge of how these ICUs do what they do to the rest of the cohort involved in the collaborative. The National Association of Children's Hospitals has been willing to open this collaborative to every pediatric ICU in the United States, not just to those within freestanding children's hospitals. This collaborative, and others like it, such as the Vermont Oxford Network for Neonatal Intensive Care and the Pediatric Inflammatory Bowel Disease Network are wonderful examples of how to improve the quality of care. The "dessert" for those critical care specialists and infectious disease consultants who are involved in the collaborative is that they have met all the requirements for part 4 of Maintenance of Certification because of the important work that they do locally.

J. A. Stockman III, MD

The catheter is stuck: complications experienced during removal of a totally implantable venous access device. A single-center study in 200 children

Wilson GJP, van Noesel MM, Hop WCJ, et al (Univ Med Centre, Rotterdam, The Netherlands; Royal Children's Hosp, Parkville, Victoria, Australia)
J Pediatr Surg 41:1694-1698, 2006

Background.—Totally implantable venous access devices (TIVAD) facilitate repeat intravenous therapy for children. Many children recover and the device may be removed. Although removal should be a simple procedure via a single incision, in our experience, this has not been the case.

Methods.—Two hundred consecutive cases of removal of TIVAD from September 2000 to January 2004 at Sophia Children's Hospital, Rotterdam, were reviewed.

Results.—Average patient age was 5.9 years. The commonest indication for placement was administration of chemotherapy (88%); commonest indication for removal was remission of disease (70%). The median duration in situ of the catheter was 29 months (range, 0.4-91 months). Complications with removal of the polyurethane catheter of the TIVAD were experienced in 16% of cases. To enable removal, a second incision was required in 28 patients, venotomy in 5; the catheter could not be removed in 3. For all complicated removals the catheter had been in situ for longer than 20 months.

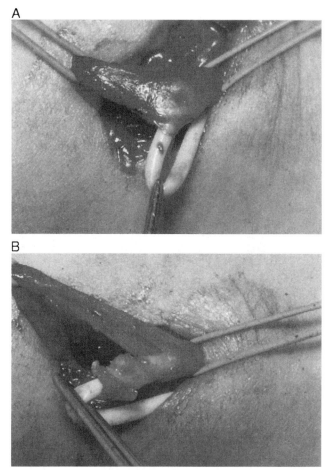

FIGURE 3.—Calcified mass (**A**) obstructing removal from vein (**B**) after venotomy; calcification densely adherent to catheter. (Courtesy of Wilson GJP, van Noesel MM, Hop WCJ, et al. The catheter is stuck: complications experienced during removal of a totally implantable venous access device. A single-center study in 200 children. *J Pediatr Surg.* 41:1694-1698. Copyright 2006, Elsevier.)

Conclusions.—Long-term implantation of TIVAD with polyurethane catheter appears unsuitable owing to a high incidence of complication at time of removal (Fig 3).

▶ In the Pronovost et al article (An intervention to decrease catheter-related bloodstream infections in the ICU) central catheter infections is discussed. In pediatrics, in addition to the temporary placement of central venous catheters in critical care units and elsewhere in hospitals, we commonly employ TIVADs such as a PORT-A-CATH Low Profile Titanium Venous Access System with a PolyFlow Polyurethane Catheter. These catheters permit repeated central venous access for delivery of medications, fluids, and nutritional fluids and for the sampling of venous blood. Their use in pediatric malignancy is routine, facilitating safe and comfortable delivery of chemotherapy. Other indications in the pediatric population include the management of children with cystic fibrosis, short gut syndrome, and some metabolic diseases. In the majority of children with these devices, the placement of the catheter is not permanent. Most of these catheters are removed in a few months or a few years depending on the reason for the placement of the catheter. Indications for removal include resolution of disease, most commonly complete remission of a malignancy, dysfunction of the catheter, or infection of the device. In most instances, these catheters can be easily and safely removed but not always so; thus, this is the reason for the article from Sophia Children's Hospital in The Netherlands.

In this study, we learn how difficult it is, in some cases, to remove a TIVAD. Some 200 consecutive cases of removal of such devices were reviewed. The average duration of the catheter placement was 29 months. About 1 in 6 individuals having the catheter removed had some problems with the removal. The basic problem in most instances related to retained catheters that were firmly adherent to a blood vessel wall, which precluded easy endovascular removal. Many times a fibrous sheath envelopes a catheter, and the sheath can become calcified. Some of these catheters were so adherent that they could not be removed, and it was believed to be less risky to leave them in place rather than for the patient to have to go through a surgical procedure such as a venotomy or a sternotomy to remove the retained pieces of a catheter. In addition to a subsequent risk of infection from a retained catheter, these catheters can be the origin of a venous thromboembolism. However, in this series with follow-up totals of 6 catheter-years, no evidence of such thromboembolism was present. The authors of this article do recommend the use of prophylactic antibiotics prior to and during procedures that may induce endocarditis if a patient is left with a piece of retained catheter.

This study shows that totally implantable venous access catheters should not be placed willy-nilly. In a small but real subset of patients, pieces of them will likely stay with the patient forever. Thus far, such retained catheters have not produced problems. However, considering the expected lifespan of the mostly cured patients who have had these catheters placed, the absence of short-term complications following completion of treatment does not preclude future harm from a retained catheter. All the catheters that were a problem in this series were catheters that were in place for 20 months or more. This leads one to wonder if such catheters, even if they are not causing problems, should be removed at about a year and a half and replaced with new ones. No firm recommendations exist, however, in this regard.

We will conclude this comment with numbers of board-certified general pediatricians and the maldistribution that currently exists within our borders. There is a remarkable variation in the numbers of board-certified generalist pediatricians throughout the United States. This is not especially unexpected, given the varying sizes of states and the numbers of children in each state. The following tables list the states with the fewest and largest numbers of board-certified generalist pediatricians (under the age of 66 and certified only in general pediatrics and not a pediatric subspecialty):

States ≤ 100 Board-Certified Generalist Pediatricians

State	# Pediatricians
Wyoming	45
North Dakota	55
South Dakota	62
Alaska	91
Montana	93
Idaho	99

States ≥ 1800 Board-Certified Generalist Pediatricians

State	# Pediatricians
California	5202
New York	4111
Texas	2633
Florida	2100
Pennsylvania	1947
Illinois	1869

More important than the numbers of pediatricians in each state is the number of children per pediatrician in each state. Which state has the largest number of children per pediatrician (the "least served" states) and which states have the fewest number of children per pediatrician (the most "highly" served states)?

Please note, that if the District of Columbia were a state, it would have the most favorable ratio of pediatricians per pediatric population at 1 pediatrician for every 622 children.

States in Which There Are ≥ 2500 Children[1] Per Pediatrician

State	# Children/# Pediatricians
Idaho	3762
Nevada	3410
South Dakota	3079
Oklahoma	2857
Mississippi	2797
Iowa	2637
Wyoming	2598

[1]The population of children is based on US Census Bureau data as of July 1, 2004, and includes children ages 0 to 18 years.

States in Which There are ≤ 1250 Children Per Pediatrician

State	# Children/# Pediatricians
Massachusetts	877
Maryland	987
Rhode Island	1003
Vermont	1054
Connecticut	1089
New York	1112
Hawaii	1144
New Jersey	1200

These data on the locales of pediatricians in the United States are available for viewing at the American Board of Pediatrics website (http://www.abp.org) in the American Board of Pediatrics 2006-2007 Workforce Data report.

J. A. Stockman III, MD

12 Musculoskeletal

Transient Paresis Associated With Cat-Scratch Disease: Case Report and Literature Review of Vertebral Osteomyelitis Caused by *Bartonella henselae*

Vermeulen MJ, Rutten GJ, Verhagen I, et al (St Elisabeth Hosp, Tilburg, The Netherlands)

Pediatr Infect Dis J 25:1177-1181, 2006

Background.—The typical presentation of cat-scratch disease (CSD) is that of a benign lymphadenitis, but in 5% to 20% of cases, an atypical presentation will occur. Nearly every organ system can be affected by hematogenous, lymphatic, or contiguous spread of the *Bartonella henselae* bacteria. In rare cases, there is neurologic involvement, with encephalitis, optic neuritis, meningitis, or myelitis being most common. A case of paresis of the arm in a child with CSD, who made a full recovery after antibiotic and neurosurgical therapy was reported.

Case Report.—Girl, 9 years, was seen with neck pain and a 3-day history of fever. Her parents reported that the neck pain might have been related to a fall on her right shoulder 2 weeks earlier. Examination revealed fever (39.6°C), torticollis, and limited flexion of the neck. There were no skin lesions or enlarged lymph nodes. Neurologic examination demonstrated normal findings. Laboratory tests revealed elevated serum C-reactive protein (CRP) and erythrocyte sedimentation rate (ESR) of 72 mg/L and 104 mm/h, respectively. However, CSF evaluation, bacterial cultures of blood and CSF, and viral studies were not diagnostic, and plain radiographs of the cervical spine were normal. It was decided to observe the patient. At 2 weeks after admission, the fever subsided and the CRP and ESR had decreased to 18 mg/L and 50 mm/h, respectively. Three days later, the patient had severe paresis of the proximal muscles of the right arm. MRI revealed a cervical paravertebral mass that extended into the foramina of the C5 and C6 roots. Abnormal signal intensities in several vertebral bodies were consistent with osteomyelitis. The patient underwent open biopsy by an anterior cervical approach, at which time purulent material in the prevertebral lesion was drained. Histopathologic analysis showed a nonspecific inflammatory reaction, with no evidence of a neoplasm. No diagnostic tests for *B henselae* were performed at that time. The patient was diagnosed with vertebral osteomyelitis and paravertebral abscess of unknown etiology and was treated successfully with a stiff neck collar and 3 weeks of IV amoxicillin/clavulanate. The patient was discharged 6 weeks after her initial symptoms, with a persisting paresis of the right arm. It later became known that the family had bought a young kitten a few weeks before manifestation of the initial symptoms. It was then hypothesized that CSD was the cause of the osteomyelitis. This was confirmed by a positive test for the presence of *B henselae* DNA in the surgically obtained material. An MRI scan at 6 weeks after discharge showed that all abnormalities had disappeared. After 3 months, the muscle strength in the affected arm had normalized.

Conclusions.—The diagnosis of CSD vertebral osteomyelitis should be considered in patients with systemic symptoms, back pain, and recent contact with cats. The prognosis for these patients is generally good.

▶ By now, most of us are familiar with the fact that CSD can present in an unusual way. Such atypical presentations occur in somewhere from 5% to 20% of those who become infected with *B henselae*. Indeed, just about every organ of the body can become involved with this infectious agent. For example, CSD can manifest itself as Parinaud oculoglandular syndrome, endocarditis, and hepatitis. Cases of encephalitis, optic neuritis, meningitis, and myelitis have been described. Osteomyelitis involving a wide assortment of bones has been estimated to occur in anywhere from 1 in 200 to 1 in 300 patients with CSD.

The case report of this 9-year-old girl with CSD is an interesting one, to say the least. She had no enlarged lymph nodes or skin manifestations. She did have fever. Neck pain was the predominant symptom. Well into the illness, and after the fever had already subsided, a severe weakness of the right proximal arm muscles developed. MRI showed a cervical paravertebral mass that extended into the foramina of the C5 and C6 nerve roots. C4, C5, and C6 vertebral bodies showed abnormal signal intensities consistent with osteomyelitis. Open biopsy revealed purulent material in the prevertebral spaces. Histopathologic analysis showed a nonspecific inflammatory reaction with no evidence of malignancy. Unfortunately, no diagnostic tests for *B henselae* were initially performed. The child was treated as if she had a routine bacterial osteomyelitis and paravertebral abscess of unknown etiology.

Some 6 weeks from the time of her symptoms, this young lady was discharged from the hospital, but had a persistent paresis of the arm. Some weeks later, it then became apparent that the family had purchased a young kitten just before the youngster's problems began. Bingo! Serology showed high titers against *B henselae*, and the surgically obtained material was looked at again and showed the presence of *B henselae* DNA by polymerase chain reaction. After 6 more weeks of appropriate therapy, the MRI returned to normal. Three months later, recovery of the weakness was observed.

This case represents the first report of proven CSD-associated vertebral osteomyelitis observed with a transient paresis. It would be hard to think of this etiology for the neurologic symptoms the child presented with, given the fact that vertebral bone infections caused by *B henselae* are so uncommon. In previous reported cases, the presenting symptom was that of back pain, not weakness. Thank goodness for MRIs. It is a shame that the authors did not take a careful history at the time of presentation since whenever there is a diagnostic dilemma, one should always round up the usual suspects. Cats are always included in the latter category.

J. A. Stockman III, MD

Changing Patterns of Acute Hematogenous Osteomyelitis and Septic Arthritis: *Emergence of Community-associated Methicillin-resistant Staphylococcus aureus*

Arnold SR, Elias D, Buckingham SC, et al (Univ of Tennessee, Memphis; Peachtree Ctr, Jesup, Ga; Cortel Clinica Ortopedica, Rio De Janeiro, Brazil; et al)
J Pediatr Orthop 26:703-708, 2006

Introduction.—An increase in the incidence and severity of acute osteoarticular infections in children was perceived after the emergence of community-associated methicillin-resistant *Staphylococcus aureus* (MRSA) in our community. This study was performed to describe changes in the epidemiology and clinical features of acute osteoarticular infections.

Methods.—The records of patients discharged from Le Bonheur Children's Medical Center with a diagnosis of acute osteoarticular infection between 2000 and 2004 were reviewed. Data regarding signs and symptoms, diagnostic testing, therapeutics, surgery, and hospital course were collected.

Results.—There were 158 cases of acute osteoarticular infection. The incidence increased from 2.6 to 6.0 per 1000 admissions between 2000 and 2004. The proportion of infections caused by methicillin-susceptible *S. aureus* (MSSA) remained constant (10%–13%) and that caused by MRSA rose from 4% to 40%. There was no difference between MRSA and MSSA patients in the duration of fever or pain before diagnosis. Seventy-one percent of patients with MRSA had subperiosteal abscesses compared with 38% with MSSA ($P = 0.02$). Ninety-one percent of MRSA patients required a surgical procedure compared with 62% of MSSA patients ($P < 0.001$). Median hospital stay was 7 days for MSSA patients and 10 days for MRSA patients ($P = 0.0001$). Three patients developed chronic osteomyelitis, 2 with MRSA. There was no association between a delay in institution of appropriate antibiotic therapy and presence of subperiosteal abscess ($P = 0.8$).

Conclusions.—There has been an increase in the incidence and severity of acute osteoarticular infections in Memphis. Patients with community-associated MRSA infections are at higher risk of subperiosteal abscess requiring surgical intervention.

▶ This report is a wake-up call to the growing trend of methicillin-resistant *Staphylococcus aureus* (MRSA) causing osteomyelitis and septic arthritis. The report catalogs a change in the epidemiology and clinical findings of children with musculoskeletal infections. Specifically, investigators compared patients with methicillin-susceptible *S. aureus* (MSSA) to those with MRSA. They noted that those children with MRSA had more subperiosteal abscesses, more frequent need for surgical procedures, longer hospital stays, and greater potential for complications such as chronic osteomyelitis. The only proposed virulence factor consistently found in these staphylococci was the extracellular toxin Panton-Valentine leukocidin, the latter having also been associated with necrotizing pneumonia and skin infections in otherwise healthy children and adolescents.

Clearly, there is an increasing prevalence of MRSA as an etiology of musculoskeletal infections in children. MRSA has become the most commonly identifiable cause of skin and soft tissue infections among patients presenting to emergency departments in many United States cities. All current evidence suggests that community-acquired MRSA infection is increasing, primarily in teenagers and particularly in young healthy boys. It can be virulent in its presentation with vasculitis, thrombophlebitis, and septic emboli to multiple organs. Early recognition and aggressive treatment is essential to prevent, or at least limit, morbidity and/or mortality. It is critical that this message gets out to all physicians and healthcare providers who deal with musculoskeletal infections such as osteomyelitis and septic arthritis.

To show you how serious an MRSA-related infection can be, recently a 13-year-old competitive soccer player was described who developed an erythematous, macular, coalescent rash over her trunk, back and all of her extremities. A day before she had developed diarrhea and abdominal pain. Her physical examination showed erythema of the buckle and labial mucosae. Her conjunctiva were reported to be injected. She was suspected of having toxic shock syndrome. Her last menstrual period had been 10 days previously, and she had never used tampons. The only significant history was that she had donned a new pair of soccer shoes and had developed friction blisters over both heals. These blisters ultimately cultured MRSA. The organism was further studied and was documented to express the toxic shock syndrome gene *TSS1*.[1]

J. A. Stockman III, MD

Reference

1. Taylor CM, Riordan FA, Graham C. New football boots and toxic shock syndrome. *BMJ*. 2006;332:1376-1378.

Family study of the inheritance of pectus excavatum

Creswick HA, Stacey MW, Kelly RE Jr, et al (Children's Hosp of The King's Daughters, Norfolk, Va)
J Pediatr Surg 41:1699-1703, 2006

Background.—The most common congenital deformity of the chest wall is pectus excavatum, a malformation that is present in between 1 in 400 and 1 in 1000 live births and causes the body of the sternum to be displaced, producing a depression. There are many different shapes of the pectus, and multiple factors probably contribute to the final form. The etiology of pectus excavatum is uncertain, but a familial tendency has been found in clinical experience, where it may be seen in more than one sibling. Pectus excavatum is commonly associated with connective tissue disorders such as Marfan and Ehlers Danlos syndromes. Extensive literature review failed to identify articles documenting families with multiple affected members.

Purpose.—The purpose of this study was to collect evidence that pectus excavatum is familial and may be an inherited disorder.

Methods.—Using the Children's Surgical Specialty Group database at Children's Hospital of The King's Daughters, families with more than one affected individual were selected. With Institutional Review Board–approved informed consent, 34 families agreed to participate. Family histories were obtained, and a 4-generation pedigree was constructed for each family. Forty questions were asked about each individual's medical history, and comprehensive systems review included features of connective tissue-related problems. Inheritance patterns for each family were determined by pedigree analysis.

Results.—A total of 14 families suggested autosomal dominant inheritance, 4 families suggested autosomal recessive inheritance, and 6 families suggested X-linked recessive inheritance. Ten families had complex inheritance patterns. Pectus excavatum occurred more frequently in males than in females (1.8:1). Long arms, legs, and fingers; high-arched palate; mitral valve prolapse; heart arrhythmia; scoliosis; double jointedness; flexibility; flat feet; childhood myopia; poor healing; and easy bruising were commonly associated with pectus excavatum.

Conclusions.—Pedigree analysis of 34 families provides evidence that pectus excavatum is an inherited disorder, possibly of connective tissue. Although some families demonstrate apparent Mendelian inheritance, most appear to be multifactorial.

▶ Pectus excavatum remains the most common congenital chest wall anomaly. It affects as many as 1 in 400 live births. Proposed theories for the development of pectus excavatum include intrauterine pressure, rickets, pulmonary restriction, abnormalities of the diaphragm that result in posterior traction on the sternum, and intrinsic failure of osteogenesis and/or chondrogenesis. Biochemical studies have shown abnormalities in collagen synthesis in some patients. Boys are affected 4 times more often than girls. This article from Virginia is important because it shows us that, in some cases at least, familial clustering of pectus excavatum is present. Before this article appeared, a familial tendency had been suggested because pectus excavatum has been seen in siblings and across multiple generations. Four-generation pedigrees on 34 families seem to provide strong evidence for a clustering of pectus excavatum in families. Although the pedigrees of several families in this study suggested simple Mendelian inheritance with possible autosomal dominant, autosomal recessive, and X-linked genes, many families demonstrate apparent multifactorial inheritance. In addition, many family members report having connective tissue peculiarities, which suggests that pectus excavatum may be due, in part, to defects in connective tissue genes affecting fibrillin, collagen, and transforming-growth factor-β.

The next time you diagnose pectus excavatum in a youngster, recognize that it would be worthwhile checking other family members for the same problem. Sooner or later, we will find the specific genetic cause, which is likely to cause a disturbance in connective tissue formation.

J. A. Stockman III, MD

Evaluation of an Algorithmic Approach to Pediatric Back Pain

Feldman DS, Straight JJ, Badra MI, et al (New York Hosp for Joint Diseases)
J Pediatr Orthop 26:353-357, 2006

Pediatric patients require a systematic approach to treating back pain that minimizes the number of diagnostic studies without missing specific diagnoses. This study reviews an algorithm for the evaluation of pediatric back pain and assesses critical factors in the history and physical examination that are predictive of specific diagnoses. Eighty-seven pediatric patients with thoracic and/or lumbar back pain were treated utilizing after this algorithm. If initial plain radiographs were positive, patients were considered to have a specific diagnosis. If negative, patients with constant pain, night pain, radicular pain, and/or an abnormal neurological examination obtained a follow-up magnetic resonance imaging. Patients with negative radiographs and intermittent pain were diagnosed with nonspecific back pain. Twenty-one (24%) of 87 patients had positive radiographs and were treated for their specific diagnoses. Nineteen (29%) of 66 patients with negative radiographs had constant pain, night pain, radicular pain, and/or an abnormal neurological examination. Ten of these 19 patients had a specific diagnosis determined by magnetic resonance imaging. Therefore, 31 (36%) of 87 patients had a specific diagnosis. Back pain of other 56 patients was of a nonspecific nature. No specific diagnoses were missed at latest follow-up. Specificity for determining a specific diagnosis was very high for radicular pain (100%), abnormal neurological examination (100%), and night pain (95%). Radicular pain and an abnormal neurological examination also had high positive predictive value (100%). Lumbar pain was the most sensitive (67%) and had the highest negative predictive value (75%). This algorithm seems to be an effective tool for diagnosing pediatric back pain, and this should help to reduce costs and patient/family anxiety and to avoid unnecessary radiation exposure.

▶ This report emanating from the pediatric orthopedic literature is an important one for those in general pediatric practice. A generation ago, we were not hearing too much about kids with back pain, now we are. In a longitudinal study that included more than 200 adolescents over a 5-year period, it was found that the annual incidence of lumbar pain ran 12% at age 12 years and slightly more than 20% at age 15 years.[1] Some have considered the complaint of back pain in a child to be a red flag and the belief exists in many that every effort should be made to reach a diagnosis. This is unlike the situation in adults where back pain is so common and is due to nonserious causes that a more laissez-faire approach is usually taken. The more we learn, however, about children is that a good bit of back pain is also benign. The difficulty, however, is separating out that group of children who have benign causes of back pain from those who have serious underlying causes. This report of Feldman et al helps us in this differentiation.

What we learn is how to use an algorithmic approach to diagnose the causes of back pain. This involves an initial workup that includes history, physical examination and plain x-ray films of the spine. If the x-ray films show positive, the patient is given a specific diagnosis on the basis of the radiographic findings and is accordingly treated. If the x-ray films show negative and no diagnostic physical signs are present, then the patient is treated as having nonspecific back pain. These patients receive observation and are symptomatically treated with rest, physical therapy and/or nonsteroidal anti-inflammatory medications. Those with negative x-ray films who experience constant pain, night pain, radicular pain, and/or have an abnormal neurologic examination will require further study with MRI. By following this algorithm, the investigators did not miss any major spinal pathology such as a tumor or infection and at the last follow-up, none of the patients who were labeled as having nonspecific back pain had a change in their diagnosis.

This report strongly suggests that history and physical examination complemented by plain x-ray films and an MRI when indicated should be the cornerstone for the evaluation of back pain. MRI clearly has supplanted bone scan as a screening tool. A bone scan is reserved to rule out metastatic disease or to determine disease activity in subjects with spondylolysis.

Try this algorithm and see if it works for you. Be reminded that constant pain, radicular pain, night pain, and an abnormal neurologic examination continue to be the red flags for important causes of back pain. Also, do not forget to query the patient about the weight of their school backpack. Be aware that more than 80% of youngsters with back pain attribute the pain to overloaded backpacks.[2]

See how you would deal with the following question posed by a teen who does not wish to develop back pain as a result of a certain form of injury. A 17-year-old young lady in your practice is planning a ski vacation with her parents. She wants to know what she might do to minimize her risk of orthopaedic injury. She has read something about the relationship of time of her menstrual cycle and orthopaedic injuries, and asks you if this relationship may in fact be true. How do you respond? Indeed there is such a relationship. Recreational alpine skiers have proved surprisingly useful in studying the relationship between menstrual cycle phase and one specific type of orthopaedic skiing injury: torn anterior cruciate ligament.[3] The likelihood of sustaining such injuries is not constant during the menstrual cycle: the risk is much greater during the pre-ovulatory phase than in the post-ovulatory phase. In fact, the relationship with timing of the menstrual cycle is sufficiently great that one wonders whether this factoid should be kept in mind when booking skiing holidays.

J. A. Stockman III, MD

References

1. Burton AK, Clarke RD, McClune TD, Tillotson KM. The natural history of low back pain in adolescents. *Spine.* 1996;21:2323-2328.
2. Skaggs DL, Early SD, D'Ambra P, Tolo VT, Kay RM. Back pain and backpacks in school children. *J Pediatr Orthop.* 2006;26:358-363.
3. Beynnon BD, Johnson RJ, Braun S, et al. The relationship between menstrual cycle phase and anterior cruciate ligament injury: a case-control study of recreational alpine skiers. *Am J Sports Med.* 2006;34:757-763.

Surgical vs Nonoperative Treatment for Lumbar Disk Herniation: The Spine Patient Outcomes Research Trial (SPORT): A Randomized Trial
Weinstein JN, Tosteson TD, Lurie JD, et al (Dartmouth Med School, Hanover, NH; Thomas Jefferson Univ, Philadelphia; Emory Univ, Atlanta, Ga; et al)
JAMA 296:2441-2450, 2006

Context.—Lumbar diskectomy is the most common surgical procedure performed for back and leg symptoms in US patients, but the efficacy of the procedure relative to nonoperative care remains controversial.

Objective.—To assess the efficacy of surgery for lumbar intervertebral disk herniation.

Design, Setting, and Patients.—The Spine Patient Outcomes Research Trial, a randomized clinical trial enrolling patients between March 2000 and November 2004 from 13 multidisciplinary spine clinics in 11 US states. Patients were 501 surgical candidates (mean age, 42 years; 42% women) with imaging-confirmed lumbar intervertebral disk herniation and persistent signs and symptoms of radiculopathy for at least 6 weeks.

Interventions.—Standard open diskectomy vs nonoperative treatment individualized to the patient.

Main Outcome Measures.—Primary outcomes were changes from baseline for the Medical Outcomes Study 36-item Short-Form Health Survey bodily pain and physical function scales and the modified Oswestry Disability Index (American Academy of Orthopaedic Surgeons MODEMS version) at 6 weeks, 3 months, 6 months, and 1 and 2 years from enrollment. Secondary outcomes included sciatica severity as measured by the Sciatica Bothersomeness Index, satisfaction with symptoms, self-reported improvement, and employment status.

Results.—Adherence to assigned treatment was limited: 50% of patients assigned to surgery received surgery within 3 months of enrollment, while 30% of those assigned to nonoperative treatment received surgery in the same period. Intent-to-treat analyses demonstrated substantial improvements for all primary and secondary outcomes in both treatment groups. Between-group differences in improvements were consistently in favor of surgery for all periods but were small and not statistically significant for the primary outcomes.

Conclusions.—Patients in both the surgery and the nonoperative treatment groups improved substantially over a 2-year period. Because of the large numbers of patients who crossed over in both directions, conclusions about the superiority or equivalence of the treatments are not warranted based on the intent-to-treat analysis.

▶ This report and the report by Weinstein et al (Surgical vs nonoperative treatment for lumbar disk herniation: the Spine Patient Outcomes Research Trial (SPORT) observational cohort) tell us about the comparison between the surgical versus the nonoperative treatment of lumbar disk herniation. The data are derived from studies of adults. Children, however, do experience the problem in question, and until we have further information specific to children, we should pay attention to the results of these adult studies. The benefit of surgical treatment for some diseases affecting the lumbar spine is not controversial in many clinical situations, such as major trauma with gross instability, unstable spondylolisthesis, persistent or complicated spinal infections, and some spinal tumors with progressive neurologic loss. The surgical treatment for complications of disk problems, however, is more debatable. Surgical treatment for primary back pain associated with disk changes (discogenic pain) is more controversial and less successful. When examination of the lumbar spine reveals only degenerative changes, which can occur as early as the teenage years, the relationship of these findings to a patient's back pain is unclear. The two studies reported from the *Journal of the American Medical Association* are from the Spine Patient Outcomes Research Trial (SPORT) on lumbar disk surgery for persistent radicular pain. These studies attempt to sort out the benefits of surgery for disk problems.

SPORT includes a multicenter, randomized, controlled trial of surgical versus nonoperative care for disk disorders. The two studies reported represent a colossal research effort and provide a fascinating snapshot of both modern patient preferences and clinical outcomes for a common clinical problem. Both surgical and nonoperative treatment are associated with clinically significant improvements over time, and differences between these treatments, as has been shown in previous studies, decrease with time. Regardless of the intervention received, most patients seem satisfied with their care. If there is a benefit to surgery it is that it tends, in those who benefit, to resolve the pain more quickly. Consequently, whether to choose a surgical approach for disk herniation depends on the individual patient's preference in addition to the commonly considered medical and surgical considerations. For example, for a self-employed carpenter with little cash reserves, for a mother of toddlers and no local resources for help, and for a salesperson working on commission, the apparently slower recovery without surgery may represent a hardship beyond physical pain. The inability to care for family, earn a living, or keep a competitive job may be the deciding factors in determining whether surgical treatment is desired. If, on the other hand, you can wait up to a year before the decision has to be made, a nonmedical approach will be as good as a surgical approach.

Again, these data apply to children only by extrapolation. Specialists in pediatric orthopedics are seasoned individuals and will help a patient make the best decision given the circumstances.

For more on the topic of surgery for spinal pain, see Zeller's excellent summary[1] describing the use of artificial spinal disks, which are proving to be superior to fusion for treating degenerative disease.

J. A. Stockman III, MD

Reference

1. Zeller JL. Artificial spinal disk superior to fusion for treating degenerative disk disease. *JAMA.* 2006;296:2665-2667.

Surgical vs Nonoperative Treatment for Lumbar Disk Herniation: The Spine Patient Outcomes Research Trial (SPORT) Observational Cohort

Weinstein JN, Lurie JD, Tosteson TD, et al (Dartmouth Med School, Hanover, NH; William Beaumont Hosp, Royal Oak, Mich; Hosp for Special Surgery, New York; et al)
JAMA 296:2451-2459, 2006

Context.—For patients with lumbar disk herniation, the Spine Patient Outcomes Research Trial (SPORT) randomized trial intent-to-treat analysis showed small but not statistically significant differences in favor of diskectomy compared with usual care. However, the large numbers of patients who crossed over between assigned groups precluded any conclusions about the comparative effectiveness of operative therapy vs usual care.

Objective.—To compare the treatment effects of diskectomy and usual care.

Design, Setting, and Patients.—Prospective observational cohort of surgical candidates with imaging-confirmed lumbar intervertebral disk herniation who were treated at 13 spine clinics in 11 US states and who met the SPORT eligibility criteria but declined randomization between March 2000 and March 2003.

Interventions.—Standard open diskectomy vs usual nonoperative care.

Main Outcome Measures.—Changes from baseline in the Medical Outcomes Study Short-Form Health Survey (SF-36) bodily pain and physical function scales and the modified Oswestry Disability Index (American Academy of Orthopaedic Surgeons/MODEMS version).

Results.—Of the 743 patients enrolled in the observational cohort, 528 patients received surgery and 191 received usual nonoperative care. At 3 months, patients who chose surgery had greater improvement in the primary outcome measures of bodily pain (mean change: surgery, 40.9 vs nonoperative care, 26.0; treatment effect, 14.8; 95% confidence interval, 10.8-18.9), physical function (mean change: surgery, 40.7 vs nonoperative care, 25.3; treatment effect, 15.4; 95% CI, 11.6-19.2), and Oswestry Disability Index (mean change: surgery, −36.1 vs nonoperative care, −20.9; treatment effect, −15.2; 95% CI, −18.5 to −11.8). These differences narrowed somewhat at 2 years: bodily pain (mean change: surgery, 42.6 vs nonoperative care, 32.4; treatment effect, 10.2; 95% CI, 5.9-14.5), physical function (mean change: surgery, 43.9 vs nonoperative care 31.9; treatment effect, 12.0; 95% CI; 7.9-16.1), and Oswestry Disability Index (mean change: surgery −37.6 vs nonoperative care −24.2; treatment effect, −13.4; 95% CI, −17.0 to −9.7).

Conclusions.—Patients with persistent sciatica from lumbar disk herniation improved in both operated and usual care groups. Those who chose operative intervention reported greater improvements than patients who elected nonoperative care. However, nonrandomized comparisons of self-reported outcomes are subject to potential confounding and must be interpreted cautiously.

Trends in Adolescent Lumbar Disk Herniation

Frino J, McCarthy RE, Sparks CY, et al (Univ of Arkansas, Little Rock; Arkansas Spine Ctr, Little Rock)
J Pediatr Orthop 26:579-581, 2006

The authors have retrospectively studied the trends in etiology, symptoms, and rate of recurrence for adolescents with disk herniations to determine the age at onset of symptoms, mechanism of injury, familial history, pattern of symptoms, level of herniation, method of treatment, and rate of recurrence. The review revealed a higher incidence of adolescent lumbar disk herniations in female patients and a higher percentage of patients with a family history than previously reported. Leg pain continues to be the primary presenting symptom in this group of patients and is often not recognized as the radicular pain of a herniated disk by the primary care physician. This reflects a lack of understanding of the relationship of the presenting symptoms to the pathology of the herniated nucleus pulposus, causing a delay in referral to the spine specialist.

▶ I'll bet that you didn't know that the first child reported to have a herniated disk was described in 1934 and that the first report of surgical management was in a 12-year-old boy in 1945. Since then, physicians caring for adolescents with low back pain have struggled to understand its cause. Although lumbar disk herniation is a common entity in the adult population, it can also be a possible cause of symptoms and significant morbidity in adolescents. This report looks at trends over time in the etiology, symptoms, rate, and recurrence in adolescents with disk herniations confirmed by magnetic resonance imaging. Quite a few interesting facts emerge, including the observation that, if a child has a lumbar disk herniation, there will be a family history of the same thing in more than 40% of cases. Also, for inexplicable reasons, adolescent girls are affected five times more frequently than adolescent boys, with the age of 15 years being the pinnacle for the development of this problem. The symptoms of herniated disk were preceded by trauma in the majority of cases (65% of the time). Presenting symptoms included low back pain with or without radiation to the buttocks, leg, foot, or ankle. Some patients presented just with leg pain or weakness.

As far as the level of herniation, adolescents and adults share the fact that the majority of disk herniations occur at low lumbar levels or at the lumbosacral junction. Only a small percentage of disk herniations are seen at L3/L4, and none are seen above this level. If one finds a spinal-canal–encroaching lesion above these levels, one would be well advised to look for other causes.

Although this report gives us much information about the "demographics" of adolescent lumbar disk herniation, it does not give us a clue to the best management approach (including surgery). A lot was written in 2006 about the "leave-well-enough-alone" approach to lumbar disk herniation; the shine is clearly off performing surgery in a reflexive manner.

J. A. Stockman III, MD

Meniscal tears in children and adolescents: results of operative treatment
Accadbled F, Cassard X, Sales de Gauzy J, et al (Children's Hosp, Toulouse, France; Clinique des Cèdres, Cornebarrieu, France)
J Pediatr Orthop B 16:56-60, 2007

The goal of this study was to evaluate the results of meniscal repair in children and adolescents by a retrospective case series. Twelve arthroscopic-assisted meniscal repairs were performed on 12 patients younger than 17 years of age (8–16 years, mean 13 years). The anterior cruciate ligament was torn in three cases. Eight lesions involved the lateral meniscus and four involved the medial meniscus; there were no discoid menisci. All patients were seen at an average of 3 years 1 month follow-up (range, 2–4 years 10 months). Three patients required subsequent surgery for partial meniscectomy. We evaluated the remaining nine patients by clinical examination, International Knee Documentation Committee clinical score, Lysholm score, Tegner's activity, and by computed tomography arthrogram or magnetic resonance imaging. Seven patients were asymptomatic at follow-up, two reported occasional pain, and none had experienced symptoms of locking. Their average Lysholm score and Tegner's activity were 96.3 and 6.6, respectively. Eight patients were International Knee Documentation Committee A and one was International Knee Documentation Committee B. Healing status was assessed at follow-up in eight patients by computed tomography arthrogram or magnetic resonance imaging: the tear was considered as completely healed in three patients. The apparent failure rate was 66%. Indications for meniscal repair in children are not actually established. The pejorative outcome of meniscectomy at a young age has led us to consider symptomatic meniscal tears for repair. Objective results of meniscal healing are poor. The method to assess healing of the repaired menisci objectively is still a matter of debate.

▶ Relatively few studies have addressed the results of meniscal repairs in children. It appears that incomplete healing is not a rare phenomenon. Furthermore, long-term outcomes of meniscectomy in childhood are not great. In fact, a significant percentage, if not the majority, of youngsters so operated on are doomed to the development of chronic arthritis of the knee and knee replacement later in life.

In this series of children and adolescents with meniscal tears, a 66% failure rate of surgical repair was found with the use of imaging criteria postsurgery. All the patients were skeletally immature at the time of operation. One in 4 of the patients wound up having no preservation of meniscal tissue, and you can bet that these are the youngsters who will require knee replacements sometime later in life for relief of chronic pain. The authors of this article believe that every attempt should be made to repair a meniscus because the alternative, meniscectomy, will clearly result in a loss of function and premature joint arthrosis. No one would disagree with this. They also caution, however, that parents should be informed of the risk of failure of this surgical procedure in the pediatric patient.

Many of the knee injuries suffered by children and adolescents are a consequence of engaging in sporting activities. Most readers of the YEAR BOOK know that I abhor all forms of exercise, but do recognize the value of sports participation . . . if only the latter were risk-free for kids.

Take for example in-line skating. Of all forms of skating, this appears to be the most risky. Virtually every child who died in more than half of children admitted to the hospital with skating injuries (almost 60%) had injuries as a result of in-line skating. It was back in 1998 that the *American Academy of Pediatrics* issued a recommendation that children and adolescents wear full protective gear, including a helmet, wrist guards, knee pads, and elbow pads while in-line skating. This recommendation has led to a decline in injuries related to in-line skating starting around 1999. This is particularly true of the use of wrist guards, which clearly are effective in reducing lower-arm injuries. To read more about the risks associated with head injury and other injuries for pediatric ice-skaters, roller-skaters, and in-line-skaters, see the superb study of Knox et al.[1]

J. A. Stockman III, MD

Reference

1. Knox CL, Comstock RD, McGeehan J, Smith GA. Differences in the risk associated with head injury for pediatric ice skaters, roller skaters, and in-line-skaters. *Pediatrics.* 2006;118:549-554.

Prevalence of Flat Foot in Preschool-Aged Children

Pfeiffer M, Kotz R, Ledl T, et al (Med Univ of Vienna; Univ of Vienna)
Pediatrics 118:634-639, 2006

Objectives.—Our aim with this study was to establish the prevalence of flat foot in a population of 3- to 6-year-old children to evaluate cofactors such as age, weight, and gender and to estimate the number of unnecessary treatments performed.

Methods.—A total of 835 children (411 girls and 424 boys) were included in this study. The clinical diagnosis of flat foot was based on a valgus position of the heel and a poor formation of the arch. Feet of the children were scanned (while they were in a standing position) by using a laser surface scanner, and rearfoot angle was measured. Rearfoot angle was defined as the angle of the upper Achilles tendon and the distal extension of the rearfoot.

Results.—Prevalence of flexible flat foot in the group of 3- to 6-year-old children was 44%. Prevalence of pathological flat foot was <1%. Ten percent of the children were wearing arch supports. The prevalence of flat foot decreases significantly with age: in the group of 3-year-old children 54% showed a flat foot, whereas in the group of 6-year-old children only 24% had a flat foot. Average rearfoot angle was 5.5° of valgus. Boys had a significant greater tendency for flat foot than girls: the prevalence of flat foot in boys was 52% and 36% in girls. Thirteen percent of the children were overweight or obese. Significant differences in prevalence of flat foot between overweight, obese, and normal-weight children were observed.

Conclusions.—This study is the first to use a three-dimensional laser surface scanner to measure the rearfoot valgus in preschool-aged children. The data demonstrate that the prevalence of flat foot is influenced by 3 factors: age, gender, and weight. In overweight children and in boys, a highly significant prevalence of flat foot was observed; in addition, a retarded development of the medial arch in the boys was discovered. At the time of the study, >90% of the treatments were unnecessary (Table 3).

TABLE 3.—Probability of the Prevalence of Flat-footedness Estimated by the Logistic-Regression Model

| | Age | | | |
	3 y, %	4 y, %	5 y, %	6 y, %
Girls, normal weight	42	31	22	15
Girls, overweight	48	37	27	19
Girls, obese	67	56	45	34
Boys, normal weight	62	51	39	29
Boys, overweight	67	57	45	34
Boys, obese	82	74	64	53

(Reproduced by permission of *Pediatrics* courtesy of Pfeiffer M, Kotz R, Ledl T, et al. Prevalence of flat foot in preschool-aged children. *Pediatrics*. 2006;118:634-639.)

▶ How many times in your practice have you been asked by a parent or parents about a child with flat feet and whether anything needs to be done about them? As frequently as such questions are asked, there appear to be few data in the literature to address such questions. This is why the report abstracted is so important. It is one of those studies from the pediatric orthopedic literature that immediately translates new information to the generalist pediatrician about a question of significant clinical relevance. What we learn is that all newborns are born with flat feet and that the longitudinal arch develops naturally during the first decade of life. A parent will notice a flat foot once a child begins to stand and the flat foot often presents concerns to a parent or parents. Traditionally, flat-footed children have been treated with arch supports or corrective shoes to improve the arch, but virtually all studies to date doubt the effectiveness of such treatment and are of the opinion that a flat foot is normal in early childhood and resolves spontaneously without treatment.

Most pediatricians don't know the definition of a flat foot because it is surrounded by confusion. The clinical diagnosis of flat foot is based on a valgus position of the heel and the formation of the medial arch on weight bearing. The report abstracted uses a generally accepted orthopedic definition of a flat foot. If the medial arch is not visible, it is graded as a moderate flat foot; classification as severe flat foot means that the medial arch of the foot is convexed. Preschool-aged children with flexible flat feet have a valgus position <20° and active correction is possible, whereas pathologic flat foot is defined by a valgus position >20°. In the study abstracted, the various anatomical measurements that determine whether feet are flat were made by using a laser surface scanner. A valgus between 0° and 4° was defined as normal, a valgus between 5° and 20° was classified as physiological flat foot, and a rearfoot valgus of ≥20° was classified as a pathological flat foot. The table shows the probability of the prevalence of flat footedness. Between 40% and 60% of 3 year olds will have this anatomical finding with overweight children having it even more commonly. Boys will have the finding half again more commonly as girls. Fewer than 1% of youngsters with flat feet have a pathological flat foot.

Thus we learn from this report just how common flat foot is in childhood and the fact that it tends to go away in the vast majority of affected children as they age. There are virtually no data to support the need for arch supports, which, along with corrective shoes, may be quite uncomfortable for a child. Add to this the enormous cost associated with special shoes and you see the burden that treatment entails. In this report, we learn that over 90% of the treatments prescribed are totally unnecessary.

The Nagai et al report (Prevalence of Charcot-Marie-Tooth disease in patients who have bilateral cavovarus feet) tells us what we should be thinking about when children present with the opposite of a flat foot, that is, a foot that has an unusually high arch, also known as a cavovarus foot.

J. A. Stockman III, MD

Prevalence of Charcot-Marie-Tooth Disease in Patients Who Have Bilateral Cavovarus Feet

Nagai MK, Chan G, Guille JT, et al (Alfred I duPont Hosp for Children, Wilmington, Del; Shriners Hosp for Children, Philadelphia)
J Pediatr Orthop 26:438-443, 2006

It is not uncommon to see a patient with bilateral cavovarus feet in the outpatient setting. A large percentage of these patients are subsequently diagnosed with an associated condition, such as Charcot-Marie-Tooth disease. The purpose of the present report was to determine the prevalence of Charcot-Marie-Tooth disease in children who have bilateral cavovarus feet. A chart review of children with bilateral cavovarus feet was done. Patients were excluded if they had an existing medical problem known to be associated with bilateral cavovarus feet. Charcot-Marie-Tooth disease was diagnosed after a clinical assessment by an orthopaedic surgeon and a neurologist. The diagnosis was confirmed by either standard nerve conduction velocity studies and/or the CMT DNA Duplication Detection Test (Athena Diagnostics Inc, Worchester, MA). A positive family history was noted only if the diagnosis had been confirmed by a nerve conduction velocity study and/or CMT DNA Duplication Detection Test. One hundred forty-eight patients met the study criteria. The probability of a patient with bilateral cavovarus feet being diagnosed with Charcot-Marie-Tooth disease, regardless of family history, was 78% (116 patients). A family history of Charcot-Marie-Tooth disease increased the probability to 91%. It is recommended that all patients with bilateral cavovarus feet, especially with a known family history, be investigated for Charcot-Marie-Tooth disease.

▶ A cavovarus foot is one that has an unusually high arch. Bilateral cavovarus feet are rarely present at birth and gradually become apparent as a child's foot grows and matures. Youngsters with this condition can present with complaints of foot and ankle pain, cosmetic deformity, and/or difficulty with shoe wear. Some youngsters with bilateral cavovarus feet are asymptomatic, and the foot finding is incidentally observed on physical examination. A specific diagnosis of a cavovarus foot is based on radiologic findings. There are normative data that determine the amount of an arch that a child should have at any given age.

This report from the Alfred I duPont Hospital for Children in Wilmington, Delaware reminds us of the many causes of bilateral cavovarus feet. The one observation of real significance is the association of bilateral cavovarus feet and Charcot-Marie-Tooth disease (an inherited progressive peripheral neuropathy). Charcot-Marie-Tooth disease presents as a slowly progressive sensory loss accompanied by weakness, muscle atrophy, and diminished deep tendon reflexes that, over time, produce a characteristic cavovarus foot deformity. The literature suggests that the prevalence of cavovarus feet in Charcot-Marie-Tooth disease can range from a low of 12% in some series to a high of 100% in other series. What we learn from the patients seen at Alfred I duPont Hospital is that for patients presenting to an orthopaedist for evaluation of bilateral cavovarus feet, the probability of reaching a diagnosis of Charcot-Marie-Tooth is 78%. The diagnosis requires either an abnormal nerve conduction velocity test or an abnormal electromyogram study.

Charcot-Marie-Tooth disease is the most common inherited disorder of peripheral nerves. Type IA is the most common subtype, accounting for slightly more than 75% of cases in this series from Delaware. The clinical manifestations of the disease may not present until adolescence or adulthood, whereas the laboratory findings are commonly present by as early as 2 years of age. To date there is no clear treatment for Charcot-Marie-Tooth disease, although large doses of ascorbic acid have improved the neuropathy in laboratory animals with the same pathophysiologic processes. DNA testing is possible given the hereditary nature of the disorder. When there is a known family history of Charcot-Marie-Tooth disease, the probability of this disease being the cause of a foot deformity is over 90%.

The authors of this report strongly recommend that all patients with bilateral cavovarus feet be assessed by an orthopaedic surgeon and neurologist, and that appropriate diagnostic tests be performed to rule out Charcot-Marie-Tooth disease. This recommendation clearly makes sense and should be followed.

Let's close this comment with a question having to do with joints. Have you ever heard the term, symphalangism? What does it refer to and how is the problem managed? It was back in 1915 that Harvey Cushing coined the term symphalangism to describe hereditary clinical stiffness of the proximal interphalangeal joint.[1] The diagnosis is currently applied most often to congenital stiffness of the interphalangeal joints and is associated with a variety of structural abnormalities. More often than not, there is a congenitally stiff metacarpophalangeal (MCP) joint of the small finger. Youngsters and adults affected with this problem look like the prototype of the individual who sticks his little finger out while sipping a cup of tea.

Please realize that those affected with symphalangism have a choice. They can leave their little fingers as they are, or if they wish to have a better range of motion of that finger, there is surgery that can be applied to this problem.[2]

J. A. Stockman III, MD

References

1. Cushing H. Hereditary achylosis of proximal phalangeal joints (symphalangism). *Proc Natl Acad Sci USA.* 1915;1:621-622.
2. Tsujii M, Hirata H, Matsumoto M, Asanuma K, Uchida A. Surgical treatment for a congenitally stiff metacarpophalangeal joint of the small finger: report of four cases. *J Hand Surg [Am].* 2006;31:1189-1192.

13 Neurology and Psychiatry

Clinical and MRI Correlates of Cerebral Palsy: The European Cerebral Palsy Study
Bax M, Tydeman C, Flodmark O (Imperial College London; Karolinska Univ Hosp, Stockholm)
JAMA 296:1602-1608, 2006

Context.—Magnetic resonance imaging (MRI) findings have been reported for specific clinical cerebral palsy (CP) subgroups or lesion types but not in a large population of children with all CP subtypes. Further information about the causes of CP could help identify preventive strategies.

Objective.—To investigate the correlates of CP in a population sample and compare clinical findings with information available from MRI brain studies.

Design and Setting.—Cross-sectional, population-based investigative study conducted in 8 European study centers (North West London and North East London, England; Edinburgh, Scotland; Lisbon, Portugal; Dublin, Ireland; Stockholm, Sweden; Tübingen, Germany; and Helsinki, Finland).

Participants.—Five hundred eighty-five children with CP were identified who had been born between 1996 and 1999; 431 children were clinically assessed and 351 had a brain MRI scan.

Main Outcome Measures.—Standardized clinical examination results, parental questionnaire responses, MRI results, and obstetric, genetic, and metabolic data from medical records.

Results.—Important findings include the high rate of infections reported by mothers during pregnancy (n = 158 [39.5%]). In addition, 235 children (54%) were born at term while 47 children (10.9%) were very preterm (<28 weeks). A high rate of twins was found, with 51 children (12%) known to be from a multiple pregnancy. Clinically, 26.2% of children had hemiplegia, 34.4% had diplegia, 18.6% had quadriplegia, 14.4% had dyskinesia, 3.9% had ataxia, and 2.6% had other types of CP. Brain MRI scans showed that white-matter damage of immaturity, including periventricular leukomalacia (PVL), was the most common finding (42.5%), followed by basal ganglia lesions (12.8%), cortical/subcortical lesions (9.4%), malformations (9.1%),

341

focal infarcts (7.4%), and miscellaneous lesions (7.1%). Only 11.7% of these children had normal MRI findings. There were good correlations between the MRI and clinical findings.

Conclusions.—These MRI findings suggest that obstetric mishaps might have occurred in a small proportion of children with CP. A systematic approach to identifying and treating maternal infections needs to be developed. Multiple pregnancies should be monitored closely, and the causes of infant stroke need to be investigated further so preventive strategies can be formulated. All children with CP should have an MRI scan to provide information on the timing and extent of the lesion.

▶ Data from the 14-center National Institute of Child Health and Human Development neonatal network of children born between 1993 and 1998 found CP rates of 19% in survivors born between 22 to 26 weeks of gestation with birth weights of less than 1000 g and 12% for children who survived after delivery at 27 to 32 weeks of gestation and weighed less than 1000 g.[1] Infants at the threshold of viability have also been followed up. These are infants with a mean birth weight of less than 750 g, a gestational age less than 24 completed weeks, and a 10-minute Apgar score of 3 or less. Three quarters of such infants did not survive, but among the survivors, 30% had clear-cut CP, and 50% had cognitive developmental disabilities.

The article by Bax et al is a major advance in our knowledge regarding CP. The study represented a multicenter collaboration that looked at clinical correlates of CP in a population sample and compared clinical findings with information available from MRI. A cross-sectional population involving more than 500 children with CP born between 1996 and 1999 was assembled from 8 major European centers. Four hundred thirty-one children with CP syndrome were clinically assessed with the use of a structured history and a systematic neurodevelopmental evaluation that included topography (ie, diplegia, hemiplegia, and quadriplegia), physiology (ie, spasticity, dyskinesia, dystonia, and ataxia), and neurologic comorbidities involving vision, hearing, and epilepsy. Of these children, 351 had a cranial MRI scanned at age 18 months or later that was systematically reviewed with the use of a consensus protocol and assessed by a single evaluator. Because MRI scans were obtained at 18 months, the completion of the early developmental stages of CNS structural integrity could be linked to the expanded list of neuromotor problems these children manifested. Thus, the study was able to provide some preliminary observations of timing, clinical risk, and functional impact on these children's neurologic development.

So what did the authors find? They observed that in terms of prenatal risk for CP, approximately 1 in 5 mothers of children with CP had a urinary tract infection during pregnancy. This represented a 6-fold increased probability of a urinary tract infection compared with mothers of children without CP. One in 3 of these youngsters was born by cesarean section, and 12% were from a multiple pregnancy. More than half of children with CP were born at term, and just 1 in 5 were born small for gestational age. More than 40% of the children who were born at term were hospitalized in a newborn special care unit for more than 5 days and were regarded as significantly ill. The children characterized as having CP had a 28% probability of having seizures, a 7.2% probability of experiencing hearing impairment, and one third of youngsters with CP had visual impairments including strabismus, restricted visual fields, and refractive errors. Just 10.9% of the children with CP were born at less than 28 weeks' gestation, and 30% were born at either 28 to 31 weeks or 32 to 36 weeks of gestational age.

So what was learned from the MRIs? White matter abnormalities were present in 43% overall and in 71% of children with diplegia, in 34% of children with hemiplegia, and in 35% of children with quadriplegia. Other important findings from neuroimaging included the appearance of basal ganglia abnormalities in 13%, brain malformations in 9.1%, cortical–subcortical abnormalities in 9.4%, and focal infarcts in 7%. Of children with basal ganglia and thalamic injuries, 76% had dystonia. Of children with hemiplegic CP, 27% had focal infarcts. The frequency of malformations was roughly as prevalent as cortical–subcortical damage. Thus, neuroimaging helped in the understanding of the timing and the extent of lesions. About 1 in 8 children with CP had a normal MRI scan.

An excellent editorial by Michael Msall accompanied this article on MRI imaging in children with CP. The editorial puts the findings of the article into perspective and should be read by everyone to understand the potential pathways leading to CP and the possible ways of modifying these pathways to minimize the risk of this devastating neurologic problem. More than three quarters of a million children and adults in the United States have a CP syndrome, and the lifetime medical cost per individual has been estimated at $1 million. This equates to $1.2 billion in direct medical costs for affected children born in 2000 alone. It is clear from the *JAMA* study that, in some respects, we have been on the wrong pathway to understanding the likely causes of CP. In retrospect, disproportionate attention to both severe perinatal hypoxemic–ischemic encephalopathy in term infants and neurodevelopmental complications in extremely premature infants has led to the erroneous perception that these 2 risk groups of children account for the majority of children with CP, when, in fact, they do not. As important as it is to do everything possible to eliminate prematurity, this alone will not wipe CP off the map.

See the Einfeld et al article (Psychopathology in young people with intellectual disability) that reminds us that young people with intellectual disabilities have been found to have levels of psychopathology approximately 3 to 4 times higher than that of typically developing children. This means that the numbers of young people with intellectual disabilities and psychopathology are actually comparable to the prevalence of schizophrenia, a disorder that is the subject of extensive research and that is well-recognized by the medical community, while the link between intellectual disability and psychopathology has been barely studied.

J. A. Stockman III, MD

Reference

1. Vohr BR, Wright LL, Poole WK, McDonald SA. Neurodevelopmental outcomes of extremely low birth weight infants <32 weeks gestation between 1993 and 1998. *Pediatrics*. 2005;116:635-643.

Psychopathology in Young People With Intellectual Disability

Einfeld SL, Piccinin AM, Mackinnon A, et al (Univ of Sydney, Australia; Pennsylvania State Univ, Univ Park; Australian National Univ, Canberra; et al)
JAMA 296:1981-1989, 2006

Context.—Comorbid severe mental health problems complicating intellectual disability are a common and costly public health problem. Although these problems are known to begin in early childhood, little is known of how they evolve over time or whether they continue into adulthood.

Objective.—To study the course of psychopathology in a representative population of children and adolescents with intellectual disability.

Design, Setting, and Participants.—The participants of the Australian Child to Adult Development Study, an epidemiological cohort of 578 children and adolescents recruited in 1991 from health, education, and family agencies that provided services to children with intellectual disability aged 5 to 19.5 years in 6 rural and urban census regions in Australia, were followed up for 14 years with 4 time waves of data collection. Data were obtained from 507 participants, with 84% of wave 1 (1991-1992) participants being followed up at wave 4 (2002-2003).

Main Outcome Measures.—The Developmental Behaviour Checklist (DBC), a validated measure of psychopathology in young people with intellectual disability, completed by parents or other caregivers. Changes over time in the Total Behaviour Problem Score and 5 subscale scores of the DBC scores were modeled using growth curve analysis.

Results.—High initial levels of behavioral and emotional disturbance decreased only slowly over time, remaining high into young adulthood, declining by 1.05 per year on the DBC Total Behaviour Problem Score. Overall severity of psychopathology was similar across mild to severe ranges of intellectual disability (with mean Total Behaviour Problem Scores of approximately 44). Psychopathology decreased more in boys than girls over time (boys starting with scores 2.61 points higher at baseline and ending with scores 2.57 points lower at wave 4), and more so in participants with mild intellectual disability compared with those with severe or profound intellectual disability who diverged from having scores 0.53 points lower at study commencement increasing to a difference of 6.98 points below severely affected children by wave 4. This trend was observed in each of the subscales, except the social-relating disturbance subscale, which increased over time. Prevalence of participants meeting criteria for major psychopathology or definite psychiatric disorder decreased from 41% at wave 1 to 31% at wave 4. Few of the participants (10%) with psychopathology received mental health interventions during the study period.

Conclusion.—These results provide evidence that the problem of psychopathology comorbid with intellectual disability is both substantial and persistent and suggest the need for effective mental health interventions.

▶ It is truly a shame that those already suffering from one disability will develop another, in this case, a psychiatric disorder. As one sees in the data from this report, the problem not only is a common one, but also a serious one. It is well worth everyone's time to read this article in some detail.

Please consider the following scenario pertaining to psychiatry as a career choice. A teen comes in for her annual sports participation examination. She too asks for some career advice. She is thinking about becoming a psychiatrist. She has heard, however, some fairly graphic and dramatic stories about psychiatrists being injured or killed on the job and wants to know if this is a real risk. How would you respond?

Psychiatrists and other mental health professionals tend, quite naturally, to deny the risk of personal injury associated with their work. Serious mental illness is already profoundly stigmatizing, so who wants to add to it as a professional by labeling patients as unpredictable and violent? Mental health professionals are however, much more likely than other professionals to be attacked at work. The latest survey from the United States Department of Justice reported an annual rate of work-related violent crime of 68 per 1000 workers for mental health professionals, compared with just 16 per 1000 for all physicians as a whole, and 12.6 per 1000 for all occupations. Although most afflicted with serious mental illness never commit a single violent act, the lifetime prevalence being 16%, mental health professionals should acknowledge the possibility of rare events and be alert to the factors that increase this risk. One of the most powerful predictors of violence is substance abuse.[1]

J.A. Stockman III, MD

Reference

1. Friedman RA. Violence and mental illness—how strong is the link? *N Engl J Med.* 2006;355:2064-2066.

Brief Maternal Depression Screening at Well-Child Visits
Olson AL, Dietrich AJ, Prazar G, et al (Dartmouth Med School, Lebanon, NH)
Pediatrics 118:207-216, 2006

Objectives.—The goals were (1) to determine the feasibility and yield of maternal depression screening during all well-child visits, (2) to understand how pediatricians and mothers respond to depression screening information, and (3) to assess the time required for discussion of screening results.

Methods.—Implementation of brief depression screening of mothers at well-child visits for children of all ages was studied in 3 rural pediatric practices. Two screening trials introduced screening (1 month) and then determined whether screening could be sustained (6 months). Screening used the 2-question Patient Health Questionnaire. Practices tracked the proportions of visits screened and provided data about the screening process.

Results.—Practices were able to screen in the majority of well-child visits (74% in trial 1 and 67% in trial 2). Of 1398 mothers screened, 17% had 1 of the depressive symptoms and 6% ($n = 88$) scored as being at risk for a major depressive disorder. During discussion, 5.7% of all mothers thought they might be depressed and 4.7% thought they were stressed but not depressed.

Pediatric clinicians intervened with 62.4% of mothers who screened positive and 38.2% of mothers with lesser symptoms. Pediatrician actions included discussion of the impact on the child, a follow-up visit or call, and referral to an adult primary care provider, a mental health clinician, or community supports. Pediatrician time needed to discuss screening results decreased in the second trial. Prolonged discussion time was uncommon (5–10 minutes in 3% of all well-child visits and >10 minutes in 2%).

Conclusions.—Routine, brief, maternal depression screening conducted during well-child visits was feasible and detected mothers who were willing to discuss depression and stress issues with their pediatrician. The discussion after screening revealed additional mothers who felt depressed among those with lesser symptoms. The additional discussion time was usually brief and resulted in specific pediatrician actions.

▶ In recent years, several reports illustrating the important role that primary care physicians play in the diagnosis and treatment of childhood depression have been published. The study of Olson et al shows that we should not be stopping with children and teens. We are in a unique position when we see mothers who are bringing their infants in for well-child visits. Maternal depression is an important problem and a common one. We are capable of screening for this during well-child visits and we should be. Read this report in detail.

J. A. Stockman III, MD

Interventions for Adolescent Depression in Primary Care

Stein REK, Zitner LE, Jensen PS (Albert Einstein College of Medicine, New York; Columbia Univ, New York)
Pediatrics 118:669-682, 2006

Background.—Depression in adolescents is underrecognized and undertreated despite its poor long-term outcomes, including risk for suicide. Primary care settings may be critical venues for the identification of depression, but there is little information about the usefulness of primary care interventions.

Objective.—We sought to examine the evidence for the treatment of depression in primary care settings, focusing on evidence concerning psychosocial, educational, and/or supportive intervention strategies.

Methods.—Available data on brief psychosocial treatments for adolescent depression in primary settings were reviewed. Given the paucity of direct studies, we also drew on related literature to summarize available evidence whether brief, psychosocial support from a member of the primary care team, with or without medication, might improve depression outcomes.

Results.—We identified 37 studies relevant to treating adolescent depression in primary care settings. Only 4 studies directly examined the impact of primary care–delivered psychosocial interventions for adolescent depression, but they suggest that such interventions can be effective. Indirect evidence from other psychosocial/behavioral interventions, including anticipatory guidance and efforts to enhance treatment adherence, and adult depression studies also show benefits of primary care–delivered interventions as well as the impact of provider training to enhance psychosocial skills.

Conclusions.—There is potential for successful treatment of adolescent depression in primary care, in view of evidence that brief, psychosocial support, with or without medication, has been shown to improve a range of outcomes, including adolescent depression itself. Given the great public health problem posed by adolescent depression, the likelihood that most depressed adolescents will not receive specialty services, and new guidelines for managing adolescent depression in primary care, clinicians may usefully consider initiation of supportive interventions in their primary care practices.

▶ Chances are you are going to be seeing many more reports such as this that examine the role of the primary care pediatrician and his or her team in the diagnosis and management of depression among pediatric-age patients, including adolescents. The reason for this is straightforward. There are an insufficient number of child psychiatrists here in the United States to deal with the emotional, psychological, and psychiatric problems of youngsters. Other care providers including primary care pediatricians, nurse clinicians, child psychologists, need to fill in the gap. It is unlikely that the situation with the workforce in child psychiatry will get better any time soon, if ever. The reasons for writing this are many, not the least of which is the unlikely scenario in which reimbursement for the child psychiatrist will improve as opposed to seeking better reimbursement arrangements at the primary care level for the required services.

What we learn from this report is that among the several dozen studies that have examined the ability of the primary care setting to provide effective care to adolescents with depression, there does appear to be a potential for successful treatment within the primary care model. For this to be effective, primary care practitioners will need to improve their skills. Anticipatory guidance will be at the heart of prevention. The primary care physician will be key in changing patient behavior and improving outcomes, especially with respect to adherence to therapeutic regimens for longer term management of ongoing problems.

As the authors of this report state, there is a clear and compelling need for more research to determine the best ways to improve primary care treatment of adolescents with depression. Nonetheless, despite the limited direct evidence for effectiveness of primary care physician's capacity to reduce depressed youths' symptoms with psychological support, the primary care setting has shown itself to be a practical, realistic, and useful setting in which to address a range of child and adolescent health issues. The primary care physician is often well respected by a youngster. Hopefully, there would be a willingness of a teen to "open up" to their primary care provider with all the problems they feel they are experiencing.

Last, when you think about it, children with psychological problems, including depression, merely represent one of many medical conditions that present in the office. A decision has to be made as to how much care can be provided by the primary care physician and what requires referral. We do that all the time when it comes to cardiac, gastrointestinal, endocrine, and other problems. As we know with the latter conditions, the vast majority of times we can care for these conditions without referral. The same should be true for most of the psychological problems that children present. It may require rearranging the way in which we practice, but if we are committed to providing high-quality effective, efficient and timely care, we have to accept the responsibility to do so.

J. A. Stockman III, MD

Depressive Symptoms as a Longitudinal Predictor of Sexual Risk Behaviors Among US Middle and High School Students

Lehrer JA, Shrier LA, Gortmaker S, et al (Univ of California, San Francisco; Harvard Med School, Boston; Harvard School of Public Health, Boston)
Pediatrics 118:189-200, 2006

Objective.—The purpose of this study was to examine whether depressive symptoms are predictive of subsequent sexual risk behavior in a national probability sample of US middle and high school students.

Methods.—Sexually active, unmarried, middle and high school students ($n = 4152$) participated in home interviews in waves I and II of the National Longitudinal Study of Adolescent Health, at an ~1-year interval. Associations between baseline depressive symptoms and sexual risk behaviors over the course of the following year were examined separately for boys and girls, adjusting for demographic variables, religiosity, same-sex attraction/behavior, sexual intercourse before age 10, and baseline sexual risk behavior.

Results.—In adjusted models, boys and girls with high depressive symptom levels at baseline were significantly more likely than those with low symptom levels to report ≥ 1 of the examined sexual risk behaviors over the course of the 1-year follow-up period. For boys, high depressive symptom levels were specifically predictive of condom nonuse at last sex, birth control nonuse at last sex, and substance use at last sex; these results were similar to those of parallel analyses with a continuous depression measure. For girls, moderate depressive symptoms were associated with substance use at last sex, and no significant associations were found between high depressive symptom levels and individual sexual risk behaviors. Parallel analyses with the continuous depression measure found significant associations for condom nonuse at last sex, birth control nonuse at last sex, ≥ 3 sexual partners, and any sexual risk behavior.

Conclusion.—In this study, depressive symptoms predicted sexual risk behavior in a national sample of male and female middle and high school students over a 1-year period.

▶ The Stein et al report (Interventions for adolescent depression in primary care) described how the primary care setting can be used to manage adolescents with depression. What we learn from this report from Boston is that when we care for middle- and high-school students with depression, that depression should be considered a marker for risky sexual behavior. In boys, for example, depressive symptoms can be predictive of noncondom use and substance abuse. Moderate depressive symptom levels seem to be associated with substance use at the time of last sexual activity in girls.

Just why do depressed youths engage in more risky sexual activity? The authors suggest that depressed youths often have impaired social relationships and diminished social support from family members and peers. Youths who are both emotionally distressed and socially isolated may be more apt to be pressured into sexual activity. This may account in part for the associations observed among girls in this study between depressive symptoms and multiple sexual partners, as well as condom and birth control nonuse. Sex in other words, is used to "please or appease" one's partner. Such sex is associated at all ages with less consistent contraception and with unwanted pregnancy.

The authors of this report also suggest another reason why depressed children engage in sexual risky activity. They propose that depressive symptoms may be associated with diminished self-efficacy (ie, confidence in one's ability to undertake a specific action in a given context) regarding factors such as resistance to sexual pressure, safer sex negotiation, mechanics of condom or other birth control use, and refusal of alcohol/other drugs. This leads to an increased likelihood of risky sexual behavior. Condom-related self-efficacy has been found to be an important predictor of youth condom use, and several studies have found self-efficacy is relevant to risky sexual behaviors and is diminished among depressed youths. This includes social self-efficacy and self-efficacy to refuse heavy drinking. In girls in particular, depression is frequently associated with low self-esteem and the need to please. Substance abuse becomes a part of the linkage as substances serve in part as self-medication for emotional distress and leave one vulnerable to engaging in risky sexual activity. Last, many teens with depressive symptoms have overt or subliminal suicidal thinking and risky sexual behavior may represent another form of self-destructive behavior. In other words, the teen sees no problem with risky sexual behavior because there are no consequences of this if they are thinking about committing suicide.

In the old days, articles such as the report of Lehrer et al from Boston would have appeared in the psychiatry or child and adolescent psychiatry literature. Kudos to these authors for publishing their report in a journal that all of us have an opportunity to see. The information provided, as does the information provided in the previous abstract, adds knowledge where knowledge is needed, at the primary care practice level. Learn from these reports and translate that knowledge into practice.

Last, even psychiatry is practiced online and eBay has jumped into the act. In Great Britain, a national health service psychiatrist is hoping to make some extra cash to pay for a Masters degree course. He has opted to try his skill on eBay, the online auction site. For a starting price of just £25, eBay customers can bid to e-mail him five questions on their chosen mental health topic, for which they will receive an online consultation. The psychiatrist has an extensive history with eBay having sold about 400 non-medical items. A search of eBay shows that no one appears to have taken him up on his clinical skills, at least at the time of this writing.[1]

J. A. Stockman III, MD

Reference

1. James A. Psychiatrist sells his skills on eBay. *Guardian.* July 19, 2006. Available at: http://society.guardian.co.uk/health/story/0,,1823202,00.html. Accessed July 21, 2007.

Self-injurious Behaviors in a College Population
Whitlock J, Eckenrode J, Silverman D (Cornell Univ, New York; Princeton Univ, NJ)
Pediatrics 117:1939-1948, 2006

Objective.—The goal was to assess the prevalence, forms, demographic and mental health correlates of self-injurious behaviors in a representative college sample.

Methods.—A random sample of undergraduate and graduate students at 2 northeastern US universities were invited to participate in an Internet-based survey in the spring of 2005. Thirty-seven percent of the 8300 invited participants responded.

Results.—The lifetime prevalence rate of having ≥1 self-injurious behavior incident was 17.0%. Seventy-five percent of those students engaged in self-injurious behaviors more than once. Thirty-six percent reported that no one knew about their self-injurious behaviors and only 3.29% indicated that a physician knew. Compared with non-self-injurers, those with repeat self-injurious behavior incidents were more likely to be female, bisexual or questioning their sexual orientation. They were less likely to be Asian/Asian American and >24 years of age. When controlling for demographic characteristics, those with repeat self-injurious behavior incidents were more likely to report a history of emotional abuse or sexual abuse, ever having considered or attempted suicide, elevated levels of psychological distress, and ≥1 characteristic of an eating disorder. A dose-response gradient was evident in each of these areas when single-incident self-injurious behaviors were compared with repeat-incident self-injurious behaviors.

Conclusions.—A substantial number of college students reported self-injurious behaviors in their lifetimes. Many of the behaviors occurred among individuals who had never been in therapy for any reason and who only rarely disclosed their self-injurious behaviors to anyone. Single self-injurious behavior incidents were correlated with a history of abuse and co-morbid adverse health conditions but less strongly than were repeat self-injurious behavior incidents. The reticence of these clients to seek help or advice renders it critical that medical and mental health providers find effective strategies for detecting and addressing self-injurious behaviors.

▶ The results of this report are astounding. It finds that the likelihood of a college-age student having inflicted harm to his or her body at some point during the college experience runs almost 20%. Although they are sometimes assumed to be a form of suicidal behavior, self-injurious behaviors, by definition, involve acts that occur without suicidal intent. The guru of this topic is Armando Favazza,[1] a child psychiatrist from Columbia, MO. In his characterization of self-injurious behaviors reflecting an impulse disorder known as the "deliberate self-harm syndrome," Favazza has identified 4 major forms of nonsocially sanctioned self-injurious behavior: major, stereotypic, compulsive, and impulsive. Although the first 3 categories are associated primarily with clinical populations, characteristics of both compulsive and impulsive self-injurious behaviors may be increasingly evident in the nonclinical populations as well. Such behaviors in clinical populations peak in middle to late adolescence. Most are associated with the term "cutting," but they actually encompass a wide variety of behaviors including but not limited to carving or cutting skin and subdermal tissue, scratching, burning, ripping or pulling skin or hair, swallowing toxic substances, bruising, and breaking bones. Individuals in clinical populations who engage in self-injurious behavior are more likely to engage in suicide-related behaviors. In this report we see that significantly more female subjects than male subjects engage in self-injurious behaviors, but these gender effects apply only to repeat incidence and are not all that strong to begin with.

Read this report in detail if you are dealing with college-age students. Read the report if you are taking care of high schoolers, because the problem frequently begins during this period of life. Currently, rates of detection of self-injurious behavior are remarkably low. A careful skin examination is likely to be the marker of the problem.

Now, here is a question related to stress-induced psychiatric difficulties. What is the origin of the term "shell shock" and how many cases are estimated to have occurred during times of war? By way of background, on October 31, 1914, a 20-year-old private soldier from Great Britain had been "rather enjoying" his day of trench warfare in northern France and had not been at all afraid of being in battle. But then German shells exploded around him and one in particular was "like a punch on the head, without any pain after it." This was the first case of shell shock to be reported.[2] This description appears to confirm one contemporaneous view that air compression from a shell or its explosion could cause various physical and mental symptoms. The initial findings, as reported in the medical literature, went against the notion that shell shock was a coverup for malingering as confirmed in a later article.[3] It soon became clear that what army doctors were seeing in World War I was not unique to soldiers coming under shellfire or unique to that conflict. "Shell shock," however, is the term that has stuck now for almost a century. Each war seems to have its own version of the problem.[4]

During World War I, summary court marshall for battlefield offenses including desertion and cowardliness commonly carried the death penalty, and was executed on the field. The estimates of the number of shell shock cases diagnosed in World War I vary from some 80,000 to 200,000, and many of these cases were given a death sentence, although this sentence was infrequently carried out. Recent data suggest that on 306 occasions, British soldiers were executed for cowardliness presumably relating to shell shock during World War I. Records also indicate that in World War I, the French and Italians had more military executions than the British. German soldiers rarely met this fate even though their stresses were likely to have been as severe. This British to German comparison calls into question the need for British commanders to have exercised their power to shoot men for offenses that would not have carried the death penalty in peacetime. By World War II, military executions of this type were banned.[5]

J. A. Stockman III, MD

References

1. Favazza AR. *Bodies under Siege: Self-mutilation and Body Modification in Culture and Psychiatry.* 2nd ed. Baltimore: Johns Hopkins University Press; 1996.
2. Myers CS. A contribution to the study of shell shock. *Lancet.* 1915;1:316-320.
3. Myers CS. Contributions to the study of shell shock. *Lancet.* 1916;1:65-69.
4. Jones E, Wessely S. *Shellshock to PTSD: Military Psychiatry from 1900 to the Gulf War.* London: Psychology Press; 2005.
5. Sharp D. Shocked, shot, and pardoned. *Lancet.* 2006;368:975-976.

Incidence, cause, and short-term outcome of convulsive status epilepticus in childhood: prospective population-based study

Chin RFM, for the NLSTEPSS Collaborative Group (Univ College London)
Lancet 368:222-229, 2006

Background.—Convulsive status epilepticus is the most common childhood medical neurological emergency, and is associated with significant morbidity and mortality. Most data for this disorder are from mainly adult populations and might not be relevant to childhood. Thus we undertook the North London Status Epilepticus in Childhood Surveillance Study (NLSTEPSS): a prospective, population-based study of convulsive status epilepticus in childhood, to obtain a uniquely paediatric perspective.

Methods.—Clinical and demographic data for episodes of childhood convulsive status epilepticus that took place in north London were obtained through a clinical network that covered the target population. We obtained these data from anonymised copies of a standardised admission proforma; accident and emergency, nursing, ambulance, and intensive-care unit notes; and interviews with parents, medical, nursing, and paramedic staff. We investigated ascertainment using capture-recapture modelling.

Findings.—Of 226 children enrolled, 176 had a first ever episode of convulsive status epilepticus. We estimated that ascertainment was between 62% and 84%. The ascertainment-adjusted incidence was between 17 and 23 episodes per 100,000 per year. 98 (56%, 95% CI 48–63) children were neurologically healthy before their first ever episode and 56 (57%, 47–66) of those children had a prolonged febrile seizure. 11 (12%, 6–18) of children with first ever febrile convulsive status epilepticus had acute bacterial meningitis. Conservative estimation of 1-year recurrence of convulsive status epilepticus was 16% (10–24%). Case fatality was 3% (2–7%).

Interpretation.—Convulsive status epilepticus in childhood is more common, has a different range of causes, and a lower risk of death than that in adults. These paediatric data will help inform management of convulsive status epilepticus and appropriate allocation of resources to reduce the effects of this disorder in childhood.

▶ None of us needs to be reminded that status epilepticus is a major medical emergency, one associated with significant morbidity and mortality. This is true despite major treatment advances. Most neurologists believe that status epilepticus in children does not differ significantly from that in adults, but this notion may be wrong. Data for adults are not necessarily directly applicable to children, and this is the importance of the study from London. Between 2002 and 2004, a total of 226 children living in northern London and aged 29 days to 15 years with status epilepticus were enrolled in this study. Of these, 176 had their first ever episode. The researchers define the disorder as tonic, clonic, or tonic-clonic seizure, two or more such attacks between which consciousness is not regained, and which last at least 30 minutes. The incidence of status epilepticus in this series was between 17 and 23 episodes per 100,000 children per year.

What we learn from the British study is that the causes of status epilepticus include 7 classes: (1) prolonged febrile seizures (32%); (2) acute symptomatic events such as meningitis (17%); (3) remote symptomatic events (pre-existing CNS abnormality in the absence of an acute insult) (16%); (4) acute on top of a remote symptomatic event (pre-existing CNS abnormality, including epilepsy, and an acute insult or febrile seizure) (16%); (5) idiopathic epilepsy (10%); (6) cryptogenic epilepsy related (2%); and (7) unclassified (7%). In the British series, half of the patients had episodes lasting more than 1 hour, which is known to be associated with significant morbidity and mortality. A small but real proportion (16%) of children with first ever episode of status epilepticus will have a recurrence within a year. The disorder is different from adult status epilepticus in that prolonged febrile seizure is the single most common cause and there is a high rate of bacterial meningitis as an etiology in comparison to adults.

While on things neurologic, what is the latest in the use of EEG devices in the legal system? On April 21, 2006, Willie Brown, Jr., was executed by lethal injection in North Carolina for the 1983 killing of a convenient-store clerk. The execution might have received little attention if not for the fact that Brown's electroencephalogram (EEG) was monitored during the procedure. This apparently unprecedented monitoring was a response to the concern that some inmates have not been properly anesthetized during executions by lethal injection and may therefore have experienced painful deaths that violated the constitutional ban on cruel and unusual punishment.[1]

The EEG device used during Brown's execution was a bispectral index (BIS) monitor made by Aspect Medical Systems of Newton, Massachusetts. This monitor works by means of a proprietary algorithm that converts the raw EEG, which is difficult to interpret in real time, into an index of hypnotic level. The compact device is used in operating rooms and intensive care units as an adjunct to other methods for monitoring the effectiveness of anesthetics and sedatives. The instrument, depending on the model, costs between $5000 and $8500. The BIS is a relatively new technology, one likely to be seen put to greater use within the legal system. Corrections officials, under pressure to prove that their execution methods are humane, are increasingly relying on medical expertise and technology. The idea is to avoid the need for medical personnel involvement because the American Medical Association, the American Society of Anesthesiologists, and others in the medical community consider any physician involvement in executions unethical. The BIS device records the EEG and converts it into a single number, ranging from zero for a flat-line, or isoelectric, tracing to 100, which is typical for a person who is awake. The target range for a patient under general anesthesia is a value of 40 to 60. During an execution by means of lethal injection, three agents are usually given: first the anesthetic sodium thiopental, then the paralytic pancuronium bromide, and finally a fatal dose of potassium chloride. The concept behind monitoring is to confirm that the sodium thiopental has rendered the inmate sufficiently unconscious so that he or she will be unaware of the subsequent injections or their effects. The supposition is that, if necessary, someone other than an anesthesiologist or other physician could rely on the BIS monitor to assess a prisoner's level of consciousness and help to insure that an execution meets constitutional standards. Unfortunately, there is no way to be certain that an executed prisoner is unaware and the concept of a humane execution would therefore be considered an oxymoron. Monitor readings may be inaccurate, particularly if the EEG signal is contaminated by artifacts, a common phenomenon.

The manufacturers of BIS have clearly stated that the use of a BIS monitor as part of an execution procedure is inconsistent with its intended use in healthcare facilities. Aspect Medical Systems will not sell a monitor for this purpose if it knows how the monitor is intended to be used. When North Carolina purchased the monitor, it gave no clear indication of its use. On April 11, 2006, a North Carolina corrections official called Aspect's toll-free sales number to purchase a monitor, which was shipped out the same day. A subsequent written purchase-order request sent from North Carolina stated, "This equipment is used to monitor vital signs and sedation scales of patients recovering from surgery."[2]. The manufacturer of the BIS device now requires that, for sales to penitentiaries, an authorized and responsible person employed by the facility must sign and date a statement assuring that sensors and monitors "will not be used on an individual or individuals during or as part of a lethal injection execution procedure."

In 2005, the United States ranked fourth in the world in numbers of executions, behind only China, Iran, and Saudi Arabia. The number of United States executions peaked at 98 in 1999. In 2005, there were 60. As of May 24, 2006, there were 20, all performed by lethal injection, according to the Death Penalty Information Center. By the way, if prison officials are denied access to bispectral index EEG monitors by the manufacturer, all they need to do is look on eBay. There are approximately 34,000 such monitors in circulation throughout the world and many are now being resold. In May 2006, one could easily find one on eBay selling for a high bid of $1,250 . . . going, going, gone.

J. A. Stockman III, MD

References

1. Koniaris LG, Zimmers TA, Lubarsky DA, Sheldon JP. Inadequate anesthesia in lethal injection for execution. *Lancet.* 2005;365:1412-1414.
2. Steinbrook R. New technology, old dilemma—monitoring EEG activity during executions. *N Engl J Med.* 2006;354:2525-2527.

Psychostimulant and other effects of caffeine in 9- to 11-year-old children
Heatherley SV, Hancock KMF, Rogers PJ (Univ of Bristol, England)
J Child Psychol Psychiatry 47:135-142, 2006

Background.—Recent research on adults suggests that 'beneficial' psychostimulant effects of caffeine are found only in the context of caffeine deprivation; that is, caffeine improves psychomotor and cognitive performance in habitual caffeine consumers following caffeine withdrawal. Furthermore, no net benefit is gained because performance is merely restored to 'baseline' levels. The effects of caffeine in children is an under-researched area, with only a handful of studies being carried out in the US where children's consumption of caffeine appears to be lower on average than in the UK.

Method.—Twenty-six children aged between 9 and 11 years completed a double-blind, placebo-controlled study. Habitual caffeine consumers (mean daily caffeine intake = 109 mg) and non/low-consumers (12 mg) were tested on two separate days following overnight caffeine abstinence. On each day measures of cognitive performance (a number search task), and self-rated mood and physical symptoms, including alertness and headache, were taken before and after administration of 50 mg of caffeine, or placebo.

Results.—At baseline (before treatment), the habitual consumers showed poorer performance on the cognitive test than did the non/low-consumers, although no significant differences in mood or physical symptoms were found between the two groups. There were significant habit by treatment (caffeine vs. placebo) interactions for accuracy of performance and headache, and a significant main effect of treatment for alertness. Post hoc comparisons showed that caffeine administration improved the consumers' accuracy on the cognitive test (to near the level displayed by the non/low-consumers at baseline), but that it had no significant effect on the non/low-consumers' performance. In the consumers, caffeine prevented an increase in headache that occurred after placebo, and it increased alertness relative to placebo. Again, however, caffeine did not significantly affect levels of headache or alertness in the non/low-consumers.

Conclusions.—These results suggest that, like adults, children probably derive little or no benefit from habitual caffeine intake, although negative symptoms associated with overnight caffeine withdrawal are avoided or rapidly reversed by subsequent caffeine consumption.

▶ Most of us do not realize it, but caffeine is the most frequently consumed drug in the world. It is also the only psychoactive drug that is legally available to children. Tea and coffee continue to account for more than 90% of the caffeine consumed worldwide. Most of the remaining caffeine is consumed via cola beverages, and these represent a larger source of caffeine that is consumed by children. Despite the ubiquitous availability of caffeine, data on the effects of caffeine on behavior, cognition, and psychomotor performance in children are virtually nonexistent as compared with the abundant data regarding this topic in adults. For these reasons, it is unclear whether the effects of caffeine observed in adults can be applied to regular or infrequent caffeine users of a much younger age. In adults, single high jolts of caffeine tend to produce negative symptoms such as anxiety and jitteriness, but moderate doses of caffeine (1 mg/kg to 3 mg/kg) have psychostimulant effects, as evidenced by a quickening of reaction time, enhanced vigilance, an increase in self-rated alertness, and improved mood. Some question these latter benefits as being more apparent than real, because it is possible that they are largely or entirely the result of "withdrawal reversal." The withdrawal reversal hypothesis proposes that caffeine does not provide net benefits for mood and performance but rather that it merely reverses the negative effects of acute caffeine withdrawal. This means that, after an overnight caffeine abstinence, caffeine consumed at breakfast merely restores performance and mood to baseline levels that would have been achieved if the individual had not previously consumed caffeine. The worry is that caffeine consumption in children might tend to put children at particular risk of experiencing the negative effects of intermittent episodes of caffeine withdrawal. The fact that some of the consequences of caffeine withdrawal, such as headache and irritability, are common in children may mean that caffeine withdrawal will exacerbate these negative symptoms.

To sort out some of these findings as they might apply to children, the authors of this report looked at 26 children between the ages of 9 and 11 years; some of these children were habitual consumers of caffeine, and some were not. It was observed that caffeine improved performance and reduced headache in the participants who were regular consumers of caffeine who had overnight caffeine abstinence but that it did not do so in participants who usually consumed little or no caffeine. In other words, caffeine only significantly affected alertness in those who were habitual users of it. These findings support the withdrawal reversal hypothesis, which suggests that caffeine merely restores performance that is degraded by withdrawal rather than providing a net benefit for the consumer. This, together with the facts that caffeine has no nutritive value and that it possibly has other negative effects, makes a case for restricting the consumption of caffeine by children.

This editor is no longer an adolescent (at least according to age criteria) and, therefore, will continue to enjoy his addiction to Starbucks' Frappuccino®, a "lowfat, creamy blend of Starbucks' coffee and milk" that contains just 180 calories and just 15 mg of cholesterol per 9.5-fluid-ounce serving. The amount of caffeine contained in this product is not stated on the label, and it would not matter if it were.

J. A. Stockman III, MD

Long-term atomoxetine treatment in adolescents with attention-deficit/hyperactivity disorder

Wilens TE, Newcorn JH, Kratochvil CJ, et al (Massachusetts Gen Hosp, Boston; Mount Sinai Med Ctr, New York; Univ of Nebraska, Omaha; et al)
J Pediatr 149:112-119, 2006

Objective.—To determine the efficacy and safety of atomoxetine in adolescent subjects treated for attention-deficit/hyperactivity disorder (ADHD) for up to 2 years.

Study Design.—Data from 13 atomoxetine studies (6 double-blind, 7 open-label) were pooled for subjects age 12 to 18 with ADHD as defined by the American Psychiatric Association's *Diagnostic and Statistical Manual of Mental Disorders IV*.

Results.—Of the 601 atomoxetine-treated subjects in this meta-analysis, 537 (89.4%) completed 3 months of acute treatment. A total of 259 subjects (48.4%) are continuing atomoxetine treatment; 219 of these subjects have completed at least 2 years of treatment. The mean dose of atomoxetine at endpoint was 1.41 mg/kg/day. Mean ADHD Rating Scale IV, parent version, investigator-administered and -scored total scores showed significant improvement ($P < .001$) over the first 3 months. Symptoms remained improved up to 24 months without dosage escalation. During the 2-year treatment period, 99 (16.5%) subjects discontinued treatment due to lack of effectiveness, and 31 (5.2%) subjects discontinued treatment due to adverse events. No clinically significant abnormalities in height, weight, blood pressure, pulse, mean laboratory values, or electrocardiography parameters were found.

Conclusions.—Two-year data from this ongoing study indicate that atomoxetine maintains efficacy among adolescents with ADHD, with no evidence of drug tolerance and no new or unexpected safety concerns.

▶ It has been only relatively recently that atomoxetine was approved by the US Food and Drug Administration for treating ADHD in youth and adults. This is a nonstimulant medication that has great appeal for use in adolescents given its once-daily administration, limited abuse potential, and long duration of action. Long-acting agents are of particular importance for adolescents compared with younger children since adolescents have more independence, extracurricular activities, homework, work and socializing opportunities, and driving responsibilities in many cases. Atomoxetine is efficacious for the long-term treatment of adolescent subjects with ADHD. Treatment improvement occurs within the first 12 weeks of therapy and is durable for at least 2 years in this report. There appear to be no new or unexpected safety concerns emerging during long-term therapy. There is no indication that growth rate deficits seen in these adolescents treated for up to 2 years would be permanent. Parents should be advised that some decrease in growth rate may be expected during the first few months of their child's treatment, but that this does not appear to be clinically significant after 2 years of continued treatment. There is no incidence of clinically significant liver dysfunction, but some have warned of at least two cases of idiosyncratic hepatic injury related to atomoxetine among 2.4 million patient exposures.

See the other 2006 Willens et al report (Do children and adolescents with ADHD respond differently to atomoxetine?) that tells us whether or not children respond differently to atomoxetine.

J. A. Stockman III, MD

Do Children and Adolescents With ADHD Respond Differently to Atomoxetine?

Wilens TE, Kratochvil C, Newcorn JH, et al (Massachusetts Gen Hosp, Boston; Nebraska Med Ctr, Omaha; Mount Sinai Med Ctr, New York; et al)
J Am Acad Child Adolesc Psychiatry 45:149-157, 2006

Objective.—Controversy exists over changes in tolerability and response to medications across the life span. Here the authors report data contrasting the efficacy and tolerability of atomoxetine between children and adolescents with attention-deficit/hyperactivity disorder (ADHD).

Method.—Data were analyzed for children ages 6–11 (510 atomoxetine, 341 placebo) and adolescents ages 12–17 (107 atomoxetine, 69 placebo) with *DSM-IV*–defined ADHD enrolled in similarly designed, double-blind, placebo-controlled trials. Efficacy measures included response rates, times to response, and mean changes from baseline to endpoint in the ADHD Rating Scale, Conners' Parent Rating Scale, and Clinical Global Impressions.

Results.—Adolescents had lower baseline ADHD scores compared with children. There were no statistically significant differences in the overall effects on ADHD symptoms, response rates, or time to response between age groups. Children, but not adolescents, had higher rates of somnolence and headache relative to placebo. No other clinically meaningful treatment differences were seen in adverse event rates, vital signs, weight, height, laboratory values, or ECG between children and adolescents.

Conclusions.—Acute atomoxetine treatment appears to be equally effective and tolerated in children and adolescents. These findings suggest that pharmacological differences in tolerability or ADHD symptom response are negligible between children and adolescents.

▶ The data from this report and the other 2006 Willens et al report (Long-term atomoxetine treatment in adolescents with attention-deficit/hyperactivity disorder) say it all when it comes to atomoxetine and its role in the management of children with ADHD, so we will shift gears and talk about some research that is currently going on in the field of neurology. Back in 2002, Paul Allen, co-founder of Microsoft, asked the question, "What is the one thing that will make the biggest difference in brain science?" The experts he was dialoging with decided that a gene expression map of the mouse brain would be of most help, and within four years, that is exactly what the science community received, all due to the philanthropy of Mr. Allen. In September 2006, the Allen Institute for Brain Science announced that it had built a three-dimensional map of the mouse brain that shows with pinpoint accuracy, where each of the mouse's 21,000 genes are expressed, a truly remarkable achievement. The atlas is made up of 85 million images of the mouse brain and contains more than 600 terabytes of information. Importantly, the atlas is freely accessible to anyone with an Internet connection and will save future researchers many hours of work and funding agencies million upon millions of dollars. Indeed, the atlas is already delivering results. A major finding to come out of the atlas is that around 80% of the mouse genome is expressed in the brain, much more than was previously thought. Very few genes are expressed in just one area and most have a broad expression profile. This is bad news because it suggests that it will be difficult to target genes or proteins therapeutically without causing some side effects. The Allen Institute now plans to collaborate with other researchers to compare healthy mouse brains with tissue from murine models of human disease. The institute will shift its focus to research on humans very shortly.[1]

J.A. Stockman III, MD

Reference

1. Butcher J. On reflection: Paul Allen 1, Bill Gates 0. *Lancet.* 2006;368:1413.

Variant Creutzfeldt-Jakob disease: prion protein genotype analysis of positive appendix tissue samples from a retrospective prevalence study
Ironside JW, Bishop MT, Connolly K, et al (Univ of Edinburgh, UK; Derriford Hosp, Plymouth, UK)
BMJ 332:1186-1188, 2006

Objective.—To perform prion protein gene (*PRNP*) codon 129 analysis in DNA extracted from appendix tissue samples that had tested positive for disease associated prion protein.

Design.—Reanalysis of positive cases identified in a retrospective anonymised unlinked prevalence study of variant Creutzfeldt-Jakob disease (vCJD) in the United Kingdom.

Study Samples.—Three positive appendix tissue samples out of 12,674 samples of appendix and tonsil tested for disease associated prion protein. The patients from whom these samples were obtained were aged 20-29 years at the time of surgery, which took place in 1996-9.

Setting.—Pathology departments in two tertiary centres in England and Scotland.

Results.—Adequate DNA was available for analysis in two of the three specimens, both of which were homozygous for valine at codon 129 in the *PRNP*.

Conclusions.—This is the first indication that the valine homozygous subgroup at codon 129 in the *PRNP* is susceptible to vCJD infection. All tested clinical cases of vCJD have so far occurred in the methionine homozygous subgroup, and a single case of probable iatrogenic vCJD infection has been identified in one patient who was a methionine/valine heterozygote at this genetic locus. People infected with vCJD with a valine homozygous codon 129 *PRNP* genotype may have a prolonged incubation period, during which horizontal spread of the infection could occur either from blood donations or from contaminated surgical instruments used on these individuals during the asymptomatic phase of the illness.

▶ This report does not focus on children, but does include young adults aged 20 to 29 years. Thus, there is a lot to be learned here by pediatric care providers about the potential risk of developing Creutzfeldt-Jakob disease. The report specifically deals with vCJD, an entity that was first described in the United Kingdom just a little over a decade ago.[1] By the mid part of this decade, more than 160 definite or highly probable cases of the disorder have been described in the United Kingdom. The study abstracted suggests that a larger epidemic may very well be brewing. The study reports a genotype analysis that has identified the presence of the homozygous valine genotype in samples of appendix tissue taken at the time of surgery in otherwise healthy young adults. The implication of this finding of most concern is that it raises the possibility that ongoing iatrogenic transmission of vCJD may prove to be the breeding ground for an epidemic of the disorder.

The concern with vCJD is that unlike the classic disease, it can be transmitted from human to human as described through its transmission via blood transfusion. Given the long incubation periods (up to 30 years) that have been described in cases of iatrogenic transmission of the classic disease, it is reasonable to consider that there are people in an extended preclinical stage of vCJD during which their tissue, in particular their blood, may pose an infectious risk to others.

Right now, Great Britain is the hotbed of both classic and vCJD. There, people should have some concern about receiving blood from another Brit, particularly in light of the new information provided by this report. There is no easy way to prevent transmission by blood transfusion. The ideal solution would be to develop a test that would identify people with presymptomatic vCJD. Unfortunately this would pose difficult ethical questions such as whether positive individuals should be informed that they have a condition which may or may not develop into a serious disease and for which there is absolutely no current treatment.

Studies such as the one by Ironside et al are key to the continuing effort to control the extent of the epidemic of vCJD overseas and highlight the urgent need for ongoing surveillance for the spread of this prion-related disorder. The "pond" that separates us from Great Britain is not a large one given international air travel.

J. A. Stockman III, MD

Reference

1. Will RG, Ironside JW, Zeidler M, et al. A new variant of Creutzfeldt-Jakob disease in the UK. *Lancet.* 1996;347:921-925.

Clinical presentation and pre-mortem diagnosis of variant Creutzfeldt-Jakob disease associated with blood transfusion: a case report
Wroe SJ, Pal S, Siddique D, et al (Natl Hosp for Neurology and Neurosurgery, London; Univ College London; Natl Blood Service, London)
Lancet 368:2061-2067, 2006

Background.—Concerns have been raised that variant Creutzfeldt-Jakob disease (vCJD) might be transmissible by blood transfusion. Two cases of prion infection in a group of known recipients of transfusion from donors who subsequently developed vCJD were identified post-mortem and reported in 2004. Another patient from this at-risk group developed neurological signs and was referred to the National Prion Clinic.

Methods.—The patient was admitted for investigation and details of blood transfusion history were obtained from the National Blood Service and Health Protection Agency; after diagnosis of vCJD, the patient was enrolled into the MRC PRION-1 trial. When the patient died, brain and tonsil tissue were obtained at autopsy and assessed for the presence of disease-related PrP by immunoblotting and immunohistochemistry.

Findings.—A clinical diagnosis of probable vCJD was made; tonsil biopsy was not done. The patient received experimental therapy with quinacrine, but deteriorated and died after a clinical course typical of vCJD. Autopsy confirmed the diagnosis and showed prion infection of the tonsils.

Interpretation.—This case of transfusion-associated vCJD infection, identified ante-mortem, is the third instance from a group of 23 known recipients who survived at least 5 years after receiving a transfusion from donors who subsequently developed vCJD. The risk to the remaining recipients of such transfusions is probably high, and these patients should be offered specialist follow-up and investigation. Tonsil biopsy will allow early and pre-symptomatic diagnosis in other iatrogenically exposed individuals at high risk, as in those with primary infection with bovine spongiform encephalopathy prions.

▶ In 2004, prion infections were identified after the deaths of 2 patients who had received blood components from donors who subsequently developed vCJD. A third patient has developed neurologic signs of the disease. The report of Wroe et al confirms a prion infection in a patient before he died, 8 years and 8 months after being given a contaminated transfusion. The inefficiency of oral transmission and the species barrier between cows and human beings have been credited with protection of human populations from a larger disease outbreak of vCJD. Nonetheless, there is evidence to suggest that the within-species transmission of the prion through transfusion is efficient and, unmanaged, could pose a serious risk of propagating the vCJD epidemic in humans.

In Great Britain, epidemiology services have been following up 66 recipients of blood products from donors who subsequently developed vCJD. Some 34 of these individuals died within 5 years of transfusion, and their deaths are not attributed to exposure because the incubation period is probably longer than 5 years. Of the 32 other recipients, 24 are alive and are at risk of developing vCJD. Of the 8 who have died, 3 were prion infected, and 2 of these developed the disease. These numbers suggest that a transfusion risk is more than remote. The potential efficacy of transmission by transfusion further increases when one notes that the recipient susceptible to developing clinical vCJD might only consist of those with the *MM* genotype in the prion protein gene.

The transfusion world is very concerned about a potential blood transfusion epidemic of vCJD based on the 3 cases that have been described. Carriers of the disease who are in their preclinical stage tend to be young adults, the very population that donates blood. There is no effective test to detect an affected donor. A recent United Kingdom policy has been put into place that refuses donations of blood from individuals who have previously received a transfusion, a policy that reduces the number of eligible blood donors by about 5% to 10%. This policy effectively prevents transfusion from propagating the vCJD epidemic. Other countries are now reassessing their policies to determine whether blood donations would be accepted from anyone who has previously received a unit or more of blood.

The punch line is clear that transmission of vCJD by transfusion is possible, and propagation of the epidemic is becoming increasingly apparent. Recognize also that animal species other than cows are developing prion-associated disease. Blood and saliva of deer with chronic wasting disease do carry infectious prions that can be easily transmitted to other deer.[1] The findings indicate that particular care should be taken when handling bodily fluids from prion-infected animals. Prion diseases, also called transmissible spongiform encephalopathies, include scrapie in sheep, bovine spongiform encephalopathy in cows, and CJD in humans. Whether chronic wasting disease is transmissible to humans, as has been shown for bovine spongiform encephalopathy, is unknown.

J. A. Stockman III, MD

Reference

1. Mathiason CK, Powers JG, Dahmes SJ, et al. Infectious prions in the saliva and blood of deer with chronic wasting disease. *Science.* 2006;314:133-136.

Symptomatic Children With Hereditary Hemorrhagic Telangiectasia: A Pediatric Center Experience

Mei-Zahav M, Letarte M, Faughman ME, et al (Univ of Toronto)
Arch Pediatr Adolesc Med 160:596-601, 2006

Objective.—To assess the clinical and genetic characteristics of symptomatic children with hereditary hemorrhagic telangiectasia (HHT).
Design.—Cross-sectional study.
Setting.—The HHT clinics in Toronto.
Participants.—All children with symptomatic HHT treated from April 1, 1996, through December 31, 2002.
Interventions.—Participants were screened for visceral arteriovenous malformations (AVMs). Molecular testing was performed in the children or their affected family members.
Main Outcome Measures.—Prevalence of epistaxis, telangiectases, pulmonary and cerebral AVMs, and genetic characteristics.
Results.—Fourteen children presented with manifestations of HHT. Seven had cardiorespiratory symptoms related to pulmonary AVMs. Three had neurological symptoms secondary to bleeding from spinal or cerebral AVMs. Two were referred because of skin telangiectases and 2, because of multiple episodes of epistaxis. Screening results revealed a cerebral AVM in 1 of 11 neurologically asymptomatic children. Of the children without respiratory symptoms, 1 was diagnosed as having definite and 1, suspected pulmonary AVMs. Four children with pulmonary AVMs carried an endoglin gene mutation (HHT type 1), and 1 carried an activin receptor–like kinase 1 gene mutation (HHT type 2). The 2 children with spinal AVMs belong to the same HHT type 2 family. No mutation was found in 1 child with pulmonary and 1 with cerebral AVMs.
Conclusions.—Visceral AVMs and mucosal telangiectases are present in children with HHT and can lead to life-threatening events. Failure to identify a disease-associated mutation for each child suggests complex mutations or novel HHT genes.

▶ When this editor was in medical school, the eponym Rendu-Osler-Weber syndrome was applied to the disorder that now is more commonly called HHT. We used to think this was a rare autosomal-dominant disorder, but most data now suggest that it has a prevalence of 1:5000 to 1:10,000 making it uncommon, but not rare. Patients with HHT usually manifest the disease by having mucocutaneous telangiectatic lesions, resulting in epistaxis in more than 90% of cases and GI bleeding in one fifth to one third of cases. In addition to this, AVMs may be found in the lungs, brain and liver.

Most of the information we have about HHT comes from detailed studies of adults with the disorder. There are very few large-scale reports of children with this entity because most diagnoses are not made until young adulthood or mid-adulthood. This series of 14 children therefore does constitute one of the largest reports of pediatric cases of HHT. Epistaxis appears to be one of the most common presentations, appearing as early as 4 years of age. The visceral

AVMs turn out to be a rare presentation in children, although if one looks for them as these authors did, one will find a cerebral AVM in about 10% of neurologically asymptomatic children. The same is true of pulmonary AVMs.

If you are uncertain about the diagnosis of HHT in a child presenting with epistaxis and who may have a positive family history, you can confirm the diagnosis by genetic analysis. You will need help from a geneticist, however, because the genetic molecular patterns of this disease tend to vary within families.

We should be grateful to the authors of this report for they tell us a great deal about HHT in the child. It is usually a heterogeneous disease. Pulmonary and cerebral AVMs can occur and can possibly lead to life-threatening complications, often as the first presentation of the disorder. Screening for visceral AVMs in asymptomatic children with a positive family history seems reasonable if for no other reason than to further elucidate the prevalence of these problems and to determine whether screening can prevent serious complications.

See the Crawford et al report (Survival probability in ataxia telangiectasia) that addresses the survival probability of those diagnosed with HHT. You will learn that the median survival in 2 large cohorts of patients with this disease, one prospective and one retrospective, is 25 and 19 years. Survival past 30 years of age seems to be quite infrequent.

J. A. Stockman III, MD

Survival probability in ataxia telangiectasia
Crawford TO, Skolasky RL, Fernandez R, et al (Johns Hopkins Hosp, Baltimore, Md; Ataxia Telangiectasia Children's Project, Deerfield Beach, Fla)
Arch Dis Child 91:610-611, 2006

Background.—Ataxia telangiectasia is a rare, multiorgan neurodegenerative disorder. Children and adults with this disease are at an increased risk of death because of lymphoreticular malignancies, infections of the respiratory system, and various rare complications. It has not been possible, with the exception of 1 large survey, to obtain a reasonable assessment of life span because ataxia telangiectasia is uncommon. However, a retrospective study conducted by the Ataxia Telangiectasia Children's Project (ATCP) and a prospective study conducted at the Ataxia Telangiectasia Clinical Center (ATCC) at Johns Hopkins have allowed for a reasonable estimate of life span in patients with ataxia telangiectasia. The purpose of this study was to assess survival probability in these patients on the basic of the ATCP and ATCC reports.

Methods.—Patients in the ATCC with a confirmed diagnosis of ataxia telangiectasia are followed up by phone contact or follow-up visits. Through the end of 2004, 24 deaths occurred. A modification of the Kaplan–Meier survival function was used to estimate the median age at death. A second cohort of patients was assembled by the ATCP. A total of 95 deaths, from 1968 to the present, were identified, along with the age at the time of death. The diagnosis of ataxia telangiectasia is unconfirmed in this cohort, but it is expected that the diagnosis will be correct for the vast majority of these patients.

Results.—In the prospective ATCC cohort, the median survival is calculated to be 25 years. In the retrospective ATCP cohort, the median survival is 19 years. In both cohorts, the age at the time of death was wide ranging. Mortality crossed the 25th and 75th centiles in the prospective ATCC cohort at ages 18 and 28 years and at ages 14 and 28 years in the retrospective ATCP cohort.

Conclusions.—Life expectancy is not well correlated with the severity of neurologic impairment in patients with ataxia telangiectasia.

Prognostic Factors for Early Severity in a Childhood Multiple Sclerosis Cohort

Mikaeloff Y, for the KIDSEP Study Group (Assistance Publique-Hôpitaux de Paris, LeKremlin-Bicêtre)
Pediatrics 118:1133-1139, 2006

Objective.—The goal was to identify prognostic factors for an early severe course in a cohort of patients with childhood-onset multiple sclerosis, for the construction of a predictive tool.

Methods.—The cohort consisted of 197 children from the French Kid Sclérose en Plaques neuropediatric cohort with relapsing/remitting multiple sclerosis beginning before the age of 16 years. Patients were included from 1990 to 2003. We used multivariate survival analysis (Cox model) to evaluate the prognostic value of clinical, MRI, and biological covariates at onset for the occurrence of a third attack or severe disability ("severity" outcome).

Results.—The cohort was monitored for a mean of 5.5 ± 3.6 years. The "severity" outcome was recorded for 144 patients (73%). The risk of severity was higher for girls, for a time between the first and second attacks of <1 year, for childhood-onset multiple sclerosis MRI criteria at onset, for an absence of severe mental state changes at onset, and for a progressive course. A derived childhood-onset multiple sclerosis potential index for early severity was found to have a positive predictive value for severity of >35% for the upper 2 quartiles.

Conclusions.—The clinical and MRI prognostic factors for early severity that were identified were used as the basis of a predictive tool, which will be validated in another cohort. This tool should make it possible to identify subgroups at risk of early severe disease and should facilitate therapeutic studies.

▶ Multiple sclerosis does occur in children. Unfortunately, it occurs with such infrequency that few studies have examined the total spectrum of illness produced by this disease. This report attempts to identify prognostic features for disease severity in children who present with multiple sclerosis. Needless to say, this study is a welcome one, because the information provided by the study helps us to understand who is likely to get into trouble more quickly and to therefore require more intensive management.

So, who is likely to have early severe problems after being diagnosed with multiple sclerosis? It is the young female, who has a short interval (less than 1 year) between the first and second attacks; it is the youngster with childhood-onset disease who demonstrates MRI criteria at the time of diagnosis, an absence of severe mental state changes at onset, and a course that seems to be out of the ordinary in terms of rapidity.

We also learn from this report that the average age of onset of multiple sclerosis in childhood is 11.9 years and that an episode of acute central nervous system inflammatory demyelination may be the first presentation of childhood-onset multiple sclerosis. The onset may mimic acute disseminated encephalomyelitis. This presentation is more common than the "typical" onset of multiple sclerosis among children who are less than 10 years old. It is very difficult to distinguish between multiple sclerosis and acute disseminated encephalomyelitis in a youngster.

Some multiple sclerosis scoring systems for adult patients were designed for diagnostic or prognostic purposes through consensus conferences, and they do not take into account the specific features of childhood-onset multiple sclerosis. We are in the early stages of creating a unique classification system for children with this terrible disease, and we hope that this one will be better than the one that has been handed down from studies of adults.

J. A. Stockman III, MD

Oral Fingolimod (FTY720) for Relapsing Multiple Sclerosis

Kappos L, for the FTY720 D2201 Study Group (Univ Hosp, Basel, Switzerland; et al)

N Engl J Med 355:1124-1240, 2006

Background.—Fingolimod (FTY720) is a new oral immunomodulating agent under evaluation for the treatment of relapsing multiple sclerosis.

Methods.—We randomly assigned 281 patients to receive oral fingolimod, at a dose of 1.25 mg or 5.0 mg, or a placebo once daily, and we followed these patients for 6 months with magnetic resonance imaging (MRI) and clinical evaluations (core study, months 0 to 6). The primary end point was the total number of gadolinium-enhanced lesions recorded on T_1-weighted MRI at monthly intervals for 6 months. In an extension study in which the investigators and patients remained unaware of the dose assignments (months 7 to 12), patients who received placebo underwent randomization again to one of the fingolimod doses.

Results.—A total of 255 patients completed the core study. The median total number of gadolinium-enhanced lesions on MRI was lower with 1.25 mg of fingolimod (1 lesion, P<0.001) and 5.0 mg of fingolimod (3 lesions, P=0.006) than with placebo (5 lesions). The annualized relapse rate was 0.77 in the placebo group, as compared with 0.35 in the group given 1.25 mg of fingolimod (P=0.009) and 0.36 in the group given 5.0 mg of fingolimod

(P=0.01). For the 227 patients who completed the extension study, the number of gadolinium-enhanced lesions and relapse rates remained low in the groups that received continuous fingolimod, and both measures decreased in patients who switched from placebo to fingolimod. Adverse events included nasopharyngitis, dyspnea, headache, diarrhea, and nausea. Clinically asymptomatic elevations of alanine aminotransferase levels were more frequent with fingolimod (10 to 12%, vs. 1% in the placebo group). One case of the posterior reversible encephalopathy syndrome occurred in the 5.0-mg group. Fingolimod was also associated with an initial reduction in the heart rate and a modest decrease in the forced expiratory volume in 1 second.

Conclusions.—In this proof-of-concept study, fingolimod reduced the number of lesions detected on MRI and clinical disease activity in patients with multiple sclerosis. Evaluation in larger, longer-term studies is warranted.

▶ The Mikaeloff et al report (Prognostic factors for early severity in a childhood multiple sclerosis cohort) dealt with information regarding the demographics of multiple sclerosis affecting children. This report largely deals with adults with the disorder, but, because multiple sclerosis is infrequent among children, we must learn from such adult experiences. Multiple sclerosis remains the most common nontraumatic cause of neurologic disability in young adults. Most believe that it is an autoimmune condition in which autoreactive T cells attack myelin sheaths, which leads to demyelination and axonal damage. Currently approved immunomodulating treatments for multiple sclerosis (interferon β and glatiramer acetate) reduce relapse rates by only about 30%. Both drugs are administered either subcutaneously or intramuscularly, and interferons are associated with a number of systemic reactions in more than 60% of patients.

Fingolimod is an oral sphingosine-1-phosphate receptor modulator. The drug acts as a superagonist of the spingosine-1-phosphate receptor on thymocytes and lymphocytes, and it induces aberrant internalization of this receptor, thus depriving the cells of a signal that is necessary to egress from secondary lymphoid tissue. This results in a majority of lymphocytes being sequestered in lymph nodes, thereby reducing peripheral lymphocyte counts and the recirculation of lymphocytes to the central nervous system. Cells that are still in lymphoid organs and those remaining in the blood continue to be functional. Fingolimod does not impair memory T-cell activation or expansion in response to systemic viral infection. In laboratory models of multiple sclerosis, the drug prevents the onset of disease, and it reduces established neurologic deficits. We see in this multicenter study the results of 255 patients who were either treated with fingolimod or a placebo. The number of MRI lesions and relapse rates remained low in the groups that received continuous fingolimod, and they were also reduced in patients who were subsequently switched from placebo to fingolimod. The drug was not without its complications. Adverse events included nasopharyngitis, shortness of breath, headache, diarrhea, and nausea. Elevations of liver enzymes occurred in about 10% of subjects.

Given the immunosuppressive effects of fingolimod, it will need to be evaluated for a longer period of time to determine the potential of this agent and similar agents to increase a patient's susceptibility to infections. Thus far, the only problem in this regard that has been observed is a more frequent number of upper respiratory tract infections in patients receiving the drug as opposed to placebo. Long-term suppression of lymphocyte migration into the central nervous system could also have additional undesired consequences. For example, recent clinical trials have shown that natalizumab (alone or in combination with interferon β-1a), although effective for the management of relapsing multiple sclerosis, does have the potential for causing a fatal opportunistic infection of the central nervous system caused by the JC polyomavirus; this problem developed in three patients. Whether this occurred as a result of the drug-induced absence of immune surveillance of the central nervous system or as a result of something else remains to be seen. Whether the long-term inhibition of lymphocyte migration caused by fingolimod treatment might carry a similar risk is not known and does require further investigation.

There were patients as young as 19 years old included in the fingolimod study. For this reason, it is possible that this drug may be beneficial for those whose disease presents during childhood and adolescence. However, more studies are needed to document this.

One concluding comment regarding multiple sclerosis. Laughing is not generally a symptom that patients go to physicians for, but pathological laughing and intractable hiccups are both recognized in a number of neurologic conditions. The most common association is with multiple sclerosis. About 10% patients with multiple sclerosis experience pathological laughing in the later chronic stages of the disease, but a recent report shows also that many of these patients have intractable hiccups as well.[1] The combination of multiple sclerosis and intractable laughing/hiccups is usually best managed with high dose intravenous steroids.

J. A. Stockman III, MD

Reference

1. de Seze J, Zephir H, Hautecoeur P, Mackowiak A, Cabaret M, Vermersch P. Pathologic laughing and intractable hiccups can occur early in multiple sclerosis. *Neurology.* 2006;67:1684-1686.

Comparison of Accidental and Nonaccidental Traumatic Head Injury in Children on Noncontrast Computed Tomography

Tung GA, Kumar M, Richardson RC, et al (Brown Med School, Providence, RI)
Pediatrics 118:626-632, 2006

Objective.—Mixed-density convexity subdural hematoma and interhemispheric subdural hematoma suggest nonaccidental head injury. The purpose of this retrospective observational study is to investigate subdural hematoma on noncontrast computed tomography in infants with nonaccidental head injury and to compare these findings in infants with accidental head trauma for whom the date of injury was known.

Patients and Methods.—Two blinded, independent observers retrospectively reviewed computed tomography scans with subdural hematoma performed on the day of presentation on 9 infant victims of nonaccidental head injury (mean age: 6.8 months; range: 1–25 months) and on 38 infants (mean age: 4.8 months; range: newborn to 34 months) with accidental head trauma (birth-related: 19; short fall: 17; motor vehicle accident: 2).

Results.—Homogeneous hyperdense subdural hematoma was significantly more common in children with accidental head trauma (28 of 38 [74%]; nonaccidental head trauma: 3 of 9 [33%]), whereas mixed-density subdural hematoma was significantly more common in cases of nonaccidental head injury (6 of 9 [67%]; accidental head trauma: 7 of 38 [18%]). Twenty-two (79%) subdural hematomas were homogeneously hyperdense on noncontrast computed tomography performed within two days of accidental head trauma, one (4%) was homogeneous and isodense compared to brain tissue, one (4%) was homogeneous and hypodense, and four (14%) were mixed-density. There was no statistically significant difference in the proportion of interhemispheric subdural hematoma, epidural hematoma, calvarial fracture, brain contusion, or subarachnoid hemorrhage.

Conclusions.—Homogeneous hyperdense subdural hematoma is more frequent in cases of accidental head trauma; mixed-density subdural hematoma is more frequent in cases of nonaccidental head injury but may be observed within 48 hours of accidental head trauma. Interhemispheric subdural hematoma is not specific for inflicted head injury.

▶ This report is an excellent primer, one worth reading in detail since it teaches all of us a great deal about the mechanisms of intracranial bleeding resulting from nonaccidental and accidental trauma. With respect to the former, in the shaken-infant, the angular acceleration-deceleration forces tend to stretch and tear cortical veins that course to the dural venous sinuses through the subarachnoid space. This results in hemorrhage into either the subdural or subarachnoid spaces. A constellation of the findings has been observed from injury by inflicted head trauma, including interhemispheric subdural hematoma (SDH), shear injuries; diffuse axonal injury, contusional white matter tears and retinal hemorrhage. In contrast, the most common mechanism of accidental head injury is a linear or translational impaction force that may cause a linear skull fracture, epidural hematoma, localized SDH, or cortical contusion. Fall from heights tends to produce higher impact forces that can produce depressed or comminuted skull fracture, subarachnoid hemorrhage, or cortical contusion. Depressed skull fracture can result from short falls when the head impacts a small surface area.

It is fairly common practice to perform a noncontrast CT scan when evaluating infants with suspected head trauma. The literature has suggested that the finding of a heterogeneous or mixed-density SDH on CT implies multiple episodes of traumatic injury and therefore, a pattern of repetitive head injury. Some have suggested that the finding of an interhemispheric SDH is pathognomonic of shaking or a shaking-impact mechanism of head injury. The purpose of the study abstracted was to investigate exactly what one would expect with a CT scan under the circumstances of nonaccidental and accidental head injury.

What we learn from this report is that homogeneous hyperdense SDH is significantly more common in cases of accidental head injury and that heterogeneous or mixed-density SDH is significantly more common in cases of nonaccidental head injury. Unfortunately, the world is not perfect and mixed-density hematoma is not specific for abuse head injury because in the early stages of accidental head injury one may see mixed-density hematomas. Also, the interhemispheric SDH turns out not to be specific for abusive head injury. Lots of expert testimony given before this report appeared will have to be debunked. It appears that nothing is sacred or pathognomonic any longer when it comes to these types of head injuries.

While on the topic of non-accidental head injury, see how you would deal with the following situation. You are seeing a teenager for his annual checkup. This one is just prior to entry into college. You ask what sports this youngster might participate in at the collegiate level. He indicates that the school he is going to is one of the few schools in the United States that has a boxing team, and he would like to try out for it. Should you tell him the latest news about the risks of boxing? What is that news?

It is well known that professional boxers are at high risk of both short-term and long-term neurologic damage. Data has shown, for example, that long-term boxers who possess the apolipoprotein epsilon 4 genotype are at significant risk of developing the Alzheimer-like illness better known as dementia pugilistica. Boxing enthusiasts, however, sometimes claim that the risk is negligible among amateurs because it is so well regulated. Au contraire. Measurements of neurofilament light protein and glial fibrillary acidic protein A in the cerebrospinal fluid of 14 amateur boxers a few days after a fight should make them think again. These markers of neural and glial injury are substantially raised in amateur boxers after a bout compared with a non-boxing control group or with repeat measurements three months later.[1]

Congratulations are in order for those who did this study of amateur boxers. Who would have ever thought that you could talk 14 young men into having spinal taps performed as part of an investigation of the risks of pugilism?

J. A. Stockman III, MD

Reference

1. Zetterberg H, Hietala MA, Jonsson M, et al. Neurochemical aftermath of amateur boxing. *Arch Neurol.* 2006;63:1277-1280.

14 Newborn

Infants' Blood Volume in a Controlled Trial of Placental Transfusion at Preterm Delivery
Aladangady N, McHugh S, Aitchison TC, et al (Queen Mother's Hosp, Glasgow, UK; Univ of Glasgow, UK; Univ of Wales, Cardiff, UK)
Pediatrics 117:93-98, 2006

Objective.—To investigate whether it was possible to promote placental blood transfer to infants at preterm delivery by (1) delaying cord clamping, (2) holding the infant below the placenta, and (3) administering an oxytocic agent to the mother, we measured the infants' blood volumes.

Design.—Randomized study.

Methods.—Forty-six preterm infants (gestational age: 24[0/7] to 32[6/7] weeks) were assigned randomly to either placental blood transfer promotion (delayed cord clamping [DCC] group, ie, ≥30 seconds from moment of delivery) or early cord clamping (ECC) with conventional management (ECC group). Eleven of 23 and 9 of 23 infants assigned randomly to DCC and ECC, respectively, were delivered through the vaginal route. The study was conducted at a tertiary perinatal center, the Queen Mother's Hospital (Glasgow, United Kingdom).

Results.—The infants' mean blood volume in the DCC group (74.4 mL/kg) was significantly greater than that in the ECC group (62.7 mL/kg; 95% confidence interval for advantage: 5.8-17.5). The blood volume was significantly increased by DCC for infants delivered vaginally. The infants in the DCC group delivered through cesarean section had greater blood volumes (mean: 70.4 mL/kg; range: 45-83 mL/kg), compared with the ECC group (mean: 64.0 mL/kg; range: 48-77 mL/kg), but this was not significant. Additional analyses confirmed the effect of DCC (at least 30 seconds) to increase average blood volumes across the full range of gestational ages studied.

Conclusions.—The blood volume was, on average, increased in the DCC group after at least a 30-second delay for both vaginal and cesarean deliveries. However, on average, euvolemia was not attained with the third-stage management methods outlined above.

▶ A lot of mystery has surrounded the topic of delayed umbilical cord clamping. For whatever reason, during labor and delivery, an infant will lose blood into the umbilical cord and placenta such that if there is an immediate clamping of the umbilical cord, it is likely that there will be some reduction in a newborn's blood volume. For example, animal studies involving foals, infant rabbits/bunnies, and puppies have shown an approximate 30% to 50% reduction in an animal's blood volume if immediate cord clamping is undertaken. In humans, at 30 weeks of gestation, approximately one half of the feto-placental blood volume of approximately 110 mL/kg remains outside the newborn circulation if the umbilical cord is clamped immediately. Despite historical controversy, the umbilical cord is now usually clamped immediately, especially after preterm delivery, for fear of delaying resuscitation or causing hypothermia. In some babies, early cord clamping results in hypovolemia and a higher severity of respiratory distress syndrome in preterm babies. Delayed cord clamping and placental transfusion might obviate these problems and reduce the need for donor blood transfusion. This report from the United Kingdom sheds new information on this topic. We see that preterm babies who undergo delayed cord clamping will have a significantly higher blood volume (74.4 mL/kg versus 62.7 mL/kg with early cord clamping). The placental transfusion was more marked after vaginal deliveries in comparison to caesarean deliveries and was more apparent for preterm babies with increasingly lower gestational ages. Interestingly, even with delayed cord clamping, euvolemia was not achieved in all babies, demonstrating the magnitude of the shifting of blood that occurs from baby to cord and placenta at the time of delivery.

It is hard to say whether this report alone will change obstetrical practices in the delivery room. The need to get babies stabilized and warm will overpower the desire to get as much blood as possible from the umbilical cord and placenta.

The following is a question that has to do with umbilical cords. More often than not, when looking at the umbilical cord of a newborn baby you will notice that the cord will have a twist or spiral to it. The question is, in what direction (clockwise or counterclockwise) do you expect this spiral to be, and what are the likely numbers of twists? Indeed, the umbilical cord is usually spiraled. A counterclockwise spiral is more frequent than a clockwise spiral with a ratio of approximately 7 to 1. Thus, if you are a betting person, you could place odds up to 7 to 1 that an umbilical cord will have a counterclockwise twist. The coiling of the umbilical vessels develops as early as 28 days after conception and is present in 95% of fetuses by 7 weeks of conception. The helices may be seen by ultrasonographic examination as early as the first trimester of pregnancy. Hypotheses for such spiraling include fetal movements, active or passive torsion of the embryo, differentiated umbilical vascular growth rates, fetal hemodynamic forces, and the arrangements of muscular fibers in the umbilical arterial wall. In other words, your guess is as good as anyone's as to why the umbilical cord does "the twist."

The umbilical coiling index (CI) represents the number of complete coils divided by the length of the cord. There are an average of 0.24 coils/centimeter. The umbilical coiling index has been shown to correlate with certain fetal problems. For example, when the index is below the 10th percentile (0.07 coils/cm), fetal death, spontaneous preterm delivery, trisomies, low five-minute Apgar scores, and single umbilical artery have been identified. Overcoiling (CI > 90th percentile, 0.30 coils/cm) is associated with asphyxia, umbilical arterial pH < 7.05, small for gestational age infants, trisomies, and single umbilical artery. Some have suggested that determination of the umbilical CI should be part of a routine examination of the placenta. Some have also suggested that unusual coiling should be looked at as part of prenatal ultrasounds. If you think this information is too much and has spiraled beyond credibility, read the report of overcoiling of an umbilical cord that recently appeared in *The Journal of Pediatrics.*[1]

J. A. Stockman III, MD

Reference

1. Trevisanuto D, Doglioni N, Zanardo V, Chiarelli S. Overcoiling of the umbilical cord. *J Pediatr*. 2007;150:112.

The premature infants in need of transfusion (PINT) study: A randomized, controlled trial of a restrictive (low) versus liberal (high) transfusion threshold for extremely low birth weight infants

Kirpalani H, for the PINT Investigators (McMaster Univ, Hamilton, Ont, Canada; et al)

J Pediatr 149:301-307, 2006

Objective.—To determine whether extremely low birth weight infants (ELBW) transfused at lower hemoglobin thresholds versus higher thresholds have different rates of survival or morbidity at discharge.

Study Design.—Infants weighing <1000 g birth weight were randomly assigned within 48 hours of birth to a transfusion algorithm of either low or high hemoglobin transfusion thresholds. The composite primary outcome was death before home discharge or survival with any of either severe retinopathy, bronchopulmonary dysplasia, or brain injury on cranial ultrasound. Morbidity outcomes were assessed, blinded to allocation.

Results.—Four hundred fifty-one infants were randomly assigned to low (n = 223) or high (n = 228) hemoglobin thresholds. Groups were similar, with mean birth weight of 770 g and gestational age of 26 weeks. Fewer infants received one or more transfusions in the low threshold group (89% low versus 95% high, $P = .037$). Rates of the primary outcome were 74.0% in the low threshold group and 69.7% in the high ($P = .25$; risk difference, 2.7%; 95% CI $-3.7%$ to 9.2%). There were no statistically significant differences between groups in any secondary outcome.

Conclusions.—In extremely low birth weight infants, maintaining a higher hemoglobin level results in more infants receiving transfusions but confers little evidence of benefit.

▶ When this editor was a fellow in training in pediatric hematology back in the early to mid 1970s, he extensively studied the issue of when premature infants required transfusional support. It is interesting that more than 30 years later studies are still appearing on this topic, underscoring that the more things change, the more they stay the same. What remains the same is that as a result of phlebotomy blood losses and inadequate erythropoiesis, very low birth weight infants still become progressively anemic. In an effort to limit the risks associated with red blood cell transfusion, many neonatal units have adopted more restrictive guidelines for transfusing preterm infants. Unfortunately, these changes in practice have not been accompanied by systematic examinations of the risks and benefits of restricting transfusions. There remains a dearth of evidence on which to base transfusion decisions for such tiny infants. More recently, several studies have suggested possible benefits from more liberal transfusion guidelines such as a reduction in the frequency of severe apnea and faster weight gain. Two additional and even more recent studies provide new information about the relative risks and benefits of using restrictive (transfusion at lower hemoglobin) rather than more liberal criteria for transfusing very low birth weight infants. These are the Iowa Trial and the PINT (Premature Infants in Need of Transfusion) Trial, an eloquent study abstracted here.[1] Both of these trials have compared the outcomes of 2 groups of infants who were randomly assigned to restrictive or liberal transfusion criteria, based on hematocrit or hemoglobin thresholds for transfusion. Despite differences in experimental design and results, these new trials together strengthen the evidence available to guide decisions about providing red blood cell transfusions to very low birth weight infants.

So what did the Iowa and PINT Trials show? The Iowa Trial was a single-center randomized clinical trial with sample size calculated to test whether using lower hematocrit thresholds for red blood cell transfusion would reduce the number of transfusions received by infants with birth weights of 500 to 1300 g. The PINT Trial was a larger multicenter randomized clinical trial designed to examine the impact of transfusion strategy on the incidence of a composite outcome—death, retinopathy of prematurity, bronchopulmonary dysplasia, or abnormal brain US—in infants with birth weight below 1000 g. The Iowa Trial found a reduction in the number of transfusions, but not the number of donor exposures in the restrictive transfusion group. The lack of difference in the number of donors presumably resulted from the use of a single-donor transfusion program. The PINT Trial found a reduction in the number of transfusions given according to study criteria in the restrictive transfusion group, but this reduction was offset by an increase in the number of transfusions given for clinical indication; consequently, the trend toward fewer total transfusions in the restrictive transfusion group was not statistically significant. The PINT Trial found no reduction in donor exposures with restrictive transfusion guidelines when all transfusions were considered, including platelet and plasma transfusions. However, when only red blood cell transfusions were compared, the number of donors was in the restrictive transfusion group was less. Perhaps the best measure of success in limiting transfusions is the number of infants who required no transfusions. The PINT Trial found that significantly more infants avoided red blood cell transfusion altogether when restrictive criteria were used, 11% versus 5%. The Iowa Trial found no such difference with 10% to 12% of infants in both groups avoiding all transfusions.

If we assume the results of both the Iowa and PINT Trials are valid, we are left with weighing the potential benefits of restrictive transfusion guidelines—more infants will avoid transfusion altogether with restrictive transfusions in the PINT Trial (but not the Iowa Trial)—against the potential benefits of liberal transfusion guidelines, especially protection against major brain injury found in the Iowa Trial (but not confirmed by the PINT Trial). A commentary on this topic does some interesting math for us that might help us decide which of these 2 studies is the more important. If we believe the finding of the PINT Trial that restrictive transfusion guidelines protect more infants from receiving 1 or more transfusions, the number needed to treat would be 17; in other words, 17 infants would have to be transfused according to the more restrictive criteria to allow 1 infant to avoid transfusions altogether.[2] If we believe the finding of the Iowa Trial that liberal transfusion guidelines reduce the risk of brain injury, the number needed to treat to achieve this benefit would be 8; in other words, 8 infants would have to be more liberally transfused to prevent 1 case of brain hemorrhage or periventricular leukomalacia. The number needed to treat to prevent 1 infant from dying or having major brain injury would be 7. Please note, however, that these calculations based on the Iowa Trial should be viewed with great caution because the study was relatively small.

So what is the punch line here? If the PINT Trial is reproducible, using a more restrictive transfusion schedule will perhaps cause infants to have fewer exposures to blood products, albeit at relatively minimal reduced levels. At the same time, it is possible that these infants may be put at an increased risk of morbidity from complications of their prematurity. Recognize that the risks of red blood cell transfusions have lessened fairly markedly with improving blood-banking methodologies and that efforts to apply more restrictive transfusion guidelines that have been driven largely by these risks of transfusion would seem to have diminishing returns.

It seems clear that we should not be pushing anemic preterm infants too far before transfusing them. The benefits of restrictive transfusion programs are there in terms of diminished blood product exposure, but these benefits seem to pale in the face of the risks associated with letting the hemoglobin get too low. That is one person's opinion, but it seems to make sense.

J. A. Stockman III, MD

References

1. Bell EF, Strauss RG, Widness JA, et al. Randomized trial of liberal versus restrictive guidelines for red blood cell transfusion in preterm infants. *Pediatrics.* 2005;115:1685-1691.
2. Bell EF. Transfusion thresholds for preterm infants: how low should we go? *J Pediatr.* 2006;149:287-289.

Changing Incidence of *Candida* Bloodstream Infections Among NICU Patients in the United States: 1995–2004

Fridkin SK, for the National Nosocomial Infections Surveillance System Hospitals (Ctrs for Disease Control and Prevention, Atlanta, Ga; et al)
Pediatrics 117:1680-1686, 2006

Objectives.—Recent reports suggest that candidemia caused by fluconazole-resistant strains is increasing in certain adult populations. We evaluated the annual incidence of neonatal candidemia and the frequency of disease caused by different species of *Candida* among neonates in the United States.

Patients.—The study included neonates admitted to 128 NICUs participating in the National Nosocomial Infections Surveillance system from January 1, 1995, to December 31, 2004 (study period).

Methods.—Reports of bloodstream infection (BSI) with *Candida* spp.; *Candida* BSIs, patient admissions, patient-days, and central venous catheter days were pooled by birth weight category. The number of *Candida* BSIs per 100 patients (attack rate) and per 1000 patient-days (incidence density) was determined. Both overall and species-specific rates were calculated; data were pooled over time to determine the differences by birth weight category and by year to determine trends over time.

Results.—From the 130,523 patients admitted to NICUs during the study period, there were 1997 *Candida* spp. BSIs reported. Overall, 1472 occurred in the <1000-g birth weight group. *Candida albicans* BSIs were most common, followed by *Candida parapsilosis*, *Candida tropicalis*, *Candida lusitaniae*, *Candida glabrata*, and only 3 *Candida krusei*. Among neonates <1000 g, incidence per 1000 patient-days decreased from 3.51 during 1995–1999 to 2.68 during 2000–2004 but remained stable among heavier neonates. No increase in infections by species that tend to demonstrate resistance to fluconazole (*C glabrata* or *C krusei*) was observed.

Conclusions.—Although *Candida* BSI is a serous problem among neonates <1000 g, incidence has declined over the past decade, and disease with species commonly resistant to azoles was extremely rare.

▶ If you are following trends in *Candida* bloodstream infections, you will recall that in the neonatal ICUs of the 1990s, the overall incidence of candidemia increased because of the increased survival and intensive care of extremely preterm infants. During that same time period, the proportion of candidemia secondary to *Candida albicans* decreased, whereas that of *C parapsilosis* increased. Few other species of *Candida* seemed to be causing problems during that period.

Candida organisms are still problematic in preterm infants. In preterm infants weighing less than 1500 g, mortality in patients with *C albicans* sepsis is as high as 44% compared with only 16% with *C parapsilosis*. What we see in this report from the Centers of Disease Control (CDC) is that in recent years there has been a significant decrease in the incidence of hospital-acquired candidemia among newborns weighing less than 1000 g. This decrease is because of a decrease in both *C albicans* and *C parapsilosis* bloodstream infections with no decrease in the incidence of *C glabrata* bloodstream infections. Nonetheless, there remains great variation in the rates of candidemia across neonatal ICUs, suggesting that significant differences exist between neonates cared for in these different neonatal ICUs. Needless to say, quality improvement collaboratives would go a long way in identifying best practices to prevent this problem.

It is not entirely clear why we have seen an overall decrease in the risk of fungal infections in our neonatal ICUs. Empiric antifungal use has been reported to be high in this population: 34% among infants with birth weight between 104 and 500 g, 28% among infants weighing 501 to 750 g, and 10% among infants weighing 751 to 1000 g.[1] Also, prophylactic fluconazole use may have increased in preterm infants as the result of publication of trials on the efficacy of this agent in preventing neonatal candidemia.

Please recognize that although the incidence of candidemia has significantly decreased among neonates less than 1000 g, this disease remains a significant problem in this vulnerable population. Recognize also that many ICUs have not experienced this decline and these units need to figure out why. Many thanks are due to the National Nosocomial Infection Surveillance System and the CDC for their vigilance in keeping an eye on this problem.

J. A. Stockman III, MD

Reference

1. Stoll B, Hansen N, Fanaroff A, et al. Late-onset sepsis in very low birth weight neonates: the experience of the NICHD Neonatal Research Network. *Pediatrics.* 2001;110:285-291.

Efficacy of phototherapy for neonatal jaundice is increased by the use of low-cost white reflecting curtains

Djokomuljanto S, Quah BS, Surini Y, et al (Universiti Sains Malaysia, Kelantan; Univ of Oslo, Norway)
Arch Dis Child Fetal Neonatal Ed 91:F439-F442, 2006

Objective.—To determine whether the addition of low-cost reflecting curtains to a standard phototherapy unit could increase effectiveness of phototherapy for neonatal jaundice.

Design.—Randomised controlled clinical trial.

Setting.—Level-one nursery of the Hospital Universiti Sains Malaysia, Kelantan, Malaysia.

Patients.—Term newborns with uncomplicated neonatal jaundice presenting in the first week of life.

Interventions.—Phototherapy with white curtains hanging from the sides of the phototherapy unit (study group, n = 50) was compared with single phototherapy without curtains (control group, n = 47).

Main Outcome Measures.—The primary outcome was the mean difference in total serum bilirubin measured at baseline and after 4 h of phototherapy. The secondary outcome was the duration of phototherapy.

Results.—The mean (standard deviation) decrease in total serum bilirubin levels after 4 h of phototherapy was significantly ($p<0.001$) higher in the study group (27.62 (25.24) μmol/l) than in the control group (4.04 (24.27) μmol/l). Cox proportional hazards regression analysis indicated that the median duration of phototherapy was significantly shorter in the study group (12 h) than in the control group (34 h; χ^2 change 45.2; $p<0.001$; hazards ratio 0.20; 95% confidence interval 0.12 to 0.32). No difference in adverse events was noted in terms of hyperthermia or hypothermia, weight loss, rash, loose stools or feeding intolerance.

Conclusion.—Hanging white curtains around phototherapy units significantly increases efficacy of phototherapy in the treatment of neonatal jaundice without evidence of increased adverse effects.

▶ What a neat little report, one that makes you wonder why you did not think of doing something like this yourself. In parts of the world where access to technology is limited, any innovative approach to economically provide alternative therapies is to be lauded. For example, several years ago, De Carvalho et al[1] showed that intensive phototherapy could be provided by a locally made unit using daylight fluorescent phototherapy lamps instead of the much more expensive blue lamps. What the authors of this report from Malaysia did was to document that single phototherapy with low-cost reflecting curtains is actually more effective than single phototherapy alone, and therefore is a valuable and inexpensive alternative to double phototherapy in the treatment of infants with jaundice. This cheap approach may be of great use to neonatal units in developing nations, where acquisition and maintenance of a sufficient number of phototherapy units might be a challenge to limited budgets. The results probably can be extrapolated to settings outside Malaysia, assuming that the response to phototherapy is similar among differing ethnic groups. In terms of cross savings, the shorter duration of therapy means that more patients can be treated with fewer phototherapy units. Also, decreasing the duration of phototherapy could translate into a shorter hospital stay, meaning less separation from the mother and less interruption of breast-feeding. Infants treated with phototherapy using curtains also seem to have considerably less rebound jaundice.

Please note that it is unlikely that we will see the approaches used in Malaysia here in the United States. The chief concern would be safety. Safety comes in a lot of different forms. The absolute safety in terms of the phototherapy itself and its effects on an infant have not been fully evaluated in the Malaysian study. Also, there could be safety concerns about the use of curtain materials that might be flammable. The bottom line is, however, that when the budget is tight, one must be innovative.

This commentary closes with a short question and answer. How many births are now attended by midwives, and where in the United States is it most likely that a birth will be attended by a midwife? The most recent information we have on this topic comes from a report that appeared in Morbility and Mortality Reports summarizing data on the percentage of births attended by midwives in 2003. In that year, approximately 8.0% of births here in the United States were attended by midwives, more than double the 1990 rate of 3.9%. In 6 states (Alaska, Georgia, New Hampshire, New Mexico, Oregon, and Vermont), rates were at least twice as high as the national rate.[2]

J. A. Stockman III, MD

References

1. De Carvalho M, De Carvalho D, Trzmielina S, Loops JM, Hansen TW. Intensified phototherapy using daylight fluorescent lamps. *Acta Pediatr.* 1999;88:768-771.
2. National Center for Health Statistics CDC Web site. Natality File 2003. Available at: http://www.cdc.gov/nchs/births.htm. Accessed June 21, 2007.

Bilirubin Measurement for Neonates: Comparison of 9 Frequently Used Methods
Grohmann K, Roser M, Rolinski B, et al (Univ Children's Hosp, Greifswald, Germany; Munich Municipal Hosp; Roche Diagnostics GmbH, Mannheim, Germany)
Pediatrics 117:1174-1182, 2006

Objective.—High blood concentrations of bilirubin are toxic to the brain and may cause kernicterus. Therefore, determination of bilirubin levels is performed for many newborns, and several different methods are available. We compared 9 frequently used methods for bilirubin determination among newborns under routine conditions, to define their sequence of use.

Methods.—In a prospective study, bilirubin concentrations were determined with 9 different methods, ie, 3 skin test devices, 3 nonchemical photometric devices (including 2 blood gas analyzers), and 3 laboratory analyzers.

Results.—A total of 124 samples were obtained. All 3 laboratory methods showed very strong correlations with each other, and their means were used as comparison values. To these comparison values, the skin test devices had correlation coefficients between 0.961 and 0.966, and the nonchemical photometric devices between 0.980 and 0.994. Bland-Altman plots demonstrated good agreement with the comparison values for all nonchemical photometric devices. All skin test devices and 1 nonchemical photometric device underestimated bilirubin levels, particularly at high concentrations.

Conclusions.—In the routine care of newborns, the first method for bilirubin testing should be a skin test. If the skin test result exceeds 200 µmol/L and other analytes are to be determined with a nonchemical photometric device, then bilirubin can be included in this analysis and the result trusted up to 250 µmol/L. If the skin test result exceeds 200 µmol/L and only bilirubin concentrations are needed, then a standard laboratory method is the first choice, to avoid repeated blood sampling. Bilirubin concentrations from nonchemical photometric devices that exceed 250 µmol/L should be confirmed with standard laboratory methods.

▶ The devices used to determine bilirubin levels in the normal newborn nursery can largely be grouped into three categories: (1) handheld point of care devices for noninvasive reading of the skin to measure transcutaneous bilirubin levels; (2) devices for nonchemical photometric measurement in blood samples; and (3) laboratory analyzers for photometric measurement of total bilirubin levels in serum or plasma after a chemical reaction. A number of different methods are available for each of these three principal groups. The clinician, however, has been left to wonder which methodologies seem best and under what circumstances. This is how the report from Germany helps us. It tells us that transcutaneous bilirubin measurements are the way to go, especially with respect to initial screening. Current transcutaneous technology allows measurement without an influence of skin pigmentation and therefore is useful in all races. Note, however, for physicians caring for neonates, it is essential to know the transcutaneous bilirubin levels up to which they can trust the skin devices and avoid total bilirubin measurements without missing an infant in need of therapeutic intervention. It is important to define a cutoff value for describing the highest measurement result at which each device correctly identifies all infants with levels above a defined bilirubin serum/plasma concentration. For 15 mg/dL total serum/plasma bilirubin, according to the data from this report, these cutoff values are between 12.2 and 13.1 mg/dL for the different devices. In other words, results from these devices up to these values need not be confirmed with a laboratory test. Using these devices, some 93% of blood sampling can be avoided.

There are a few words of caution regarding the approaches used in this study. The study subjects were white, term infants. Also, bilirubin measurements were performed on the third day of life, on average. Thus, the conclusions should be used with care for low birth weight or preterm infants. These transcutaneous devices can be used not only in the hospital setting, but also in the outpatient setting. They will not uniformly replace measured plasma/serum total bilirubin measurements, but do seem to be useful at lower levels of bilirubin in avoiding unnecessary blood sampling.

Please note, the differential diagnosis of yellow discoloration of the skin includes carotenemia, hypothyroidism, diabetes mellitus, liver disease, and renal disease. Recently a 55-year-old man presented with a 1-month history of yellow discoloration of his palms and soles. Diabetes mellitus had been diagnosed 1 month previously. His conjunctiva were not icteric. He was not ingesting excessive amounts of carotene-rich fruits or vegetables, such as carrots, squash, or green beans. This fellow typified the fact that not all that is yellow in somebody with clear eyes has carotenemia. Once the chap's diabetes was under control, his yellow discoloration improved.[1] Remember the differential diagnosis of yellow skin.

J. A. Stockman III, MD

Reference

1. Lin J-N. Images in clinical medicine. Yellow palms and soles in diabetes mellitus. *N Engl J Med.* 2006;355:1486.

Neonatal hyperbilirubinemia in African American males: The importance of glucose-6-phosphate dehydrogenase deficiency

Kaplan M, Herschel M, Hammerman C, et al (Hebrew Univ, Jerusalem; Univ of Chicago; Ben Gurion Univ of the Negev, Be'er Sheva, Israel; et al)
J Pediatr 149:83-88, 2006

Objective.—To perform risk factor analysis for the prediction of hyperbilirubinemia in an African American male neonatal cohort.

Study Design.—A database of 500 previously published term and near-term African American male neonates was further analyzed to determine the role of risk factors for hyperbilirubinemia. Factors studied included birth weight ≥ 4.0 kg, gestational age ≤ 37 weeks, breast-feeding, glucose-6-phosphate dehydrogenase (G-6-PD) deficiency, and predischarge bilirubin $\geq 75^{th}$ percentile. Hyperbilirubinemia was defined as any bilirubin value $\geq 95^{th}$ percentile on the hour-of-life-specific bilirubin nomogram.

Results.—Forty-three (8.6%) neonates developed hyperbilirubinemia. At 48 ± 12 hours, median transcutaneous bilirubin was 8.3 mg/dL, 75th percentile 10.0 mg/dL, and 95th percentile 12.6 mg/dL. Of the risk factors, only exclusive breast-feeding, G-6-PD deficiency and predischarge bilirubin $\geq 75^{th}$ percentile were significant (Adjusted Odds Ratios [95% Confidence Intervals; CI] 3.15 [1.39-7.14], $P = .006$; 4.96 [2.28-10.80], $P = .001$; and 7.47 [3.50-15.94], $P < .0001$, respectively). G-6-PD-deficient neonates who were also premature and breast-feeding had the highest incidence of hyperbilirubinemia (60%).

Conclusions.—African American male neonates may be at higher risk for hyperbilirubinemia than previously thought. Screening for G-6-PD deficiency and predischarge bilirubin determination may be useful adjuncts in hyperbilirubinemia prediction in these newborns.

▶ Normally we think that infants with a black ancestry in fact are at low risk for the development of neonatal hyperbilirubinemia compared with their white infant peers. This in fact is broadly true except in the subset of the population with G-6-PD deficiency. Somewhere between 11% and 13% of black male newborn infants will have G-6-PD deficiency. There are many case reports of kernicterus here in the United States that have involved G-6-PD-deficiency affected neonates. Slightly more than 20% of infants in the US kernicterus registry have been documented to have G-6-PD deficiency.

The report of Kaplan et al represents a study designed to determine what the risk factors are for the development of hyperbilirubinemia in the newborn black population. The only significant risk factors observed for term infants were exclusive breast-feeding and the presence of G-6-PD deficiency. If one removes the population of infants with G-6-PD deficiency from the overall population of black newborn infants, it turns out that black neonates do have a lower risk of neonatal hyperbilirubinemia, an observation that has relatively little clinical significance in that not knowing the G-6-PD status requires all of us to assume that a black infant may be affected with this disorder given its high prevalence.

So what do these data mean? In the aggregate, it can be concluded that the black neonatal population may not be at as low a risk for hyperbilirubinemia as it was previously thought because of the problem of G-6-PD deficiency. Ideally, hospitals serving the black communities here in the United States (essentially all communities) should consider setting up a G-6-PD screening system with a rapid predischarge turnaround time. This is possible. Infants with G-6-PD deficiency should get extra attention in terms of postnatal follow-up if there is an early discharge.

See the Beal et al report (The changing face of race: risk factors for neonatal hyperbilirubinemia) that tells us a bit more about the use of maternal race as a risk factor for the development of neonatal hyperbilirubinemia. A mother's answer on an admission record as to what her race is often is an inaccurate reflection of what that race actually is. If a mother is only given 1 choice to check off regarding race, mothers of multiracial infants tend to over select black in their newborn infant's ancestry. This may artificially lower one's thinking about the risk for development of hyperbilirubinemia. At the same time it might cause an unnecessary screening for G-6-PD deficiency, if there is no black ancestry.

J. A. Stockman III, MD

The Changing Face of Race: Risk Factors for Neonatal Hyperbilirubinemia
Beal AC, Chou S-C, Palmer RH, et al (Harvard School of Public Health, Boston; Henry Ford Health System, Detroit)
Pediatrics 117:1618-1626, 2006

Objectives.—Race is a predictor of health outcomes and risk for some clinical conditions, for example, mother's race predicts risk for hyperbilirubinemia in newborns, with blacks at lowest risk. Little is known about the correlation of race as recorded in medical records with self-reported race. Also, use of maternal race to predict newborn risk for hyperbilirubinemia has not been tested for multiracial mothers and newborns. We sought to examine how maternal race documented in medical records correlates with self-reported race and to examine the correlation between mothers' and newborns' race in the context of risk for neonatal hyperbilirubinemia, focusing on multiracial mothers and newborns.

Design.—A cohort study with 3021 newborns at ≥ 35 weeks gestation discharged from normal nursery between January 2001 and October 2002 with a telephone survey of their mothers within 6 months of birth.

Setting.—The study was conducted in the Neonatology Department of Henry Ford Hospital.

Patients.—There were 1773 mothers (58%) with incorrect telephone numbers. Of 1248 mothers contacted, 866 (69%) completed the interview.

Outcome Measures.—We measured mother's race in hospital database and mother's reported race for herself, her newborn, and the father, allowing ≤ 5 responses for each.

Results.—Of mothers documented in the medical record as white, 64% self-reported as white. Among mothers recorded as black, 70% self-reported as black. Mothers identified 93 newborns as ≥2 races with primary race matching both parents for 41%, father for 25%, mother for 23%, and neither parent for 11%. Of 70 newborns whose parents were not the same race, mothers identified 45 (64%) as ≥2 races.

Conclusions.—There is incomplete overlap between racial identification in medical records versus self-report. Given 1 choice, mothers of multiracial infants overselect black in their newborns' ancestry. Because black race is the lowest risk category for neonatal hyperbilirubinemia, this may lead to underestimating their risk.

Outcomes among Newborns with Total Serum Bilirubin Levels of 25 mg per Deciliter or More

Newman TB, for the Jaundice and Infant Feeding Study Team (Univ of California, San Francisco; et al)
N Engl J Med 354:1889-1900, 2006

Background.—The neurodevelopmental risks associated with high total serum bilirubin levels in newborns are not well defined.

Methods.—We identified 140 infants with neonatal total serum bilirubin levels of at least 25 mg per deciliter (428 micromol per liter) and 419 randomly selected controls from a cohort of 106,627 term and near-term infants born from 1995 through 1998 in Kaiser Permanente hospitals in northern California. Data on outcomes were obtained from electronic records, interviews, responses to questionnaires, and neurodevelopmental evaluations that had been performed in a blinded fashion.

Results.—Peak bilirubin levels were between 25 and 29.9 mg per deciliter (511 μmol per liter) in 130 of the newborns with hyperbilirubinemia and 30 mg per deciliter (513 μmol per liter) or more in 10 newborns; treatment involved phototherapy in 136 cases and exchange transfusion in 5. Follow-up data to the age of at least two years were available for 132 of 140 children with a history of hyperbilirubinemia (94 percent) and 372 of 419 controls (89 percent) and included formal evaluation at a mean (±SD) age of 5.1±0.12 years for 82 children (59 percent) and 168 children (40 percent), respectively. There were no cases of kernicterus. Neither crude nor adjusted scores on cognitive tests differed significantly between the two groups; on most tests, 95 percent confidence intervals excluded a 3-point (0.2 SD) decrease in adjusted scores in the hyperbilirubinemia group. There was no significant difference between groups in the proportion of children with abnormal neurologic findings on physical examination or with documented diagnoses of neurologic abnormalities. Fourteen of the children with hyperbilirubinemia (17 percent) had "questionable" or abnormal findings on neurologic examination, as compared with 48 controls (29 percent; $P=0.05$; adjusted odds ratio, 0.47; 95 percent confidence interval, 0.23 to 0.98; $P=0.04$). The frequencies of parental concern and reported behavioral problems also were not significantly different between the two groups. Within the hyperbilirubinemia group, those with positive direct antiglobulin tests had lower scores on cognitive testing but not more neurologic or behavioral problems.

Conclusions.—When treated with phototherapy or exchange transfusion, total serum bilirubin levels in the range included in this study were not associated with adverse neurodevelopmental outcomes in infants born at or near term.

▶ If one looks back over the past 4 decades of literature dealing with newborn infants, there is probably more written about neonatal hyperbilirubinemia than any other single newborn entity. The reason why is that as much as we learn about neonatal hyperbilirubinemia, there seems to be lingering doubts about what we already know. The worry with hyperbilirubinemia, of course, is the development of bilirubin encephalopathy evolving into kernicterus, a devastating chronic debilitating condition characterized by the clinical findings of choreoathetoid cerebral palsy, central neural hearing loss, palsy of the vertical gaze and tooth enamel hypoplasia resulting from bilirubin-induced cell toxicity. Early on, most newborn infants described with kernicterus had it as the result of Rh hemolytic disease, but kernicterus has been reported in apparently healthy term and near-term breastfed infants without documented hemolysis. In fact, reported cases of kernicterus have been on the rise for the past 20 years, a rise directly correlated with the increasing rates of breastfeeding seen here in the United States.

The study of Newman et al is one of the most important to have appeared in the last year and a half in the pediatric literature. The investigators report on a large prospective, blinded study of neurodevelopmental outcomes in 140 term and near-term newborn infants with total bilirubin levels of 25 mg/dL (428 µmol/L) or more. No cases of kernicterus developed in this patient population and no significant differences between the 2 groups in intelligence or visual-motor integration were observed. Developmental follow-up data were available for almost all children through at least 2 years and formal evaluations were performed for the majority of those in the hyperbilirubinemia group at a mean of 5.1 years.

In the group of extreme hyperbilirubinemia babies that were part of this report, almost all (135 of 140 infants) were able to be managed with phototherapy alone. Just 5 received an exchange transfusion.

So what do the data from this report truly mean? Do they provide assurance that total bilirubin levels between 20 mg/dL and 25 mg/dL are unlikely to put an infant at risk for acute bilirubin encephalopathy in the absence of other contributing factors? The answer is yes. The data also demonstrate that the presence of mild cognitive, behavioral, and motor impairment in children with a history of total bilirubin levels within this range should not be attributed to hyperbilirubinemia. Some caution should be reserved in interpreting all the data, however. One subset of infants with hyperbilirubinemia did have outcomes significantly different from those of controls. These were infants with total bilirubin levels above 25 mg/dL who had a positive direct antiglobulin test for immune-mediated hemolytic disease. This subset of babies did have lower IQ scores, suggesting that hemolysis probably enhances the risk of bilirubin-induced central nervous system injury. It is on this basis that the American Academy of Pediatrics (AAP) recommends that infants with hemolysis should be treated more aggressively. Likewise, the data from the report are consistent with the recommendations of the AAP that treatment should be given to all babies to keep the total bilirubin levels from ever exceeding 25 mg/dL.

If you want to read more about neonatal hyperbilirubinemia and its associated risk, see the superb editorial that accompanied the Newman article, an editorial by Jon Watchko.[1] Dr Watchko reminds us that about 1 in 700 newborn infants will have a total serum bilirubin level of 25 mg/dL or more and about 1 in 10,000 will have a level of 30 mg/dL or more. Despite the encouraging conclusions of the report of Newman et al, kernicterus still occurs in some infants, particularly those with risk factors such as reduced albumin binding of bilirubin, low gestational age, glucose-6-phosphate dehydrogenase deficiency, acidosis, and possibly other risk factors. Many of these risk factors are not recognized or easily detectable, thus there will always be a lingering problem with kernicterus if we do not follow infants carefully for the development of hyperbilirubinemia. This means timely postnatal follow-up before bilirubin levels can become harmful. No infant should go home from the nursery without the ability to be seen within a reasonable period. A report that follows reminds us that black male neonates should be watched even more carefully for the development of hyperbilirubinemia given the high prevalence in this population of glucose-6-phosphate dehydrogenase deficiency.

J. A. Stockman III, MD

Reference

1. Watchko JF. Neonatal hyperbilirubinemia—What are the risks? *N Engl J Med.* 2006;1947-1949.

Interobserver variability of the 5-minute Apgar score

O'Donnell CPF, Kamlin COF, Davis PG, et al (Univ of Melbourne; Murdoch Children's Research Inst, Melbourne)
J Pediatr 149:486-489, 2006

Objectives.—To assess interobserver variability of Apgar scores assigned with video recordings of neonatal resuscitation (AS_{video}) and compare the scores assigned by observers of videos to the Apgar score given by staff attending the delivery (AS_{del}).

Study Design.—Ten-second clips of 30 newborns taken at 5 minutes were shown to observers. Infants were 23 to 40 weeks' gestation, received varying degrees of resuscitation, and were monitored with pulse oximetry. Forty-two observers (neonatal/obstetric medical/nursing staff) scored infants' respiratory effort, muscle tone, reflex irritability, and color. The value for heart rate was assigned from the oximeter, which was masked in all clips. All 42 AS_{video} and the AS_{del} were represented graphically for each infant. Interobserver reliability was assessed by use of a variance components model.

Results.—AS$_{video}$ varied widely between observers. Variability was large for all 4 elements of the score observers assigned and was seen irrespective of the infant's level of illness. AS$_{del}$ was greater than AS$_{video}$ in most cases, on average by 2.4 points. There was no evidence that the level of discrepancy was substantially different between groupings of staff.

Conclusion.—The Apgar score has poor interobserver reliability. More objective and precise measures of newborns' condition are required.

▶ It has been 55 years since Virginia Apgar reported "a simple, clear classification or grading of newborn infants, which can be used as a basis for discussion and comparison of the results of obstetric practices, types of maternal pain relief, and the effects of resuscitation."[1] You would think after 55 years that we would have gotten it right, but as we see in this very interesting report, there is still some significant variation in how the Apgar scoring is done, even in excellent medical centers. In their study, O'Donnell et al assessed the assignment of 5-minute Apgar scores in a tertiary care setting. Post hoc assessments using video recordings taken 5 minutes after delivery were compared with the clinical assessments made by a neonatal care provider team. Color, which Apgar felt was the least useful score component, was not used. A maximum score under these circumstances, therefore, was 8. The variability among the 42 video scorers was substantial, and the reliability was poor for all four elements of the score. The standard deviation of the total video scores was 1.9. The scores determined clinically varied significantly from the video assessments. Twenty of the 30 clinical assessments were two or more points higher than the corresponding video assessment with greater standard deviation at lower scores.

The results of this report are really not all that surprising because previous studies have shown similar findings.[2] So is it time to euthanize the Apgar score or possibly replace it with something better? As of now, there really is not anything better. Nonetheless, the demise of the Apgar score has been predicted, such as in an editorial in *The Lancet*, which called for the Apgar score to "be pensioned off."[3]

It is time to work on a more refined neonatal scoring system for the delivery room. We could start by adding a simple pulse oximeter to the evaluation of every newborn. Let's not, however, forget to honor Virginia Apgar and her contribution to the vulnerable and venerable scoring system we now use. Perhaps the next generation of assessments will be called the "Super Apgar."

Before closing this commentary, we ask a question. What is one way to increase birth rates in countries that have demonstrated a decline? A possible answer is to pay mothers who have babies! Maternity payments of $3000 have been credited with increasing the birth rate in Australia — by an extra 10,000 babies. A total of 268,667 parents in 2005-2006 claimed the stipend, showing a significantly greater than expected rise in birth rates once subsidy payments became available for new mothers in the land down under.[4]

J. A. Stockman III, MD

References

1. Apgar V. A proposal for a new method of evaluation of the newborn infant. *Curr Res Anesth Analg.* 1953;32:260-267.
2. Clark DA, Hakanson DO. The inaccuracy of Apgar scoring. *J Perinatol.* 1998;8:203-205.
3. Is the Apgar score outmoded? *Lancet.* 1989;1:591-592.
4. Payments brought prompt baby boom in Australia [editorial]. *BMJ.* 2006;333:618.

Effect of light reduction on the incidence of retinopathy of prematurity

Braz RRT, Moreira MEL, de Carvalho M, et al (Oswaldo Cruz Found, Rio de Janeiro, Brazil; Laranjeiras Perinatal Clinic, Rio de Janeiro, Brazil)

Arch Dis Child Fetal Neonatal Ed 91:F443-F444, 2006

Background.—Clinical studies thus far have yielded conflicting results on the effects of light on retinopathy of prematurity (ROP). A Cochrane review and meta-analysis has concluded that it is unlikely that the ambient luminosity affects the incidence of ROP, but this review also stressed the large confidence intervals in the combined data, which were due to the small number of threshold or prethreshold diseases. Additional evidence was provided that exposure to light does not affect the incidence of ROP.

Methods.—The study group included all infants born at a gestational age of less then 32 weeks or a birth weight of less than 1600 g at 2 neonatal ICUs. The infants were randomly assigned to 2 groups, trial and control, and stratified by birth weight (>1000 g or <1000 g). Infants in the trial group received ocular protection against the ambient light in both eyes, from birth until 35 weeks of corrected gestational age. Infants in the control group did not receive ocular protection and were kept under the regular light conditions. Indirect ophthalmoscopy was performed within 4 to 6 weeks of birth and thereafter every 1 or 2 weeks. The diagnosis of ROP was confirmed in at least 2 examinations according to the criteria of the CRYO-ROP study. Statistical analysis was performed by using the χ^2 test, Student t test, and logistic regression.

Results.—The final study group included 95 newborns in the trial group and 93 in the control group. The mean luminosity was 383 lux (range, 188-540 lux). There were no significant differences between the groups in terms of body weight, gestational age, and the main maternal and neonatal morbidities. There were no significant differences in terms of respiratory assistance between the 2 groups. The incidence of ROP of any grade was 46% in both groups.

Conclusions.—The reduction of ambient light had no effect on the incidence of ROP.

▶ There has been a lot written about the potential harm that ambient light might have on infants with respect to the development of ROP. One meta-analysis that reviewed existing articles on the topic concluded that it was unlikely ambient brightness would affect the incidence of ROP.[1] This same meta-analysis, however, pointed out that large confidence intervals in the combined databases made conclusions in this regard somewhat tentative, thus the value of this study performed in Brazil on almost 200 newborns.

In this study, half of a group of infants had eye patches, and the other half were left exposed to room light (mean luminosity, 383 lux). The infants were followed up throughout their nursery stay and after discharge with indirect ophthalmoscopy. The results were pretty straightforward. Reduction of ambient light does not have any effect on the incidence of retinopathy in infants born significantly prematurely.

And on the third day, God created light. Let there be light in the nurseries.

J. A. Stockman III, MD

Reference

1. Phelps DL, Watts JL. Early light reduction for preventing retinopathy of prematurity in very low birthweight infants. *Cochrane Database Syst Rev.* 2001;1:CD000122.

The Contribution of Preterm Birth to Infant Mortality Rates in the United States

Callaghan WM, MacDorman MF, Rasmussen SA, et al (Ctrs for Disease Control and Prevention, Atlanta, Ga; Ctrs for Disease Control and Prevention, Hyattsville, Md)
Pediatrics 118:1566-1573, 2006

Objective.—Although two thirds of infant deaths in the United States occur among infants born preterm (<37 weeks of gestation), only 17% of infant deaths are classified as being attributable to preterm birth with the standard classification of leading causes of death. To address this apparent discrepancy, we sought to estimate more accurately the contribution of preterm birth to infant mortality rates in the United States.

Methods.—We identified the top 20 leading causes of infant death in 2002 in the US linked birth/infant death file. The role of preterm birth for each cause was assessed by determining the proportion of infants who were born preterm for each cause of death and by considering the biological connection between preterm birth and the specific cause of death.

Results.—Of 27,970 records in the linked birth/infant death file for 2002, the 20 leading causes accounted for 22,273 deaths (80% of all infant deaths). Among infant deaths attributable to the 20 leading causes, we classified 9596 infant deaths (34.3% of all infant deaths) as attributable to preterm birth. Ninety-five percent of those deaths occurred among infants who were born at <32 weeks of gestation and weighed <1500 g, and two thirds of those deaths occurred during the first 24 hours of life.

Conclusions.—On the basis of this evaluation, preterm birth is the most frequent cause of infant death in the United States, accounting for at least one third of infant deaths in 2002. The extreme prematurity of most of the infants and their short survival indicate that reducing infant mortality rates requires a comprehensive agenda to identify, to test, and to implement effective strategies for the prevention of preterm birth.

Trends in cerebral palsy among infants of very low birthweight (<1500 g) or born prematurely (<32 weeks) in 16 European centres: a database study
Platt MJ, Cans C, Johnson A, et al (Univ of Liverpool, England; Pavillion Taillefer, Grenoble, France; Univ of Oxford, England; et al)
Lancet 369:43-50, 2007

Background.—The risk of cerebral palsy, the commonest physical disability of children in western Europe, is higher in infants of very low birthweight (VLBW)—those born weighing less than 1500 g—and those from multiple pregnancies than in infants of normal birthweight. An increasing proportion of infants from both of these groups survive into childhood. This paper describes changes in the frequency and distribution of cerebral palsy by sex and neurological subtype in infants with a birthweight below 1000 g and 1000–1499 g in the period 1980–96.

Methods.—A group of 16 European centres, Surveillance of Cerebral Palsy in Europe, agreed on a standard definition of cerebral palsy and inclusion and exclusion criteria. Data for children with cerebral palsy born in the years 1980–96 were pooled. The data were analysed to describe the distribution and prevalence of cerebral palsy in VLBW infants. Prevalence trends were expressed as both per 1000 livebirths and per 1000 neonatal survivors.

Findings.—There were 1575 VLBW infants born with cerebral palsy; 414 (26%) were of birthweight less than 1000 g and 317 (20%) were from multiple pregnancies. 1426 (94%) had spastic cerebral palsy, which was unilateral (hemiplegic) in 336 (24%). The birth prevalence fell from 60.6 (99%CI 37.8–91.4) per 1000 liveborn VLBW infants in 1980 to 39.5 (28.6–53.0) per 1000 VLBW infants in 1996. This decline was related to a reduction in the frequency of bilateral spastic cerebral palsy among infants of birthweight 1000–1499 g. The frequency of cerebral palsy was higher in male than female babies in the group of birthweight 1000–1499 g (61.0 [53.8–68.2] *vs* 49.5 [42.8–56.2] per 1000 livebirths; p=0.0025) but not in the group of birthweight below 1000 g.

Interpretation.—These data from a large population base provide evidence that the prevalence of cerebral palsy in children of birthweight less than 1500 g has fallen, which has important implications for parents, health services, and society.

▶ Until the late 1990s, cerebral palsy was defined as a nonprogressive disorder of movement, posture, or both. No reliable measure of the severity of the motor disability was available nor were other cognitive or neurosensory problems considered. The current definition of cerebral palsy includes not only motor disorders but also disturbances of sensation, cognition, communication, perception and behavior, and seizures.[1] These important advances in diagnosis and assessment have improved the classification of children with cerebral palsy. The current classification includes anatomical and radiologic findings and causation and timing of the lesion. This classification aids comparison of the frequency of cerebral palsy and its correlates and enables a multidisciplinary approach to treatment.

Most preterm babies who develop cerebral palsy have it in association with periventricular leukomalacia, with or without severe periventricular hemorrhaging or infarction. Many factors may cause cerebral palsy, including perinatal ischemia, anoxia, perinatal infections, and the iatrogenic effects of drugs such as steroids in the postnatal period. Cerebral palsy is also significantly more common in multiple births. The prevalence of cerebral palsy, especially in infants less than 28 weeks' gestation, mainly reflects the aggressiveness of perinatal care. Thus, in the 1990s, the concern was that the prevalence of cerebral palsy would, in fact, continue to increase. As it turns out, we finally have some good news about cerebral palsy from the Surveillance of Cerebral Palsy in Europe. This group found that the prevalence of cerebral palsy in VLBW infants and those born at less than 32 weeks' gestation has decreased significantly from 6% of live births in 1980 to just 4% by the turn of the century. This improvement has occurred despite an increase in VLBW live births, a decrease in neonatal deaths, an increase in multiple births, and a decrease in the mean viable birth weight and gestational age. This decrease in cerebral palsy prevalence occurred mainly in VLBW infants (1000-1499 g). The prevalence of cerebral palsy for infants of VLBW weighing less than 1000 g did not change, although its incidence decreased for survivors born after 1990. The Surveillance of Cerebral Palsy in Europe study observed children up to 4 years of age, when a diagnosis of cerebral palsy would be able to be reliably made. Measurements of intelligence, vision, hearing, and walking were assessed.

So is the battle won? Obviously, there is no cause for complacency when it comes to cerebral palsy. In the European report, some 35% of children with bilateral spastic cerebral palsy were unable to walk, and almost a quarter of children had severe mental retardation (ie, an IQ less than 50). Furthermore, data from Europe and the United States suggest that, while the frequency of cerebral palsy may be decreasing, the number of live-born VLBW babies is increasing; thus, the absolute number of youngsters with cerebral palsy may, in fact, not be on the decline. The key here is the prevention of preterm birth and its associated brain injury.

J. A. Stockman III, MD

Reference

1. Stanley F, Blair E, Alberman E. *Cerebral Palsies: Epidemiology and Causal Pathways.* London: MacKeith Press; 2000.

Cerebral Palsy in a Term Population: Risk Factors and Neuroimaging Findings

Wu YW, Croen LA, Shah SJ, et al (Univ of California, San Francisco; Kaiser Permanente Division of Research, Oakland, Calif)
Pediatrics 118:690-697, 2006

Objective.—The purpose of this work was to study risk factors and neuroimaging characteristics of cerebral palsy in term and near-term infants.

Patients and Methods.—Among a cohort of 334 339 infants ≥36 weeks' gestation born at Kaiser Permanente Medical Care Program in northern California in 1991–2003, we identified infants with cerebral palsy and obtained clinical data from electronic and medical charts. Risk factors for cerebral palsy among infants with different brain abnormalities were compared using polytomous logistic regression.

Results.—Of 377 infants with cerebral palsy (prevalence: 1.1 per 1000), 273 (72%) received a head computed tomography or MRI. Abnormalities included focal arterial infarction (22%), brain malformation (14%), and periventricular white matter abnormalities (12%). Independent risk factors for cerebral palsy were maternal age >35, black race, and intrauterine growth restriction. Intrauterine growth restriction was more strongly associated with periventricular white matter injury than with other neuroimaging findings. Nighttime delivery was associated with cerebral palsy accompanied by generalized brain atrophy but not with cerebral palsy accompanied by other brain lesions.

Conclusions.—Cerebral palsy is a heterogeneous syndrome with focal arterial infarction and brain malformation representing the most common neuroimaging abnormalities in term and near-term infants. Risk factors for cerebral palsy differ depending on the type of underlying brain abnormality.

▶ By now, all of us in the profession know that cerebral palsy is not one entity, but rather represents a group of nonprogressive motor impairment syndromes caused by lesions of the brain arising early in development. The significant majority of cases of children with cerebral palsy have no described cause. Despite advances in obstetrics and neonatal care, the prevalence of cerebral palsy has remained the same or may in fact be slightly increasing in recent decades. Statistics show that about 8,000 children are born annually here in the United States with cerebral palsy. More than half of these affected children are born at term.

This report from California adds important new information on the type of anatomic problems seen in the brains of children with cerebral palsy and also tells us something about the risk factors for this problem. Among infants born at or near term at Kaiser Permanente Medical Care Program in northern California, the most important risk factors for the development of cerebral palsy were maternal age greater than 35 years, black race, and intrauterine growth restriction. Intrauterine growth restriction was strongly associated with the presence of periventricular white matter injury when neuroimaging studies are undertaken. Other abnormalities in these youngsters include focal arterial infarction and brain malformation.

Please note that 1 risk factor for the development of cerebral palsy is being delivered at night. The authors speculate that this is a result of birth asphyxia leading to brain atrophy for reasons that need further study. See the Abdel-Latif ME et al report (Mortality and morbidities among very premature infants admitted after hours in an Australian neonatal intensive care unit network) that gives us more information on night-time deliveries. It is pretty clear that, except for pizza, it is better to have a delivery while the sun shines.

J. A. Stockman III, MD

Mortality and Morbidities Among Very Premature Infants Admitted After Hours in an Australian Neonatal Intensive Care Unit Network

Abdel-Latif ME, for the Australian Capital Territory Neonatal Intensive Care Audit Group (Royal Hosp for Women, New South Wales, Australia; et al)
Pediatrics 117:1632-1638, 2006

Objectives.—To assess risk-adjusted early (within 7 days) mortality and major morbidities of newborn infants at <32 weeks' gestation who are admitted after office hours to a regional Australian network of NICUs where statewide caseload is coordinated and staffed by on-floor registrars working in shift rosters. We hypothesize that adverse sequelae are increased in these infants.

Designs.—We conducted a database review of the records of infants ($n =$ 8654) at <32 weeks' gestation admitted to a network of 10 tertiary NICUs in New South Wales and the Australian Capital Territory from 1992 to 2002. Multivariate logistic regression analysis was performed to adjust for case-mix and significant baseline characteristics.

Outcomes.—Sixty-five percent of infants were admitted to the NICUs after hours. These infants did not have an increase in early neonatal mortality or major neonatal sequelae compared with their office-hours counterparts. Admissions during late night hours after midnight or fatigue risk periods before the end of a medical 12-hour shift were not associated with higher early mortality. Risk factors significantly predictive of early neonatal death were lack of antenatal steroid treatment, Apgar score <7 at 5 minutes, male gender, gestation age, and being small for gestation.

Conclusions.—Current staffing levels, specialization, and networking are associated with lower circadian variation in adverse outcomes and after-hours admission to this NICU network and have no significant impact on early neonatal mortality and morbidity.

▶ The Wu et al report (Cerebral palsy in a term population: risk factors and neuroimaging findings) was from the Kaiser Permanente Medical Care Program in northern California. This report suggested that there was an increased risk of the development of cerebral palsy in infants who were born at night. In fact, other studies have shown that infants delivered at night have an increased risk of asphyxia-related neonatal deaths.[1-3] This has been documented here in the United States, and also in Great Britain and Germany. What we see, however, in Australia is that there seems to be no diurnal variation in neonatal morbidity or mortality rates in that country. No evidence was found that the quality of perinatal care in New South Wales or the Australian capital territory varied by time of the day or night. Being born after hours did not seem to compromise anyone, neither mother nor child. This seems to suggest that models of staffing that had been introduced into that country have lowered circadian variation in deaths among high-risk infants.

There seems to be a lesson or two we can learn from our colleagues down under. It is time to pay attention to what they seem to have done right in their provision of staffing services in NICUs.

J. A. Stockman III, MD

References

1. Heller G, Misselwitz B, Schmidt S. Early neonatal mortality, asphyxia related deaths, and timing of low risk births in Hesse, Germany, 1990-8: observational study. *BMJ.* 2000;321:274-275.
2. Stewart JH, Andrews J, Cartlidge PH. Numbers of deaths related to intrapartum asphyxia and timing of birth in all Wales perinatal survey, 1993-5. *BMJ.* 1998;316:657-660.
3. Gould JB, Qin C, Chavez G. Time of birth and the risk of neonatal death. *Obstet Gynecol.* 2005;106:352-358.

Neurosensory Impairment after Surgical Closure of Patent Ductus Arteriosus in Extremely Low Birth Weight Infants: Results from the Trial of Indomethacin Prophylaxis in Preterms

Kabra NS, and the Trial of Indomethacin Prophylaxis in Preterms (TIPP) Investigators (McMaster Univ, Hamilton, Ont, Canada; et al)
J Pediatr 150:229-234, 2007

Objectives.—To determine whether surgical closure of a patent ductus arteriosus (PDA) is a risk factor for bronchopulmonary dysplasia (BPD), severe retinopathy of prematurity (ROP), and neurosensory impairment in extremely low birth weight (ELBW) infants.

Study Design.—We studied 426 infants with a symptomatic PDA, 110 of whom underwent PDA ligation and 316 of whom received medical therapy only. All infants participated in the multicenter Trial of Indomethacin Prophylaxis in Preterms (TIPP) and were observed to a corrected age of 18 months.

Results.—Of the 95 infants who survived after PDA ligation, 50 (53%) had neurosensory impairment, compared with 84 of the 245 infants (34%) who survived after receiving only medical therapy (adjusted odds ratio, 1.98; 95% CI, 1.18-3.30; $P = .0093$). BPD (adjusted odds ratio, 1.81; 95% CI, 1.09-3.03; $P = .023$) and severe ROP (adjusted odds ratio, 2.20; 95% CI, 1.19-4.07; $P = .012$) were also more common after surgical PDA closure.

Conclusions.—PDA ligation may be associated with increased risks of BPD, severe ROP, and neurosensory impairment in ELBW infants.

▶ Surgery to close a PDA is commonly performed in premature infants. In such babies, a persistent PDA is the result in large part of alterations in prostaglandin metabolism. Inhibition of prostaglandin production with the use of indomethacin has been the cornerstone of pharmacologic closure of PDAs in tiny babies and has been so for the past 30 or more years. Not all babies, however, respond and then a decision has to be made whether more needs to be done. Preterm babies do have a high rate of spontaneous PDA closure during the first 2 years of life. It is questionable whether pharmacologic attempts at closure are needed in most of these babies. The study of Kabra et al adds to our understanding about this problem. The investigators undertook a study to determine whether surgical PDA closure was a risk factor for neurosensory impairment at 18 months in children who were enrolled in TIPP. The data suggest that babies who are operated on have roughly twice the risk of neurosensory impairment compared with babies receiving only medical therapy for their PDAs. In addition, there was an added risk for the development of severe ROP in surgically treated babies.

In addition to the problems with surgery as noted by Kabra et al, surgical ligation of a PDA is known to be associated with its own specific set of morbidities: the need for thoracotomy, the risk of pneumothorax, chylothorax, infection, and vocal cord paralysis. As many as half of tiny babies require pharmacologic support to maintain blood pressure during the postoperative period after a PDA closure.

One should consider the findings of the Kabra et al study to be preliminary. In head-to-head comparisons of surgical closure of PDA versus pharmacologic closure, rather than sequential surgical closure after a pharmacologic failure, surgically ligated babies did have longer durations of continuous positive airway pressure than those treated with indomethacin. More studies are needed to validate these findings.

There is an excellent review of PDA and its management by Clyman and Chorne.[1] They suggest that pharmacologic treatment of PDA in the newborn period offers measurable benefits without an increase in clinically-significant adverse effects, but should be used early since it works best when administered early. Further investigations are clearly needed to determine which infants are most likely to benefit from one form of therapy versus another and, as importantly, which babies are better left untreated altogether.

J. A. Stockman III, MD

Reference

1. Clyman RI, Chorne N. Patent ductus arteriosus: evidence for and against treatment. *J Pediatr.* 2007;150:216-219.

Treatment of Periodontal Disease and the Risk of Preterm Birth

Michalowicz BS, for the OPT Study (Univ of Minnesota, Minneapolis; et al)

N Engl J Med 355:1885-1894, 2006

Background.—Maternal periodontal disease has been associated with an increased risk of preterm birth and low birth weight. We studied the effect of nonsurgical periodontal treatment on preterm birth.

Methods.—We randomly assigned women between 13 and 17 weeks of gestation to undergo scaling and root planing either before 21 weeks (413 patients in the treatment group) or after delivery (410 patients in the control group). Patients in the treatment group also underwent monthly tooth polishing and received instruction in oral hygiene. The gestational age at the end of pregnancy was the prespecified primary outcome. Secondary outcomes were birth weight and the proportion of infants who were small for gestational age.

Results.—In the follow-up analysis, preterm birth (before 37 weeks of gestation) occurred in 49 of 407 women (12.0%) in the treatment group (resulting in 44 live births) and in 52 of 405 women (12.8%) in the control group (resulting in 38 live births). Although periodontal treatment improved periodontitis measures (P<0.001), it did not significantly alter the risk of preterm delivery (P=0.70; hazard ratio for treatment group vs. control group, 0.93; 95% confidence interval [CI], 0.63 to 1.37). There were no significant differences between the treatment and control groups in birth weight (3239 g vs. 3258 g, P=0.64) or in the rate of delivery of infants that were small for gestational age (12.7% vs. 12.3%; odds ratio, 1.04; 95% CI, 0.68 to 1.58). There were 5 spontaneous abortions or stillbirths in the treatment group, as compared with 14 in the control group (P=0.08).

Conclusions.—Treatment of periodontitis in pregnant women improves periodontal disease and is safe but does not significantly alter rates of preterm birth, low birth weight, or fetal growth restriction.

▶ There are lots of risk factors for preterm births. These include multiple gestation, black race, low socioeconomic status, low maternal body mass index (<19.8), and short cervical length (<25 mm as measured on US). Chorioamnionitis, asymptomatic bacteriuria, bacterial vaginosis, and infections at other sites (eg, appendicitis, pneumonia, and periodontal disease) have all been associated with preterm birth. Indeed, periodontal disease has been identified as a risk factor for heart disease, rheumatoid arthritis, and other medical conditions, perhaps via the pathway of increased inflammation. Periodontal disease may lead to preterm birth through seeding of the placenta or amniotic fluid by oral pathogens. However, only a very small percentage of preterm births are associated with intrauterine infection with oral flora. On the other hand, systemic inflammation that is initiated by periodontal disease may lead to both preterm labor and membrane rupture.

Michalowicz et al report the results of a multicenter trial in which 823 pregnant women with periodontal disease were randomly assigned to undergo scaling and root planing either early in the second trimester or after delivery.

The latter was the control group. Periodontal treatment during pregnancy did not result in a significant reduction in the rate of preterm birth before 37 weeks of gestation (12% in the treatment group and 12.8% in the control group), nor did it result in an upward shift in the gestational age distribution.

It is hard to explain the findings observed in this report. One could hypothesize that waiting until pregnancy to deal with periodontal disease is like closing the barn door after the horse is out—the inflammation is already underway, and it is too late to accomplish anything during the pregnancy. It is possible that treatment either before pregnancy (nulliparous women) or in the period between pregnancies (for multiparous women, especially those with a history of preterm birth) might yield more promising results.

There are other ongoing studies looking at the relationship between periodontal disease and preterm delivery. These studies involve more patients than those included in the report by Michalowicz et al. The results of these studies will help clarify whether periodontal treatment has a role in reducing the rate of preterm birth. In the meantime, we have no evidence to support the provision of periodontal treatment for pregnancy for the purposes of reducing preterm birth.

One final comment having to do with dental work and dental bacteremia. Serial blood samples before and after dental extraction in 500 children have shown that bacteria are cleared from the blood within 12 minutes of an extraction, more rapidly than previously assumed. Fifteen preextraction samples have shown evidence of bacteria, as have 102 of the samples taken after extraction. Bacteremia is highest for the first 7.5 minutes postextraction, then diminishes rapidly.[1]

J. A. Stockman III, MD

Reference

1. Roberts GJ, Jaffray EC, Spratt DA, et al. Duration, prevalence and intensity of bacteraemia after dental extractions in children. *Heart.* 2006;92:1274-1277.

Oxygen Saturation Trends Immediately After Birth

Rabi Y, Yee W, Chen SY, et al (Univ of Calgary, Alta, Canada; Partnership for Research and Education in Mothers and Infants Inst, Calgary, Alta, Canada; Calgary Health Region, Alta, Canada)
J Pediatr 148:590-594, 2006

Objective.—To describe the changes in oxygen saturation (SpO_2) in healthy infants during the first 10 minutes of life.

Study Design.—In this observational study, infants ≥35 weeks gestation at birth who did not require supplemental oxygen had continuous recordings taken of the preductal SpO_2 over the first 10 minutes of life.

Results.—A total of 115 infants were analyzed. On average, infants delivered by cesarean delivery had a 3% lower SpO_2 than infants delivered by vaginal delivery (95% confidence interval [CI] = −5.8 to −0.7; $P = .01$). Infants born by cesarean delivery also took longer (risk ratio, 1.79) to reach

a stable $SpO_2 \geq 85\%$ (95% CI = 1.02 to 3.14; P = .04). At 5 minutes of age, median SpO_2 values (interquartile range) were 87% (80% to 95%) for infants delivered vaginally and 81% (75% to 83%) for those delivered through cesarean section. The median SpO_2 did not reach 90% until 8 minutes of age in either group.

Conclusions.—The process of transitioning to a normal postnatal oxygen saturation requires more than 5 minutes in healthy newborns breathing room air.

▶ In recent years, there has been growing interest in using SpO_2 monitoring to routinely guide resuscitation management in the delivery room. The data from the study abstracted, however, suggest that early oximetry readings must be interpreted in light of what normal findings may be in populations of otherwise healthy babies. Essentially, all newborns are "cyanotic" at birth. Recognize that the arterial SpO_2 in the normal fetus is only 20 mm Hg, equivalent to an SpO_2 of only about 60%. Several studies using pulse oximetry in the delivery room have documented that it takes more than 5 minutes for a newborn undergoing normal postnatal transition to attain an SpO_2 of greater than 80%. On average, it takes up to 10 minutes for a baby to reach 90% SpO_2. Administering 100% oxygen to a spontaneously breathing neonate, based only on visual assessment of cyanosis, may be not only unnecessarily invasive, but could lead to potential complications related to hyperoxia. When supplemental oxygen is used, it would be ideal to use an amount, and in a manner, that essentially mimics the normal rate of increase in SpO_2 observed in otherwise healthy newborns. Also note that infants born by cesarean section do have modestly lower SpO_2 levels and will require a longer period of time to reach a stable $SpO_2 \geq 85\%$ in the immediate newborn period in comparison with infants born vaginally.

J. A. Stockman III, MD

Achieved Versus Intended Pulse Oximeter Saturation in Infants Born Less Than 28 Weeks' Gestation: The AVIOx Study

Hagadorn JI, for the AVIOx Study Group (Connecticut Children's Med Ctr, Hartford; et al)
Pediatrics 118:1574-1582, 2006

Objective.—The objective of this study was to document pulse oximeter saturation levels achieved in the first 4 weeks of life in infants who were born at <28 weeks' gestation, compared with the levels that were targeted by local policy, and examine factors that are associated with compliance with the target range.

Methods.—Infants who were <28 weeks' gestation and ≤96 hours of age were enrolled in a prospective, multicenter cohort study. Oximetry data were collected with masked signal-extraction oximeters for a 72-hour period in each of the first 4 weeks of life. Data were compared with the pulse oximeter saturation target range prescribed by local institutional policy.

Factors that were associated with intended range compliance were identified with hierarchical modeling.

Results.—Fourteen centers from 3 countries enrolled 84 infants with mean ± SD birth weight of 863 ± 208 g and gestational age of 26 ± 1.4 weeks. Oxygen saturation policy limits ranged between 83% and 92% for lower limits and 92% and 98% for upper limits. For infants who received respiratory support, median pulse oximeter saturation level achieved was 95%. Center-specific medial levels were within the intended range at 12 centers. Centers maintained infants within their intended range 16% to 64% of the time but were above range 20% to 73% of the time. In hierarchical modeling, wider target ranges, higher target range upper limits, presence of a policy of setting oximeter alarms close to the target range limits, and lower gestational age were associated with improved target range compliance.

Conclusions.—Success with maintaining the intended pulse oximeter saturation range varied substantially among centers, among patients within centers, and for individual patients over time. Most noncompliance was above the intended range. Methods for improving compliance and the effect of improved compliance on neonatal outcomes require additional research.

▶ There is an old saying that you can never have too much of a good thing. However, we certainly learned that was not the case when it came to supplying oxygen to preterm babies. After learning that, however, we also learned that walking the thin line of not giving too much oxygen also resulted in periods of hypoxemia in some babies. This resulted in poor growth, cardiopulmonary complications of chronic lung disease, neurodevelopmental disabilities, and increased mortality. What the report by Hagadorn and colleagues shows us is just how difficult it is to navigate the complexities of adequate oxygen targeting in preterm babies. Opinions still seem to vary widely about whether we should be shooting for an oxygen saturation between 85% and 90% during the first weeks of life for babies in our neonatal intensive care units. However, no one argues about trying to avoid oxygen saturations of more than 95%. The rub is that babies seem to do their own thing. They vary with regard to their oxygen requirements despite our best efforts to provide sustained safe levels of oxygen. This report tells us that, half the time, we are missing the "sweet zone" of desired oxygen saturations. For infants who are receiving respiratory support, the median pulse oximeter saturation level ran 95%. Centers maintained infants within their intended range, varying from a low of 16% in some locales to a high of 64%, with the latter being the "best" in the group.

You may also want to read the commentary by Greenspan and Goldsmith[1]; it provides us with some suggestions for improving this situation. We need improved saturation monitors, and we need to apply performance-improvement principles to the process of oxygen monitoring. The commentary also suggests that providers need to understand that cumulative oxygen saturations over time represent a bell-shaped curve and that the role of the healthcare team is to minimize the tails of the curve in both directions. That is what quality improvement is all about: narrowing the variation.

Hopefully, someday we will have better technologies that will allow us to automatically vary oxygen saturations on the basis of numbers as they are

coming from pulse oximeters. Even with such technology, careful monitoring of the monitoring would be necessary. In the meantime, reducing fluctuations in oxygen saturation requires personnel who are highly trained and totally dedicated to the purpose of fine-tuning these babies.

While on the topic of oxygen, here is a group of little known facts about mountain climbing and oxygenation. At one time, it was thought that it would be physiologically impossible to climb Everest with or without oxygen. In 1953, Hillary and Tenzing proved that it was possible to reach the summit with oxygen and in 1978, Messner and Habler demonstrated that it was possible without oxygen. It would seem logical to assume that climbing Everest might have become an altogether less deadly activity. However, by mid 2006, the body count for that year had already reached 15, the most since the disaster of 1996 when 16 people died, 8 in one night following an unexpected storm. An analysis of the death rate on Mount Everest between 1980 and 2002 has found that the death rate has not changed over the years with about one death for every 10 successful ascents. A sobering statistic for anyone who reaches the summit is that you have approximately a one in 20 chance of not making it down.

So why are so many people dying on Mount Everest? The main reasons that people die while climbing Mount Everest (or other high altitude sites) are injuries and exhaustion. However, there is also a large proportion of climbers who die from altitude-related illness, specifically from high altitude cerebral edema and high altitude pulmonary edema. Part of the problem relates to the fact that unfortunately it is difficult to gain experience of what it is like climbing above camp 3 of Everest (8,300 meters) without actually climbing Mount Everest. Climbers invariably do not know what their actual abilities are above 8,300 meters until they try it. High altitude climbers going above 8,300 meters are now being told there is a very good rule of thumb that they should follow in trying to decide whether they are going to make it or should turn around. In general, one's rate of ascent should be no longer than 1 to 1.5 hours per 100 meters. If you are too slow, this means that something is wrong and your chances of not making it off the mountain are greatly increased. Unfortunately, when the summit is in sight, advice such as this is often ignored.[2]

J. A. Stockman III, MD

References

1. Greenspan JS, Goldsmith JP. Oxygen therapy in preterm infants: hitting the target. *Pediatrics*. 2006;118:1740-1741.
2. Sutherland AI. Why are so many people dying on Everest? *BMJ* 2006;333:452.

Inhaled Nitric Oxide in Preterm Infants Undergoing Mechanical Ventilation

Ballard RA, for the NO CLD Study Group (Children's Hosp of Philadelphia; et al)
N Engl J Med 355:343-353, 2006

Background.—Bronchopulmonary dysplasia in premature infants is associated with prolonged hospitalization, as well as abnormal pulmonary and neurodevelopmental outcome. In animal models, inhaled nitric oxide improves both gas exchange and lung structural development, but the use of this therapy in infants at risk for bronchopulmonary dysplasia is controversial.

Methods.—We conducted a randomized, stratified, double-blind, placebo-controlled trial of inhaled nitric oxide at 21 centers involving infants with a birth weight of 1250 g or less who required ventilatory support between 7 and 21 days of age. Treated infants received decreasing concentrations of nitric oxide, beginning at 20 ppm, for a minimum of 24 days. The primary outcome was survival without bronchopulmonary dysplasia at 36 weeks of postmenstrual age.

Results.—Among 294 infants receiving nitric oxide and 288 receiving placebo birth weight (766 g and 759 g, respectively), gestational age (26 weeks in both groups), and other characteristics were similar. The rate of survival without bronchopulmonary dysplasia at 36 weeks of postmenstrual age was 43.9 percent in the group receiving nitric oxide and 36.8 percent in the placebo group (P=0.042). The infants who received inhaled nitric oxide were discharged sooner (P=0.04) and received supplemental oxygen therapy for a shorter time (P=0.006). There were no short-term safety concerns.

Conclusions.—Inhaled nitric oxide therapy improves the pulmonary outcome for premature infants who are at risk for bronchopulmonary dysplasia when it is started between 7 and 21 days of age and has no apparent short-term adverse effects.

Early Inhaled Nitric Oxide Therapy in Premature Newborns with Respiratory Failure

Kinsella JP, Cutter GR, Walsh WF, et al (Univ of Colorado, Denver; Children's Hosp, Denver; Univ of Alabama at Birmingham; et al)
N Engl J Med 355:354-364, 2006

Background.—The safety and efficacy of early, low-dose, prolonged therapy with inhaled nitric oxide in premature newborns with respiratory failure are uncertain.

Methods.—We performed a multicenter, randomized trial involving 793 newborns who were 34 weeks of gestational age or less and had respiratory failure requiring mechanical ventilation. Newborns were randomly assigned to receive either inhaled nitric oxide (5 ppm) or placebo gas for 21 days or until extubation, with stratification according to birth weight (500 to 749 g, 750 to 999 g, or 1000 to 1250 g). The primary efficacy outcome was a composite of death or bronchopulmonary dysplasia at 36 weeks of postmenstrual age. Secondary safety outcomes included severe intracranial hemorrhage, periventricular leukomalacia, and ventriculomegaly.

Results.—Overall, there was no significant difference in the incidence of death or bronchopulmonary dysplasia between patients receiving inhaled nitric oxide and those receiving placebo (71.6 percent vs. 75.3 percent, P=0.24). However, for infants with a birth weight between 1000 and 1250 g, as compared with placebo, inhaled nitric oxide therapy reduced the incidence of bronchopulmonary dysplasia (29.8 percent vs. 59.6 percent); for the cohort overall, such treatment reduced the combined end point of intracranial hemorrhage, periventricular leukomalacia, or ventriculomegaly (17.5 percent vs. 23.9 percent, P=0.03) and of periventricular leukomalacia alone (5.2 percent vs. 9.0 percent, P=0.048). Inhaled nitric oxide therapy did not increase the incidence of pulmonary hemorrhage or other adverse events.

Conclusions.—Among premature newborns with respiratory failure, low-dose inhaled nitric oxide did not reduce the overall incidence of bronchopulmonary dysplasia, except among infants with a birth weight of at least 1000 g, but it did reduce the overall risk of brain injury.

▶ Bronchopulmonary dysplasia, commonly also called chronic lung disease of prematurity, remains a significant problem for premature infants. More than one third of those surviving with a birthweight of less than 1250 g will have this problem as defined by the need for supplemental oxygen at 36 weeks of postmenstrual age. Most of these infants are ones who have required mechanical ventilation for at least 1 week postpartum.

There are a variety of maneuvers that neonatologists have used to treat the respiratory distress syndrome so commonly seen in premature infants to decrease the prevalence of the subsequent development of bronchopulmonary dysplasia. Selective pulmonary vasodilatation with inhaled nitric oxide clearly has been shown to improve oxygenation and to reduce the need for extracorporeal membrane oxygenation in term infants with persistent pulmonary hypertension. Early reports have shown improved oxygenation in preterm infants with severe respiratory failure. These early studies have also suggested that early treatment with nitric oxide might decrease the risk of chronic lung injury, although the data have been conflicting, at least until the report abstracted appeared by Ballard et al (Inhaled nitric oxide in preterm infants undergoing mechanical ventilation) and another by Kinsella et al (Early inhaled nitric oxide therapy in premature newborns with respiratory failure). In the clinical trial undertaken by Kinsella et al, infants who were less than 48 hours of age receiving mechanical ventilation were randomly assigned to receive inhaled nitric oxide at a dose of 5 ppm or nitrogen placebo for 21 days or until they no longer required mechanical ventilation. Consistent with several other trials, the results indicated no overall difference between the groups in the combined primary outcome (death or bronchopulmonary dysplasia), which occurred in approximately three quarters of the infants. If one looks at the group of infants with a birthweight of 1000 g to 1250 g, however, inhaled nitric oxide treatment did reduce the combined primary outcome and bronchopulmonary dysplasia rates. A lower rate of severe intracranial hemorrhage was also seen.

In the study of Ballard et al, infants were enrolled who were ventilator-dependent at 7 to 21 days of age. Infants were assigned to a 24-day course of nitrogen placebo or inhaled nitric oxide at an initial dose of 20 ppm for 48 to 96 hours, with the dose reduced at weekly intervals to 10, 5, and 2 ppm. Nitric oxide treatment improved survival at 36 weeks postmenstrual age and reduced the duration of oxygen therapy and hospitalization.

So the question is, does inhaled nitric oxide now have a role in the treatment of preterm infants with respiratory failure? This question was addressed in a commentary that accompanied the Ballard et al article.[1] It is proposed that in the most critically ill infants with extremely low birthweights, inhaled nitric oxide does not seem to improve survival or the development of bronchopulmonary dysplasia, and since such treatment may be associated with brain injury or increased mortality in some groups, it cannot be recommended. Nonetheless, the reports of Ballard et al and Kinsella et al suggest the possibility of benefit in less critically ill infants. Unfortunately, there are many unknown issues here involving the appropriate effective dose, duration of therapy, time of initiation and the appropriate selection of infants who might benefit from this approach.

Clearly we need more studies of nitric oxide and its use in preterm babies with respiratory distress. Long-term follow-up will be needed especially given the experience with postnatal dexamethasone treatment, which showed early promise in terms of short-term benefits, but then was found to be associated with an increased risk of neurodevelopmental impairment. One should also factor in cost for nitric oxide therapy, which runs about $3000 per day. You can bet that payors are not going to shell out big bucks for this therapy on a routine basis until we know more about its benefits.

J. A. Stockman III, MD

Reference

1. Stark AR. Inhaled NO for preterm infants—getting to yes? *N Engl J Med.* 2006;355:404-406.

The Epidemiology of Meconium Aspiration Syndrome: Incidence, Risk Factors, Therapies, and Outcome

Dargaville PA, for the Australian and New Zealand Neonatal Network (Royal Hobart Hosp, Australia; et al)
Pediatrics 117:1712-1720, 2006

Objective.—We sought to examine, in a large cohort of infants within a definable population of live births, the incidence, risk factors, treatments, complications, and outcomes of meconium aspiration syndrome (MAS).

Design.—Data were gathered on all of the infants in Australia and New Zealand who were intubated and mechanically ventilated with a primary diagnosis of MAS (MAS$_{INT}$) between 1995 and 2002, inclusive. Information on all of the live births during the same time period was obtained from perinatal data registries.

Results.—MAS_{INT} occurred in 1061 of 2,490,862 live births (0.43 of 1000), with a decrease in incidence from 1995 to 2002. A higher risk of MAS_{INT} was noted at advanced gestation, with 34% of cases born beyond 40 weeks, compared with 16% of infants without MAS. Fetal distress requiring obstetric intervention was noted in 51% of cases, and 42% were delivered by cesarean section. There was a striking association between low 5-minute Apgar score and MAS_{INT}. In addition, risk of MAS_{INT} was higher where maternal ethnicity was Pacific Islander or indigenous Australian and was also increased after planned home birth. Uptake of exogenous surfactant, high-frequency ventilation, and inhaled nitric oxide increased considerably during the study period, with >50% of infants receiving ≥ 1 of these therapies by 2002. Risk of air leak was 9.6% overall, with an apparent reduction to 5.3% in 2001–2002. The duration of intubation remained constant throughout the study period (median: 3 days), whereas duration of oxygen therapy and length of hospital stay increased. Death related to MAS occurred in 24 infants (2.5% of the MAS_{INT} cohort; 0.96 per 100,000 live births).

Conclusions.—The incidence of MAS_{INT} in the developed world is low and seems to be decreasing. Risk of MAS_{INT} is significantly greater in the presence of fetal distress and low Apgar score, as well as Pacific Islander and indigenous Australian ethnicity. The increased use of innovative respiratory supports has not altered the duration of mechanical ventilation.

▶ At least one third of infants with meconium aspiration syndrome will require intubation and mechanical ventilation. Some will go on to require high-frequency ventilation, inhaled nitric oxide, and surfactant administration. Over the past couple of decades, we have begun to recognize which infants are at highest risk for meconium aspiration syndrome. The presence of fetal compromise, indicated by abnormalities of fetal heart rate tracings and/or poor Apgar scores, is known to increase the risk of this problem. Cesarean delivery is also associated with a greater incidence of the problem. In addition, there is an apparent relationship between maternal ethnicity and risk of meconium-stained amniotic fluid and the suggestion in several reports of an increased risk of meconium aspiration syndrome in black Americans or Africans and Pacific Islanders. It has been known for some time that advanced gestation is a risk factor both for meconium-stained amniotic fluid and for meconium aspiration syndrome.

The report abstracted comes from a collaborative database of the Australian and New Zealand Neonatal Network, supplemented by data from other perinatal data registries. The data show that the low incidence of meconium aspiration syndrome and its apparent reduction during the period of study have declined and do confirm that modern obstetric practices can, for the most part, interrupt the chain of events that results in significant aspiration of meconium. This reduction in incidence cannot be ascribed to more zealous delivery room management, in particular, tracheal suctioning. In fact, routine intubation of the trachea after the observation of meconium-stained amniotic fluid has been largely abandoned in Australia and New Zealand largely on the basis of the publication of a randomized, controlled trial finding no benefit from this intervention in an infant who is otherwise born vigorous.[1] Careful attention to the risk factors for meconium aspiration syndrome seems to have been the reason why there has been a reduction in the prevalence of this problem in New Zealand and Australia, and most likely in other developed countries as well.

Despite the fact that the incidence of meconium aspiration syndrome requiring intubation is low and may be decreasing, it is still a problem. In this report, we see that the mortality risk for ventilated infants with meconium aspiration syndrome remains significant with an overall mortality rate of 6.6%. Pneumothorax continues to be one of the most important complications of the syndrome occurring in almost 10% of ventilated infants.

One final note about meconium aspiration syndrome and that is that its prevalence seems to be higher with home deliveries, a reminder that home delivery should be reserved for pizza.

J. A. Stockman III, MD

Reference

1. Wiswell TE, Gannon CM, Jacob J, et al. Delivery room management of the apparently vigorous meconium-stained neonate: results of the multicenter, international collaborative trial. *Pediatrics.* 2000;105:1-7.

Inhibition of Meconium-Induced Cytokine Expression and Cell Apoptosis by Pretreatment With Captopril

Zagariya A, Bhat R, Navale S, et al (Michael Reese Hosp, Chicago; Univ of Illinois at Chicago)
Pediatrics 117:1722-1728, 2006

Objective.—To study whether pretreatment of newborn lungs by captopril inhibits meconium-induced lung injury and inflammatory cytokine expression.

Design.—Four groups of 2-week-old rabbit pups were used for the study: group 1, saline instilled rabbits; group 2, captopril-pretreated rabbits; group 3, meconium-instilled rabbits; and group 4, captopril-pretreated and then meconium-instilled rabbits. Each group was studied at different time points: 0, 2, 4, 8, and 24 hours after instillation of meconium. Experiments were done at the University of Illinois and Michael Reese Hospital at Chicago. After treatment and instillation of meconium, the right lung was fixed with formalin, and 2-μm slices were obtained for immunohistochemistry. The left lung was used for obtaining of lung lavage and measurement of total proteins (for enzyme-linked immunosorbent assay) and mRNA (for reverse transcription-polymerase chain reaction) purification.

Results.—We found that meconium induces inflammatory cytokine expression and apoptotic lung cell death. In situ end labeling revealed a dramatic DNA fragmentation in the meconium group, which supports the presence of apoptosis. Using enzyme-linked immunosorbent assay, we demonstrated increase of interleukin 6 and interleukin 8 cytokines in meconium-instilled lungs, which were significantly decreased in captopril-pretreated lungs. Captopril pretreatment also decreased meconium-induced cell death and angiotensinogen expression. We believe this effect is explained by the ability of captopril to decrease processing of ANGEN to angiotensinogen (ANG) I and finally to ANG II. It suggests that captopril inhibits ANG II-induced lung cell apoptosis.

Conclusion.—Our results demonstrate that captopril pretreatment significantly inhibits meconium-induced lung cell death, cytokine, and ANGEN expression in newborn lungs.

▶ The Dargaville et al report (The epidemiology of meconium aspiration syndrome: incidence, risk factors, therapies, and outcome) gives us information on the current prevalence of meconium aspiration syndrome. This report from Chicago tells us a great deal about the pathophysiology of the disorder including specifics about the way in which it does damage to a newborn infant's lungs. Previously, these investigators showed that expression of cytokines and cell death by apoptosis in the lungs of newborn infants are the consequences of meconium aspiration. Apoptosis refers to programmed cell death as opposed to cell death that occurs from other causes. Programmed cell death specifically means that some mechanism causes a cell to trigger its own machinery to kill itself. Cell apoptosis is usually accompanied by significant cell loss, loss of cell-cell contacts, aggregation of chromatin, and the appearance of apoptotic bodies, which are phagocytized by macrophages and are shed into the lumen of the lung.

The importance of this report is that it shows that captopril, an angiotensin-converting enzyme inhibitor may be helpful in the management of meconium aspiration syndrome. Meconium-induced apoptosis is activated by a strong vasoconstrictor, angiotensin II, which is a final step of angiotensinogen degradation in the cell. Apoptosis is modulated by 2 types of angiotensin II receptors. ACE inhibitors such as captopril, or selective antagonists of these receptors, will decrease levels of angiotensin II or limit its action and therefore may significantly inhibit apoptotic cell death. The work of the investigators in Chicago shows that meconium induces expression of inflammatory cytokines and expression of angiotensinogen genes resulting in massive cell lung death by apoptosis. Pretreatment with captopril inhibits these findings leading to the suggestion that captopril may play an important role in reducing meconium-induced inflammatory lung injury and further supports its potential use a new therapeutic intervention for meconium aspiration syndrome.

Sure as shooting you will see clinical trials of angiotensin-converting enzyme inhibitors and also of selective receptor antagonists sometime in the not widely distant future.

J. A. Stockman III, MD

Laparotomy versus Peritoneal Drainage for Necrotizing Enterocolitis and Perforation

Moss RL, Dimmitt RA, Barnhart DC, et al (Yale Univ, New Haven, Conn; Univ of Alabama, Birmingham; Stanford Univ, Calif; et al)
N Engl J Med 354:2225-2234, 2006

Background.—Perforated necrotizing enterocolitis is a major cause of morbidity and mortality in premature infants, and the optimal treatment is uncertain. We designed this multicenter randomized trial to compare outcomes of primary peritoneal drainage with laparotomy and bowel resection in preterm infants with perforated necrotizing enterocolitis.

Methods.—We randomly assigned 117 preterm infants (delivered before 34 weeks of gestation) with birth weights less than 1500 g and perforated necrotizing enterocolitis at 15 pediatric centers to undergo primary peritoneal drainage or laparotomy with bowel resection. Postoperative care was standardized. The primary outcome was survival at 90 days postoperatively. Secondary outcomes included dependence on parenteral nutrition 90 days postoperatively and length of hospital stay.

Results.—At 90 days postoperatively, 19 of 55 infants assigned to primary peritoneal drainage had died (34.5 percent), as compared with 22 of 62 infants assigned to laparotomy (35.5 percent, P=0.92). The percentages of infants who depended on total parenteral nutrition were 17 of 36 (47.2 percent) in the peritoneal-drainage group and 16 of 40 (40.0 percent) in the laparotomy group (P=0.53). The mean (±SD) length of hospitalization for the 76 infants who were alive 90 days after operation was similar in the primary peritoneal-drainage and laparotomy groups (126±58 days and 116±56 days, respectively; P=0.43). Subgroup analyses stratified according to the presence or absence of radiographic evidence of extensive necrotizing enterocolitis (pneumatosis intestinalis), gestational age of less than 25 weeks, and serum pH less than 7.30 at presentation showed no significant advantage of either treatment in any group.

Conclusions.—The type of operation performed for perforated necrotizing enterocolitis does not influence survival or other clinically important early outcomes in preterm infants.

▶ Necrotizing enterocolitis is a risk that low birth weight infants entertain. Although necrotizing enterocolitis has many causes, the final common pathway leading to intestinal necrosis and perforation is thought to be intestinal ischemia and the invasion of bacteria through an immature mucosal barrier. When perforation occurs, it is followed by peritonitis and systemic sepsis resulting in a high risk of death. The usual management of this problem has been a laparotomy with resection of all necrotic intestine and intestinal diversion. Such an approach is a hand-me-down from adult surgery, where it is considered unthinkable to leave necrotic intestine in place.

It was more than 3 decades ago that surgeons in Canada reported on a series of 6 infants with extremely low birth weights who were in desperate shape and who were treated with a temporizing primary peritoneal-drainage procedure. Three of the infants survived and 2 of these infants did not require a second operation.[1] The idea here was that in a critically ill infant, it would be safer simply to relieve increased intra-abdominal pressure, drain the infection, and allow the physiologic status of an infant to improve before a more definitive operative procedure. As you might suspect, many viewed this approach with disdain. It hardly caught on, although there were a small number of reports with similar rates of success in the interval 3 decades.

The study by Moss et al represents a multi-institutional, randomized, controlled trial comparing primary peritoneal drainage with laparotomy and bowel resection for the treatment of intestinal perforation among 117 premature infants with birth weights less than 1500 g. The primary outcome of the study was survivorship at 90 days postoperatively. Secondary outcomes included dependence on parenteral nutrition 90 days postoperatively and lengths of the hospital stay. No significant differences were observed between the groups in any of these outcomes. This would, at first blush, appear to imply that because primary peritoneal drainage is less invasive, simpler and less costly in comparison with laparotomy, it should be used in all infants with birth weights of less than 1500 g who have intestinal perforation secondary to necrotizing enterocolitis.

Before embracing the results of this study, it would be important to read the commentary that accompanied it in the *New England Journal of Medicine*.[2] The commentary suggests that the Moss study is not the final word on the debate about whether to operate or not operate. One hundred seventeen patients is a lot of patients, but when one breaks these patients down by subcategories, one finds an inability to provide clear guidance for patients within certain weight ranges. Also, the follow-up was insufficient to permit comparisons of neurodevelopmental outcomes between the 2 groups of patients. These limitations not withstanding, the results support the conclusion that, at least among neonates with birth weights of less than 1000 g, there is no apparent difference in short-term survival, length of hospitalization, or requirement for parenteral nutrition between infants who undergo primary peritoneal drainage and those who undergo laparotomy. Thus, as far as we know, primary peritoneal drainage is a reasonable treatment approach particularly in very tiny infants with tenuous health.

All of us should laud the study of Moss et al. It is hard to put together large numbers of patients with these types of problems and it is only by such an approach that we can develop critical evidence to help guide decision making. Thank you Dr Moss, et al.

J. A. Stockman III, MD

References

1. Ein SH, Marshall DG, Girvan D. Peritoneal drainage under local anesthesia for perforations from necrotizing enterocolitis. *J Pediatr Surg.* 1977;12:963-967.
2. Flake AW. Necrotizing enterocolitis in preterm infants—is laparotomy necessary? *N Engl J Med.* 2006;354:2275-2276.

Palliative care for prenatally diagnosed lethal fetal abnormality

Breeze ACG, Lees CC, Kumar A, et al (Addenbrooke's Hosp, Cambridge, England)

Arch Dis Child Fetal Neonatal Ed 92:56-58, 2007

Diagnosis of lethal fetal abnormality raises challenging decisions for parents and clinicians. Most parents opt for termination, which may include feticide. Advances in imaging seem unlikely to lead to earlier diagnoses. Perinatal palliative care offers an alternative. Parental decision making and the clinical aspects of perinatal palliative care were studied after a prenatal diagnosis of lethal fetal abnormality in 20 pregnancies. 40% of parents chose to continue the pregnancy and pursue perinatal palliative care. Six of these eight babies were liveborn and lived for between 1 ½ h and 3 weeks.

▶ The dilemma that a couple must face when presented with the fact that their unborn child has a lethal fetal abnormality is incomprehensible. Whereas some couples will request termination of the pregnancy, some parents would rather continue the pregnancy, particularly if the diagnosis is made late in the second trimester, since the ending of the pregnancy could involve feticide as the alternative. The decision to carry a pregnancy to term in such circumstances obviously is not an easy one given the potential complications associated with delivery and the anticipated care and inevitable death of the newborn.

In this report from Cambridge, England, we see that about 40% of couples who learn during a pregnancy that their baby has a fatal anomaly or abnormality will make a positive decision not to terminate the pregnancy, preferring to pursue perinatal palliative care. The reasons for this decision are probably multiple. For these couples it may help them to avoid feelings of guilt and allow them and other family members to spend time with, and prepare for, the baby's death. If the decision is to allow the pregnancy to naturally end and then to begin palliative care, this should be prepared for with an advanced individualized care plan with discussions to include obstetricians, neonatal staff, parents, and family. Guidelines for such palliative care have been described.[1]

Data from this report and others show that most babies with lethal abnormalities are born alive when parents decide to continue a pregnancy. When looking at the experience in retrospect, parents who choose this approach seem to give positive feedback about their decision and the care that is provided. Needless to say, it is critical that perinatal staff receive the support that they also require, psychological and otherwise.

Palliative perinatal care in the circumstances described really does not represent a moral or ethical dilemma, but rather a choice that parents and families face, fortunately infrequently. More frequent, however, are the moral and ethical choices families deal with every day when working with a severely disabled youngster within the family. Take, for example, the case of Ashley X. In 2006, this 9-year-old with static encephalopathy—who is in an infant state and cannot sit up, roll over, hold an object, walk or talk—received national attention. In a radical move, she has been receiving growth attenuation treatment designed to keep her the size of a 6-year-old with the goal to improve her quality of life and make it easier for her parents to continue to care for her at home. More controversially, the girl also had a hysterectomy to eliminate the menstrual cycle and associated cramps as well as breast bud removal to avoid the development of large breasts. Ashley's case history was published in the *Archives of Pediatrics and Adolescent Medicine.*[2] Ashley's management created a worldwide debate within the medical community, and this debate motivated Ashley's parents, a professional couple from Seattle, to go public, naming their daughter and posting family photographs on the Internet explaining the basis of the family's circumstances (http://ashleytreatment.spaces.live.com/blog/). The Internet site took a million hits in the first 48 hours of 2007 and topped the health section of Google News for several days. More than 400 press articles worldwide were published related to the moral and ethical circumstances of Ashley's care. Ashley is expected to stay at about 4'5" all her life and to continue to weigh 75 pounds. Her parents' actions appear to be motivated only by a desire to improve her quality of life.

To read more about difficult moral choices such as the care being provided to Ashley X, read the important editorial in the *British Medical Journal* on this topic.[3]

J. A. Stockman III, MD

References

1. Calhoun BC, Napolitano P, Terry M, Bussey C, Hoeldtke NJ. Perinatal hospice. Comprehensive care for the family of the fetus with a lethal condition. *J Reprod Med.* 2003;48:343-348.
2. Gunther DF, Diekema DS. Attenuating growth in children with profound developmental disability: a new approach to an old dilemma. *Arch Pediatr Adolesc Med.* 2006;160:1013-1017.
3. Coombes R. Ashley X: a difficult moral choice. *BMJ.* 2007;334:72-73.

Provision of taped conversations with neonatologists to mothers of babies in intensive care: randomised controlled trial
Koh THHG, Butow PN, Coory M, et al (Inst of Women's and Children's Health, Douglas, QLD, Australia; James Cook Univ, Douglas, QLD, Australia; Univ of Sydney; et al)
BMJ 334:28-31, 2007

Objective.—To determine whether providing mothers of babies in neonatal intensive care units with audiotapes of their conversations with a neonatologist improves recall of information and psychological wellbeing.

Design.—Randomised, single blinded trial.

Setting.—Neonatal intensive care unit, North Queensland, Australia.

Participants.—200 mothers of babies in a neonatal intensive care unit.

Interventions.—Mothers given (n=102) or not given (n=98) audiotapes of their conversations with a neonatologist.

Main Outcome Measures.—Recall of information, attitudes to and use of the tape, satisfaction with conversations, postnatal depression, anxiety, general health, and stress about parenting, at 10 days and four and 12 months.

Results.—91% (n=93) of mothers in the tape group listened to the tape (once by day 10, twice by four months, and three times by 12 months; range 1-10). At 10 days and four months, mothers in the tape group recalled significantly more information about diagnosis, treatment, and outcome than mothers in the control group. At four months mothers in the tape group were 75% more likely to recall all of the information about treatment than mothers in the control group (59% *v* 34%; risk ratio 1.75, 95% confidence interval 1.27 to 2.4). Six mothers, all in the control group, could not recall their conversations. No statistically significant differences were found between the groups in satisfaction with conversations (10 days), postnatal depression and anxiety scores (10 days, four and 12 months), and stress about parenting (12 months).

Conclusion.—Providing the mothers of babies in neonatal intensive care units with audiotapes of conversations with a neonatologist enhanced their recall of information (up to four months). The taped conversations did not affect the mothers' wellbeing or satisfaction with the neonatologist.

▶ If there is one component of the movement to improve the quality of care here in the United States that deserves more attention than anything else, it is communication. We see in this report a randomized controlled trial by Koh et al that investigates whether providing mothers of babies in a neonatal intensive care unit with audiotapes of their conversations with a neonatologist improves recall of information and psychological wellbeing. Mothers receiving these audiotapes definitely do recall significantly more information about diagnosis, treatment, and outcome than women in the control group when assessed at 10 days and at four months after their babies' discharge from the nursery.

Any communication strategy in any setting has to be effective, practical, and affordable. You will have to decide whether recording your conversations with a family and giving the family that recording makes sense. There are a number of practical issues here. Cassette tapes are becoming increasingly obsolete in today's technologically advanced society. At the same time, however, more recent formats like compact discs and MP3 files are perhaps more appropriate but hardly universally used. Here in the United States, any lawyer worth his or her salt would tell you that a taped conversation is technically a part of a medical record and therefore absolutely confidential with respect to HIPPA compliance and requirements for storage and retrieval of the information. In reality, according to our legal system, a taped conversation, once created, may need to be stored indefinitely for medical legal reasons in this bummer of a world in which we live.

Before there were tape recorders, compact discs, and MP3 players, in addition to the spoken word, we often gave parents written materials. Most of us still do. If we need to improve communication in this regard, we need to improve our written forms of communication as well. The written word will always remain a practical tool and one worthy of assessment for the purposes of quality improvement.

Let's close this comment with a query about gender and birth rates. Historical data show that during times of societal crises, fewer boys than girls seem to be born. Why might this be? At times of stress, it may very well be that the weaker, male fetuses miscarry more often than the more "naturally stronger" females, perhaps explaining why live male births decline at times of societal crises, such as natural disasters and economic recessions. Rather than putting this phenomenon down to a stress response that ends up damaging unborn babies, Swedish researchers say research data support an alternative hypothesis that stressed mothers actively "cull" weaker fetuses.[1] The occurrences associated with September 11, 2001 provide an opportunity to study the relationship between stress and not only birth rate, but also birth gender. Anxiety and stress in New York City in the aftermath of the terrorist attack on the World Trade Center may have resulted in the birth of fewer boys months later, the research shows. Based on more than 700,000 births in New York City between January 1996 and June 2002, a study shows that the birth-sex ratio for the city dropped to below 1 in the January after the attacks—its lowest level ever.[2] One theory is that the stress of the attack, particularly in women in the second and early trimesters of their pregnancy, resulted in a disproportionate loss of male fetuses, thus lowering the odds of a male birth. Previous research has suggested that the sex ratio falls in populations subjected to external stressors, with the odds of a male birth falling with earthquakes, political and social upheavals, and economic downturns. Another explanation is that stress may reduce the conception of boys.[3]

J. A. Stockman III, MD

References

1. Catalano R, Bruckner T. Secondary sex ratios and male lifespan: damaged or culled cohorts. *Proc Natl Acad Sci USA.* 2006;103:1639-1643.
2. Catalano R, Bruckner T, Marks AR, Eskenazi B. Exogenous shocks to the human sex ratio: the case of September 11, 2001 in New York City. *Hum Reprod.* 2006;21:3127-3131.
3. Dobson R. Fewer boys born in New York after 9/11 attacks. *BMJ.* 2006;333:516.

15 Nutrition and Metabolism

Folic acid supplements and risk of facial clefts: national population based case-control study
Wilcox AJ, Lie RT, Solvoll K, et al (NIH, Durham, NC; Univ of Bergen, Norway; Univ of Oslo, Norway; et al)
BMJ 334:464-467, 2007

Objective.—To explore the role of folic acid supplements, dietary folates, and multivitamins in the prevention of facial clefts.

Design.—National population based case-control study.

Setting.—Infants born 1996-2001 in Norway.

Participants.—377 infants with cleft lip with or without cleft palate; 196 infants with cleft palate alone; 763 controls.

Main Outcome Measures.—Association of facial clefts with maternal intake of folic acid supplements, multivitamins, and folates in diet.

Results.—Folic acid supplementation during early pregnancy ($\geq$400 µg/day) was associated with a reduced risk of isolated cleft lip with or without cleft palate after adjustment for multivitamins, smoking, and other potential confounding factors (adjusted odds ratio 0.61, 95% confidence interval 0.39 to 0.96). Independent of supplements, diets rich in fruits, vegetables, and other high folate containing foods reduced the risk somewhat (adjusted odds ratio 0.75, 0.50 to 1.11). The lowest risk of cleft lip was among women with folate rich diets who also took folic acid supplements and multivitamins (0.36, 0.17 to 0.77). Folic acid provided no protection against cleft palate alone (1.07, 0.56 to 2.03).

Conclusions.—Folic acid supplements during early pregnancy seem to reduce the risk of isolated cleft lip (with or without cleft palate) by about a third. Other vitamins and dietary factors may provide additional benefit.

▶ Everyone knows about the need for dietary fortification with folic acid to prevent pregnancies affected by a neural tube defect (eg, spina bifida and anencephaly). Fortification of enriched cereal grain became mandatory in the United States in January 1998. Data from the 1999 to 2000 National Heath and Nutrition Examination Survey (NHANES) indicate that median serum folate concentrations in nonpregnant women of childbearing age increased substantially compared with concentrations before fortification was mandated. The US Public Health Service recommends that all women of childbearing age who are capable of becoming pregnant consume 400 µg of folic acid daily to reduce the number of cases of neural tube defect. Folic acid has been added to a range of enriched cereal-grain products (eg, breads, rolls, macaroni products, rice, corn meal, corn grits, and farina). In addition to improved dietary habits in folic acid fortification, the Public Health Service also has recommended the use of dietary supplements containing folic acid. The Centers for Disease Control and Prevention (CDC) now reports that the average serum folate level here in the United States has increased from 4.1 ng/mL to 13.0 ng/mL during the last 20 years.

This abstracted report from Norway underscores the need for folic acid supplementation, not only to prevent neural tube defects, but now also to reduce the risk of facial clefts. The risk of cleft lip with or without cleft palate is substantially reduced by folic acid supplementation during the month before becoming pregnant and in the first 2 months of pregnancy. The evidence is that folic acid supplementation in the amount of 40 µg or more a day definitively reduces the risk of isolated cleft lip with or without cleft palate by about one third. The evidence continues to mount about the need for folic acid supplementation. In some parts of the world, such as Europe, such supplementation is not routine and should be.

To close this commentary, here are a couple of questions regarding nutrition. You are in Great Britain on a sabbatical and have just given birth. The question is, where in Britain is the least friendliest place to breastfeed? Where is the friendliest place to breastfeed? Interestingly, McDonald's fast food chain was awarded the Boobie Prize for being the least friendly place in Britain to breastfeed in 2006. Ikea was awarded the prize for being the best. The Boobie Prize was launched by the National Childbirth Trust to give to companies for either appalling or outstanding treatment of breastfeeding mothers. Nominations were invited from anywhere in the United Kingdom.[1] Companies in Scotland, which has a law protecting a woman's right to breastfeed in public, received very few nominations for the worst place to breastfeed.

J. A. Stockman III, MD

Reference

1. Boobie Prize Web site. Available at: http://www.boobieprize.ncl.org.uk. Accessed June 21, 2007.

Effect of zinc supplementation on mortality in children aged 1–48 months: a community-based randomised placebo-controlled trial

Sazawal S, Black RE, Ramsan M, et al (Johns Hopkins Univ, Baltimore, Md; Public Health Lab-Ivo de Carneri, Wawi, Chake-Chake, Pemba, Zanzibar, Tanzania; UNICEF Tanzania, United Republic of Tanzania; et al)
Lancet 369:927-934, 2007

Background.—Studies from Asia have suggested that zinc supplementation can reduce morbidity and mortality in children, but evidence from malarious populations in Africa has been inconsistent. Our aim was to assess the effects of zinc supplementation on overall mortality in children in Pemba, Zanzibar.

Methods.—We enrolled 42,546 children aged 1–36 months, contributing a total of 56,507 child-years in a randomised, double-blind, placebo-controlled trial in Pemba, Zanzibar. Randomisation was by household. 21,274 children received daily supplementation with zinc 10 mg (5 mg in children younger than 12 months) for mean 484.7 days (SD 306.6). 21,272 received placebo. The primary endpoint was overall mortality, and analysis was by intention to treat.

Findings.—Overall, there was a non-significant 7% (95% CI −6% to 19%; $p = 0.29$) reduction in the relative risk of all-cause mortality associated with zinc supplementation.

Interpretation.—We believe that a meta-analysis of all studies of mortality and morbidity, will help to make evidence-based recommendations for the role of zinc supplementation in public health policy to improve mortality, morbidity, growth, and development in young children.

▶ Although vitamin A supplementation is not much of an issue here in the United States, it is worldwide. Deficiency of a few essential nutrients is recognized to greatly increase the risk of morbidity and mortality from infectious diseases in developing countries. Evidence for zinc as one such important micronutrient has emerged. Zinc supplementation has been shown to produce significant reduction in rates and severity of diarrhea and pneumonia. Reports from several clinical trials in Asian populations have noted that zinc supplementation significantly reduces child mortality rate. The same is true of studies from sub-Saharan Africa. It should be noted that the protective effects of zinc are not restricted to children with low baseline concentrations of zinc in plasma or serum.

In this study reported from Zanzibar, zinc supplementation did not result in a significant reduction in overall mortality rate in children 1 to 48 months in a population with a high rate of malaria. The effect did vary somewhat by age, however, with no effect on mortality rate in infants and a marginally significant 18% reduction in mortality in children 12 to 48 months old. This effect was mainly a consequence of fewer deaths from malaria and other infections. The results of this study should not diminish the importance of zinc as an agent to diminish the rate of infection. In Zanzibar, the principal problem has not been with the types of infections that zinc is most potent against as a preventative.

The World Health Organization has designed a strategy to focus on introduction of zinc for the treatment of diarrhea, not just for its prevention. The administration of zinc with oral rehydration salts for diarrhea has already shown some promising results. To read more about exactly how zinc does its job in improving a baby's immunity, read this report in detail. After iron, zinc is the second most abundant trace element in the body. It mediates many different physiologic functions. It is a necessary component of many metalloproteins, including those important for DNA replication and cell division and is crucial for maintenance of immunologic integrity. In studies of zinc deficiency, the production of tumor necrosis factor-α, interferon-C and interleukin-2 made by peripheral blood mononuclear cells is decreased, whereas products of certain other factors are unaffected. These immunologic changes are easily reversed with zinc supplementation. Because of its role in maintenance of cell integrity and immunity, zinc is thought to play a critically important role in the prevention of infectious diseases of a wide variety. The effect of zinc on diarrhea might also be related to its role in water and electrolyte transport, intestinal permeability, enzyme functions of enterocytes, enhanced intestinal tissue repair, or enhanced local immunity restricting bacterial overgrowth and causing early pathogen clearance.

J. A. Stockman III, MD

Fast Food Consumption and Breakfast Skipping: Predictors of Weight Gain from Adolescent to Adulthood in a Nationally Representative Sample

Niemeier HM, Raynor HA, Lloyd-Richardson EE, et al (Brown Med School, Providence, RI)
J Adolesc Health 39:842-849, 2006

Purpose.—To investigate whether fast food consumption and breakfast skipping are associated with weight gain during the transition from adolescence to adulthood.

Methods.—A prospective study of 9919 adolescents participating in Waves II (age range 11–21 years) and III (age range 18–27 years) of the National Longitudinal Study of Adolescent Health. BMI z scores (zBMI) were computed using the 2000 Centers for Disease Control and Prevention growth charts. Multivariate regression models assessed the relationship between Wave II fast food and breakfast consumption and change in fast food and breakfast consumption between Waves II and III and weight gain during the transition to adulthood.

Results.—Marked increases in fast food consumption and decreases in breakfast consumption occurred over the 5-year interval. Greater days of fast food consumption at Wave II predicted increased zBMI at Wave III. Fewer days of breakfast consumption at Wave II and decreases in breakfast consumption between Waves II and III predicted increased zBMI at Wave III.

Conclusions.—Fast food consumption and breakfast skipping increased during the transition to adulthood, and both dietary behaviors are associated with increased weight gain from adolescence to adulthood. These behaviors may be appropriate targets for intervention during this important transition.

▶ The Continuous Survey of Food Intake by Individuals found that in 1977-1978, the proportions of foods consumed from restaurants and fast food outlets was just 6.5%, and that in 1994-1996 the proportion had increased to 19.3%.[1] In a sample of almost 5000 students aged 11 to 18 years, approximately three quarters reported eating at a fast food restaurant within the prior 7 days.[2] All studies to date have shown that obese children and adolescents consume more fast food than their nonobese counterparts.

At the same time there has been a rising trend in fast food consumption by teens, there has also been a decline in breakfast consumption. This decline has coincided with an increase in the prevalence of obesity. Thus, it has been theorized that skipping breakfast may contribute to excess energy intake. Children who regularly eat breakfast consume a lower proportion of energy from fat and eat snacks that are lower in fat than children who skip breakfast. A number of studies have consistently found a positive relationship between breakfast skipping and measures of adiposity in children. There have been very few longitudinal studies of fast food and breakfast consumption and the effect of these behaviors on weight change over time, and no longitudinal studies have examined these behaviors during the important transition from adolescence to adulthood—thus, the purpose and value of the study reported from Rhode Island. The data from this nationally representative study are the first to show increases in fast food consumption and breakfast skipping during the transition from adolescence to adulthood. Importantly, greater fast food consumption and breakfast skipping during adolescence and increases in breakfast skipping from adolescence to young adulthood were definitively associated with increased weight gain during this transition. During the transition, there was about a 25% increase in the consumption of fast foods. Study subjects also reported that they had consumed breakfast on an average of 4 to 5 days during adolescence, but this dropped to just 3 days per week by young adulthood.

It is pretty obvious why the above trends result in obesity. Fast food consumption means the consumption of food items that are high in energy density, predominantly because of their high dietary fat content. Those who regularly skip breakfast consume a greater percentage of energy from fat and snacks that are higher in fat. Skipping breakfast may also lead to greater levels of hunger later in the day, producing overeating, or may lead to choices to consume foods that are higher in energy density, producing greater overall intake. Those who eat breakfast also tend to be more physically active for some reason.

Thus it is that the family that dines together, at home, including at breakfast, is the fitter of families here in the United States. On a side note, have you ever wondered who is able to better correctly assess the caloric content of large meals: a trim person or an obese person? The answer is neither. We all tend to underestimate the caloric content of what we eat. It has been clear for some time that people who are overweight tend to underestimate more than people of normal weight, a bias that has been disastrous for weight control. Providers have always assumed that overweight people are simply lying to themselves about what they eat and by extension, lying to the people trying to help them. Two recent experiments, however, show that it is meal size, not food psychology that counts. Both indicate that people, whatever their weight, find it harder to guess the caloric content of large portions by comparison to small ones. A sample of diners in fast food outlets here in the United States were almost exactly right when assessing small portions, but significantly underestimated the caloric content of larger portions by almost 40%. University students given 15 pre-prepared meals to estimate did the same thing, underestimating the larger portions by a huge amount.

One solution to the problem would be a calorie count beside each meal on the menu. Alternatively, it would be easier, say the authors of the report, to advise people to take each small meal item separately (chips, burger, drink), rather than trying to guess the calorie count of the whole meal all at once. Some fast food restaurants have taken this message to heart and do publish the number of calories that one will eat if one purchases a food item.[3]

J. A. Stockman III, MD

References

1. Nielsen SJ, Siega-Riz AM, Popkin BM. Trends in food locations and sources among adolescents and young adults. *Prev Med.* 2002;35:107-113.
2. Whalen CK, Kliewer W. Social influences on the development of cardiovascular risk during childhood and adolescence. In: Czajkowski SM, Shumaker SA, eds. *Social Support and Cardiovascular Disease.* New York,NY: Springer;, 1994:223-257.
3. Wansink B, Chandon P. Meal size, not body size, explains errors in estimating the calorie content of meals. *Ann Intern Med.* 2006;145:326-332.

The Burden of Diabetes Mellitus Among US Youth: Prevalence Estimates From the SEARCH for Diabetes in Youth Study
Liese AD, for the SEARCH for Diabetes in Youth Study Group (Univ of South Carolina, Columbia; et al)
Pediatrics 118:1510-1518, 2006

Objective.—Our goal was to estimate the prevalence of diabetes mellitus in youth <20 years of age in 2001 in the United States, according to age, gender, race/ethnicity, and diabetes type.

Methods.—The SEARCH for Diabetes in Youth Study is a 6-center observational study conducting population-based ascertainment of physician-diagnosed diabetes in youth. Census-based denominators for 4 geographically based centers and enrollment data for 2 health plan-based centers were used to calculate prevalence. Age-, gender-, and racial/ethnic group-specific prevalence rates were multiplied by US population counts to estimate the total number of US youth with diabetes.

Results.—We identified 6379 US youth with diabetes in 2001, in a population of ~3.5 million. Crude prevalence was estimated as 1.82 cases per 1000 youth, being much lower for youth 0 to 9 years of age (0.79 cases per 1000 youth) than for those 10 to 19 years of age (2.80 cases per 1000 youth). Non-Hispanic white youth had the highest prevalence (1.06 cases per 1000 youth) in the younger group. Among 10- to 19-year-old youth, black youth (3.22 cases per 1000 youth) and non-Hispanic white youth (3.18 cases per 1000 youth) had the highest rates, followed by American Indian youth (2.28 cases per 1000 youth), Hispanic youth (2.18 cases per 1000 youth), and Asian/Pacific Islander youth (1.34 cases per 1000 youth). Among younger children, type 1 diabetes accounted for ≥80% of diabetes; among older youth, the proportion of type 2 diabetes ranged from 6% (0.19 cases per 1000 youth for non-Hispanic white youth) to 76% (1.74 cases per 1000 youth for American Indian youth). We estimated that 154,369 youth had physician-diagnosed diabetes in 2001 in the United States.

Conclusions.—The overall prevalence estimate for diabetes in children and adolescents was ~0.18%. Type 2 diabetes was found in all racial/ethnic groups but generally was less common than type 1, except in American Indian youth.

▶ This report and the Anand et al report (Diabetes mellitus screening in pediatric primary care) both appeared in *Pediatrics,* and they both had the same goals: to describe the prevalence of diabetes among United States youth and to determine how effectively we are screening for the disease. The first report is from SEARCH. The SEARCH for Diabetes in Youth Study Group is a population-based, observational study of physician-diagnosed diabetes among youth less than 20 years old. SEARCH was initiated in 2000, and it collects data from a total of six centers in the United States. What we see in the report from SEARCH are estimates of the prevalence of diabetes among children in the pediatric population (<20 years old) that are based on findings from 2001. It is clear that these population-based estimates made by SEARCH represent the largest surveillance effort in diabetes in youth conducted to date in this country. The data are about as accurate as data can get, and they show that physician-diagnosed diabetes runs at a prevalence of about 1 in every 523 youths. This converts to a prevalence rate of 1.82 cases per 1000 individuals who are less than 20 years old. By comparison, cancer rates in this age group run 1.2 per 1000, and asthma rates run 120 per 1000. If one converts the diabetes diagnosis to dollars and cents, for all ages, the tab in the United States is about $132 billion annually. There are no specific figures for children and adolescents.

In addition to giving us fairly solid evidence about the prevalence of diabetes overall among youth in the United States, SEARCH also gives us information by race and ethnicity. For example, prevalence estimates of 1.29 cases per 1000 Hispanic children and adolescents compares with just 0.83 cases per 1000 Asian-Pacific youth. For black youth, the SEARCH estimate is 1.93 cases per 1000 youth, which is slightly higher than that reported in other small studies. Among 10- to 19-year-old youth, 64% of blacks and 74% of Hispanic youths had type 1 diabetes. The problem is more prevalent among girls than boys in all races and ethnicities. Among older youth, the proportion of diabetes accounted for by type 2 diabetes does seem to vary dramatically across racial/ethnic groups, varying from just 6% for non-Hispanic white youth to 76% among American-Indian youth.

The Anand et al report shows that, although pediatricians are screening for diabetes mellitus, in many instances, this screening is not conducted in accordance with the guidelines of the American Diabetes Association. These guidelines suggest the following: (1) testing for type 2 diabetes at the onset of puberty or at the age of 10 years, whichever occurs first; and (2) testing children of any age who are overweight (>85th percentile for age and gender) and who have any two of the following risk factors: family history of type 2 diabetes in a first- or second-degree relative; race/ethnicity of American Indian, black, Hispanic, or Asian/Pacific Islander; and signs of insulin resistance or conditions that are associated with insulin resistance, such as acanthosis nigricans, hypertension, high lipids, or polycystic ovarian syndrome. After it has been started, the testing for type 2 diabetes is recommended to be carried out every 2 years. A fasting blood glucose is the preferred test, and pediatricians are encouraged to test for type 2 diabetes in any high-risk patient who does not seem to meet these American Diabetes Association recommended guidelines.

J. A. Stockman III, MD

Diabetes Mellitus Screening in Pediatric Primary Care
Anand SG, Mehta SD, Adams WG (Boston Univ)
Pediatrics 118:1888-1895, 2006

Objective.—The goal was to determine the rates of diabetes screening and the prevalence of screening abnormalities in overweight and nonoverweight individuals in an urban primary care clinic.

Methods.—This study was a retrospective chart review conducted in a hospital-based urban primary care setting. Deidentified data for patients who were 10 to 19 years of age and had ≥ 1 BMI measurement between September 1, 2002, and September 1, 2004, were extracted from the hospital electronic health record.

Results.—A total of 7710 patients met the study criteria. Patients were 73.0% black or Hispanic and 47.0% female; 42.0% of children exceeded normal weight, with 18.2% at risk for overweight and 23.8% overweight. On the basis of BMI, family history, and race, 8.7% of patients met American Diabetes Association criteria for type 2 diabetes mellitus screening, and 2452 screening tests were performed for 1642 patients. Female gender, older age group, and family history of diabetes were associated with screening. Increasing BMI percentile was associated with screening, exhibiting a dose-response relationship. Screening rates were significantly higher (45.4% vs 19.0%) for patients who met the American Diabetes Association criteria; however, less than one half of adolescents who should have been screened were screened. Abnormal glucose metabolism was seen for 9.2% of patients screened.

Conclusions.—This study shows that, although pediatricians are screening for diabetes mellitus, screening is not being conducted according to the American Diabetes Association consensus statement. Point-of-care delivery of consensus recommendations could increase provider awareness of current recommendations, possibly improving rates of systematic screening and subsequent identification of children with laboratory evidence of abnormal glucose metabolism.

▶ This report and the Liese et al report (The burden of diabetes mellitus among US youth: prevalence estimates from the SEARCH for Diabetes in Youth Study) have provided us with much information about the prevalence of diabetes mellitus here in the United States. The prevalence here is substantially higher than in certain parts of the world, especially Asia. In Japan, for example, the consumption of certain dietary elements such as green tea is pervasive. There, about 80% of the population drinks green tea and the average consumption per capita is in excess of 2 cups per day. In western populations, it has been shown that coffee consumption is associated with a reduced risk for type 2 diabetes. Based on this, investigators were interested to see what the effect was of green tea in this regard. A total of 17,413 persons who had no history of type 2 diabetes were followed for a 5 year period. Consumption of green tea and coffee was definitively inversely associated with a risk for diabetes after adjustments for age, sex, body mass index, and other risk factors. Those drinking 6 or more cups of green tea per day or more than 3 cups of coffee per day had a 33% and 42% reduction, respectively, in the risk of developing diabetes mellitus compared with those who drank less than one cup per week of either brew. Black tea did not appear to offer any protection. If one equates the caffeine content of the coffee and green teas, it appears that total caffeine intake from these beverages is associated with a 33% reduced risk for diabetes.

Thus, it is that consumption of green tea, coffee and total caffeine may indeed be associated with a decreased risk for type 2 diabetes.[1] Now if somebody could just change the color of green tea, some of us might think about imbibing it.

J. A. Stockman III, MD

Reference

1. Iso H, Date C, Waki K, et al. The relationship between green tea and total caffeine intake and risk for self-reported type 2 diabetes among Japanese adults. *Ann Intern Med.* 2006;144:554-562.

Effect of Youth-Onset Type 2 Diabetes Mellitus on Incidence of End-Stage Renal Disease and Mortality in Young and Middle-Aged Pima Indians

Pavkov ME, Bennett PH, Knowler WC, et al (NIH, Phoenix, Ariz)
JAMA 296:421-426, 2006

Context.—The long-term outcome of persons with youth-onset type 2 diabetes mellitus has not been well described.

Objective.—To compare incidence of diabetic end-stage renal disease (ESRD) and mortality in Pima Indians with youth- and older-onset type 2 diabetes mellitus.

Design, Setting, and Participants.—Longitudinal population-based study conducted between 1965 and 2002 in Pima Indians from the state of Arizona. Participants were divided into 2 groups: (1) youth-onset type 2 diabetes mellitus (onset <20 years of age) and (2) older-onset type 2 diabetes mellitus (onset ≥20 - <55 years of age). Events and person-years of follow-up were stratified in a time-dependent fashion by decades of age. End-stage renal disease was defined as dialysis attributed to diabetic nephropathy or death from diabetic nephropathy.

Main Outcome Measures.—Incidence rate of diabetic ESRD and mortality between 25 and 55 years of age, according to age at onset of type 2 diabetes mellitus.

Results.—Among the 1856 diabetic participants, 96 had youth-onset type 2 diabetes mellitus. The age-sex-adjusted incidence of diabetic ESRD was 25.0 cases per 1000 person-years (95% confidence interval [CI], 6.7-43.1) in youth-onset diabetes mellitus and 5.4 cases per 1000 person-years (95% CI, 4.4-6.4) in older-onset diabetes mellitus (incidence rate ratio, 4.6; 95% CI, 2.2-9.8). Age-specific incidence rates were higher in participants with youth-onset diabetes mellitus at all ages. Between 25 and 55 years of age, the age-sex-adjusted death rate from natural causes was 15.4 deaths per 1000 person-years (95% CI, 0.2-30.5) in participants with youth-onset diabetes mellitus and 7.3 deaths per 1000 person-years (95% CI, 5.9-8.7) in individuals with older-onset diabetes mellitus (death rate ratio, 2.1; 95% CI, 0.8-5.7). Compared with nondiabetic participants, the death rate was 3.0 times as high in individuals with youth-onset diabetes mellitus (95% CI, 1.1-8.0) and 1.4 times as high in individuals with older-onset diabetes mellitus (95% CI, 1.1-1.8). In a subset of 1386 participants with complete data for all covariates who were observed from the onset of diabetes mellitus, the age at onset of diabetes mellitus was not associated with the incidence of ESRD (hazard ratio, 1.0; 95% CI, 0.9-1.2) after adjusting for sex, mean arterial pressure, body mass index (calculated as weight in kilograms divided by height in meters squared), plasma glucose concentration, smoking, hypoglycemic medicines, and blood pressure medicines in a Cox proportional-hazards model.

Conclusions.—Early-onset type 2 diabetes mellitus is associated with substantially increased incidence of ESRD and mortality in middle age. The longer duration of diabetes mellitus by middle age in individuals diagnosed younger than age 20 years largely accounts for these outcomes.

▶ The Pima Indian population represents an interesting and important group of youngsters to study. In Pima Indians, youth-onset type 2 diabetes mellitus is associated with a lower frequency of retinopathy for a given duration of diabetes mellitus than adult-onset type 2 diabetes, but with a similar frequency of overt nephropathy, suggesting that youth does not offer the same protection from progressive diabetic kidney disease as it does from diabetic retinopathy. This finding strongly suggests that youngsters who have diabetes mellitus develop and who have diabetic kidney disease develop will have a higher mortality during their peak productive years and will require extensive use of healthcare services.

This report tells us that onset of type 2 diabetes mellitus in youngsters is associated with a nearly 5-fold increase in the incidence of end-stage renal disease between 25 and 54 years of age compared with later onset of diabetes mellitus. The Pima Indian population is an important one for learning a lot about this problem because information on long-term outcomes of persons with childhood onset type 2 diabetes in other populations is very limited because of the small number of cases and the absence of long-term follow-up. These data cannot be unequivocally applied to all populations, however, given the differing genetic makeup of various populations. For example, if one looks at long-term micro- and macrovascular complications in the Japanese population with the onset of type 2 diabetes mellitus in early life, just 5% have end-stage renal disease after 20 years duration of diabetes. On the other hand, in the Japanese population, atherosclerotic vascular disease, including cerebrovascular, cardiac and peripheral artery disease is the leading cause of death with childhood onset of type 2 diabetes.

The bottom line here is that it is not good to develop diabetes mellitus when you are a child. This equally applies to the teenage population. Although the data of Pima Indians cannot be applied to all here in the United States, it is highly likely that there will be some similarities. We do need better management techniques for this disorder. See the Shojania report (Effects of quality improvement strategies for type 2 diabetes on glycemic control: a meta-regression analysis) that looks at quality improvement strategies for type 2 diabetes. One key ingredient in the success of interventions appears to be the ability of case managers to make medication changes without waiting for physician approval. There is nothing magical about many aspects of the management of type 2 diabetes, but the sooner the better when changing glycemic control approaches.

J. A. Stockman III, MD

Effects of Quality Improvement Strategies for Type 2 Diabetes on Glycemic Control: A Meta-Regression Analysis

Shojania KG, Ranji SR, McDonald KM, et al (Univ of Ottawa, Ont, Canada; Univ of California, San Francisco; Stanford Univ, Palo Alto, Calif)
JAMA 296:427-440, 2006

Context.—There have been numerous reports of interventions designed to improve the care of patients with diabetes, but the effectiveness of such interventions is unclear.

Objective.—To assess the impact on glycemic control of 11 distinct strategies for quality improvement (QI) in adults with type 2 diabetes.

Data Sources and Study Selection.—MEDLINE (1966-April 2006) and the Cochrane Collaboration's Effective Practice and Organisation of Care Group database, which covers multiple bibliographic databases. Eligible studies included randomized or quasi-randomized controlled trials and controlled before-after studies that evaluated a QI intervention targeting some aspect of clinician behavior or organizational change and reported changes in glycosylated hemoglobin (HbA_{1c}) values.

Data Extraction.—Postintervention difference in HbA_{1c} values were estimated using a meta-regression model that included baseline glycemic control and other key intervention and study features as predictors.

Data Synthesis.—Fifty randomized controlled trials, 3 quasi-randomized trials, and 13 controlled before-after trials met all inclusion criteria. Across these 66 trials, interventions reduced HbA_{1c} values by a mean of 0.42% (95% confidence interval [CI], 0.29%-0.54%) over a median of 13 months of follow-up. Trials with fewer patients than the median for all included trials reported significantly greater effects than did larger trials (0.61% vs 0.27%, $P = .004$), strongly suggesting publication bias. Trials with mean baseline HbA_{1c} values of 8.0% or greater also reported significantly larger effects (0.54% vs 0.20%, $P = .005$). Adjusting for these effects, 2 of the 11 categories of QI strategies were associated with reductions in HbA_{1c} values of at least 0.50%: team changes (0.67%; 95% CI, 0.43%-0.91%; n = 26 trials) and case management (0.52%; 95% CI, 0.31%-0.73%; n = 26 trials); these also represented the only 2 strategies conferring significant incremental reductions in HbA_{1c} values. Interventions involving team changes reduced values by 0.33% more (95% CI, 0.12%-0.54%; $P = .004$) than those without this strategy, and those involving case management reduced values by 0.22% more (95% CI, 0.00%-0.44%; $P = .04$) than those without case management. Interventions in which nurse or pharmacist case managers could make medication adjustments without awaiting physician authorization reduced values by 0.80% (95% CI, 0.51%-1.10%), vs only 0.32% (95% CI, 0.14%-0.49%) for all other interventions ($P = .002$).

Conclusions.—Most QI strategies produced small to modest improvements in glycemic control. Team changes and case management showed more robust improvements, especially for interventions in which case managers could adjust medications without awaiting physician approval. Estimates of the effectiveness of other specific QI strategies may have been limited by difficulty in classifying complex interventions, insufficient numbers of studies, and publication bias.

Clinical and Molecular Genetic Spectrum of Congenital Deficiency of the Leptin Receptor

Farooqi IS, Wangensteen T, Collins S, et al (Addenbrooke's Hosp, Cambridge, England; Wellcome Trust Sanger Inst, Cambridgeshire, England; Inst of Child Health, London; et al)
N Engl J Med 356:237-247, 2007

Background.—A single family has been described in which obesity results from a mutation in the leptin-receptor gene (*LEPR*), but the prevalence of such mutations in severe, early-onset obesity has not been systematically examined.

Methods.—We sequenced *LEPR* in 300 subjects with hyperphagia and severe early-onset obesity, including 90 probands from consanguineous families, and investigated the extent to which mutations cosegregated with obesity and affected receptor function. We evaluated metabolic, endocrine, and immune function in probands and affected relatives.

Results.—Of the 300 subjects, 8 (3%) had nonsense or missense *LEPR* mutations—7 were homozygotes, and 1 was a compound heterozygote. All missense mutations resulted in impaired receptor signaling. Affected subjects were characterized by hyperphagia, severe obesity, alterations in immune function, and delayed puberty due to hypogonadotropic hypogonadism. Serum leptin levels were within the range predicted by the elevated fat mass in these subjects. Their clinical features were less severe than those of subjects with congenital leptin deficiency.

Conclusions.—The prevalence of pathogenic *LEPR* mutations in a cohort of subjects with severe, early-onset obesity was 3%. Circulating levels of leptin were not disproportionately elevated, suggesting that serum leptin cannot be used as a marker for leptin-receptor deficiency. Congenital leptin-receptor deficiency should be considered in the differential diagnosis in any child with hyperphagia and severe obesity in the absence of developmental delay or dysmorphism.

▶ All of us have seen children presenting very early in life with morbid obesity. When this occurs, we should think about some of the genetic obesity syndromes. Patients with genetic obesity syndromes have largely been identified in childhood as the result of associated mental retardation and developmental abnormalities. Several monogenic disorders have now been identified in which obesity itself is the sole predominant presenting feature. Such disorders result from disruption of the hypothalamic leptin–melanocortin signaling pathway. As of early 2007, 12 subjects with congenital leptin deficiency due to loss-of-function mutations in the gene encoding leptin had been identified. Characteristic features include hyperphagia, obesity, hypogonadism, and impaired T-cell–mediated immunity. Treatment with recombinant human leptin reverses all aspects of the presentation. So far, only one mutation in the leptin-receptor gene (*LEPR*) has been reported, this in 3 severely obese adult siblings from a consanguineous family of Algerian origin. This mutation results in abnormal splicing of the leptin-receptor transcripts and generates a mutant leptin receptor that lacks both transmembrane and intracellular domains. The mutant receptor circulates at high concentrations, binding leptin and resulting in very elevated serum leptin levels.

The authors of this report decided to look at several hundred severely obese individuals who had early-onset obesity to determine the actual prevalence of pathogenic mutations in the *LEPR* gene. It turns out that the prevalence of pathogenic *LEPR* mutations in early, severe-onset obesity runs about 3%. This figure may be a bit high given that many of the patients studied were distantly related to each other (the study was performed in Great Britain).

Congenital leptin-receptor deficiency is characterized by severe, early-onset obesity associated with selective deposition of fat mass. Most subjects have hyperphagia from a very early age. Children with leptin-receptor deficiency seem to have normal linear growth during childhood. However, because of the lack of a pubertal growth spurt, the final height of adult subjects with leptin-receptor deficiency is reduced. There is little in the literature about why these youngsters turn out to be short adults. Assessment of the growth hormone–insulin-like growth factor axis is difficult in obese children and adults, because obesity by itself is associated with abnormal results of basal and dynamic tests of this axis. Some children also fail to fully develop secondary sexual characteristics.

Please recognize that congenital leptin-receptor deficiency cannot be ruled out simply by measuring serum leptin levels. This diagnosis must be considered in all patients with severe obesity and hyperphagia in the absence of developmental delay and dysmorphic features. The diagnosis has implications for the care of these patients, both in terms of genetic counseling of the affected families and in terms of future prospects for treatment, because these patients would be predicted to have a favorable response to drugs targeted at pathways downstream of the leptin receptor.

To say all this differently, the next time you see a morbidly obese child, at least think of the possibility of leptin-receptor deficiency as a potential cause of the problem. The diagnosis is more common than we thought a few years ago.

J. A. Stockman III, MD

Evaluating the Validity of a Bedside Method of Detecting Hypoglycemia in Children

Elusiyan JBE, Adeodu OO, Adejuyigbe EA (Obafemi Awolowo Univ, Ile-Ife, Nigeria)
Pediatr Emerg Care 22:488-490, 2006

Background.—Hypoglycemia in the pediatric age group is a common finding associated with a wide variety of disorders. It often presents urgent diagnostic and therapeutic challenges. In the tropics where facilities for laboratory evaluation are inadequate and inefficient, there is need to evaluate alternative methods of diagnosis.

Aims and Objectives.—The aim of the study was to validate the glucometer method of assessing hypoglycemia in pediatric patients.

Methodology.—Four hundred fifty-three consecutively admitted patients were recruited into the study. After a detailed history and thorough physical examination, 2 mL of blood was obtained from each patient. A drop was put on the test strip, and plasma glucose level read off a glucometer. The remainder was sent to the laboratory for comparative plasma glucose determination by the glucose oxidase method. Hypoglycemia was defined as plasma glucose less than 2.5 mmol/L (<45 mg/dL).

Results.—Out of the 453 studied, only 392 (86.5%) had complete results and were included in the analysis. Thirty-eight (9.7%) were hypoglycemic by the glucometer method, but only 25 (6.4%) of them were hypoglycemic by the laboratory method. The glucometer was found to be highly sensitive and specific, and its results compare favorably with the laboratory values. The glucometer gave a predictive index of a positive test as 63.12% and of a negative test as 99.72%. It however leads to overdiagnosis of hypoglycemia.

Conclusions.—The glucometer was found to be highly sensitive and specific, and its result correlates significantly well with the laboratory method. The glucometer method for blood sugar determination in emergency cases is highly recommended in children.

▶ A laboratory is not always around when we need it to tell whether a patient may have hypoglycemia. This report from Nigeria gives us information about how accurate bedside glucometers are in telling us whether a patient is hypoglycemic. In older infants and children, a whole blood glucose concentration of less than 40 mg/dL (2.2 mmol/L) or a plasma glucose less than 45 mg/dL (2.5 mmol/L) represents hypoglycemia whether or not clinical manifestations are present. Obviously prolonged hypoglycemia can have significant long-term sequelae.

So just how good are modern glucometers when it comes to picking up hypoglycemia? The data from this report give us the answer. The glucometer method has a sensitivity of 96.00% and a specificity of 96.19% when compared with laboratory methods in detecting low blood sugar levels. These figures represent findings that are substantially better than earlier studies and imply that a normal run-of-the-mill, off-the-shelf glucometer is useful for ruling out hypoglycemia. Furthermore, the results are available very rapidly in comparison to laboratory testing. The authors go so far as to recommend using a glucometer in an emergency room setting for the detection of hypoglycemia in children.

J. A. Stockman III, MD

Outcome of neonatal screening for medium-chain acyl-CoA dehydrogenase deficiency in Australia: a cohort study

Wilcken B, Haas M, Joy P, et al (Children's Hosp at Westmead, Sydney, Australia; Univ of Sydney, Australia; Univ of Technology, Sydney, Australia; et al)
Lancet 369:37-42, 2007

Background.—Medium-chain acyl-CoA dehydrogenase (MCAD) deficiency is the disorder thought most to justify neonatal screening by tandem-mass spectrometry because, without screening, there seems to be substantial morbidity and mortality. Our aim was to assess the overall effectiveness of neonatal screening for MCAD deficiency in Australia.

Methods.—We identified MCAD-deficient patients from a total population of 2,495,000 Australian neonates (810,000 screened) born between April 1, 1994, and March 31, 2004. Those from a cohort of 1,995,000 (460,000 screened) were followed up for at least 4 years, and we recorded number of deaths and severe episodes, medical and neuropsychological outcome, and hospital admissions within the screened and unscreened groups.

Findings.—In cohorts aged at least 4 years there were 35 MCAD-deficient patients in those not screened (2.28 per 100,000 total population) and 24 in the screened population (5.2 per 100,000). We estimated that patients with this disorder in the unscreened cohort remained undiagnosed. Before 4 years of age, three screened patients had an episode of severe decompensation (including one neonatal death) versus 23 unscreened patients (including five deaths). At the most conservative estimate, relative risk of an adverse event was 0.44 (95% CI 0.13–1.45). In the larger cohort the relative risk (screened *vs* unscreened) of an adverse event by age 2 years was 0.26 (95% CI 0.07–0.97), also a conservative estimate. 38 of 52 living patients had neuropsychological testing, with no suggestions of significant differences in general cognitive outcome between the groups.

Interpretation.—Screening is effective in patients with MCAD deficiency since early diagnosis reduces deaths and severe adverse events in children up to the age of 4 years.

▶ Here is another article on neonatal screening for MCAD deficiency. Together with phenylketonuria, MCAD is the disorder most frequently diagnosed by neonatal screening with tandem mass spectrometry. MCAD deficiency is an inherited disorder caused by mutations on the *ACADM* gene that cause enzyme deficiency or inactivity and can result in severe acute metabolic decompensation during fasting or in association with infection or catabolic stress. Affected individuals risk episodes of hypoketotic hypoglycemia that lead to coma or death. In reports of subjects diagnosed clinically with the disorder, some 20% to 25% die, usually during a first episode, and another 20% sustain neurologic damage. A retrospective neonatal-screening study of some 100,000 stored samples reported that 1 in 8 patients had died and that many had learning difficulties.

The aim of newborn screening for MCAD is to prevent episodes of metabolic decompensation in association with stress. Although the detection of MCAD deficiency is a primary justification for the expanded screening programs that are being implemented in some countries, no population-based data exist for long-term outcomes. As the first study to provide such data in screened and unscreened birth cohorts in the same country, the article by Wilcken et al shows findings that lend support to an important health care policy question.

Wilcken et al studied almost 2.5 million children born in Australia between 1994 and 2004, a third of whom were screened at 2 to 3 days of age for MCAD deficiency. In an analysis confined to those born before 2003 and for whom at least 4 years' follow-up existed, the researchers now report death in 17% of those with the disorder who were diagnosed through clinical presentation or after diagnosis of a sibling compared with just 4% of those diagnosed through neonatal screening. As importantly, these investigators also report preliminary results of cognitive testing in surviving children who were at least 4 years of age. Test scores were normal in both screened and unscreened children with MCAD deficiency. Because previous studies had shown that children with repeated episodes of decompensation had developmental problems, the current article from Australia suggests that improved clinical awareness of MCAD deficiency in that country has led to these improved neurologic outcomes.

The Australian study provides the best evidence so far that MCAD deficiency outcomes are different for screened and unscreened populations. The findings suggest that screening for the disorder is associated with fewer episodes of decompensation and death. If one runs the math, at least in Australia, about 1 in 10 children with the deficiency will have their death prevented by neonatal screening. When everything is taken together, it does appear that neonatal screening is cost-effective for this disease. Does your state screen for MCAD deficiency?

While on the topic of things metabolic, recent data has appeared that may explain the secret of Lance Armstrong's sporting prowess as a racing cyclist. The secret may have to do with his liver.[1] It has been suggested that the enormous amount of lactic acid produced by muscle cells during endurance sporting activity is removed by hepatic enzymes converting it to glucose. Armstrong's enhanced gluconeogenesis could be constitutional, but it is more likely to be due to his heavy training program. From the age of 12, he has indicated that he swam 12,000 meters and cycled 32 km every day. It may also explain how he made such a good recovery from testicular cancer. Testicular cancer cells are known to produce extremely high levels of lactic acid.

J. A. Stockman III, MD

Reference

1. Bongaerts GP, Wagener DJ. Increased hepatic gluconeogenesis: the secret of Lance Armstrong's success. *Med Hypotheses.* 2007;68:9-11.

The incidence of inherited metabolic disorders in the West Midlands, UK

Sanderson S, Green A, Preece MA, et al (Univ of Cambridge, England; Public Health Genetics Unit, Cambridge, England; Birmingham Children's Hosp, England)

Arch Dis Child 91:896-899, 2006

Background.—Inherited metabolic disorders (IMDs) are a heterogeneous group of genetic conditions mostly occurring in childhood. They are individually rare but collectively numerous, causing substantial morbidity and mortality.

Aims.—To obtain up-to-date estimates of the birth prevalence of IMDs in an ethnically diverse British population and to compare these estimates with those of other published population-based studies.

Methods.—Retrospective data from the West Midlands Regional Diagnostic Laboratory for Inherited Metabolic Disorders (Birmingham, UK) for the 5 years (1999–2003) were examined. The West Midlands population of 5.2 million is approximately 10% of the UK population. Approximately 11% of the population of the region is from black and ethnic minority groups compared with approximately 8% for the the UK.

Results.—The overall birth prevalence was 1 in 784 live births (95% confidence interval (CI) 619 to 970), based on a total of 396 new cases. The most frequent diagnoses were mitochondrial disorders (1 in 4929; 95% CI 2776 to 8953), lysosomal storage disorders (1 in 5175; 95% CI 2874 to 9551), amino acid disorders excluding phenylketonuria (1 in 5354; 95% CI 2943 to 9990) and organic acid disorders (1 in 7962; 95% CI 3837 to 17 301). Most of the diagnoses (72%) were made by the age of 15 years and one-third by the age of 1 year.

Conclusions.—These results are similar to those of the comparison studies, although the overall birth prevalence is higher in this study. This is probably due to the effects of ethnicity and consanguinity and increasing ascertainment. This study provides useful epidemiological information for those planning and providing services for patients with IMDs, including newborn screening, in the UK and similar populations.

▶ Bet you are not aware of the origins of the term "inborn errors of metabolism." The term comes from Archibald Garrod,[1] who did some classic studies on alkaptonuria, cystinuria, and pentosuria more than a century ago. Actually, Archibald used a somewhat different term than inborn errors of metabolism, one that quickly was recognized as socially unacceptable. He had coined the term "inborn freaks of metabolism." At the turn of the last century, the word freak simply meant anything with some significant rarity. IMDs are indeed quite infrequent. As we see in this report from the United Kingdom, the prevalence of phenylketonuria (PKU) runs in the neighborhood of 1 in 12,000 live births. More frequent are the mitochondrial disorders, which have a prevalence of about 1 in 5000. If one looks at all the metabolic disorders together, however, they are not rare given their prevalence of 1 in 700 or so live births. Any large nursery will see a few infants each year with a metabolic disorder.

As a reminder, PKU is a good example of how the application of new advances, diagnostically and therapeutically, can have a dramatic effect on outcomes. PKU was first described by Folling in the 1930s. Biochemical diagnosis could then be made on urine samples from infants with developmental and neurologic problems. Two decades passed before others showed that a phenylalanine-restrictive diet could be safely given to affected children, although they remain severely impaired and dependent. Many were institutionalized for life. It required the development by Robert Guthrie in the 1960s of a cheap, sensitive, and specific screening test that could be applied to large populations before a true effect on outcome could be shown. Since then, further technologic improvements have provided accurate quantitative measurements of phenylalanine, and an explosion of phenylalanine-free nutritional products means that a newborn with PKU diagnosed today can expect a normal or near-normal life. Management of PKU is certainly one of the success stories of 20th century medicine. The addition of tandem mass spectrometry to newborn screening opened up an entire new world of possibilities for detecting additional metabolic disorders including those of organic acid metabolism. Not only are infants and children being diagnosed with IMDs, but more adults are now diagnosed with these disorders for the first time. The data from the United Kingdom suggest that more than a quarter of patients are now diagnosed after 14 years of age, sometimes even as late as in the eighth decade. Suddenly prevalence figures for these disorders have increased remarkably by virtue of the detection of adults. With better screening detection and the recognition of metabolic disorders affecting adults, what was once a search for a needle in a haystack no longer requires such a large search party to ferret out disease.

J. A. Stockman III, MD

Reference

1. Garrod AE. The incidence of alkaptonuria: a study in chemical individuality. 1902 [classic article]. *Yale J Biol Med.* 2002;4:221-231.

Clinical, Biochemical, and Genetic Heterogeneity in Short-Chain Acyl-Coenzyme A Dehydrogenase Deficiency

van Maldegem BT, Duran M, Wanders RJA, et al (Univ of Amsterdam; Univ of Groningen, The Netherlands; Univ Med Ctr Nijmegen, The Netherlands)
JAMA 296:943-952, 2006

Context.—Short-chain acyl-coenzyme A (CoA) dehydrogenase (SCAD) deficiency (SCADD) is an autosomal recessive, clinically heterogeneous disorder with only 22 case reports published so far. Screening for SCADD is included in expanded newborn screening programs in most US and Australian states.

Objectives.—To describe the genetic, biochemical, and clinical characteristics of SCADD patients in The Netherlands and their SCADD relatives and to explore the genotype to phenotype relation.

Design, Setting, and Participants.—Retrospective study involving 31 Dutch SCADD patients diagnosed between January 1987 and January 2006 and 8 SCADD relatives. SCADD was defined by the presence of (1) increased butyrylcarnitine (C4-C) levels in plasma and/or increased ethylmalonic acid (EMA) levels in urine under nonstressed conditions on at least 2 occasions, in combination with (2) a mutation and/or the c.511C>T or c.625G>A susceptibility variants on each SCAD-encoding (*ACADS*) allele. Patients were included only if the SCAD-encoding (*ACADS*) was fully sequenced and if current clinical information could be obtained. Relatives were included when they carried the same *ACADS* genotype as the proband, and had increased C4-C and/or EMA.

Main Outcome Measures.—Prevalence, genotype (mutation/mutation, mutation/variant, variant/variant), C4-C and EMA levels, clinical signs and symptoms, and clinical course.

Results.—A birth-prevalence of at least 1:50,000 was calculated. Most patients presented before the age of 3 years, with nonspecific, generally uncomplicated, and often transient symptoms. Developmental delay, epilepsy, behavioral disturbances, and hypoglycemia were the most frequently reported symptoms. The *ACADS* genotype showed a statistically significant association with EMA and C4-C levels, but not with clinical characteristics. Seven out of 8 SCADD relatives were free of symptoms.

Conclusions.—SCADD is far more common than assumed previously, and clinical symptoms in SCADD are nonspecific, generally uncomplicated, often transient, and not correlated with specific *ACADS* genotypes. Because SCADD does not meet major newborn screening criteria, including a lack of clinical significance in many patients and that it is not possible to differentiate diseased and nondiseased individuals, it is not suited for inclusion in newborn screening programs at the present time.

▶ This report of van Maldegem et al raises some interesting questions about newborn screening programs. SCADD is an autosomal recessive inborn error of mitochondrial fatty acid β-oxidation presenting usually with a variety of clinical signs and symptoms. Developmental delay, hyper- and hypotonia, ketotic hypoglycemia, and epilepsy are most frequently reported. Various metabolites accumulate in blood and SCADD may be able to be screened for in the newborn period. The diagnosis of SCADD is confirmed by enzyme activity measurements in muscle, fibroblasts and/or lymphocytes, and by DNA studies. SCADD is a rare disorder with only 22 genetically confirmed cases having been reported in the literature. Apart from the case report of one patient who appeared to benefit from riboflavin therapy, the efficacy of any therapy has never been systematically studied in a group of SCADD patients. There is no evidence indicating that early detection of SCADD is clinically useful. Nonetheless, many, if not most, neonatal screening panels are designed to detect the various metabolites that would be increased in SCADD-affected infants.

Doubts about the indication for screening for SCADD have been expressed by the Newborn Screening Expert Group of the American College of Medical Genetics, acknowledging the lack of evidence related to the availability of a treatment and a poorly understood natural history. This report from The Netherlands was designed to calculate the prevalence of SCADD in that country and to document and summarize the genetic, biochemical, and clinical characteristics of the largest group of SCADD patients and their relatives published so far. The importance of this study goes well beyond an analysis of a rare disorder, for it tells us much information about the pros and the cons of our current neonatal screening programs.

Here in the United States, 4 million newborn infants will receive expanded neonatal screening for metabolic disorders each year; 12,000 will receive a false-positive screening result and just 1000 will be diagnosed with an actual metabolic disorder. Although frequent hospitalizations, developmental delay, and mental retardation and death will be prevented in many of these diagnosed children, many others will have a disorder that is mild or benign. Despite uncertainty, expanded newborn screening for a wide variety of rare disorders appears to be here to stay. Currently, 47 states mandate or offer expanded screening. At one time, to qualify for neonatal screening, a condition had to be sufficiently common to warrant inclusion. The rationale that a condition be common no longer seems warranted, given the ease with which disorders can be added when screening is conducted using tandem mass spectrometry. There is clear evidence that the public considers learning disabilities, speech delay, and behavioral difficulties to be serious enough to warrant screening even if some of the disorders causing these things are not readily treatable. When it comes to very rare disorders such as SCADD, it is clear that there will be many more false-positive identifications than there are actually affected individuals, which will cause parent distress and possibly even altered parent-child relationships in some families. The conclusion of the study from The Netherlands is that SCADD does not meet major newborn screening criteria and is not suited for inclusion in newborn screening programs at this time. This seems to make sense for 2 reasons: a high rate of false-positive results and the fact that the disorder, even if diagnosed early, does not seem to have any adequate treatments. These are good criteria to use for any similar disorder when trying to decide whether such disorders should be included in newborn screening panels.

J. A. Stockman III, MD

Long-term Outcome and Clinical Spectrum of 73 Pediatric Patients With Mitochondrial Diseases

Debray F-G, Lambert M, Chevalier I, et al (Université de Montreal; McGill Univ, Montreal; Univ of Toronto)
Pediatrics 119:722-733, 2007

Objectives.—We sought to determine the clinical spectrum, survival, and long-term functional outcome of a cohort of pediatric patients with mitochondrial diseases and to identify prognostic factors.

Methods.—Medical charts were reviewed for 73 children diagnosed between 1985 and 2005. The functional status of living patients was assessed prospectively by using the standardized Functional Independence Measure scales.

Results.—Patients fell into 7 phenotypic categories: neonatal-onset lactic acidosis (10%), Leigh syndrome (18%), nonspecific encephalopathy (32%), mitochondrial (encephalo)myopathy (19%), intermittent neurologic (5%), visceral (11%), and Leber hereditary optic neuropathy (5%). Age at first symptoms ranged from prenatal to 16 years (median: 7 months). Neurologic symptoms were the most common (90%). Visceral involvement was observed in 29% of the patients. A biochemical or molecular diagnosis was identified for 81% of the patients as follows: deficiency of complex IV (27%), of pyruvate dehydrogenase or complex I (25% each), of multiple complexes (13%), and of pyruvate carboxylase (5%) or complexes II+III (5%). A mitochondrial DNA mutation was found in 20% of patients. At present, 46% of patients have died (median age: 13 months), 80% of whom were <3 years of age. Multivariate analysis showed that age at first symptoms was a major independent predictor of mortality: patients with first symptoms before 6 months had a highly increased risk of mortality. Cardiac or visceral involvement and neurologic crises were not independent prognostic factors. Living patients showed a wide range of independence levels that correlated positively with age at first symptoms. Among patients aged >5 years (*n* = 32), 62% had Functional Independence Measure quotients of >0.75.

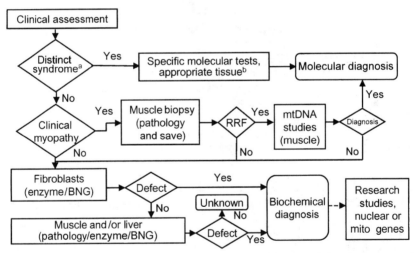

FIGURE 5.—Algorithm of investigations for patients suspected of MD. [a] Including Kearns-Sayre and Pearson syndrome, MELAS, Leber, NARP, and mitochondrial encephalopathy with RRF (MERRF). [b] LHON and NARP mutations are easily identified in leukocyte DNA, and some patients with MELAS can be diagnosed in this fashion; mtDNA deletions in Kearns-Sayre syndrome require analysis of muscle DNA. The T8993G/C (NARP) mutations should be tested in blood from any patients with Leigh syndrome. We also test French-Canadian infants with lactic acidosis for the founder mutation for Saguenay-Lac St-Jean cytochrome oxidase deficiency. (Online Mendelian inheritance in Man No. 220111). BNG indicates blue native gel; pathology, light microscopic or ultrastructural findings suggestive of MD (eg, RRFs or mitochondrial dysmorphology and inclusions); mito genes, genes encoded by the mitochondrial gene. (Courtesy of Debray F-G, Lambert M, Chevalier I, et al. Long-term outcome and clinical spectrum of 73 pediatric patients with mitochondrial diseases. *Pediatrics.* 2007;119:722-733. Reproduced by permission of *Pediatrics.*)

Conclusions.—Mitochondrial diseases in children span a wide range of symptoms and severities. Age at first symptoms is the strongest predictor of mortality. Despite a high mortality rate in the cohort, 62% of patients aged >5 years have only mild impairment or normal functional outcome (Fig 5).

▶ Mitochondrial diseases are sufficiently rare that most of us have a hard time remembering all of the details related to their presentation. This is why the article by Debray et al is so terribly important. Given the diversity of clinical presentations of what are a vast group of inherited disorders of energy metabolism and the difficulty in establishing a diagnosis, many affected youngsters are diagnosed too late to be of much help to them. This is unfortunate. Debray et al describe the phenotypic spectrum of these patients on the basis of a long-term follow-up and report the first standardized evaluation of the functional independence level of pediatric patients with metabolic disorders. Some 73 patients have been followed up in Montreal, and the data from this report are an analysis of these patients.

It is learned that the first manifestations of metabolic disease occur at an average of 7 months after birth. Obviously, some babies have this at birth. The oldest observation of a manifestation of metabolic disease was in a 16-year-old teenager. A wide range of symptoms were noted, including nonspecific psychomotor delay (38%), metabolic acidosis (14%), failure to thrive (10%), acute or subacute developmental regression (9%), visceral involvement (liver dysfunction, 4%; hypertrophic cardiomyopathy, 3%) and various combinations of focal neurologic symptoms (22%), including seizures, ataxia, extrapyramidal signs, muscle weakness or pain, ptosis and headache. For those showing metabolic diseases in the immediate neonatal group, most were diagnosed immediately at birth with fulminant lactic acidosis and neurologic distress. All died in the first few months (median age at death, 4 days).

The authors of this report remind us that nearly any pediatric specialist may be confronted with the initial diagnosis of a metabolic disease, to which the mnemonic "any age, any symptom, any organ" has been applied.[1] To say this differently, all physicians need a high level of suspicion to pick up a diagnosis that is seen in only 1 in about 7500 children. Beyond the neonatal period, a tip off to a possible diagnosis may be the development of an acute acidotic crisis in association with what otherwise is a benign infectious disease. This life-threatening complication, little emphasized in the literature, is a major issue in patient management, requiring ICU admission for IV bicarbonate administration and other supportive measures. Despite management, the mortality rate remains nearly 50%. Most crises coming in this manner occur during infancy but beyond the neonatal period.

Figure 5 has been provided by the authors as a proposed algorithm to approach patients with lactic acidosis or presumed metabolic disease. Because most of these conditions are currently untreatable, the authors suggest starting with the least-invasive techniques (fibroblast culture and blood DNA testing for specific etiologies as indicated) before performing muscle and/or liver biopsy. Minimally invasive tests have a substantial yield. In some cases, the strategy of sequential testing eliminates the need for risky procedures.

We know fairly little about the long-term outcome of pediatric patients with metabolic diseases. In this abstracted report, age at first symptom was positively correlated with poor outcome. Encouragingly, substantial portion of patients older than 5 years had no or mild impairment.

This editor considers the report of Debray et al to be one of the most important articles of 2007. It adds substantially to our understanding about a group of largely orphan diseases and encourages us all to think about them as a cause of obscure signs and symptoms.

We close this last commentary with a series of little known facts related to a particular food, the common chili and its impact, medical and otherwise. It is an unpleasant thought, but probably a true fact, that when the French were involved militarily in Mexico in the 19th century, the corpses of their dead were fed upon by wolves, but local soldiers bodies were left alone by animals because of the high chili content of the Mexican diet.[2] In the intervening years, there has been a lot in the medical literature about *Capsicum spp.* In fact, on April 1, 2006, the world's hottest chili was identified.[3] The chili in question was farmed in England, not in Central or South America, and the chili rated a 900,000 on the Scoville scale on independent testing. If you are not familiar with the Scoville scale, in 1912, while working for Parke Davis Pharmaceutical Company, Wilbur Scoville devised a dilution test for rating the heat of chilies. Prior to the description of the Dorset Naga chili, the previous record holder for Scoville scale for chilies was held by Habanero, scoring just 570,000 Scoville units. Medicinal grade capsaicin comes in at a scale of 15 million Scoville units. Regarding capsaicin and its close relatives (the main one being the dihydrocapsaicin), these are vanillylnoneamides with minor modifications in the nine-carbon chain, whereas the red coloring comes from the carotene-like capsanthin and capsorubin. Capsaicin receptors have long been a topic of research by pharmacologists for their possible role in the management of prostatic cancer. They are also frequently instilled in inflamed, painful bladders where they literally "burn" nerve endings, producing pain relief after a brief period of intense pain (usually managed with heavy sedation). More and more medical uses are being found for capsaicin.

For growers of the powerful Dorset Naga chili, the future does not look very bright because the chili is so hot one needs to use rubber gloves to handle it. Some of us cannot even handle hot wings at our local Chili's. To read more about the history of chilies in medicine, see the review by Sharp.[4]

J. A. Stockman III, MD

References

1. Munnich A, Rötig A, Chretien D, et al. Clinical presentation of mitochondrial disorders in childhood. *J Inherit Metab Dis.* 1996;19:521-527.
2. Davidson A. *The Oxford Companion to Food.* Oxford: Oxford University Press; 1999:171.
3. de Bruxelles S. The chili so hot you need gloves. *Times Online* [serial online]. April 1, 2006. Available at: http://www.timesonline.co.uk/tol/news/uk/article 700700.ece. Accessed: April 11, 2006.
4. Sharp D. Some like it hottest. *Lancet.* 2006;367:1804.

16 Oncology

The Incidence Peaks of the Childhood Acute Leukemias Reflect Specific Cytogenetic Aberrations
Forestier E, for the Nordic Society of Paediatric Haematology and Oncology NOPHO (Univ of Umeå, Sweden; et al)
J Pediatr Hematol Oncol 28:486-495, 2006

The correlation between age and karyotype was studied in 1425, 0 to 14.9 years old children who were diagnosed with acute lymphoblastic leukemia (ALL) or acute myeloblastic leukemia. Almost 80% of the non-Down B-cell precursor ALL cases in the 2 to 7 years frequency peak group who had aberrant cytogenetic results had either a high-hyperdiploid clone (51 to 61 chromosomes) or a translocation t(12;21)(p13;q22). Among B-cell precursor ALL cases, high white blood cell counts correlated with earlier age at diagnosis ($r_S = -0.23$; $P < 0.001$) being most evident for 11q23/MLL-aberrations, translocation t(12;21)(p13;q22), and high-hyperdiploidy. Among acute myeloblastic leukemia patients, frequency peaks were found for those with MLL/11q23 rearrangements (peak: first year), Down syndrome (peak: second to third year), or cytogenetic abnormalities other than translocations t(8;21), t(15;17), and inv(16)/t(16;16) (peak: first to third year). The epidemiology of the cytogenetic subsets of acute leukemias questions whether age as a disease-related prognostic parameter has any relevance in childhood leukemia clinical research beyond being a surrogate marker for more important, truly biologic features such as cytogenetic aberrations and white cell count at diagnosis. Further research is needed to explore whether the 2 to 7 years age incidence peak in childhood ALL harbor yet unidentified cytogenetic subsets with the same natural history as the high-hyperdiploid and t(12;21)-positive leukemias.

▶ This report reminds us of the origins of childhood acute leukemias. The age-related incidence pattern of ALL has been interpreted to support a prenatal origin. The possibility of a prenatal origin is underscored by the fact that many cases of ALL and acute myeloblastic leukemia (AML) have been shown in retrospect to demonstrate clone-specific 11q23-, t(12;21)-, and t(8;21)-translocations, hyperdiploidy, or clone-specific immune gene rearrangements at birth. This is when Guthrie cards are examined in retrospect. On the basis of these and other findings, the natural history of the majority of childhood ALL cases has been proposed to reflect in utero emergence of preleukemic cells and crucial—but rare—postnatal interactions between these, the immune system, and common childhood infections. In contrast, little is known about the etiology of AML except for those with secondary leukemia and those with a known predisposing disorder, such as Down syndrome.

In this study from Norway, we see an improved understanding of childhood acute leukemia epidemiology and the clarification of the cytogenetic backbone for etiologic research that is based on analyzed data from the Nordic Society of Paediatric Haematology and Oncology population-based cytogenetic registry. This leukemia registry contains data from all children diagnosed before the age of 15 years in Denmark, Finland, Iceland, Norway, and Sweden. During a recent 10-year period, more than 1000 cases of ALL and some 350 cases of AML have been entered into the registry. The data from this study break down the prevalence for acute childhood leukemias into several categories. Infant leukemias are characterized by an inferior outcome, whereas the larger cohort of children with leukemia have a peak incidence in the 2- to 7-year age group, with the latter age group having a much more favorable outcome. The remainder of children are an inhomogeneous group that have a fairly stable incidence during childhood. Among the latter are T-cell leukemias and more rare subsets of various chromosomal aberrations. It is clear that 11q23-translocated leukemias are the leukemia of infancy. When these leukemias appear in very early infancy, their prenatal origin is well proven, and close to 100% concordance rates are seen in monozygous infant twins. These mutations are present at birth and almost invariably lead to overt leukemia. With respect to those who manifest their leukemia at 2 to 7 years of age and who generally have a better prognosis, a significant proportion of this peak incidence leukemia is not explained by t(12;21)-positive and high-hyperdiploid leukemias.

As for ALL, childhood AML encompasses several well-defined cytogenetic subgroups that each have their characteristic age and incidence curve. The incidence peak of AML in the first 3 years of life primarily reflects AML in children affected with Down's syndrome. Later, classic AML shows specific chromosomal abnormalities that are fairly evenly distributed throughout childhood. The incidence patterns of AML in children with Down's syndrome makes it the second largest single group of all patients with AML.

If there is a bottom line to all of this, it is not that age specifically predicts prognosis; instead, age at presentation with leukemia reflects certain cytogenetic patterns of abnormalities, and it is the latter pattern display that better predicts prognosis. To say this differently, there is no substitute, any longer, for obtaining cytogenetic profiles on all newly diagnosed leukemia patients. This is sophisticated material and involves studies that can only be undertaken at referral centers.

J. A. Stockman III, MD

Toxicity and efficacy of 6-thioguanine versus 6-mercaptopurine in childhood lymphoblastic leukaemia: a randomised trial

Vora A, for the Medical Research Council/National Cancer Research Network Childhood Leukaemia Working Party (Sheffield Children's Hosp, England; et al)

Lancet 368:1339-1348, 2006

Background.—6-mercaptopurine has been a standard component of long-term continuing treatment for childhood lymphoblastic leukaemia, whereas 6-thioguanine has been mainly used for intensification courses. Since preliminary data have shown that 6-thioguanine is more effective than 6-mercaptopurine, we compared the efficacy and toxicity of the two drugs for childhood lymphoblastic leukaemia.

Methods.—Consecutive children with lymphoblastic leukaemia diagnosed in the UK and Ireland between April, 1997, and June, 2002, were randomly assigned either 6-thioguanine (750 patients) or 6-mercaptopurine (748 patients) during interim maintenance and continuing therapy. All patients received 6-thioguanine during intensification courses. We analysed event-free and overall survival on an intention-to-treat basis. We obtained toxicity data using an adverse-event reporting system, with follow-up questionnaires to seek detailed information for specific toxicities. This trial is registered with the International Standard Randomised Controlled Number 26727615 with the name ALL97.

Findings.—After a median follow up of 6 years, there was no difference in event-free or overall survival between the two treatment groups (Fig 5). Although 6-thioguanine conferred a significantly lower risk of isolated CNS

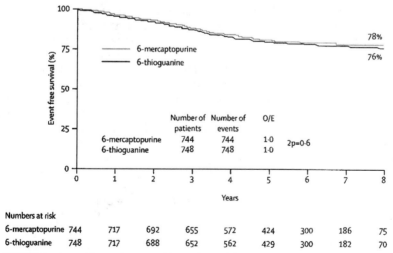

FIGURE 5.—Actuarial event-free survival by randomized thipurine. O/E = observed events divided by expected events. (Courtesy of Vora A, Mitchell CD, Lennard L, et al. Toxicity and efficacy of 6-thioguanine versus 6-mercaptopurine in childhood lymphoblastic leukaemia: a randomised trial. *Lancet.* 368:1339-1348. Copyright 2006 by Elsevier.)

relapse than did 6-mercaptopurine (odds ratio [OR] 0.53, 95% CI 0.30–0.92, p=0.02), the benefit was offset by an increased risk of death in remission (2.22, 1.20–4.14, p=0.01), mainly due to infections during continuing therapy. Additionally, 95 patients developed veno-occlusive disease of the liver. Of these, 82 were randomly assigned 6-thioguanine, representing 11% of all 6-thioguanine recipients. On long-term follow-up, about 5% of 6-thioguanine recipients have evidence of non-cirrhotic portal hypertension due to periportal liver fibrosis or nodular regenerative hyperplasia.

Interpretation.—Compared with 6-mercaptopurine, 6-thioguanine causes excess toxicity without an overall benefit. 6-mercaptopurine should remain the thiopurine of choice for continuing therapy of childhood lymphoblastic leukaemia.

▶ For some time now, contemporary first-line treatment for childhood acute lymphoblastic leukemia (ALL) has been based on serial multidrug phases of therapy delivered over 2 to 3 years. Appropriate therapy leads to survival rates of about 80% over the long haul and patients at that point are overwhelmingly likely to remain free of disease. Traditional management of ALL involves treatment that includes induction of remission, consolidation as well as reinduction to prevent emergence of a drug-resistant leukemic clone, extra compartment therapy to treat the central nervous system and the testes, and maintenance therapy to eradicate residual leukemic cells.

The report of Vora et al comes from the United Kingdom where the investigators compared the toxicity and efficacy of 6-thioguanine with 6-mercaptopurine for maintenance of childhood ALL. Both agents are thiopurines and both have played important roles in leukemia protocols. 6-mercaptopurine is largely used in lymphoblastic leukemias and 6-thioguanine is used mainly in acute myeloid leukemia or relapsed ALL. First-line treatment for childhood ALL most often includes several cycles of 6-mercaptopurine, starting as early consolidation treatment up to about 36 months after diagnosis. Vora et al challenge this tradition by randomly assigning almost 1500 children to receive either 6-thioguanine or 6-mercaptopurine. The results were a mixed blessing. After 6 years, event-free survival did not differ between the 2 groups. There was a large reduction in the recurrence in CNS disease by 6-thioguanine (OR 0.53), but this advantage was offset by an increased risk of death in remission (OR 2.22), mainly caused by infections. Also, some 11% of patients in the 6-thioguanine group had nonfatal liver toxicity develop with features of veno-occlusive disease compared with fewer than 2% in the 6-mercaptopurine group. If you are not familiar with veno-occlusive disease of the liver, symptoms and signs include tender enlargement of the liver, hyperbilirubinemia with raised levels of liver enzymes, a decreased platelet count, and portal hypertension. One or more of these signs and symptoms occur in 85% of 6-thioguanine–treated patients during maintenance therapy.

Thus, it is that the more we learn about the management of childhood ALL, the more the traditional approaches for standard-risk patients seem to be a fine balance between outcomes versus risks. Pending conclusive evidence of greater efficacy of 6-thioguanine compared with 6-mercaptopurine, and a better understanding of the mechanisms of liver toxicity to allow identification of patients who can be given the drug safely, 6-mercaptopurine should remain the standard thiopurine in the continuing therapy of childhood ALL.

J. A. Stockman III, MD

Chronic Health Conditions in Adult Survivors of Childhood Cancer
Oeffinger KC, for the Childhood Cancer Survivor Study (Mem Sloan-Kettering Cancer Ctr, New York; et al)
N Engl J Med 355:1572-1582, 2006

Background.—Only a few small studies have assessed the long-term morbidity that follows the treatment of childhood cancer. We determined the incidence and severity of chronic health conditions in adult survivors.

Methods.—The Childhood Cancer Survivor Study is a retrospective cohort study that tracks the health status of adults who received a diagnosis of childhood cancer between 1970 and 1986 and compares the results with those of siblings. We calculated the frequencies of chronic conditions in 10,397 survivors and 3034 siblings. A severity score (grades 1 through 4, ranging from mild to life-threatening or disabling) was assigned to each condition. Cox proportional-hazards models were used to estimate hazard ratios, reported as relative risks and 95% confidence intervals (CIs), for a chronic condition.

Results.—Survivors and siblings had mean ages of 26.6 years (range, 18.0 to 48.0) and 29.2 years (range, 18.0 to 56.0), respectively, at the time of the study. Among 10,397 survivors, 62.3% had at least one chronic condition;

TABLE 3.—Relative Risk of Selected Severe (Grade 3) or Life-Threatening or Disabling (Grade 4) Health Conditions among Cancer Survivors, as Compared with Siblings

Condition	Survivors (N = 10,397)	Siblings (N = 3034)	Relative Risk (95% CI)
	percent		
Major joint replacement*	1.61	0.03	54.0 (7.6-386.3)
Congestive heart failure	1.24	0.10	15.1 (4.8-47.9)
Second malignant neoplasm†	2.38	0.33	14.8 (7.2-30.4)
Cognitive dysfunction, severe	0.65	0.10	10.5 (2.6-43.0)
Coronary artery disease	1.11	0.20	10.4 (4.1-25.9)
Cerebrovascular accident	1.56	0.20	9.3 (4.1-21.2)
Renal failure or dialysis	0.52	0.07	8.9 (2.2-36.6)
Hearing loss not corrected by aid	1.96	0.36	6.3 (3.3-11.8)
Legally blind or loss of an eye	2.92	0.69	5.8 (3.5-9.5)
Ovarian failure‡	2.79	0.99	3.5 (2.7-5.2)

*For survivors, major joint replacement was not included if it was part of cancer therapy.
†For both groups, this category excludes basal-cell and squamous-cell carcinoma (grade 2). For siblings, this category includes a first cancer.
‡Values are for women only.
Reprinted by permission from Oeffinger KC, Mertens AC, Sklar CA, et al, for the Childhood Cancer Survival Study. Chronic health conditions in adult survivors of childhood cancer. N Engl J Med. 355:1572-1582. Copyright 2006, Massachusetts Medical Society. All rights reserved.

27.5% had a severe or life-threatening condition (grade 3 or 4). The adjusted relative risk of a chronic condition in a survivor, as compared with siblings, was 3.3 (95% CI, 3.0 to 3.5); for a severe or life-threatening condition, the risk was 8.2 (95% CI, 6.9 to 9.7). Among survivors, the cumulative incidence of a chronic health condition reached 73.4% (95% CI, 69.0 to 77.9) 30 years after the cancer diagnosis, with a cumulative incidence of 42.4% (95% CI, 33.7 to 51.2) for severe, disabling, or life-threatening conditions or death due to a chronic condition.

Conclusions.—Survivors of childhood cancer have a high rate of illness owing to chronic health conditions (Table 3).

▶ This report is one of the most important to ever appear in *The New England Journal of Medicine* with respect to its implications for pediatrics. It was also in *The New England Journal of Medicine* back in 1948 that an article by Sydney Farber and his colleagues reported that they had successfully used aminopterin to induce temporary remission in children with lymphoid leukemia.[1] This exciting article suggested that what had been a uniformly fatal disease might be amenable to treatment and, some dared to hope, cure. By 1970, De Vita et al at the National Cancer Institute showed that a combination of non–cross-reactive chemotherapeutic agents, the MOPP regimen, could induce sustained remission in patients with advanced Hodgkin's disease.[2] From such beginnings, an extraordinary success story unfolded, and today, more than 75% of children with cancer are being cured of their disease. Nearly 20,000 patients under the age of 21 years receive a diagnosis of cancer each year in the United States, and more than 15,000 per year enter the ranks of the cured and live into adulthood. Some would say that the "war on cancer" might have already been won. Au contraire as we see, however, in the report abstracted from *The New England Journal of Medicine*, which shows that those who are cured of childhood cancer may later experience a host of adverse events, some of which may not appear for many years after treatment. These findings suggest the need for vigorous and long-term monitoring of young cancer survivors, accompanied by early intervention when problems arise.

So what is the dark side to being cured of childhood cancer? Oeffinger et al report the latest follow-up from a remarkable long-term study that does for the survival of childhood cancer what the Framingham Heart Study did for the natural history of cardiovascular disease. The Childhood Cancer Survivor Study (CCSS), established in 1994, is conducted by a consortium of 25 pediatric oncology treatment centers that have pooled data on their survivors, who were treated between 1970 and 1986, when significant strides were first made in the treatment of the most common types of cancer in children. Although several previous studies documented the substantial incidence of specific long-term side effects of treatment faced by cancer survivors, no study has approached the sheer number of patients followed by the CCSS. This group is clearly the standard by which all future studies should be measured.

So what do the data tell us about the health of long-term cancer survivors? There is an extraordinarily high incidence of late and often permanent complications arising from intensive treatment with combination chemotherapy and ionizing radiation. The long-term risks are cumulative, with no evidence so far of a plateau. This is worrisome news. Almost two thirds of patients report at least one chronic health problem, and one quarter have a severe condition. Almost one quarter report having three or more chronic health problems. By any criteria, these results are alarming and bespeak a significant level of complications in a population in which only a minority of patients receive follow-up from specialists. Only time will tell how, for example, the preexisting myocardial damage from anthracycline exposure or heart irradiation for Hodgkin's disease will affect cardiac risk factors in combination with the normal risk factors that all of us have (eg, hypolipidemia, hypertension, diabetes, and kidney disease).

One of the major unsolved problems in American medicine is how to effectively transition care from pediatric providers to adult providers. It would seem to be incumbent on us to ensure that survivors of childhood cancer in particular are followed closely by physicians who understand the effects and outcomes of cancer treatment—who know what these patients have been through and what future complications to look for. Sadly, such follow-up is the exception rather than the rule. Historically, most of these patients, especially the adolescents and younger adults, have been cared for by pediatric oncologists. Over time, however, most of these patients drift away from the specialty clinic as they age. It is clear that the complications, both known and unknown, that will develop in survivors can demand a level of knowledge that is beyond the range of the general internist or family physician, or even the adult medical oncologist. In an interesting commentary on the follow-up of childhood cancer survivors, Rosoff[3] proposes incorporation of specific training in this area into our residency programs in internal medicine, pediatrics, and family medicine, and as an alternative, the development of a postgraduate fellowship in an adult subspecialty, analogous to the fellowships in adult congenital heart disease that are common in most major academic medical centers. Part of the solution is also to empower patients to recognize that they have a responsibility to monitor their health as well. Empowerment means providing this patient population with current and potential future knowledge about what conditions they have an increased risk for developing. Because the number of childhood cancer survivors has risen substantially, the development of follow-up clinics is not beyond the pale. Such clinics could easily be staffed using a multidisciplinary approach.

J. A. Stockman III, MD

References

1. Farber S, Diamond LK, Mercer RD et al. Temporary remissions in acute leukemia in children produced by folic acid antagonist 4-aminopsteroly-glulanic acid (aminopsterin). *N Engl J Med*. 1948;238:787-793.
2. Neville HR. Vincent De Vita receives first Pezcoller Award. *J Natn Cancer Inst*. 1988;80:719.
3. Rosoff PM. The two-edged sword of curing childhood cancer. *N Engl J Med*. 2006;355:1522-1523.

Hypertension in Childhood Cancer: A Frequent Complication of Certain Tumor Sites

Madre C, Orbach D, Baudouin V, et al (Institut Curie, Paris; Hopital Robert Debré-APHP, Paris)
J Pediatr Hematol Oncol 28:659-664, 2006

The clinical features and management of severe hypertension (HT) (blood pressure > 99th percentile + 5 mm Hg) have been rarely described in pediatric oncology.

Objectives.—Retrospective descriptive study of the case files of 31 patients followed in the Institut Curie Department of Pediatric Oncology between 1999 and 2004 and presenting severe HT at the time of diagnosis of their tumor.

Results.—The median age was 2 years 1 month (range: 3 mo to 6 y 8 mo). Median blood pressure was 99th percentile + 30 mm Hg (range: 99th percentile + 7 mm Hg to 99th percentile + 62 mm Hg). The tumors presented by these children were: Wilms tumor (n = 17, ie, 20% of all Wilms tumors treated during this period), neuroblastoma (n = 12, ie, 10% of all neuroblastomas treated during this period) or other tumors (n = 2). HT was asymptomatic in all children. Initial management consisted of etiologic treatment by primary chemotherapy and/or surgical resection of the tumor, associated with antihypertensive therapy, initially administered by intravenous injection for 12 children (nicardipine, labetalol) and then orally in all children (calcium channel blockers, n = 23; angiotensin-converting enzyme inhibitor, n = 16; β-blockers, n = 4; α/β-blockers, n = 2; diuretics, n = 1). Dual therapy was necessary in 7 cases and triple therapy was necessary in 1 case. The median duration of antihypertensive therapy was 40 days (range: 9 to 195). No child developed a serious complication of HT.

Conclusions.—Initial HT is a frequent complication of Wilms tumor and neuroblastoma and affects young children (< 2.5 y). It is often severe, asymptomatic, but needs specific treatment and resolves after treatment of the tumor.

▶ Anyone who cares for children with cancer recognizes the fact that hypertension is not a rare finding at presentation or during the course of disease treatment. This study from Paris underscores this point and confirms the high prevalence of hypertension in childhood cancer, a complicating factor in some 10% to 20% of children being treated for certain forms of malignancy. For example, almost 20% of children with a neurogenic tumor will have hypertension. Other series have reported a 25% to 60% frequency of hypertension in children with Wilms tumor. This hypertension is often severe. Brain tumors are also associated with the presence of hypertension. Fortunately, most children with a malignancy and hypertension do not have clinical signs and symptoms directly related to elevated blood pressure.

The pathophysiologic mechanism causing hypertension in children afflicted with a cancer remains largely unexplained. The presumed mechanisms for hypertension include stretching of a renal pedicle, compression of the healthy renal parenchyma, secretion of catecholamines, a renal vein or inferior vena cava thrombosis, or associated renal disease. Many times those with Wilms tumor will not have a specific identifiable cause for their hypertension. The hypertension is likely induced by excessive renin secretion by the tumor or compression of the healthy renal parenchyma. Excessive renin secretion caused by activation of the renin-angiotensin system may coexist with these other causes of hypertension, although a recent study has shown elevated plasma renin activity in children with Wilms tumor and hypertension in only 56% of subjects.[1]Fortunately, children with malignancy and hypertension will have the latter adequately treated by management of their malignancy. Antihypertensive therapy is usually required only for a brief period until the chemotherapy takes effect. It should be remembered that in children with retroperitoneal tumors responsible for bilateral renal pedicle compression as a cause of hypertension, ACE inhibitors should be avoided or administered cautiously with regular Doppler surveillance of renal vessels and monitoring of renal function. These examinations are needed to detect renal hypoperfusion related to the glomerular postcapillary vasodilator action of ACE inhibitors.

Although no untoward effects were seen as a consequence of hypertension in the patients reported here, this is only because the hypertension was aggressively managed. Early treatment of hypertension is needed to prevent immediate serious complications. In this series, one-third of youngsters required urgent intravenous antihypertensive therapy because of their age and the magnitude of the elevation in blood pressure.

See the Olgar et al report (Can renal leukemic infiltration cause hypertension in children?) that explains that acute lymphoblastic leukemia (ALL) can also be a cause of hypertension in children. Just over 6% of ALL patients at presentation will be hypertensive, and it is this group of patients that has twice the likelihood of developing the tumor lysis syndrome. The hypertension is presumably due to renal leukemic infiltration. Fortunately, hypertension resolves within about 2 weeks of institution of conventional chemotherapy.

J. A. Stockman III, MD

Reference

1. Hadley GP, Mars M. Hypertension in a cohort of African children with renal tumours. *Pediatr Surg Int.* 2006;22:219-223.

Can Renal Leukemic Infiltration Cause Hypertension in Children?
Olgar S, Yetgin S, Cetin M, et al (Hacettepe Univ, Ankara, Turkey)
J Pediatr Hematol Oncol 28:579-584, 2006

Out of 334 children with acute lymphoblastic leukemia who were treated with St Jude Total XI and Total XIII chemotherapy protocols were investigated and 21 (6.3%) were hypertensive. The incidence of tumor lysis syndrome was higher in the hypertensive group than in the nonhypertensive group (28.6% vs. 11.5%) ($P = 0.035$). There were no differences between patients treated with high-dose methylprednisolone and prednisolone St

Jude Total XI and Total XIII, St Jude Total XIII LR and St Jude Total XIII HR groups in respect of the above-mentioned parameters. Central nervous system involvement, skeletal system involvement, abdominal lymphadenopathy, elevated lactate dehydrogenase and leukocyte count, French-American-British types and immunophenotypes were not found to be statistically significant to the development of hypertension ($P > 0.05$). We found that renal leukemic infiltration is a risk factor in hypertension development ($P = 0.04$) and hypertension is a risk factor for renal parenchymal disorder in the follow-up period ($P = 0.0001$). Six patients presenting with hypertension in the first week of disease therapy were evaluated for renal parenchymal disorder and glomerular filtration rate abnormality in the follow-up period. Glomerular filtration rate abnormality was found in 1 and renal scintigraphic dimercaptosuccinic acid abnormalities (reduced uptake and dilated hypoactivity) were found in 4 patients. Hypertension was also found to be a risk factor for renal parenchymal disorder in the follow-up period.

▶ Anything at all that helps children with malignancies fare better with their disease is a welcome addition to our treatment regimens. Recently, something that we normally decry seems to be of some benefit in this regard. Specifically, we are speaking of chewing gum. Prolonged gum chewing has been shown to increase salivary flow 3-fold to 10-fold, with a peak after a few minutes and a plateau thereafter. In addition, the habitual use of sugar-free chewing gum is associated with enhanced saliva stimulation responsible for increases in plaque buffering power and remineralization, with no fall in plaque pH resulting from the gum itself, no enhanced plaque acidogenicity in response to dietary carbohydrates, and improved salivary gland function. The chewing of gum has also been studied as a possible aid in reducing the complications of oral mucositis in children receiving chemotherapy.[1] While finding no evidence that chewing 5 to 6 pieces of gum per day decreases the risk of severe oral mucositis in children receiving chemotherapy, this study does suggest benefits from chewing gum in reducing low-grade oral mucositis. This same study found a significant reduction in the time on parenteral nutrition in children chewing gum in comparison to those who were not when receiving chemotherapy. This suggests that increasing saliva clearance may be associated with a faster recovery period.

Chances are we will be hearing more about this "Wrigley Effect" in children receiving chemotherapy. Stay tuned.

J.A. Stockman III, MD

Reference

1. Gandemer V, Le Deley MC, Dollfus C, et al. Multicenter randomized trial of chewing gum for preventing oral mucositis in children receiving chemotherapy. *J Pediatr Hematol Oncol.* 2007;29:86-94.

The prevalence of overweight and obesity in pediatric survivors of cancer
Nathan PC, Jovcevska V, Ness KK, et al (Hosp for Sick Children, Toronto; Univ of Minnesota, Minneapolis; Univ Health Network, Toronto)
J Pediatr 149:518-525, 2006

Objective.—To compare the prevalence of overweight in a cohort of pediatric survivors of cancer with that in the general population.

Study Design.—We reviewed the charts of 441 cancer survivors followed at a Canadian tertiary care pediatric hospital and calculated their most recent body mass index. We compared this cohort with population data generated from the Canadian Community Health Survey.

Results.—At a median age of 14.7 years (range, 3.4 to 19.5 years) and a median time from diagnosis of 9.7 years (range, 3.4 to 19.2 years), 140 of 441 patients (31.7%) were overweight or obese. Only 12 of the 441 patients (2.7%) were underweight. Males age 6 to 11 years (odds ratio [OR] = 2.29; 95% confidence interval [CI] = 1.36 to 3.86; $P < .001$) and male survivors of acute lymphoblastic leukemia (OR = 1.55; 95% CI = 1.03 to 2.52; $P = .04$) were more likely to be overweight than the general population. No other age or diagnostic group had an increased risk of overweight.

Conclusions.—The prevalence of overweight was not increased in this cohort compared with the general population. However, almost ⅓ of these patients are overweight, necessitating a clinical and research focus on preventing and combating overweight in childhood cancer survivors.

▶ Much of the research on obesity in childhood cancer survivors has focused on patients who received cranial irradiation for acute lymphoblastic leukemia (ALL) or brain tumors. These populations are considered at particular risk because irradiation, surgery, and the tumor itself can all damage the hypothalamic-pituitary axis. Direct damage to the satiety center in the ventro-medial hypothalamus, insensitivity to leptin, and deficiency of growth hormone have been proposed as specific mechanisms for overweight in these patients. What has not been well studied are the patterns of overweight, however, in survivors of other types of childhood cancer. Although direct damage to the hypothalamic-pituitary axis is not likely, these patients may be susceptible to overweight because of risk factors common in the general population, including poor dietary choices and increased sedentary behavior. It is the latter group of patients who survived childhood cancers other than leukemia and brain tumors that this report focuses on.

If there is good news to report from the findings of this study, it is that the prevalence of overweight (20.9%) and obesity (10.9%) among pediatric survivors of childhood cancer does not differ from that observed in the general population. However, cancer therapy increases the long-term risk of morbidity and mortality in survivors of childhood cancer, and a clinical concern is that one third of this population exacerbates this risk by being overweight. Although they are no different than their peers, this group should be vigilant about maintaining their health better than the peer group that they associate with. Overweight in survivors of childhood cancer has been linked to several risk factors for cardiovascular disease, including hyperlipidemia, glucose intolerance, and hypertension. Combine this with prior exposure to cardiotoxic anthracycline chemotherapy (received by more than 60% of cancer survivors) and you have a lethal brew later in life.

The data of this report clearly demonstrate that the only diagnosis associated with an increased prevalence of overweight or obesity is ALL, and this association is statistically significant only in boys. Survivors of ALL treated with cranial irradiation therapy do not seem to be at increased risk of overweight or obesity compared with those who have been treated with chemotherapy alone. The increased body mass index observed in ALL patients is found as early as the end of their initial treatment for malignancy. This means that management of weight will fall within the purview of the pediatric oncologist as well as the generalist pediatrician.

The punch line here is pretty straightforward. Survivors of ALL need extraordinary attention to manage their weight and to prevent long-term consequences of being both overweight and a cancer survivor. Additionally, although the overall prevalence of overweight is not increased in other childhood cancer survivors, its potential impact is magnified by the risk of comorbid conditions. Therefore any childhood cancer survivor should be rigorously followed and managed to prevent overweight and obesity.

The Oeffinger report (Chronic health conditions in adult survivors of childhood cancer) is a landmark study that reveals alarming rates of chronic disease among adult survivors of childhood cancer. The findings of that report underscore the many health hazards that children may run into when they survive cancer.

J. A. Stockman III, MD

Symptoms Affecting Children With Malignancies During the Last Month of Life: A Nationwide Follow-up

Jalmsell L, Kreicbergs U, Onelöv E, et al (Karolinska Institutet, Stockholm; Dana Farber Cancer Inst, Boston; Sahlgrenska Academy, Gothenburg, Sweden)
Pediatrics 117:1314-1320, 2006

Objective.—In a population-based nationwide survey, we aimed to study symptoms in children with malignancies during the last month of their lives. Understanding which symptoms affect children in the terminal phase of disease is crucial to improve palliative care.

Methods.—We attempted to contact all parents in Sweden who had lost a child to cancer during a 6-year period. The parents were asked, through an anonymous postal questionnaire, about symptoms that affected the child's sense of well-being during the last month of life.

Results.—Information was supplied by 449 (80%) of 561 eligible parents. The symptoms most frequently reported with high or moderate impact on the child's well-being were: physical fatigue (86%), reduced mobility (76%), pain (73%), and decreased appetite (71%). Irrespective of the specific malignancy, physical fatigue was the most frequently reported symptom, and pain was among the 3 most frequently reported. Children who died at 9 to 15 years of age were reported to be moderately or severely affected, by a number of symptoms, significantly more often than other children. The gender of the reporting parent had no significant bearing on any of the symptoms reported.

Conclusions.—The most frequently reported symptoms in children with malignancies to be aware of and possibly address during the terminal phase are physical fatigue, reduced mobility, pain, and decreased appetite. Children aged 9 to 15 years are reported to be moderately or severely affected by more symptoms than children in other age groups. Mothers and fathers report a similar prevalence of symptoms.

▶ In early 2006 the American Board of Medical Specialties approved subcertification in the field of palliative medicine. The American Board of Pediatrics was among a number of certifying boards that petitioned for such subcertification. It is an unfortunate fact that children with cancer do not uniformly survive and some will need palliative care; thus the importance of the report from Sweden that gives us useful information about what symptoms are likely to be problematic during the last month of life in children who will die from a malignancy. We see that the most frequently recognized symptom in the terminally ill child has been pain and many studies have identified pain and pain relief as one of the main concerns for the child and his or her family. However, there are many other symptoms that contribute to the suffering of the child and for which we need to find better management approaches. The authors of this report have analyzed the symptoms that moderately or severely affect the sense of well being of children with malignancies during the last month of their lives as reported by the parents in a population-based, nationwide study. We see that the symptoms most frequently reported to affect well-being include physical fatigue (86%), reduced mobility (76%), pain (73%), and poor appetite (71%). These symptoms, as well as weight loss, vomiting, and sleepiness during the day, are all symptoms that more than half of parents reported as having a moderate or high impact on the child's well-being. These symptoms were present largely irrespective of the diagnosis of the child's specific malignancy.

Perhaps the knowledge provided by this report will help to improve the care to further minimize suffering at the end of a child's life. That is the least we can do for these kids who have been through so much.

J. A. Stockman III, MD

ac Disease and Childhood Cancer

Cereda S, Cefalo G, Spreafico F, et al (Istituto Nazionale per lo Studio e la Cura dei Tumori, Milano, Italy)
J Pediatr Hematol Oncol 28:346-349, 2006

Background.—Celiac disease (CD) is a genetically determined condition characterized by malabsorption, abnormal small-bowel structure, and gluten intolerance. CD is one of the most common inherited disorders and has a worldwide distribution. Patients with CD have been shown to have an increased frequency of serum histocompatibility antigens, in particular HLA-DQ2 and DQ8. It has been hypothesized that genetic factors such as these may predispose individuals to intolerance of dietary proteins such as the peptides in gluten. Thus, patients with CD are treated with a life-long gluten-free diet. Cancer is primarily a disease of aging and is very rare in childhood. A higher rate of malignancy in adult patients with CD has been confirmed in several studies, particularly for lymphoma, adenocarcinoma of the small intestine, and squamous cell carcinomas of the esophagus, mouth, and pharynx. Several studies have also shown that a gluten-free diet is also protective against the onset of malignancy in this setting. Few cases of CD have been associated with pediatric malignancies in the literature. Three such cases are presented.

> *Case 1.*—Boy, 5 years, with Burkitt's lymphoma was treated with 3 months of chemotherapy. Six years after completing the cancer treatment, he was given a diagnosis of CD because of evidence of poor growth. At the diagnosis of malignancy, he was seen with abdominal pain, a mass, and ascites. He is now alive, cancer free, and restricted from gluten.
>
> *Case 2.*—Boy, 4 years, was given a diagnosis of ependymoma 2 years after a diagnosis of CD. The symptoms of CD at diagnosis were anorexia, diarrhea, and growth arrest; the symptoms of malignancy were a headache and vomiting persisting for 2 weeks. He has undergone radical surgery, radiotherapy at the disease site, and 3 months of chemotherapy.
>
> *Case 3.*—Girl, 6 years, was given a diagnosis of Ewing sarcoma 1.5 years after receiving a diagnosis of CD. At CD diagnosis, she had neurologic symptoms as well as dermatitis on the legs and chest and around the mouth, persisting for 4 months. Ewing sarcoma arose on the left leg and was treated with radical surgery and 6 months of chemotherapy.

Conclusions.—Both patients 2 and 3 started a gluten-restricted diet after the diagnosis of CD. Several studies on the possible association between CD and cancer have revealed a greater risk of malignancy in adults with CD than in the general population, particularly in cases of small-bowel cancer, esophageal carcinoma, and lymphoma. The mechanism responsible for the development of cancer in patients with CD is not known, but a greater intestinal permeability to environmental carcinogens, chronic inflammation, chronic antigenic stimulation, the release of proinflammatory cytokines, immune surveillance problems, and nutritional deficiencies due to CD have been suggested.

▶ A high rate of malignancy in adult patients with CD has been confirmed in several studies. In particular, an increased risk for small-bowel cancer, esophageal carcinoma, and lymphoma exists. Patients with CD have a significantly increased odds ratio of 2.6 for non-Hodgkin's lymphoma. The association relates to 2 infrequent types of lymphoma: small-bowel non-Hodgkin's lymphoma (odds ratio, 11.8) and enteropathy-associated T-cell lymphoma (odds ratio, 28). Although this rare T-cell lymphoma occurs approximately 20 times more frequently in patients with CD, the overall association of all non-Hodgkin's lymphomas with CD is less common than thought. The odds ratios associated with CD are 10 for small-bowel adenocarcinoma, 4.2 for esophageal cancer, 2.3 for oropharyngeal cancer, and 1.5 for colorectal cancer.

We do not know what the mechanism is behind the development of cancer in patients with CD. A greater intestinal permeability to environmental carcinogens, chronic inflammation, chronic antigenic stimulation, the release of proinflammatory cytokines, immune surveillance problems, and nutritional deficiencies due to CD have all been suggested as possibilities. Sticking to a gluten-free diet for 5 consecutive years or more diminishes the risk of malignancy to that of control subjects without CD.

Few cases in the literature report the association between CD and pediatric cancer. In Europe, about 2 dozen cases of CD and cancer in children have been reported throughout history. If you take all reported cases worldwide, the most prevalent type of pediatric cancer in a patient with CD is non-Hodgkin's lymphoma (30%), followed by sarcoma (20%), medulloblastoma (10%), carcinoma (10%), leukemia (7%), neuroblastoma (7%), Wilms' tumor (3.2%), ependymoma (3.2%), hepatoblastoma (3.2%), craniopharyngioma (3.2%), and Hodgkin's lymphoma (3.2%). It is worth noting that 10% of cancers were diagnosed before a diagnosis of CD was made, and in another 13%, it was diagnosed at the same time as the CD. In the pediatric population reported in this study, the mean time from a diagnosis of CD to the appearance of cancer in those not on a gluten-restricted diet was 7.1 years. In these patients, the most common tumor was a non-Hodgkin's lymphoma (37%), and all the non-Hodgkin's lymphomas originated from the small bowel. On the other hand, the mean time to cancer onset in the pediatric patients on a gluten-free diet was 6.5 years, and the prevalent type of neoplasm was brain cancer (26%), of which 20% was medulloblastoma. Sarcomas of bone and soft tissue and non-Hodgkin's lymphoma accounted for 20%. All these non-Hodgkin's lymphomas originated from the lymphoreticular system.

It is obvious that an association exists between CD and childhood cancer, but the risk of developing the latter during childhood is much, much less than at older ages. Nonetheless, vigilance is still important. Many of the malignancies that are associated with CD are quite treatable and, in a significant percentage of patients, curable.

J. A. Stockman III, MD

Increasing Incidence of Thyroid Cancer in the United States, 1973-2002

Davies L, Welch HG (Dept of Veterans Affairs Med Ctr, White River Junction, Vt; Darmouth Med School, Hanover, NH)
JAMA 295:2164-2167, 2006

Context.—Increasing cancer incidence is typically interpreted as an increase in the true occurrence of disease but may also reflect changing pathological criteria or increased diagnostic scrutiny. Changes in the diagnostic approach to thyroid nodules may have resulted in an increase in the apparent incidence of thyroid cancer.

Objective.—To examine trends in thyroid cancer incidence, histology, size distribution, and mortality in the United States.

Methods.—Retrospective cohort evaluation of patients with thyroid cancer, 1973-2002, using the Surveillance, Epidemiology, and End Results (SEER) program and data on thyroid cancer mortality from the National Vital Statistics System.

Main Outcome Measures.—Thyroid cancer incidence, histology, size distribution, and mortality.

Results.—The incidence of thyroid cancer increased from 3.6 per 100,000 in 1973 to 8.7 per 100,000 in 2002—a 2.4-fold increase (95% confidence interval [CI], 2.2-2.6; $P<.001$ for trend). There was no significant change in the incidence of the less common histological types: follicular, medullary, and anaplastic ($P>.20$ for trend). Virtually the entire increase is attributable to an increase in incidence of papillary thyroid cancer, which increased from 2.7 to 7.7 per 100,000—a 2.9-fold increase (95% CI, 2.6-3.2; $P<.001$ for trend). Between 1988 (the first year SEER collected data on tumor size) and 2002, 49% (95% CI, 47%-51%) of the increase consisted of cancers measuring 1 cm or smaller; 87% (95% CI, 85%-89%) consisted of cancers measuring 2 cm or smaller. Mortality from thyroid cancer was stable between 1973 and 2002 (approximately 0.5 deaths per 100,000).

Conclusions.—The increasing incidence of thyroid cancer in the United States is predominantly due to the increased detection of small papillary cancers. These trends, combined with the known existence of a substantial reservoir of subclinical cancer and stable overall mortality, suggest that increasing incidence reflects increased detection of subclinical disease, not an increase in the true occurrence of thyroid cancer.

▶ You might ask why this pediatric editor includes an article dealing with the increasing incidence of thyroid cancer here in the United States when this is a disease that rarely affects children. The disease can affect a child. As important, the roots of adult thyroid cancer may find themselves in the soil of childhood exposure to various entities that can trigger the later development of thyroid cancer. Data do show that the average age of diagnosis for thyroid cancer is 45 years with women being affected more than men by a ratio of 2.7 to 1. The distribution of histological categories for thyroid cancer is as follows: 88% papillary, 9% follicular, and 3% poorly differentiated (medullary and anaplastic).

What we learn from the Surveillance, Epidemiology, and End Results (SEER) program is that the incidence of thyroid cancer has increased more than 2.4 fold in the past 30 years. Most of this increase (87%) relates to a diagnosis of small papillary cancers. Fortunately, mortality has remained stable during this three-decade period. This suggests that the rise in incidence of cancer reflects an increased detection of subclinical thyroid disease, not an increase in the true occurrence of thyroid cancer, but this is speculative.

The American Thyroid Association has established evidence-based management guidelines for subjects found to have thyroid nodules. Whether these recommendations apply down into the childhood age group remains to be seen, but it is worth reminding ourselves what these recommendations are. The first recommendation is that thyroid sonography should be the initial study in anyone with one or more suspected thyroid nodules. Second, fine needle aspiration biopsy is the procedure of choice for evaluating thyroid nodules. Third, when several nodules larger than 1 cm to 1.5 cm are present, a biopsy should be performed on those with a suspicious sonographic appearance. Patients with nodules that are 8 mm to 9 mm and that have suspicious ultrasonographic findings (eg, blurred margins, mixed echogenicity, intranodular calcification, or Doppler flow), suspicious cervical lymph nodes, or a history of radiation exposure or familial thyroid cancer should be considered for ultrasound-guided fine needle aspiration biopsy. In adults, smaller nodules most likely can be followed up over several years without biopsy if they are not increasing in size. To read more on the topic of managing small thyroid cancers, albeit in adults, see the review by Mazzaferri.[1]

Having a thyroid disorder is one of the most common reasons why one undergoes a radionuclide scan. As we close this commentary having to do with thyroid disease, see how you would address the following fictitious scenario. A parent of one of your patients asks you for some "free" advice. This fellow wants to know if there is anything about the treatment of his illness that might produce some difficulty for his family, including several young children in the family, because they will soon be flying off to Disney World in Florida. It seems that this 40-year-old man had a history of weight loss, sweating, diarrhea, and tachycardia. His internist did thyroid studies and diagnosed him with hyperthyroidism. Because of difficulty with medical management, he was recently treated with radioiodine. The amount used was 400MBq of I[131]. What suggestions might you have for this man? The advice you would give has to do with the fact that individuals who are treated with radiopharmaceuticals may pose an environmental hazard to those around them. For this reason, all individuals so treated are given radionuclide instruction cards highlighting the usual precautions to be taken with respect to how bodily fluids should be handled in order to not expose others, particularly young children, to radioactive materials. You recommend to this fellow that he follow such precautions.

It is possible that you might forget one other important piece of information related to a case report of a 46-year-old man from Great Britain, who was also managed with I[131] for hyperthyroidism.[2] Six weeks after being treated for hyperthyroidism, this individual went to the United States for a holiday to Disney World. At the Orlando Airport, he set off the security alarms at check-in. He was immediately detained and strip-searched. Sniffer dogs were also used. A prolonged period of interrogation ensued. Luckily, he was carrying his radionuclide warning card with him. He was released after a long delay and much embarrassment. This fellow's case report represents the fifth such triggering of radiation alarms after radionuclide treatment. In the first report of such a circumstance back in 1986, two people tried to enter the White House for a public tour four days after exercise stress testing with a thallium scan. They set off the radiation alarm and were detained until the cause of the security breech was established.[3] In 1988, the day after having a thallium stress test, a 65-year-old patient went to his bank to examine the contents of his safety box. The security alarm sounded when he entered the bank vault. He continued to set off the alarm on subsequent visits to the vault until the ninth day after his thallium stress test.[4] In 2004, 25 days after having been treated with 150MBq of radioiodine for toxic multinodular goiter, a 76-year-old man set off the radiation alarm at Vienna International Airport and was investigated thoroughly. After this, a radiation protection certificate was designed and given to all patients receiving radionuclide treatment in Austria in order that similar problems are avoided.

Back in 2004, two days after having thallium-201 myocardial profusion scan, a 55-year-old pilot triggered the radiation detector alarms while traveling as a crew member to Moscow. After extensive investigations, he was released later that day. Four days later he set off the security alarm again at the same airport and was again detained, but was later released.[5]

It appears that security radiation detectors commonly found in airports and other high-risk places have varying sensitivity. One study has found that after receiving radioisotopes, patients might trigger radiation alarms for a varying number of days depending on the radioisotope.

Airports worldwide are deploying more sensitive radiation detection systems, and one would therefore expect additional such cases to be reported unless the medical community takes the responsibility of forewarning patients about the problem. Patients should receive a document verifying that there is a reason why they might set off a radiation detector.[6]

J. A. Stockman III, MD

References

1. Mazzaferri EL. Managing small thyroid cancers. *JAMA*. 2006;295:2179-2182.
2. Gangopadhyay KK, Sundram F, De P. Trigging radiation alarms after radioiodine treatment. *BMJ*. 2006;333:293-294.
3. Toltzis RJ, Morton DJ, Gerson MC. Problems on Pennsylvania Avenue. *N Engl J Med*. 1986;315:836-837.
4. Levin ME, Fischer KC. Thallium stress test and bank vaults. *N Engl J Med*. 1988;315:587.
5. Iqbal MB, Sharma R, Underwood SR, Kaddoura S. Radioisotopes and airport security. *Lancet*. 2005;366:342.
6. Zuckier L, Stabin M, Garetano G, Monetti M, Lanka V. Sensitivity of personal homeland security radiation detectors to medical radionuclides and implications for counseling of nuclear medicine patients. Radiological Soc North America 2004 Web site. Available at: http://rsna2004.rsna.org/rsna2004/V2004/conference/event_display.cfm?em_id=4407767&id=66601&p_navID=272. Accessed June 7, 2006.

Rituximab (anti-CD20) Adjunctive Therapy for Opsoclonus-Myoclonus Syndrome

Pranzatelli MR, Tate ED, Travelstead AL, et al (Southern Illinois Univ, Springfield; All Children's Hosp, St Petersburg, Fla; St John's Mercy Med Ctr, St Louis; et al)
J Pediatr Hematol Oncol 28:585-593, 2006

Purpose.—To determine if rituximab, an anti-CD20 monoclonal antibody, reduces cerebrospinal fluid (CSF) B-cell expansion in opsoclonus-myoclonus syndrome (OMS) and results in clinical improvement.

Methods.—Sixteen children with OMS and increased % CD20+ B-cells in CSF received 4 rituximab infusions (375 mg/m^2 IV) as add-on therapy to corticotropin (ACTH), intravenous immunoglobulins, or both, and were reevaluated 6 months later. Outcome measures were clinical (motor function, behavior, sleep) and immunologic (CSF and blood immunophenotype and Ig levels). Controls were 16 age-matched and sex-matched children, who did not have OMS.

Results.—After rituximab, 81% of OMS had a lower motor severity score, and 44% improved one severity category. Mean total score decreased by 44% ($P = 0.0005$). Rituximab reduced rage score, nighttime awakenings, and the number of children with opsoclonus, action myoclonus, drooling, gait ataxia, and rage. Despite a 51% reduction in ACTH dose, 9 of 11 children on ACTH did not relapse. The percentage of CSF CD19+ (and CD20+) B-cells was lowered in all children (undetectable in 6), with a 90% reduction in the group mean ($P = 0.00003$). CSF B-cells were no longer expanded compared with controls. In blood, CD19+ B-cells decreased (-90%, $P = 0.0003$), as did the CSF:blood CD19+ B-cell ratio ($P = 0.00003$). Serum IgM fell by 69% (below reference range), with no statistically significant change in IgG or IgA.

Conclusions.—Rituximab seems efficacious and safe as adjunctive therapy for OMS. Selective targeting of CSF B lymphocytes represents a novel and valuable paradigm shift in the therapy for centrally mediated paraneoplastic disorders.

▶ Opsoclonus-myoclonus syndrome (OMS), a serious neurologic complication of neuroblastoma is another possible indication for therapeutic management with rituximab. Rituximab, you will recall, is a chimeric IgG monoclonal antibody directed against B-cells. It binds to the CD20 antigen on the surface of mature B-cells. This targets the cells for apoptosis and immune-mediated destruction but does not affect stem cells or pro-B-cells. Once given, rituximab depletes circulating B-cells for 6 to 9 months, presumably eliminating B-cell clones, and binds to lymphoid cells in the spleen, thymus, and lymph nodes. Although rituximab was approved by the US Food and Drug Administration in 1997 to treat B-cell non-Hodgkin lymphomas, successful off-label treatment of several autoimmune disorders has been reported. Almost half a million subjects, mostly adults, have been treated with rituximab worldwide.

So what does all this have to do with treatment of the OMS? Cerebrospinal fluid (CSF) B-cell overrepresentation or "expansion" is a biomarker of disease activity in OMS, persisting in children with lingering symptoms, corresponding with clinical severity, and resisting conventional treatment. Although small numbers of B-cells are found in the CSF of healthy individuals, expansion of CSF B-cells indicates B-cell recruitment to the central nervous system with possible proliferation, inflammation, and production of potentially pathogenic anti-neural autoantibodies, such as those already reported in youngsters with OMS. The authors of this study figured that eliminating these B-cells with rituximab might help to control OMS, which can be virtually incapacitating in some children. Their hunch was correct in that rituximab was found to be efficacious and safe as an adjunctive therapy for OMS.

OMS joins a growing list of autoimmune disorders involving various organ systems for which rituximab seems to hold promise, including red cell aplasia, cold agglutinin disease, hemolytic anemia, idiopathic thrombocytopenia, thrombotic thrombocytopenic purpura, paraneoplastic pemphigus, rheumatoid arthritis, graft-versus-host disease, and Wegener granulomatosis. Rituximab has also been used to treat disorders with neurologic manifestations, such as polyneuropathy associated with anti-myelin-associated IgM antibodies and lupus, and is currently being evaluated in myasthenia gravis.

The neat part about rituximab when used to manage the paraneoplastic complications of malignancy is that it appears to be compatible to conventional therapies and is not associated with serious reactions. Recognize, however, that rituximab is genetically engineered from murine cells, the proteins of which can cause hypersensitivity. Infusion-related symptoms, such as fever, chills, nausea, hives, fatigue, headache, and itching—largely due to cytokine release—usually resolve with slowing of the infusion or the addition of antihistamines. Rarely, rituximab can cause more serious hypersensitivity reactions, such as hypotension, bronchospasm, and angioedema. Symptomatic treatment with antipyretics, antihistamines, and steroids controls severe reactions in most cases.

One would think that rituximab might significantly increase one's risk of severe and life-threatening infection. Actually, the low incidence of such complications may be due to the sparing of plasma cells, which lack CD20, or the antimicrobial effects of IVIG and the trimethoprim/sulfamethoxazole, which were co-administered to most of the patients in this series. Other studies of rituximab in children seem to favor the risk/benefit ratio of the drug when used to manage autoimmune disorders. Rituximab does not produce the severe myelosuppression seen with standard chemotherapeutic agents.

The opsoclonus-myoclonus syndrome is just one of a number of unusual ways in which childhood malignancies may present. See how you would handle the following real life situation. You receive a call from the college where one of your patients is enrolled. That patient is a competitive weightlifter who has achieved several important wins to his credit during his college years. The reason for the call is that the college's dean's office has received a report that this student has not passed an illicit drug use screen. Specifically, the student has tested positive for beta-human chorionic gonadotropin (HCG) on urine screening. The student swears that he has never engaged in any illicit drug use and demands to be seen by his own physician for examination.

Would you politely indicate that there is no reason for such an examination, believing that it is likely that this student did in fact use drugs, or would you go ahead and see your patient for further examination?

This case is a real one of a competitive weightlifter who was ultimately referred to an endocrinologist after a positive urine beta-human chorionic gonadotropin result was found. The 17-year-old was asymptomatic and denied illicit drug use. Blood tests confirmed an increase in beta-HCG levels, and further study showed decreased lutenizing hormone and follicle stimulating hormone levels and increased testosterone levels. Examination, including testicular assessment with ultrasonography, was unremarkable leading the care provider to believe that there may be an extragonadal germ cell tumor causing the findings. A computed tomographic scan of the chest, abdomen and pelvis was performed that demonstrated a 33-mm anterior mediastinal mass, which showed fluoro-deoxy glucose avidity on positron emission tomography. Following surgery, his beta-HCG levels rapidly declined and have remained normal.[1]

This is one lucky fellow. HCG is a hormone produced in large quantities by germ cell tumors of different origins. Less than 5% of seminomas are extragonadal and are therefore not readily detectable on physical examination. Also, just 40% of seminomas of this type produce increased levels of beta-HCG. This tumor can metastasize, as do testicular seminomas, although this occurs late.

As much as this editor abhors exercise, it was the very fact that this young fellow was engaging in a sporting activity that may very well have saved his life. Win one for exercise.

J. A. Stockman III, MD

Reference

1. Newcomb AE, Clarke CP, Chiang CY, Jerums G. Urine drug testing in an athlete leads to the diagnosis of unsuspected mediastinal germ cell tumor. *J Thorac Cardiovasc Surg.* 2006;132:722-723.

Use of Sentinel Lymph Node Biopsy and High-dose Interferon in Pediatric Patients With High-risk Melanoma: The Hospital for Sick Children Experience
Shah NC, Gerstle JT, Stuart M, et al (Univ of Toronto)
J Pediatr Hematol Oncol 28:496-500, 2006

Background.—Melanoma comprises less than 3% of all cancers seen in children. Sentinel lymph node biopsy (SLNBX) is an important predictor of outcome in adult melanoma and has not been widely used in pediatrics. Furthermore, adjuvant interferon has only been rarely used in childhood high-risk disease.

Objective.—To review our experience with high-risk melanoma, the feasibility of SLNBX and the tolerance of high-dose interferon (HDI) therapy.

Methods.—We retrospectively reviewed the medical records of patients with the diagnosis of cutaneous melanoma at our center over a 10-year period.

Results.—Eleven patients were identified (median age of 12 y). Six of 10 patients who underwent SLNBX had disease in the lymph nodes and no complications from this procedure were observed. After complete lymph node dissection in these 6 patients, 1 developed wound infection and 2 had chronic lymph edema. Five patients were treated with adjuvant HDI of whom 2 patients required dose modification due to myelosuppression and liver toxicity. After a median follow-up of 26 months, 10 out of 11 patients are in remission.

Conclusions.—SLNBX is feasible and safe in pediatric melanoma and offers the potential to identify patients at high risk for disease progression who could benefit from HDI.

▶ As time passes, we are learning a good deal more about childhood melanoma. In the first 10 years of life, melanoma accounts for only 0.9% of all cancers. During adolescent years, however, melanoma accounts for 7% of all childhood cancers. During the last 30 years, the incidence of melanoma in children younger than 20 years old has increased at a rate of about 3% per year after adjustment for age, race, sex, and ambient UV radiation. The incidence of melanoma is significantly less in blacks, Asians, and Native Americans compared with that of white patients. The incidence of melanoma in males is significantly less than in females, largely because of the differing rates of melanoma occurring in the extremities. To say this differently, boys are more covered up than girls and perhaps at less risk to UV exposure. There are some who clearly have an increased risk of melanoma. These include those with pre-existing conditions, such as giant congenital melanocytic nevus, maternal transmission, acquired melanocytic nevi, DNA repair disorders, immunodeficiency disorders, and familial melanoma.

The British Isles have the highest rates of skin cancer in children and adolescents in Europe.[1] The incidence of malignant melanoma in adolescents is increasing faster in the British Isles than in other European regions, based on analysis of data from 20 European nations. The incidence in Europe increased annually in adolescents by 4.1% for melanoma and 2.5% for other skin cancers between 1978 and 1997. Increases in skin cancer incidence over time have been observed only in adolescents, possibly reflecting a change in risk factors relevant to adolescents and adults, but not to children. The results of the study show that in the 19- to 20-year period of the study, the age standardized rate of malignant melanoma per million for adolescents in the British Isles increased from 5.31 to 22.9, a rise of more than four-fold. For Europe as a whole, these rates increased from 6.3 to 14.

The article from Canada is important because it helps us understand the prognosis for clinical outcome in melanoma. The main determinant of clinical outcome is the stage of the disease. For patients with localized disease, the thickness of the primary tumor, the presence or absence of ulceration, and nodal status are the most important predictors of clinical outcome. Five-year melanoma survival rate for pediatric cases is 100% for in situ disease, 77.2%

for regional disease, and 57.3% for those with distant metastases. SLNBX is a reliable and accurate method to identify nodal metastases. Biopsy of such nodes has proven to be an important prognostic tool and avoids the potential morbidity of complete lymph node dissection. These statements, however, are based on adult melanoma, and the use of SLNBX in pediatric melanoma patients has been limited to small case series. Its prognostic importance has not been fully explored in the young age group, thus this report from Canada is important. We see that SLNBX is 95% sensitive in detecting metastatic disease at the draining regional nodal basin. Patients with a negative SLNBX have a 5-year disease-free survival of 90% compared with those with a positive SLNBX in which the survival rate at 5 years is just 50%. The conclusion is that SLNBX is a safe and accurate procedure for the identification of nodal metastases in children with melanoma. Immediate complete lymph node dissection after a positive SLNBX has a high event-free survival rate although complete lymph node dissection in children has a relatively high rate of complications. The use of HDI in patients with lymph node metastases for melanoma is associated with predictable but manageable toxicity and also adds to the survival rate.

J. A. Stockman III, MD

Reference

1. de Vries E, Steliarova-Foucher E, Spatz A, Ardanaz E, Eggermont AM, Coebergh JW. Skin cancer incidence and survival in European children and adolescents (1978-1997). Report from the Automated Childhood Cancer Information System project. *Eur J Cancer.* 2006;42:2170-2182.

Colorectal Carcinoma in Childhood: A Retrospective Multicenter Study
Kravarusic D, Feigin E, Dlugy E, et al (Tel Aviv Univ, Tel Aviv; Hebrew Univ, Jerusalem, Israel)
J Pediatr Gastroenterol Nutr 44:209-211, 2007

Objectives.—Colorectal carcinoma, a common adult malignancy, has an estimated childhood incidence of 0.3 to 1.5/million in Western countries and 0.2/million in Israel. Diagnosis is difficult because adult screening measures are unfeasible in children. The tumor is frequently associated with predisposing genetic factors, aggressive biological behavior, and poor prognosis. The aim of this multicenter study was to document the clinical profile, treatment and prognosis of colorectal carcinoma in children in Israel.

Patients and Methods.—The clinical, laboratory, therapeutic, and prognostic parameters of all 7 children from 4 medical centers in Israel who were diagnosed with colorectal carcinoma over a 25-y period were reviewed.

Results.—Patients presented with rectal bleeding (4 of 7), abdominal pain (2 of 7), and abdominal distension (2 of 7). Average time to diagnosis was 6 months. Six patients underwent surgery (1 refused), and 5 received chemotherapy. Histopathological studies showed poorly differentiated mucinous adenocarcinoma, signet-ring type, in 4 cases, moderately differentiated adenocarcinoma in 2, and well-differentiated carcinoma in 1. Three patients died of the disease, 2 shortly after diagnosis. One patient with recurrent metastatic disease was lost to follow-up.

Conclusion.—Colorectal carcinoma in children is characterized by aggressive tumor behavior and delayed diagnosis, resulting in a worse prognosis than in adults. Heightened physician awareness of the possibility of this disease in children, with special attention to adolescents with predisposing factors and rectal bleeding, could help to improve outcome.

▶ This report from Israel was one of the most important publications in 2007 that related to colorectal cancer because it actually tells us about this particular form of cancer, specifically, in childhood. In previous reports, we learned about the hereditary risk of this problem, but now we see the exact nature of the illness when it does affect the youngest of our population. Colorectal carcinoma is a common adult malignancy but is extremely rare in children and adolescents. It has been suggested that the incidence ranges from a low of 0.3 to 1.5 per million. While the disease usually has a good prognosis in adults when caught early, the situation in children is different. The rarity of the tumor and its high potential for dissemination are usually responsible for a late diagnosis and poor outcome. In this series from Israel, about two thirds of affected individuals were born to families that met the definition of hereditary nonpolyposis colon cancer genotype. Among the other hereditary forms of colorectal carcinoma found in this series were familial adenomatous polyposis, juvenile polyposis syndrome, and Peutz-Jeghers syndrome. Some of the reported cases were the consequence of intermediate or longstanding inflammatory bowel disease, particularly ulcerative colitis.

Unfortunately, the children in this series, as is true of reported children in other studies, tended to have a poor prognosis as a result of diagnostic delay. The latter is explained by the nonspecific symptomatology of abdominal pain, distention, constipation, vomiting, nausea, rectal bleeding, anemia, and weight loss, all of which are seen in a whole host of common other gastrointestinal disorders. It is fairly rare for a child who has rectal bleeding to have it on the basis of a malignancy. Thus, a high index of suspicion is necessary for an early diagnosis. In this series, the average patient had symptoms for at least 6 months before the diagnosis was made.

It appears that colorectal cancer in children is somewhat different than the disease seen in adults. The aggressive nature of the malignancy is probably attributable to the high rate of mucinous histology in youngsters. Mucinous carcinoma of the colon accounts for only 5% to 10%, at best, of all adult cancers, but as we see in this study from Israel, it is actually more common than not as the histology found in affected children.

As far as actual prognosis is concerned, it is poor. Most series of patients involve only small numbers of children, but it is clear that the 5-year survival is not much better than 10%. Given the fact that we are learning more and more about predisposition conditions, including those that have a molecular predilection for the development of colon cancer, we should be able to do a better job of screening those at highest risk among our childhood population of patients. This means taking a very careful family history, the tip-off in most cases.

As of now, recommendations regarding screening colonoscopy in children are vague in exactly who should undergo periodic screening and how often. We need desperately collaborative studies to tighten up these recommendations so that we know what to do to prevent or detect early these rare, but all-too-lethal, cancers in children.

J. A. Stockman III, MD

Inheritance of a Cancer-Associated *MLH1* Germ-Line Epimutation
Hitchins MP, Wong JJL, Suthers G, et al (St Vincent's Hosp, Sydney, Australia; Univ of New South Wales, Sydney, Australia; Victor Chang Cardiac Research Inst, Sydney, Australia; et al)
N Engl J Med 356:697-705, 2007

Background.—Hereditary nonpolyposis colorectal cancer is caused by germ-line sequence mutations in mismatch-repair genes, particularly *MLH1* and *MLH2*. Persons who have hypermethylation of one allele of *MLH1* in somatic cells throughout the body have a predisposition for the development of cancer in a pattern typical of hereditary nonpolyposis colorectal cancer. This study sought evidence for transmission between generations because the presence of an *MLH1* epimutation in the germ line implies a potential for inheritance.

Methods.—A group of 24 patients in whom colorectal or endometrial cancer had developed before age 50 years was studied. From these 24 patients, 2 unrelated women were identified, each of whom had the typical molecular and clinical characteristics of persons with germ-line *MLH1* epimutations.

Results.—In both women there was dense methylation of 1 allele of the *MLH1* and *EPM2AIP* promoters in somatic cells from the 3 embryonic germ layers. Both women had metachronous carcinomas that had microsatellite instability and lacked *MLH1* expression. To identify *MLH1* epimutations within families of the probands, combined bisulfite restriction analysis was performed on constitutional DNA from 9 first-degree relatives, none of whom had a history of cancer. Partial methylation of *MLH1* was found in one of Patient A's 4 sons. However, the epimutation was erased in his spermatazoa. The affected maternal allele was inherited by 3 other siblings from these 2 families, but in those offspring the allele had reverted to the normal active state.

Conclusions.—This study found evidence of germ-line epimutation of *MLH1* in a woman with cancer and in her son, which is supportive of the concept of trans-generational epigenetic inheritance. The *MLH1* epimutation that predisposed the mother to multiple tumors with microsatellite instability has increased the risk of cancer in her son. The findings from this study and others have provided insights into the pattern of inheritance of germ-line epimutations. An alternative explanation for our findings is that epimutations are not inherited per se but instead are erased in gametogenesis but reestablished in successive generations because of *cis*-acting or *trans*-acting genetic factors that increase susceptibility to *MLH1* epimutations.

▶ This entry has to do with germ-line mutations related to *MLH1* and *MSH2*. Persons with a germ-line epimutation, like those with hereditary nonpolyposis colorectal cancer, have only 1 functional allele of the *MLH1* gene from conception. Cancers typical of the hereditary nonpolyposis colorectal cancer syndrome have developed in all such cases described to date. Colorectal and other tumors in persons with *MLH1* germ-line epimutations do not express the *MLH1* protein and have microsatellite instability (the hallmark of failed mismatched repair function), accompanied in some cases by somatic loss of the wild-type allele. The findings from the families in this report, as well as from previous studies, offer insights into the pattern of inheritance of germ-line epimutations. Offspring of patients with *MLH1* epimutations must be regarded as being at risk for cancer until proven otherwise. The broader implication of this report is that disease states in humans may be the consequence of nonmendelian inheritance of epigenetic changes in 1 or more genes.

Although germ-line sequence mutations are faithfully transmitted from 1 generation to the next in a mendelian pattern, epimutations do not involve changes in the DNA sequence and are relatively unstable, perhaps as the result of epigenetic reprogramming in primordial germ cells and gametes, this in the male genome in the zygote and in the preimplantation embryo. The findings from this report are consistent with germ-line transmission of a silent epigenetic state that confers disease susceptibility in humans. Thus, hereditary germ-line related cancers can be transmitted in typical mendelian fashion or in alternative genetic ways.

J. A. Stockman III, MD

A Proposed Score for Predicting Severe Infection Complications in Children With Chemotherapy-induced Febrile Neutropenia

Rondinelli PIP, Ribeiro Kde C, de Camargo B (Hosp do Câncer A C, Camargo, São Paulo, Brazil)
J Pediatr Hematol Oncol 28:665-670, 2006

Background.—Febrile neutropenia (FN) is one of most common complications in patients with cancer during chemotherapy. Identifying factors associated with severe infectious complications (SICs) at time of admission for fever and neutropenia is necessary for better treatment.

Procedure.—We revised all medical charts of patients under 18 years old who developed a first episode of FN present from January 2000 to December 2003. Criteria for a SIC were defined. These included the presence of bacteremia or fungemia, sepsis, septic shock, and/or death from infection. To identify risk factors SIC was associated with the first FN episode.

Results.—Factors identified in univariate analysis were female sex, age less than 5 years old, acute myeloid leukemia, baseline disease activity, use of central venous catheter, hemoglobin level < 7 g/dL, leukocytes count < 500 cells/mm³, granulocytes count < 500 cells/mm³, monocytes count < 100 cells/mm³, platelets < 20,000, and body temperature > 38.5°C, a chemotherapy interval < 7 days, presence of mucositis, pneumonia, absence of upper respiratory tract infection, or the presence of any clinical focus on first physical examination. In multivariate analysis the variables that remained as independent predictive risk factors for SIC were age less than 5 years, use of central venous catheter, body temperature > 38.5°C, hemoglobin level < 7 g/dL, any clinical focus of infection on first examination and absence of upper respiratory tract infection. The FN population was than divided among 3 different risk groups as follows: group 1 (low risk), group 2 (intermediate risk), with a 13 (4.4 to 38.3)-fold risk for SIC; and group 3 (high risk) with a 50 (16.4 to 149.2)-fold risk for SIC.

Conclusions.—This study suggests that patients with FN can be stratified for risk of SIC using clinical parameters at hospital admission.

Effects of Acute Exercise on Neutrophils in Pediatric Acute Lymphoblastic Leukemia Survivors: A Pilot Study

Ladha AB, Courneya KS, Bell GJ, et al (Univ of Alberta, Edmonton, Canada)
J Pediatr Hematol Oncol 28:671-677, 2006

Purpose.—This nonrandomized controlled trial was designed to investigate the effects of acute exercise on neutrophil count and function in children and adolescents receiving maintenance treatment for acute lymphoblastic leukemia (ALL) compared to matched controls.

Methods.—Participants (n = 10; 4 ALL patients and 6 healthy matched controls) were males between the ages of 7 to 18 years. On visit 1, participants completed an incremental exercise test to volitional exhaustion on a treadmill to determine peak aerobic fitness (VO_{2peak}). On visit 2, participants completed a 30-minute exercise session consisting of an intermittent run-walk on a treadmill at 70% to 85% of VO_{2peak} with blood sampling completed at 5 time points: fasting, preexercise, postexercise, 1-hour postexercise, and 2-hour postexercise.

Results.—A significant increase in absolute neutrophil count from preexercise to postexercise was observed in both groups ($P = 0.011$). Neutrophil oxidative capacity was significantly depressed in the ALL group at the basal level ($P = 0.029$), however, it increased in both groups after exercise and stimulation.

Conclusions.—This preliminary study suggests that 30 minutes of moderate intensity exercise in ALL patients receiving maintenance therapy provides a similar neutrophil response to that of healthy age and sex-matched controls.

▶ This editor likes exercise about as much as Britney Spears likes having her picture taken while driving an SUV with her baby on her lap. Nonetheless, I'll eat crow when it comes to the good news that exercise has a beneficial effect in children being treated for acute lymphoblastic leukemia (ALL). Before the report from Canada appeared, there had been only one study that examined the immune responses to exercise in pediatric cancer patients. A case series by Shore and Shepard in 1999 investigated the effects of a 12-week exercise training program in children receiving chemotherapy for various types of cancer and found reduced immunity after training and in comparison to normal children.[1] The latter paper suggested some potential risk factors cautioning against exercise that might impair a child's immune system, one already compromised by the effects of anticancer treatment. The findings from the Shore and Shepard paper, however, were of marginal, if any, clinical significance.

The Canadian study investigated the effects of an acute bout of moderate intensity exercise on neutrophil count and function in children and adolescents undergoing maintenance therapy for ALL. It was designed specifically to explore if exercise-induced neutrophil responses differ for ALL patients versus healthy age-sex–matched controlled individuals. It is during the maintenance phase of treatment that children are returning to the classroom or playing with fellow peers and trying to regain some normalcy to childhood, and it was during the maintenance phase that this study was carried out. The principal findings of the study were that acute exercise resulted in a significant change in the absolute neutrophil count and that there was no significant difference between ALL patients and healthy control subjects. The ALL group of youngsters did have a significantly depressed basal neutrophil oxidative burst of activity compared with controls following exercise. This is likely because they were immunosuppressed, an effect unrelated to the exercise itself.

So what does all this mean? An increase in circulating neutrophils in blood as a consequence of exercise can do nothing other than be of some potential benefit to youngsters with a compromised immune system resulting from chemotherapy. This benefit can be seen at just 60% of maximum oxygen uptake during periods of exercise, an amount quantitatively similar to normal sporting activity. Perhaps 30 minutes of moderate to vigorous intermittent exercise is as good as granulocyte-stimulating factor in terms of theoretical therapeutic benefit.

We will close this comment with a question. Can you catch breast cancer from your dog? The answer is found in interesting data that has recently appeared. Compared with controls, significantly more patients with breast cancer own dogs rather than cats.[2] Even more striking, more than twice the number of patients compared with controls had kept dogs throughout the past 10 years. The nature of breast cancer in dogs seems to support the role of a zoonotic factor in the development of cancer because dogs have a protracted course of disease, similar to human breast cancer, whereas the disease is very short in cats.

J. A. Stockman III, MD

References

1. Shore S, Shepard RJ. Immune responses to exercise in children treated for cancer. *J Sports Med Phys Fitness*. 1999;39:240-243.
2. Laumbacher B, Fellerhoff B, Herzberger B, Wank R. Do dogs harbour risk factors for human breast cancer? *Med Hypotheses*. 2006;67:21-26.

17 Ophthalmology

Exclusion of Students With Conjunctivitis From School: Policies of State Departments of Health
Ohnsman CM (Wills Eye Inst)
J Pediatr Ophthalmol Strabismus 44:101-105, 2007

Purpose.—To use current state department of health regulations regarding exclusion of students with conjunctivitis from school as a starting point in developing uniform recommendations for schools.

Methods.—State departments of health were asked to state their policy regarding when a child with conjunctivitis may return to school. This information was collated and examined for trends. The results were compared with current literature on infectious conjunctivitis.

Results.—Of the 43 states that responded, 7 allow children with conjunctivitis to remain in school, 8 allow their return once antibiotic treatment is initiated, 12 allow their return 24 hours after antibiotics are initiated, 13 exclude them until the disease is noncommunicable, and 16 require the approval of a physician for return to school. Seventeen states gave multiple recommendations, which were often contradictory.

Conclusions.—Although no current consensus exists among state health officials regarding students with conjunctivitis, the literature supports excluding children with conjunctivitis from school until they are asymptomatic. When patients are treated with fourth-generation fluoroquinolones, the length of exclusion may be as little as 24 hours in cases of bacterial conjunctivitis, and longer in cases of viral conjunctivitis. Following these guidelines may prevent epidemics of bacterial and viral conjunctivitis.

▶ No one can argue that both bacterial and viral types of conjunctivitis are mainly self-limited diseases, lasting at most from 5 to 14 days before spontaneous resolution occurs. During this period, however, the disease can be spread by contact with an infected individual. The need for exclusion of a student with acute conjunctivitis from school is based on this potential concern of spread, but such exclusion is truly controversial. Some authorities recommend allowing school attendance, stating that those with conjunctivitis are no more or less infectious than anyone else with a viral or bacterial respiratory illness. The purpose of the report abstracted from the Wills Eye Institute in Philadelphia was to query the Departments of Health of the 50 states to review their policies with respect to exclusion from school of students with conjunctivitis. Interestingly, 43 of the 50 states responded. Alabama, California, Florida, Maine, Michigan, Montana, New Jersey, North Dakota, Oregon, Tennessee, Vermont, and Wisconsin reported no official policy on exclusion. Seven states recommended no exclusion from school for conjunctivitis: Iowa (if nonpurulent), Kansas (if viral), Kentucky (if mild), Massachusetts (if viral), Minnesota (usually), Oklahoma and Pennsylvania (if viral). Connecticut and Kentucky (if bacterial), Minnesota, North Dakota, and West Virginia allow students with conjunctivitis to return to school once antibiotic treatment is started. In South Dakota, students with conjunctivitis may return to school after antibiotic treatment is initiated or with a physician's written prescription. In Indiana, students are excluded until antibiotic treatment is started, until the disease is noncommunicable, or until a physician approves a return to school. A number of states require exclusion from school until 24 hours after the initiation of antibiotic treatment. These include Delaware, Montana, Ohio, Rhode Island, and Vermont, as well as Kansas, Massachusetts, and Pennsylvania if the conjunctivitis is bacterial. Arizona and Virginia also exclude students until 24 hours after antibiotics have been started or until the disease is noncommunicable. In Illinois, students may return to school after 24 hours of antibiotic treatment or with a physician's approval. Maryland requires 24 hours of antibiotic treatment, noncommunicable status, or physician approval before the student returns to school.

Needless to say, there is little uniformity or agreement among states regarding their policies on school exclusion for youngsters with conjunctivitis. It is clear that some health departments must think highly of a physician's diagnostic skills in that they seem to differentiate between viral and bacterial conjunctivitis when most of us have a difficult time doing this. As far as the American Academy of Pediatrics' position on this issue, the Red Book states the following: "Except when viral or bacterial conjunctivitis is accompanied by systemic signs of illness, infected children should be allowed to remain in school once any indicated therapy is implemented, unless their behavior is such that close contact with other students cannot be avoided."

As of now, no effective treatment has been found for viral conjunctivitis. On the other hand, topical antibiotics have been demonstrated to reduce the duration of acute bacterial conjunctivitis. Most clinicians therefore prescribe antibiotic drops or ointment to empirically treat presumed bacterial conjunctivitis. However, the choice of antibiotic remains unclear, leading many to select the least expensive medication. Many of the older antibiotics no longer are effective, however, for *Streptococcus pneumoniae* and *Haemophilus influenzae*. Because it is not always possible to differentiate between viral and bacterial conjunctivitis, in equivocal cases, current standards say that it is reasonable to begin treatment with a fourth-generation fluoroquinolone, given its safety and lack of propensity for bacterial resistance.

As of now, most schools will dismiss a child who has evidence of acute infectious conjunctivitis. Once a diagnosis of infectious conjunctivitis has been confirmed, the child, given a fourth-generation fluoroquinolone, preferably moxifloxacin, may return to school, once treated, and symptoms start to resolve, which is usually the next day.

Needless to say, the recommendations noted above, consistent with this abstracted report, are hardly based on solid evidence-based medicine. It would be thought that something as simple as the infectivity of conjunctivitis would be amenable to a collaborative study.

J. A. Stockman III, MD

A Community Outbreak of Conjunctivitis Caused by Nontypeable *Streptococcus pneumoniae* in Minnesota

Buck JM, Lexau C, Shapiro M, et al (Minnesota Dept of Health, St Paul; Ctrs for Disease Control and Prevention, Atlanta, Ga)
Pediatr Infect Dis J 25:906-911, 2006

Background.—The Minnesota Department of Health (MDH) was notified of an outbreak of conjunctivitis in city A with cultures positive for *Streptococcus pneumoniae*.

Methods.—MDH staff contacted clinics and schools in city A and city B regarding conjunctivitis cases, reviewed clinical findings of conjunctivitis cases in city A, and collected isolates for subtyping.

Results.—Between September 1 and December 12, 2003, cities A and B reported 735 conjunctivitis cases. Fifty-one percent of the cases were reported from schools, childcare centers and colleges. Adults were more likely to report itching, burning or swelling of the eye(s); children were more likely to report crusty eyes ($P < 0.05$). Forty-nine percent of conjunctival cultures (71 of 144) were positive for *S. pneumoniae*. All isolates were nontypeable by serotyping. Pulsed field gel electrophoresis identified 3 clonal groups with 84% of isolates belonging to one clonal group. Multilocus sequence typing revealed that isolates had the same multilocus sequence type as isolates from a 2002 outbreak at a New England college.

Conclusions.—This outbreak was widespread in the community and conjunctivitis clinical presentation varied by age. The predominant strains in this outbreak were related to a pneumococcal strain implicated in prior conjunctivitis outbreaks, suggesting these strains have a predilection for causing conjunctivitis.

▶ This report underscores the fact that outbreaks of conjunctivitis can be caused by nontypeable *Streptococcus pneumoniae* and that such infections can spread rapidly within a community. In this case, two towns, each with population of 20,000, near Minneapolis, reported an outbreak of more than 700 cases of conjunctivitis, mostly in schools, child health centers and colleges. In this outbreak, conjunctivitis spread widely among members of the community. The outbreak was already well underway in the 2 cities before it was detected and reported.

Nontypeable *S. pneumoniae* strains have been implicated previously in sporadic cases of outbreaks of conjunctivitis. These have occurred in many areas of the United States and largely are focused in schools or colleges. Reported

Main Outcome Measures.—Severity of symptoms on days 1-3 after consultation, duration of symptoms, and belief in the effectiveness of antibiotics for eye infections.

Results.—Prescribing strategies did not affect the severity of symptoms but duration of moderate symptoms was less with antibiotics: no antibiotics (controls) 4.8 days, immediate antibiotics 3.3 days (risk ratio 0.7, 95% confidence interval 0.6 to 0.8), delayed antibiotics 3.9 days (0.8, 0.7 to 0.9). Compared with no initial offer of antibiotics, antibiotic use was higher in the immediate antibiotic group: controls 30%, immediate antibiotics 99% (odds ratio 185.4, 23.9 to 1439.2), delayed antibiotics 53% (2.9, 1.4 to 5.7), as was belief in the effectiveness of antibiotics: controls 47%, immediate antibiotics 67% (odds ratio 2.4, 1.1 to 5.0), delayed antibiotics 55% (1.4, 0.7 to 3.0), and intention to reattend for eye infections: controls 40%, immediate antibiotics 68% (3.2, 1.6 to 6.4), delayed antibiotics 41% (1.0, 0.5 to 2.0). A patient information leaflet or eye swab had no effect on the main outcomes. Reattendance within two weeks was less in the delayed compared with immediate antibiotic group: 0.3 (0.1 to 1.0) v 0.7 (0.3 to 1.6).

Conclusions.—Delayed prescribing of antibiotics is probably the most appropriate strategy for managing acute conjunctivitis in primary care. It reduces antibiotic use, shows no evidence of medicalisation, provides similar duration and severity of symptoms to immediate prescribing, and reduces reattendance for eye infections.

▶ This report from Great Britain reminds one of the analogies that can be drawn with the management of acute otitis media. Although upper respiratory tract infections and acute infective conjunctivitis are minor illnesses that are usually self-limiting, the use of antibiotics in these disorders is high. Randomized controlled trials and meta-analyses of such trials have shown that antibiotics provide mainly short-term benefits, and the reduction in symptoms is in fact too limited to justify the use of antibiotics for such a minor problem as conjunctivitis. This randomized trial by Everitt and colleagues found that acute infective conjunctivitis is similar to otitis media in that patients with conjunctivitis who receive antibiotics immediately fare no better than those who have watchful waiting. The average score for severity of symptoms on days 1 to 3 did not differ significantly between those treated and those who were not treated. Unfortunately, immediate prescribing seems to medicalize patients with conjunctivitis in as much as patients receiving immediate antibiotics are more likely to state that they would come back again for eye infections than those assigned to no antibiotic therapy. The middle ground, of course, is delayed antibiotic administration for those whose disease is not resolving on their own and in whom an organism is found on culture. Compared with no antibiotics, delayed prescribing has the advantage of reduced antibiotic use, no evidence of medicalization, similar symptom control to that of immediate prescribing, and reduced reattendance for minor eye infections that require no treatment.

J. A. Stockman III, MD

ReNu with MoistureLoc. The majority of these patients reported using poor contact lens hygiene practices, including overnight daily use of contact lenses and the use of contact lenses past the replacement date. Most patients were not initially correctly diagnosed as having a fungal keratitis, and the majority developed sight-threatening lesions requiring inpatient management of their infections. Unfortunately, many patients were left with diminished visual acuity. When the Singapore study was published, it was too early to speculate as to the role of the ReNu line of products as a cause of the outbreak.

Chang et al summarized the multistate outbreak of *Fusarium* keratitis here in the United States. The investigators were clearly able to pinpoint ReNu with MoistureLoc contact lens solution as the culprit. The report outlined the cases of 164 patients in 33 states and 1 United States territory. The authors were not specifically able to document the mechanism for the association of the *Fusarium* keratitis with the use of ReNu MoistureLoc solution, which was introduced into the marketplace in the fall of 2004. It does not seem that the problem was caused by intrinsic contamination of the solution itself. Samples of unopened bottles of relevant lots were tested by the Centers for Disease Control and Prevention (CDC) during their investigation of the epidemic, and all were sterile. Bausch & Lomb also routinely cultured their products during the manufacturing process and found no apparent contamination. Extrinsic contamination originating at the manufacturing plant or nearby warehouse also appears to be unlikely as the cause of the outbreak. This leaves as the possible cause extrinsic contamination of the contact lens solution bottles or lens cases occurring outside of the manufacturing or storage processes, perhaps in patients' homes. It appears that this outbreak may have been caused by a complex and, as yet, undetermined interaction between MoistureLoc, *Fusarium*, and, possibly, the lens case or the contact lens. The MoistureLoc formula contains 2 ingredients not found in other soft contact lens solutions currently on the market: alexidine (a disinfectant) and polyquarterium-10 (a moisture-retaining polysaccharide that holds water close to the contact lens surface). Although in vitro studies have demonstrated that the formulation meets all the current biocidal standards against *Fusarium*, persistence of this activity in a variety of environments, including simulated noncompliant use, is not customarily tested and is currently unknown. In addition, the effect of polysaccharides and surfactants on the growth or survival of *Fusarium* is not well understood.

The *Fusarium* keratitis outbreak here in the United States had a high degree of morbidity. Most patients were young and had no immune-compromising illness, yet corneal transplantation was required or planned for more than one third of infected patients. The requirement for corneal transplant was much higher here than in Singapore.

Needless to say, as soon as the problem was identified, Bausch & Lomb quickly withdrew their formulation solution from the market. Given the many unknowns related to this miniepidemic, it is clear that soft contact lens users should use meticulous hygiene, including washing and drying hands before handling lenses, storing lenses in new contact lens solution after each use, and carefully following the directions for use of their contact lenses and lens solution products.

J. A. Stockman III, MD

An Outbreak of *Fusarium* Keratitis Associated With Contact Lens Wear in Singapore

Khor W-B, Aung T, Saw S-M, et al (Singapore Eye Research Inst; Singapore Natl Eye Centre; Natl Univ of Singapore; et al)
JAMA 295:2867-2873, 2006

Context.—Fungal keratitis is a potentially blinding condition that is rarely seen with contact lens wear.

Objective.—To describe a nationwide outbreak of fungal keratitis caused by *Fusarium* species among contact lens wearers in Singapore.

Design, Setting, and Patients.—Nationwide, hospital-based case series. All cases of fungal keratitis among contact lens wearers in all ophthalmology departments in Singapore were reviewed along with the charts of all contact lens wearers with culture-proven fungal keratitis from March 2005 through May 2006. A standardized telephone interview was conducted to obtain additional clinical information.

Main Outcome Measure.—Diagnosis of *Fusarium* keratitis associated with contact lens wear.

Results.—During the study period, 66 patients (68 affected eyes) were diagnosed with *Fusarium* keratitis associated with contact lens wear; the estimated annual national incidence is 2.35 cases per 10,000 contact lens wearers (95% confidence interval, 0.62-7.22). Patients ranged in age from 13 to 44 years (mean [SD], 27.1 [8.4] years), of which 32 (48.5%) were men. The vast majority (65 patients; 98.5%) wore soft, disposable contact lenses; 62 patients (93.9%) reported using 1 brand of contact lens cleaning solution (ReNu, Bausch & Lomb, Rochester, NY), including 42 patients (63.6%) who recalled using ReNu with MoistureLoc. Most patients (81.8%) reported poor contact lens hygiene practices, including overnight use of daily wear contact lenses (19.7%), and use of contact lenses past the replacement date (43.9%). The final best-corrected visual acuity ranged from 20/20 to 20/80. Five patients (5 eyes; 7.4%) required emergency therapeutic or tectonic corneal transplantation.

Conclusions.—A new and evolving epidemic of *Fusarium* keratitis associated with contact lens wear was found in Singapore. Physicians and eye care practitioners worldwide need to be aware of the likelihood of similar outbreaks emerging among contact lens wearers.

▶ The problem of contact lens keratitis reminds us of a comment made by Jenner more than 2 centuries ago: "The deviation of man from the state in which he was originally placed by nature seems to have provided him with a prolific source of diseases" (Edward Jenner, English surgeon and discoverer of small pox vaccine, 1749-1823).

J. A. Stockman III, MD

The clinical features, MRI findings, and outcome of optic neuritis in children

Wilejto M, Shroff M, Buncic JR, et al (Univ of Toronto)
Neurology 67:258-262, 2006

Background.—Optic neuritis (ON) in childhood is thought to be more likely bilateral and less likely to lead to multiple sclerosis (MS) vs ON in adults.

Methods.—The authors evaluated clinical features, maximal visual deficit and recovery, visual evoked potentials (VEPs), neuroimaging, and outcome in a cohort of children with ON.

Results.—Records of 36 children (female/male ratio 1.6), ages 2.2 to 17.8 (mean 12.2) years, were reviewed. ON was unilateral in 58% and bilateral in 42%. Maximal visual deficit was severe in 69%, but full recovery occurred in 39 of 47 affected eyes (83%). VEPs were abnormal in 88%. Neurologic abnormalities in addition to those associated with ON were documented in 13 children. Neuroimaging studies of the optic nerve were abnormal in 55%. Brain MRI in 35 children demonstrated white matter lesions separate from the optic nerves in 54%. Follow-up is 2.4 years (0.3 to 8.3 years). To date, 13 children (36%) have been diagnosed with MS and 1 has Devic disease. Bilateral ON was more likely to be associated with MS outcome ($p = 0.03$). All 13 children with MS had white matter lesions on brain MRI. None of the children with a normal brain MRI have developed MS to date.

Conclusions.—Contrary to expectations, optic neuritis (ON) in childhood was more likely to be unilateral, multiple sclerosis (MS) risk was high (36% at 2 years), and bilateral rather than unilateral ON was associated with a greater likelihood of MS. Clinical findings extrinsic to the visual system on baseline examination ($p < 0.0001$) and MRI evidence of white matter lesions outside the optic nerves ($p < 0.0001$) were strongly correlated with MS outcome.

▶ Although ON is an infrequently made diagnosis in children, it does put a chill up the spines of those who make such a diagnosis because of the fact that ON has been considered to be a harbinger for the development of MS. Prior to the publication of the report abstracted, we have actually had little information to tell us about the clinical features and outcomes of ON in children. Now we know.

What we learn from this report is that ON presenting in childhood has at least a 36% risk for the subsequent diagnosis of multiple sclerosis, within a 2-year period. These data suggest a prevalence of MS that is significantly higher than suspected, based on previous studies. Children with bilateral ON seem to be more likely to have an abnormal MRI than those with unilateral ON. Contrary to expectations, bilateral ON was found to be associated with a higher risk for MS in children. MRI evidence of one or more brain white matter lesions is indeed the most significant marker for the development of MS. On the other hand, not a single child with a normal brain MRI was later shown to have MS.

All of the 13 children eventually diagnosed with MS had at least one white matter lesion identified on MRI.

Last, please note that optic neuritis may also represent the first attack of Devic disease, an inflammatory, demyelinating condition in which clinical disease is referable to the optic nerves and spinal cord, but without involvement of the remaining central nervous system white matter. Devic disease is associated with a high mortality (30%) in adults. It is possible that the same process may produce milder manifestations in children. Soon we may have a specific diagnostic tool to detect Devic disease. Recently, a serum antibody that targets the aquaporin 4 molecule has been identified in adults with Devic disease. Studies of the aquaporin 4 antibody in children are currently underway.

J. A. Stockman III, MD

Severe cough and retinal hemorrhage in infants and young children
Goldman M, Dagan Z, Yair M, et al (Assaf Harofeh Med Ctr, Zerifin, Israel; Tel Aviv Univ, Israel)
J Pediatr 148:835-836, 2006

Background.—Significant mortality and morbidity rates are associated with child abuse. Up to 1% of the children in the United States are reported to be abused or neglected, and the mortality rate among the patients is 5% to 20%. Retinal hemorrhage is a common finding in child abuse, often associated with the shaken baby syndrome, and has been reported in 38% to 100% of children with nonaccidental head injury. Other reported causes of this injury in children are accidental trauma, bleeding disorders, infections, and vaginal delivery in newborns. In adults there have been reports of retinal hemorrhage after performance of a Valsalva maneuver. The rapid rise in intraabdominal and intrathoracic pressure can also be observed in coughing, vomiting, and weight lifting. The purpose of this study was to investigate whether severe coughing might cause retinal hemorrhage in young children.

Methods.—All children age 3 months to 2 years admitted to the Department of Pediatrics at an Israeli hospital with severe coughing were eligible for the study. Severe coughing was defined as coughing that persisted for 3 or more days, was the primary reason for referral to the emergency department, and required hospitalization. Children were excluded if there was any history of child abuse or a history of vomiting or other diseases or conditions in which bleeding is a prominent feature, including cardiopulmonary resuscitation and accidental trauma. All children underwent an ocular examination by an experienced pediatric ophthalmologist within 48 hours of admission.

Results.—Of the 100 children enrolled in the study, 65 were male. The patients ranged in age from 3 to 24 months, with a median age of 7 months. The duration of coughing before the ocular examination ranged from 3 to 31 days, with a median of 6 days. The clinical diagnoses at discharge included pertussis, pertussis-like syndrome, upper respiratory tract infection, asthma exacerbation, bronchiolitis, acute laryngitis or tracheobronchitis, lobar or bronchopneumonia, and unspecified cough. No retinal hemorrhages were detected in any of the 100 patients examined (95% confidence interval, 0% to 3%).

Conclusions.—There was no evidence of retinal hemorrhage in 100 consecutive children with severe coughing. Therefore, child abuse must be excluded when retinal hemorrhage is found in infants and young children with cough.

▶ One of the key markers of the abuse of young children may be the occurrence of retinal hemorrhages. Child abuse, however, is not the only cause of retinal hemorrhage. Accidental trauma, bleeding disorders, infections, and vaginal delivery can also produce similar findings, although the latter resolves within a few weeks. In adults, there are several reports of retinal hemorrhage after a Valsalva maneuver, a phenomenon termed Valsalva retinopathy or maculopathy. The authors of this report decided to see whether persistent coughing might be a cause of retinal hemorrhage in young children. Severe coughing was defined as coughing for 3 or more days. Children were excluded if they had a history of vomiting, cardiopulmonary resuscitation, trauma, leukemia, bleeding disorders, rickets, or malaria (the study was performed in Israel). Out of 100 children with serious coughing episodes, not a single case of retinal hemorrhage was observed.

You can bet that those who are expert in the field of child abuse will seize on this report to validate the belief that, until proven otherwise, retinal hemorrhage in infants and young children equals child abuse until the latter is excluded.

All too often expert testimony, frequently given in cases related to child abuse, comes from non-experts as opposed to those who are highly skilled not only in the definitions of what child abuse consists of, but also in knowing the details of the law. Those who are not such experts can in many senses be called "quacks." If you are not familiar with the origins of the word quack, it comes from the Dutch *quaken*: to prattle, chatter, and perhaps to sound like a duck. The word seems to have been first applied to physicians around the 17th century when the term "quack-solving physicians" entered the lexicon. More or less interchangeable with "empiric," "mountebank," and "charlatan," the label was often deployed by university-educated medical practitioners as a way to distinguish themselves from, and disparage as dangerous, those who advertised medicinal products on traveling stages or on street corners.[1] Those who provide expert testimony who are not experts are in fact selling their products on traveling stages. They might do better by themselves by performing on street corners.

J. A. Stockman III, MD

Reference

1. Wear A. Quack. *Lancet.* 2005;366:1157.

Prevalence of Visual Impairment in the United States

Vitale S, Cotch MF, Sperduto RD (NIH, Bethesda, Md)
JAMA 295:2158-2163, 2006

Context.—The prevalence of visual impairment in the US public has not been surveyed nationally in several decades.

Objective.—To estimate the number of US individuals aged 12 years or older who have impaired distance vision due to uncorrected refractive error.

Design, Setting, and Participants.—The National Health and Nutrition Examination Survey (NHANES), using a multistage probability sampling design, included a vision evaluation in a mobile examination center. Visual acuity data were obtained from 13,265 of 14,203 participants (93.4%) who visited the mobile examination center in 1999-2002. Visual impairment was defined as presenting distance visual acuity of 20/50 or worse in the better-seeing eye. Visual impairment due to uncorrected refractive error was defined as (presenting) visual impairment that improved, aided by automated refraction results, to 20/40 or better in the better-seeing eye.

Main Outcome Measures.—Presenting distance visual acuity (measured with usual corrective lenses, if any) and distance visual acuity after automated refraction.

Results.—Overall, 1190 study participants had visual impairment (weighted prevalence, 6.4%; 95% confidence interval [CI], 6.0%-6.8%), and of these, 83.3% could achieve good visual acuity with correction (95% CI, 80.9%-85.8%). Extrapolating these findings to the general US population, approximately 14 million individuals aged 12 years or older have visual impairment (defined as distance visual acuity of 20/50 or worse), and of these, more than 11 million individuals could have their vision improved to 20/40 or better with refractive correction.

Conclusions.—Visual impairment due to uncorrected refractive error is a common condition in the United States. Providing appropriate refractive correction to those individuals whose vision can be improved is an important public health endeavor with implications for safety and quality of life.

▶ The National Health and Nutrition Examination Survey (NHANES) continues to provide important information of a diverse nature, including the prevalence of visual impairment here in the United States. What we learn from the most recent NHANES study is that uncorrected refractive error is a common condition here in the United States and one that does cause significant visual impairment. Approximately 14 million individuals do have visual impairment (defined as a distance visual acuity of 20/50 or worse) and of these, more than 11 million individuals could have their vision improved to 20/40 or better with refractive correction.

Please note that NHANES does include in its analysis youngsters as young as 12 years. Among those age 12 to 19 years, visual impairment was observed in just under 10% (a figure that is almost 50% higher than in older age groups). Of the 9.7% of teens with visual impairment, almost all are due to uncorrected refractive error (93.1%). One wonders how important a role such refractive errors are as a cause of learning disability among high school aged children.

Because this commentary is about visual loss, let's close with a query having to do with something that can cause visual loss. What medical problem arose in Great Britain following an advertising stunt by a major supermarket that labelled its eggs as "mischief eggs" for Halloween? Well, it turns out that some 13 individuals in Liverpool, England sustained eye injuries from eggs thrown at them over Halloween. The apparently fashionable Halloween "trick" resulted in 4 of these patients having long-term ophthalmologic sequelae, including retinal detachment, corneal scarring, and in two cases, a continuing risk of glaucoma. All of this followed a peculiar advertising campaign of a supermarket chain. You can bet a lawsuit or two was instituted as a result of this series of misadventures.[1]

J. A. Stockman III, MD

Reference

1. Stewart RM, Durnian JM, Briggs MC. "Here's egg in your eye": a prospective study of blunt ocular trauma resulting from thrown eggs. *Emerg Med J.* 2006;23:756-758.

18 Respiratory Tract

Effect of exposure to traffic on lung development from 10 to 18 years of age: a cohort study
Gauderman WJ, Vora H, McConnell R, et al (Univ of Southern Calif, Los Angeles; Sonoma Technology Inc, Petaluma, Calif; Institut Municipal d'Investigació Mèdica, C Doctor Aiguader, Barcelona; et al)
Lancet 369:571-577, 2007

Background.—Whether local exposure to major roadways adversely affects lung-function growth during the period of rapid lung development that takes place between 10 and 18 years of age is unknown. This study investigated the association between residential exposure to traffic and 8-year lung-function growth.

Methods.—In this prospective study, 3677 children (mean age 10 years [SD 0.44]) participated from 12 southern California communities that represent a wide range in regional air quality. Children were followed up for 8 years, with yearly lung-function measurements recorded. For each child, we identified several indicators of residential exposure to traffic from large roads. Regression analysis was used to establish whether 8-year growth in lung function was associated with local traffic exposure, and whether local traffic effects were independent of regional air quality.

Findings.—Children who lived within 500 m of a freeway (motorway) had substantial deficits in 8-year growth of forced expiratory volume in 1 s (FEV$_1$, -81 mL, p=0.01 [95% CI -143 to -18]) and maximum midexpiratory flow rate (MMEF, -127 mL/s, p=0.03 [-243 to -11]), compared with children who lived at least 1500 m from a freeway. Joint models showed that both local exposure to freeways and regional air pollution had detrimental, and independent, effects on lung-function growth. Pronounced deficits in attained lung function at age 18 years were recorded for those living within 500 m of a freeway, with mean percent-predicted 97.0% for FEV$_1$ (p=0.013, relative to >1500 m [95% CI 94.6–99.4]) and 93.4% for MMEF (p=0.006 [95% CI 89.1–97.7]).

Interpretation.—Local exposure to traffic on a freeway has adverse effects on children's lung development, which are independent of regional air quality, and which could result in important deficits in attained lung function in later life.

▶ In the past year, I've seen several reports dealing with air pollution. One, that of Gauderman et al (Effect of exposure to traffic on lung development from 10 to 18 years of age: a cohort study), deals with children. Another, Miller et al (Long-term exposure to air pollution and incidence of cardiovascular events in women), deals with women. With respect to children, evidence is provided that living close to highways (in this case freeways since the report emanates from California) leads to reduced lung development in children. In a longitudinal study, more than 3600 children, 10 to 18 years old, were followed up, with yearly measurements of lung function. Children living less than 500 m from freeways had reduced lung-function growth, compared with that of those living more than 1500 m away. This finding is important because it shows that within communities, some children are at higher risk than others, leading to the interesting question of environmental equity since in many communities, more affluent families tend to be located at greater distances from busy highways. At the same time, at least around Los Angeles, there is a propensity for schools to be built near highways. This is for accessibility reasons.

Thus far, it is not entirely clear which pollutants emanating from motor vehicles are worse than others. Diesel-engine exhaust contains large quantities of nanoparticles with organic hydrocarbon components on their surface. Primary emissions also include organic vapors and nanoparticles in the nucleation mode. Indeed, a number of human experimental studies with dilute diesel-exhaust show extensive inflammatory effects on the bronchial wall with adverse functional consequences. The underlying mechanisms proposed for the abnormal lung function in childhood related to exposure to such emissions include oxidative stress and activation of several mitogen-activated protein kinases and transcription factors and disturbances in cell function by the physical and chemical characteristics of diesel exhaust. Diesel-exhaust reactions have been reported to extend to disturbances in vascular tone and coagulation.

The report of Gauderman et al, and also previous epidemiologic studies on adverse health effects of traffic focus on traffic emissions and risks of living close to major highways. The findings lead to important questions for society about the structure of our transportation systems, engines, fuels, combustion and road dust in urban areas. As of this writing, the only diesel automobile approved for sale in California is the latest version of the diesel engine manufactured by Mercedes Benz ("Bluetooth"). Unfortunately, the real problem lies with commercial vehicles, specifically heavy-duty trucks that spew their vile exhaust into the air.

J. A. Stockman III, MD

Air Pollution and Infant Death in Southern California, 1989-2000

Ritz B, Wilhelm M, Zhao Y (Univ of California, Los Angeles)
Pediatrics 118:493-502, 2006

Objective.—We evaluated the influence of outdoor air pollution on infant death in the South Coast Air Basin of California, an area characterized by some of the worst air quality in the United States.

Methods.—Linking birth and death certificates for infants who died between 1989 and 2000, we identified all infant deaths, matched 10 living control subjects to each case subject, and assigned the nearest air monitoring station to each birth address. For all subjects, we calculated average carbon monoxide, nitrogen dioxide, ozone, and particulate matter < 10 μm in aerodynamic diameter exposures experienced during the 2-week, 1-month, 2-month, and 6-month periods before a case subject's death.

Results.—The risk of respiratory death increased from 20% to 36% per 1-ppm increase in average carbon monoxide levels 2 weeks before death in early infancy (age: 28 days to 3 months). We also estimated 7% to 12% risk increases for respiratory deaths per 10-μg/m^3 increase in particulate matter < 10 μm in aerodynamic diameter exposure experienced 2 weeks before death for infants 4 to 12 months of age. Risk of respiratory death more than doubled for infants 7 to 12 months of age who were exposed to high average levels of particulates in the previous 6 months. Furthermore, the risk of dying as a result of sudden infant death syndrome increased 15% to 19% per 1-part per hundred million increase in average nitrogen dioxide levels 2 months before death. Low birth weight and preterm infants seemed to be more susceptible to air pollution-related death resulting from these causes; however, we lacked statistical power to confirm this heterogeneity with formal testing.

Conclusions.—Our results add to the growing body of literature implicating air pollution in infant death from respiratory causes and sudden infant death syndrome and provide additional information for future risk assessment.

▶ This study emanates from California where the investigators examined the influence of outdoor air pollution on infant death in the South Coast Air Basin (SoCAB) of southern California during the period 1989 to 2000. This region encompasses 6745 square miles of nondesert area around Los Angeles, San Bernardino, Riverside, and Orange Counties. There are approximately 15 million people who live in SoCAB. The investigators found that there was a direct correlation between levels of carbon monoxide and nitrogen dioxide during certain periods associated with an increase in infant deaths. Whether there was a direct correlation between this pollution and an increased rate of mortality remains to be proven, but where there is smoke there certainly is fire. The findings corroborate earlier studies inside and outside the United States. Previous short-term exposure studies examining pollution increases within days before infant deaths have provided some evidence for possible associations between gaseous pollutants and respiratory deaths in infants and young children.

Exactly how air pollution might increase mortality, particularly in the young, remains to be documented. Studies elsewhere have suggested that such deaths are due to respiratory problems triggered by the air pollution. See the Rogers and Dunlop report (Air pollution and very low birth weight infants: a target population?) that presents data on air pollution and very low birthweight preterm delivery.

J. A. Stockman III, MD

Air Pollution and Very Low Birth Weight Infants: A Target Population?

Rogers JF, Dunlop AL (Ctrs for Disease Control and Prevention, Atlanta, Ga; Emory Univ, Atlanta, Ga)
Pediatrics 118:156-164, 2006

Objective.—The goal was to examine systematically the association between maternal exposure to particulate matter of <10 µm and very low birth weight (<1500 g) delivery for evidence of an effect on duration of gestation and/or intrauterine growth restriction.

Methods.—This case-control study took place between April 1, 1986, and March 30, 1988, in Georgia Health Care District 9 and included 128 mothers of very low birth weight infants, all of whom were preterm and were classified as either small for gestational age or appropriate for gestational age, and 197 mothers of term, appropriate-for-gestational-age infants weighing ≥2500 g. Maternal exposure to particulate matter of <10 µm was estimated with 2 exposure measures, namely, a county-level measure based on residence in a county with an industrial point source and an environmental transport model based on the geographic location of the birth home.

Results.—Considering preterm/appropriate-for-gestational-age infants as cases and term/appropriate-for-gestational-age infants as controls, adjusted odds ratios for maternal exposure to particulate matter of <10 µm were statistically significant (adjusted odds ratio for county-level model: 4.31; adjusted odds ratio for environmental transport model: 3.68). Although elevated, no statistically significant association was found between maternal exposure and preterm/appropriate-for-gestational-age delivery when compared to preterm/small-for-gestational-age delivery.

Conclusions.—There are increased odds of maternal exposure to ambient particulate matter of <10 µm for very low birth weight preterm/appropriate-for-gestational-age delivery, compared with term/appropriate-for-gestational-age delivery, which suggests that the observed association between maternal exposure to air pollution and low infant birth weight (particularly <1500 g) is at least partially attributable to an effect on duration of gestation.

▶ The role of air pollution in postnatal infant death has been well studied and documented. Less well studied is the impact of air pollution on adverse birth outcomes, the subject of this report emanating from Georgia. The study demonstrates a significant increase in the odds of maternal exposure to air pollution and the delivery of very low birthweight infants. Across the United States, the prevalence of exposure to ambient air pollution among pregnant women, particularly in urban settings or settings near a point source of pollution, is quite appreciable. Thus, even a small increase in the risk of adverse birth outcomes resulting from maternal exposure to air pollution could translate into substantial adverse health events. There are many unanswered questions regarding the role of specific components of air pollution and their effects on birth outcomes, so future studies will need to address these deficiencies.

On a related topic, new evidence has appeared that prenatal exposure to air pollution may cause congenital heart defects. Investigators in the Research Triangle Park of North Carolina have compared pollution statistics and records of birth between 1997 and 2000 in 7 Texas counties. The researchers focused on the quality of the air that women were breathing during their first 2 months of pregnancy. In Texas, women who had been exposed early in their pregnancies to relatively high concentrations of carbon monoxide, sulfur dioxide, or particulate matter were much more likely than other women to have infants with certain heart defects. This finding strengthens the hypothesis that pollution and birth defects are indeed linked.[1]

J. A. Stockman III, MD

Reference

1. Harder B. Can polluted air cause birth defects? *Sci News*. 2005;168:158.

Long-Term Exposure to Air Pollution and Incidence of Cardiovascular Events in Women

Miller KA, Siscovick DS, Sheppard L, et al (Univ of Washington, Seattle; Fred Hutchinson Cancer Research Ctr, Seattle)
N Engl J Med 356:447-458, 2007

Background.—Fine particulate air pollution has been linked to cardiovascular disease, but previous studies have assessed only mortality and differences in exposure between cities. We examined the association of long-term exposure to particulate matter of less than 2.5 μm in aerodynamic diameter ($PM_{2.5}$) with cardiovascular events.

Methods.—We studied 65,893 postmenopausal women without previous cardiovascular disease in 36 U.S. metropolitan areas from 1994 to 1998, with a median follow-up of 6 years. We assessed the women's exposure to air pollutants using the monitor located nearest to each woman's residence. Hazard ratios were estimated for the first cardiovascular event, adjusting for age, race or ethnic group, smoking status, educational level, household income, body-mass index, and presence or absence of diabetes, hypertension, or hypercholesterolemia.

Results.—A total of 1816 women had one or more fatal or nonfatal cardiovascular events, as confirmed by a review of medical records, including death from coronary heart disease or cerebrovascular disease, coronary revascularization, myocardial infarction, and stroke. In 2000, levels of $PM_{2.5}$ exposure varied from 3.4 to 28.3 µg per cubic meter (mean, 13.5). Each increase of 10 µg per cubic meter was associated with a 24% increase in the risk of a cardiovascular event (hazard ratio, 1.24; 95% confidence interval [CI], 1.09 to 1.41) and a 76% increase in the risk of death from cardiovascular disease (hazard ratio, 1.76; 95% CI, 1.25 to 2.47). For cardiovascular events, the between-city effect appeared to be smaller than the within-city effect. The risk of cerebrovascular events was also associated with increased levels of $PM_{2.5}$ (hazard ratio, 1.35; 95% CI, 1.08 to 1.68).

Conclusions.—Long-term exposure to fine particulate air pollution is associated with the incidence of cardiovascular disease and death among postmenopausal women. Exposure differences within cities are associated with the risk of cardiovascular disease.

▶ Miller et al report on data from the Women's Health Initiative observational study, which greatly expands our understanding of how fine particulate pollution affects health. While the Women's Health Initiative study has been unisex, there is little reason not to believe that the seeds of a virtually identical problem would also be found in children. Although earlier long-term prospective studies have shown an association between levels of air pollutions consisting of particulate matter less than 2.5 µm in aerodynamic diameter and an increased risk of death from all causes, and from cardiovascular disease in particular, the Women's Health Initiative broadens the scope of findings in that it demonstrates that nonfatal cardiovascular events are also strongly associated with fine particulate concentrations in the community. Although earlier work relied solely on death certificates to define the rate of death from cardiovascular disease, in the Women's Health Initiative, cardiovascular events and mortality rate were defined by objective review of medical records.

Perhaps the most important finding of the Women's Health Initiative is the establishment of a solid and strong statistical association between fine particulate air pollution and death from coronary artery disease as well as an increase in morbidity related to coronary artery disease. Specifically, Miller et al found an increased relative risk of 1.76 for deaths for cardiovascular disease for every 10 µg per cubic meter increase in the mean concentration of air pollutants.

Please do not think that men are completely off the hook when it comes to the effects of air pollution. Associations between fine particulate concentrations and abnormal variability in heart rate were reported several years ago in asymptomatic men exposed to air pollution.[1] Interestingly, studies have shown that statins significantly improve the risk associated with exposure to air pollution, suggesting that the antiinflammatory effect of statins is what allows them to be beneficial in such circumstances.

To read more about the cardiovascular risk associated with fine particulate air pollution, as well as the consequences of air pollution on lung development in children, see the editorials by Dockery et al and Sandström et al.[2,3] Last, if all this sounds like bad news, it is, but realize that eating an appropriate amount of fish while pregnant will benefit your child's development, clearly showing that not everything that gets into our body is bad for our kids.

J. A. Stockman III, MD

References

1. Chen JC, Stone PH, Verrier RL, et al. Personal coronary risk profiles modify autonomic nervous system responses to air pollution. *J Occup Environ Med.* 2006;48:1133-1142.
2. Dockery DW, Stone PH. Cardiovascular risks from fine particulate air pollution. *N Engl J Med.* 2007;356:511-513.
3. Sandström T, Brunekreef B. Traffic-related pollution and lung development in children. *Lancet.* 2007;369:535-537.

Environmental Tobacco Smoke Exposure: Prevalence and Mechanisms of Causation of Infections in Children

Kum-Nji P, Meloy L, Herrod HG (Virginia Commonwealth Univ, Richmond; Univ of Tennessee, Memphis)
Pediatrics 117:1745-1754, 2006

Background and Objectives.—Environmental tobacco smoke (ETS) exposure is probably one of the most important public health hazards in our community. Our aim with this article is to (1) review the prevalence of ETS exposure in the United States and how this prevalence is often measured in practice and (2) summarize current thinking concerning the mechanism by which this exposure may cause infections in young children.

Methods.—We conducted a Medline search to obtain data published mainly in peer-reviewed journals.

Results.—There is still a very high prevalence of ETS exposure among US children ranging from 35% to 80% depending on the method of measurement used and the population studied. The mechanism by which ETS may be related to these infections is not entirely clear but may be through suppression or modulation of the immune system, enhancement of bacterial adherence factors, or impairment of the mucociliary apparatus of the respiratory tract, or possibly through enhancement of toxicity of low levels of certain toxins that are not easily detected by conventional means.

Conclusions.—The prevalence of ETS exposure in the United States is still very high, and its role in causing infections in children is no longer in doubt even if still poorly understood. Research, therefore, should continue to focus on the various mechanisms of causation of these infections and how to best reduce the exposure levels.

▶ Just how bad is environmental smoke on the health of infants and children? Obviously, this question is somewhat rhetorical. The literature is replete with studies on the role of ETS exposure on asthma. Within the past decade, such exposure is being increasingly associated with behavioral and cognitive problems in children. Furthermore, ETS exposure has been shown in a number of studies to adversely affect physical growth in young children. Such exposure has also been shown to be unequivocally associated with a higher incidence of upper and lower respiratory infections, including the common cold, middle-ear disease, respiratory syncytial virus infection, bronchitis, pneumonia, and other serious bacterial infections. Any one of a number of studies has directly linked ETS with sudden infant death syndrome.

Despite the strong associations between ETS exposure and the prevalence of infections in children, the mechanism by which tobacco smoke causes this problem has not been well studied, at least until this report, which suggests that smoke may suppress or modulate the immune system and very well may enhance bacterial adherence factors and impair the mucociliary apparatus of the respiratory tract. It is also possible that very low levels of toxins in smoke, levels that are not readily measurable, may potentiate these harmful effects.

This report helps us better understand some of the potential mechanisms by which tobacco smoke exposure can be harmful to children. Despite the overwhelming epidemiologic evidence linking tobacco smoke to an increased rate of infections in children, it is still not entirely clear exactly how smoke does these evil things. Most studies that have attempted to evaluate the problem have used laboratory animal models and the results from these studies have not been particularly convincing. We need more human studies. For all we know, it is prenatal exposure that is the first trigger for a problem that may not show itself for some months or years after birth.

Mothers who smoke are much less likely to either start or sustain breastfeeding. Prolonged breastfeeding is known to diminish the risk of infection in an infant and toddler and perhaps one of the mechanisms of action of smoke in the environment on an increased risk of infection is simply the result of the fact that infants born of mothers who smoke are much less likely to be breastfed.

We here in the United States are not the only ones that have put on a big push to ban public smoking. A similar trend, albeit later, is taking place in the European Union. France was one of the first countries in Europe to introduce anti-smoking controls in 1992, but that attempt was widely seen as a failure because there was no effective information campaign to support it. On February 1, 2007, smoking was banned in all public places in France except bars and restaurants (which had a one-year's grace). The early indications are that people are complying. Germany has been dragged kicking and screaming into the fresh air, but its struggle has had as much to do with the country's constitutional structure as with Germans' pension for nicotine. After much wrangling, the federal government and the 16 states that make up the country have now agreed on how to divide up their obligations to the World Health Organization treaty. The federal government will be responsible for public buildings and public transport, whereas the states will regulate smoking in bars and restaurants. The federal government seems to be committed to a comprehensive ban. Currently, 1 in 3 German adults smoke, which is high for Western Europe, but attitudes among Germans seem to be changing. The number of German children between the ages of 12 to 17 years who smoke fell between 2001 and 2005 from 28% to 20%.

Spain introduced a part smoking ban (bars under 100 square meters could decide to allow smoking, for example) in January 2006. A significant reduction in smoking rates has already been observed in Spain. In England, it is anticipated new bans in place will result in a 20% to 30% reduction among English smokers within several years. The cigarette manufacturer, Imperial Tobacco, has already seen a 4% decline in tobacco sales in Great Britain.

Thus, things are finally on the move when it comes to the ban on public smoking throughout the world, or at least some parts of the world.[1]

J. A. Stockman III, MD

Reference

1. Spinney L. Public smoking bans shows sign of success in Europe. *Lancet.* 2007;369:1507-1508.

Effects of parental smoking and level of education on initiation and duration of breastfeeding

Di Napoli A, Di Lallo D, Pezzotti P, et al (Agency for Public Health of Lazio Region, Rome; Local Health Authority RM/E, Rome)
Acta Paediatr 95:678-685, 2006

Aim.—To evaluate the effects of parental smoking and level of education on the initiation and duration of breastfeeding in a prospective cohort study on mother–infant pairs.

Methods.—We studied 543 mother–infant pairs enrolled after delivery at a hospital in Rome. Information about parents' characteristics were obtained from a questionnaire administered in hospital; the outcome of the study was the infant's feeding habits in the preceding 24 h, assessed by telephone every 2 wk. The effects of parental smoking and level of education on initiation and duration of breastfeeding were evaluated through multivariate logistic regression models and time-dependent Cox models.

Results.—After controlling for confounding factors, we found a negative effect for mothers' smoking both on breastfeeding initiation (odds ratio 2.19, 95% CI 1.05–4.55) and duration (hazard ratio 3.37, 95% CI 1.85–6.13) when at least one parent had a low level of education.

Conclusion.—Our study shows that maternal smoking, particularly when one of the parents has a low level of education, determines a negative effect on the initiation and duration of breastfeeding. Public health policy should promote educational programmes for both parents focused on quitting smoking, which could have positive effects on the initiation and duration of breastfeeding.

▶ The data from this report speak for itself. As mentioned in the commentary for the Kum-Nji et al report (Environmental tobacco smoke exposure: prevalence and mechanisms of causation of infections in children), the march is on to ban smoking. Ireland has been a country that has adored its cigarettes and beer, but even there, change is underway. Surveys of a cohort of Irish smokers before and after the ban on smoking in public places have shown that the Irish have largely accepted the new law. Compliance was very high 9 months after the institution of the ban, with smoking continuing in just 5% of public houses,

3% of restaurants, and 14% of workplaces. Some 83% of Irish workers regard the law as "good" or "very good." Nearly half report visiting pubs less often than before the ban, and those that do go spend less time there. The study did not investigate the economic consequences but quotes the experience of New York City. In New York, the number of smokers dining out declined, but this decline was completely offset by the rise in visits of the majority of the population that is now non-smoking.[1]

Interestingly, a study from Norway, where smoking was banned in restaurants, bars, and hotels in 2004, shows that Norwegian waiters and barmen now cough and wheeze remarkably less than before the institution of the smoking ban.[2]

J. A. Stockman III, MD

References

1. Fong GT, Hyland A, Borland R, et al. Reductions in tobacco smoke pollution and increases in support for smoke-free public places following the implementation of comprehensive smoke-free workplace legislation in the Republic of Ireland: findings from the ITC Ireland/UK Survey. *Tob Control*. 2006;15:51-58.
2. Eagan TM, Hetland J, Aarø LE. Decline in respiratory symptoms in service workers five months after a public smoking ban. *Tob Control*. 2006;15:242-246.

Teen Smokers Reach Their Mid Twenties
Patton GC, Coffey C, Carlin JB, et al (Murdoch Children's Research Inst, Parkville, Victoria, Australia; Univ of Melbourne, Australia)
J Adolesc Health 39:214-220, 2006

Purpose.—Most outcome studies of adolescent smokers have focused on tobacco use in the short term. Few have reported on the health of adolescent smokers as they reach young adulthood.

Methods.—The design was a 10-year, eight-wave cohort study of a statewide community sample of 1943 participants in Victoria, Australia. Participants were initially aged 14 to 15 years. Tobacco use was assessed with self-reported frequency of use and a seven-day retrospective diary. The Fagerstrom Test for Nicotine Dependence was used to define nicotine dependence in young adulthood. A computerized interview assessment was used during the teens and in young adulthood.

Results.—Former daily smokers in adolescence accounted for most cases of nicotine dependence and high-dose (10+ cigarettes per day) smoking in young adulthood. Other substance abuse and psychiatric morbidity in young adulthood were also markedly elevated in this group. This was most clearly evident for cannabis dependence, where close to two-thirds of all cases were formerly daily tobacco smokers. Male smokers were more likely to continue as young adults. Persistent symptoms of depression and anxiety during the teens predicted progression to nicotine dependence, as did having a parent smoking daily.

Conclusions.—The poor health outcomes of daily adolescent smokers as they reach young adulthood provide a rationale for greater tobacco control initiatives directed at early users. Clinical interventions might usefully consider factors such as psychiatric morbidity and parental smoking.

▶ The data from this report are appalling in the sense that it is clear that once one starts smoking as a teenager, one is likely to continue to smoke. These data remain factual even though there has been a fall in adult smoking here in the United States as well as some other countries.[1] Data from the United States National Health Interview Surveys from the 1960s onward suggest that adolescent smokers persist in smoking for many years, with the median cessation age only being in the mid 30s.[2]

In 2000, the United States Supreme Court threw out regulations on tobacco advertising and cigarette sales to minors imposed in 1996 by former Food and Drug Administration (FDA) Commissioner, David Kessler. Since then, the campaign for Tobacco-Free Kids has led an effort to lobby for the passage of federal legislation that would put all tobacco products under a single regulatory roof. If enacted, the Family Smoking Prevention and Tobacco Control Act would give the FDA regulatory authority over tobacco products and would be the first federal legislation on tobacco since the 1988 airline-smoking ban. It does not appear that Congress is on the verge, however, of standing up to Big Tobacco. Interestingly, one of the most vocal champions of this proposed bill has turned out to be none other than the nation's largest cigarette company, Philip Morris, maker of Marlboro, the top cigarette brand in the United States and throughout the world. The latter company now marches shoulder-to-shoulder with the campaign for Tobacco-Free Kids, the American Cancer Society, and the American Heart Association, among others, in lobbying for passage of this legislation while all the other major tobacco companies have at one time or another opposed the proposed legislation. If you are other than an optimist, you might think that Philip Morris' support for the bill should prompt skepticism that the legislation's public-health benefits are marginal at best. This just may be true. First, the measure would stringently regulate new and potentially less hazardous tobacco products, but would not apply these same regulatory standards to the most irredeemably harmful form of tobacco existing, cigarettes. Second, although the bill would require the FDA to prevent the introduction of new cigarette brands for which "there is a lack of a showing that permitting such tobacco products to be marketed would be appropriate for the production of the public health," the bill permits Marlboro and the other most popular existing cigarette brands to remain on the market, even though these products are one of the leading threats to the public's health. Third, the bill bans the use of strawberry, grape, chocolate, and other similar flavoring additives in cigarettes, but does not require the FDA to eliminate (or even reduce the levels of) toxic gases, including hydrogen cyanide or the more than 40 known cancer-causing constituents of cigarette smoke such as benzopyrene, benzine, and radioactive polonium.

Any historian will tell you that history has shown that the tobacco industry has outwitted public-health advocates at every attempt to impose meaningful federal tobacco legislation. The main goal of the Federal Cigarette Advertising and Labeling Act of 1970 was to remove ubiquitous cigarette advertisements from the broadcast media, yet no sooner had overt commercials for cigarettes left the airways than televised sports events, such as the Marlboro Grand Prix, the Virginia Slims Tennis Circuit, and Winston Cup Racing, began to proliferate. The Master Settlement Agreement of 1998 has resulted in only a tiny fraction of settlement monies from cigarette companies being directed toward smoking prevention and cessation. Only 4 states currently are allocating to tobacco prevention the minimum amount recommended by the Centers for Disease Control and Prevention. All told, only approximately 2.6% of tobacco revenues are being spent on tobacco prevention and cessation.

Wisdom says that one should never look a gift horse in the mouth, but the very fact that Philip Morris is supporting legislation to control tobacco use should create skepticism that legislation of this type is in any way sufficient to diminish the tobacco pandemic and should prompt concern that, once again, public-health groups may have been outsmarted by the "Marlboro Man."

J. A. Stockman III, MD

References

1. Pierce JP, Fiore MC, Novotny TE, Hatziandreu EJ, Davis RM. Trends in cigarette smoking in the United States. Projections to the year 2000. *JAMA.* 2000;261:61-65.
2. Pierce JP, Gilpin E. How long will today's new adolescent smoker be addicted to cigarettes? *Am J Public Health.* 1996;86:253-256.

Reduced Lung Function at Birth and the Risk of Asthma at 10 Years of Age
Håland G, for ORAACLE (Ullevål Univ, Oslo, Norway; et al)
N Engl J Med 355:1682-1689, 2006

Background.—Reduced lung function in early infancy has been associated with later obstructive airway diseases. We assessed whether reduced lung function shortly after birth predicts asthma 10 years later.

Methods.—We conducted a prospective birth cohort study of healthy infants in which we measured lung function shortly after birth with the use of tidal breathing flow-volume loops (the fraction of expiratory time to peak tidal expiratory flow to total expiratory time [t_{PTEF}/t_E]) in 802 infants and passive respiratory mechanics, including respiratory-system compliance, in 664 infants. At 10 years of age, 616 children (77%) were reassessed by measuring lung function, exercise-induced bronchoconstriction, and bronchial hyperresponsiveness (by means of a methacholine challenge) and by conducting a structured interview to determine whether there was a history of asthma or current asthma.

Results.—As compared with children whose t_{PTEF}/t_E shortly after birth was above the median, children whose t_{PTEF}/t_E was at or below the median were more likely at 10 years of age to have a history of asthma (24.3% vs. 16.2%, P=0.01), to have current asthma (14.6% vs. 7.5%, P=0.005), and to have severe bronchial hyperresponsiveness, defined as a methacholine dose of less than 1.0 μmol causing a 20% fall in the forced expiratory volume in 1 second (FEV₁) (9.1% vs. 4.9%, P=0.05). As compared with children whose respiratory-system compliance was above the median, children with respiratory compliance at or below the median more often had a history of asthma (27.4% vs. 14.8%; P=0.001) and current asthma (15.0% vs. 7.7%, P=0.009), although this measure was not associated with later measurements of lung function. At 10 years of age, t_{PTEF}/t_E at birth correlated weakly with the maximal midexpiratory flow rate (r=0.10, P=0.01) but not with FEV₁ or forced vital capacity.

Conclusions.—Reduced lung function at birth is associated with an increased risk of asthma by 10 years of age.

▶ This report from Oslo, Norway shows that reduced lung-function values within a few days after birth, as measured by tidal flow-volume loops and passive respiratory mechanics, are significant risk factors for asthma in the first 10 years of life. This extends previous findings relating early lung function to the presence or absence of childhood respiratory illness. The study included children who were representative of the native population of urban Oslo. The study design was prospective. Parents, children, and those who evaluated the children 10 years of age were unaware of the measurements of lung function shortly after birth. These results suggest that alterations of airway function associated with later asthma may be present a few days after birth. It is important to note, however, that the clinical implications of reduced lung function shortly after birth at an individual level are unclear. Variations of lung function between individuals as well as within an individual a few days after birth are well recognized. The results of this study indicate that these lung-function measures are predictive for later asthma, but the correlation coefficient for this prediction remains modest. Thus, the data from the Norwegian study do not support the use of neonatal measurement of lung function as a screening test for the subsequent risk of asthma.

J. A. Stockman III, MD

Neonatal Screening for Cystic Fibrosis Does Not Affect Time to First Infection With *Pseudomonas aeruginosa*

Baussano I, Tardivo I, Bellezza-Fontana R, et al (Univ of Turin, Italy; ASO OIRM-Sant'Anna, Turin, Italy)
Pediatrics 118:888-895, 2006

Objective.—Newborn screening for cystic fibrosis was introduced in the Piedmont region of Italy in the year 2000. Our aim with this study was to estimate the effect of newborn screening on the risk of *Pseudomonas aeruginosa* infection at the regional cystic fibrosis pediatric reference center.

Methods.—The time to first infection with *P aeruginosa* within the historical cohort of cystic fibrosis children diagnosed between January 1, 1997, and June 30, 2004, was investigated, comparing survival functions and the adjusted hazard ratio of children diagnosed before and after newborn screening introduction. The role of pancreatic insufficiency was also concurrently investigated.

Results.—Overall, 71 children diagnosed with cystic fibrosis were identified, 27 cases were clinically diagnosed before newborn screening introduction, and 5 of them presented with meconium ileus, whereas 44 were identified by newborn screening. Among them 35 needed pancreatic enzyme supplementation, whereas 34 children were infected with *P aeruginosa*. Both the nonparametric and semiparametric survival estimates failed to show any significant increase in the risk of *P aeruginosa* infection among screened children compared with historical controls. However, the median time from cystic fibrosis diagnosis to *P aeruginosa* infection among screened children was significantly shorter (183 vs 448 days). Children with impaired pancreatic function were at high risk of *P aeruginosa* infection.

Conclusions.—The results of the study suggest that health authorities should regard newborn screening for cystic fibrosis as an opportunity to improve care and outcomes among affected children and shift the focus from whether it is appropriate to screen to how to optimize biomedical and psychosocial outcomes of screening.

▶ The report from Italy asks the question of whether neonatal screening detection of cystic fibrosis helps prevent the onset of time to first infection with *Pseudomonas aeruginosa*. The diagnosis of cystic fibrosis by screening anticipates clinical diagnosis by more than a year in about half of patients with cystic fibrosis. This anticipation may translate into the exposure of asymptomatic children to nosocomial transmission of respiratory infections, unless infection control policies are strictly implemented. Because early infection with *P aeruginosa* is associated with a progressive deterioration of pulmonary function and increased mortality risks, it is of some value to evaluate the role of cystic fibrosis newborn screening as a risk factor for the transmission of *P aeruginosa* infection.

What we learn from this report is that the study in Italy failed to show any significant relationship between the nature of the diagnostic approach to cystic fibrosis and the risk of the first respiratory infection being caused by *P aeruginosa*. On the other hand, it revealed a relationship between the need for pancreatic enzyme supplementation and the occurrence of the *P aeruginosa* infection. This suggests that early screening may result in affected individuals coming to centers where children are exposed nosocomially to *P aeruginosa* infection. Needless to say, the latter is a preventable circumstance suggesting that the strict adoption of infection-transmission-control measures are critical in patients who had the infection newly diagnosed.

Italy is not the only country overseas that is looking at the benefits of screening newborns for cystic fibrosis. Recent data from the United Kingdom are also quite interesting. A cost of illness study used data from the United Kingdom's cystic fibrosis database for the year 2002 to compare treatment costs of 184 children diagnosed with cystic fibrosis as newborns through screening and 950 children diagnosed clinically when age 1 to 9 years. The mean cost of treatment for children diagnosed through screening was $7228.00, compared with $12,008.00 for children diagnosed later in life (mean $352 versus $2442). Even greater financial benefits would probably have been shown if indirect savings had been included, such as time off work, travel to medical centers, etc. Since the 1980s, evidence has accumulated to support the value of early screening of newborns for cystic fibrosis. Early diagnosis by screening and early treatment have benefits for nutrition, growth, cognitive function, lung function, and longevity in individuals with cystic fibrosis in Great Britain as has been found in the rest of the world.

Perhaps more governments throughout the globe will now be persuaded to implement screening for cystic fibrosis. Currently, Australia and New Zealand screen all newborns. Twenty-six programs have been implemented in Europe, and currently in the United States, 27 states have mandated screening for newborns for cystic fibrosis.[1]

J. A. Stockman III, MD

Reference

1. Sims EJ, Mugford M, Clark A, et al. Economic implications of newborn screening for cystic fibrosis: a cost of illness retrospective cohort study. *Lancet.* 2007;369:1187-1195.

Potential impact of newborn screening for cystic fibrosis on child survival: A systematic review and analysis
Grosse SD, Rosenfeld M, Devine OJ, et al (Ctrs for Disease Control and Prevention, Atlanta, Ga; Children's Hosp and Regional Med Ctr, Seattle; Univ of Wisconsin, Madison)
J Pediatr 149:362-366, 2006

Objective.—To estimate the population impact of child mortality as a result of cystic fibrosis (CF) potentially preventable by newborn screening.

Study Design.—A systematic literature review of mortality in children with classic CF without meconium ileus (MI) in screened and unscreened cohorts was extended by contacting investigators for unpublished data. In addition, survival in US states with and without newborn screening (NBS) programs for CF was compared using data from the Cystic Fibrosis Foundation Patient Registry (CFFPR).

Results.—Among non-US studies, CF-related mortality risk to approximately 10 years of age was lower by 5 to 10 per 100 in screened cohorts. Unpublished US data from a trial of NBS for CF indicate no CF-related deaths to 10 years of age in either cohort. CFFPR data suggest improved survival among children with CF born in US states with NBS, with a CF-related mortality difference to 10 years of age between the screened and unscreened groups between 1.5 and 2 per 100 children with CF without MI.

Conclusion.—In addition to improving nutritional outcomes, newborn screening for CF may result in improved child survival. The absolute differential in mortality risk, although modest in size, appears comparable to NBS for certain other genetic disorders.

▶ Most of us have been reading about neonatal screening for CF for more than a decade or two. It seems clear that early diagnosis and treatment of classic CF has been shown to result in improved nutrition and growth. What has remained somewhat debatable is the potential benefits of neonatal screening on the onset of lung disease and ultimate survivorship. Policy makers have tended to focus neonatal screening programs on diseases for which life-saving intervention can be most helpful. Mortality among children with CF is low here in the United States. Fewer than 3% of affected children without MI born between 1987 and 1991, died before reaching the age of 10 years. Nonetheless, this important systematic review clearly indicates that CF NBS is unequivocally associated with an absolute differential in the cumulative risk of child death by age 10 years among children with CF without MI. The relative risk of CF-related death among children before their 10th birthday was 3½ times higher in states without screening programs compared with states with screening for CF.

Although screening newborns for CF are mandated by a growing number of states on the basis of evidence of nonfatal endpoints such as malnutrition, we now see that there are some mortality differences in screened versus nonscreened CF populations. One can compare this with sickle cell disease screening, which will produce a reduction in mortality of somewhere between 1.0 per 100 to 2.4 per 100 children, this reduction resulting from earlier initiation of antibiotic prophylaxis and the prevention of sepsis. Approximately 1000 children are born each year here in the United States with sickle cell anemia compared with approximately 800 children born with CF without MI. If one looks at mortality differentials of 2 per 100 for both disorders, this would imply approximately 20 sickle cell-related deaths and 15 CF-related deaths each year among children preventable by NBS. By comparison, classic galactosemia presents in about 75 newborn infants each year and is associated with a mortality of perhaps 20% without screening. Most of the projected 15 annual deaths related to galactosemia are averted by NBS for this disorder. One can therefore conclude that CF may be comparable to sickle cell anemia and galactosemia in the numbers of deaths preventable by NBS.

See the van den Akker-van Marle et al report (Cost-effectiveness of 4 neonatal screening strategies for cystic fibrosis) that tells us about the cost effectiveness of four neonatal screening strategies for CF.

J. A. Stockman III, MD

Cost-effectiveness of 4 Neonatal Screening Strategies for Cystic Fibrosis
van den Akker-van Marle ME, Dankert HM, Verkerk PH, et al (Netherlands Organization for Applied Scientific Research, Quality of Life, Leiden, Netherlands; Atrium Med Centre, Heerlen, Netherlands)
Pediatrics 118:896-904, 2006

Objectives.—The purpose of this work was to assess the costs of 4 neonatal screening strategies for cystic fibrosis in relation to health effects. In each strategy, the first test was the measurement of serum concentration of immunoreactive trypsin. The second step consisted of either a second immunoreactive trypsin test (strategy 1) or a multiple mutation analysis (strategy 2). In strategies 3 and 4, a third step was added to strategy 2: a second immunoreactive trypsin test (strategy 3) or an extended mutation analysis of the cystic fibrosis gene, that is, a denaturing gradient gel electrophoresis analysis (strategy 4).

Methods.—We conducted an economic-modeling exercise in the Netherlands based on published data and expert opinions. Subjects were a hypothetical cohort of 200 000 neonates, the approximate number of children born annually in the Netherlands, and we assessed the costs and number of life-years gained as a result of neonatal screening for cystic fibrosis. The costs and effects of changes in reproductive decisions because of neonatal screening were also assessed.

Results.—Immunoreactive trypsin + immunoreactive trypsin had the most favorable cost-effectiveness ratio of €24 800 per life-year gained. Immunoreactive trypsin + DNA + denaturing gradient gel electrophoresis achieved more health effects than immunoreactive trypsin + DNA + immunoreactive trypsin at lower cost. The incremental costs per life-year gained of the immunoreactive trypsin + DNA + denaturing gradient gel electrophoresis strategy compared with the immunoreactive trypsin + immunoreactive trypsin strategy were €130 700, whereas the incremental costs of the immunoreactive trypsin + DNA strategy compared with the immunoreactive trypsin + DNA + denaturing gradient gel electrophoresis strategy were €2 154 300. When changes in reproductive decisions as a result of neonatal screening are also taken into account, neonatal screening for cystic fibrosis may lead to financial savings of approximately €1.8 million annually, depending on the screening strategy used.

Conclusions.—Cystic fibrosis screening for neonates is a good economic option, and positive health effects can also be expected. Immunoreactive trypsin + immunoreactive trypsin and immunoreactive trypsin + DNA + denaturing gradient gel electrophoresis are the most cost-effective strategies.

▶ The Grosse et al report (Potential impact of newborn screening for cystic fibrosis on child survival: a systematic review and analysis) and commentary demonstrated the clear effectiveness of neonatal screening for cystic fibrosis in terms of prevention of significant mortality in the first decade of life. This report from The Netherlands tells us which methods commonly used to screen for cystic fibrosis in the newborn period are most cost-effective. The study examined 3 screening strategies. In each screening strategy, the first test consists of measuring serum concentrations of immunoreactive trypsin. The second step is either a second immunoreactive trypsin (IRT) test or a single/multiple mutation analysis (IRT + DNA strategy). A third step can be added to strategy 2: a second IRT test (IRT + DNA + IRT strategy) or an extended mutation analysis of the cystic fibrosis gene performed by gel electrophoresis. In all the strategies, infants with a positive screening test are referred for sweat testing to confirm or exclude the cystic fibrosis diagnosis. The IRT + IRT strategy had the best cost-effectiveness ratio with €24,800 per life-year gained. Other strategies could cost as much as €154,300 per life-year gained.

When this editor was growing up, he was taught by his parents about knowing the price of everything and the value of nothing. When it comes to newborn screening for cystic fibrosis, fortunately, the more money you spend does not necessarily result in more lives saved. It was more than 20 years ago that some states, Colorado in particular, began pancreatitis-associated protein testing as a screen for cystic fibrosis in the newborn period. Inclusion of this type of testing and retesting for positives continues to remain the mainstay of adequate screening despite more costly technologies being available in recent years.

Since the introduction of cystic fibrosis newborn screening, the benefits and risks of the procedure have been debated. In 1992, the American Society of Human Genetics did not recommend cystic fibrosis newborn screening unless individuals had a positive family history of cystic fibrosis. In 1997, however, a systematic review of the scientific evidence on cystic fibrosis newborn screening led the Centers for Disease Control and Prevention to draw up recommendations on pilot screening programs. Since that time, evidence has clearly accumulated in support of the beneficial role of cystic fibrosis newborn screening to patients with cystic fibrosis and their families. It has therefore been suggested that public health authorities should shift their attention from the legitimacy of screening procedures to optimizing how these screening procedures are carried out and what outcomes result from screening.

Let's close this comment with a peripheral question having to do with cystic fibrosis and other diseases similar to cystic fibrosis and air transport. The question is, what are the problems and pitfalls to successful aeromedical evacuation?

There are a number of patient hazards related to air transport. The first that comes to mind is the risk of hypoxia. Cabin pressures in modern passenger aircraft are maintained at an altitude equivalent to that of 5,000 to 8,000 feet above sea level. At this level, passengers without serious medical problems typically have an oxygen saturation of approximately 94%. In patients with poor profusion, oxygen saturation can drop into the precarious range of the hemoglobin oxygen dissociation curve. Patients in such situations will need supplemental oxygen, possibly ventilation, and if anemic, pre-flight transfusion should be accomplished. Patients with pulmonary compromise obviously are at greatest risk.

Another problem with air transport is gas expansion. The latter accounts for the majority of contraindications to aeromedical travel. A change from sea level to 8,000 feet of altitude will expand the volume of trapped gas by 35%. In vulnerable patients, this can provoke a tension pneumothorax, dehiscence of some surgical wounds as a result of expansion of intraabdominal gas, intracranial hemorrhage, and irreversible ocular damage. Whereas hypoxia can be detected with pulse oximetry and mitigated with supplemental oxygen, the consequences of gas expansion are difficult to recognize and also to reverse aboard an aircraft. Recent surgery and head and chest trauma impose the greatest risks of such gas expansion. Those who have had diving-related injuries will have decompression sickness problems exacerbated by air transport. If you get into trouble in the air, please instruct the pilot, if at all possible, to lower the altitude of the aircraft to as near ground level as is safe.[1]

Please note that no private air carrier or commercial airline will perform an air evacuation without securing a payment commitment in the form of a guarantee from an insurance or medical assistance company or a preflight transfer funds from the private account of a patient or family member. All forms of aeromedical transport are expensive, but air ambulance services especially so, with some transoceanic retrievals topping $100,000.

J. A. Stockman III, MD

Reference

1. Teichman PG, Donchin Y, Kot RJ. International aeromedical evacuation. *N Engl J Med.* 2007;356:262-270.

19 Therapeutics and Toxicology

Effect of reducing caffeine intake on birth weight and length of gestation: randomised controlled trial

Bech BH, Obel C, Henriksen TB, et al (Univ of Aarhus, Denmark; Aarhus Univ Hosp, Skejby, Denmark; Univ of California, Los Angeles)

BMJ 334:409-412, 2007

Objective.—To estimate the effect of reducing caffeine intake during pregnancy on birth weight and length of gestation.

Design.—Randomised double blind controlled trial.

Setting.—Denmark.

Participants.—1207 pregnant women drinking at least three cups of coffee a day, recruited before 20 weeks' gestation.

Interventions.—Caffeinated instant coffee (568 women) or decaffeinated instant coffee (629 women).

Main Outcome Measures.—Birth weight and length of gestation.

Results.—Data on birth weight were obtained for 1150 liveborn singletons and on length of gestation for 1153 liveborn singletons. No significant differences were found for mean birth weight or mean length of gestation between women in the decaffeinated coffee group (whose mean caffeine intake was 182 mg lower than that of the other group) and women in the caffeinated coffee group. After adjustment for length of gestation, parity, prepregnancy body mass index, and smoking at entry to the study the mean birth weight of babies born to women in the decaffeinated group was 16 g (95% confidence interval −40 to 73) higher than those born to women in the caffeinated group. The adjusted difference (decaffeinated group-caffeinated group) of length of gestation was −1.31 days (−2.87 to 0.25).

Conclusion.—A moderate reduction in caffeine intake in the second half of pregnancy has no effect on birth weight or length of gestation.

▶ I read this report from Denmark in Los Angeles swigging down my second cup of coffee one morning. Although some may like their coffee black and others white, whether it is wise to drink coffee in pregnancy is not a black and white issue. Some studies report that the consumption of more than a modest amount of caffeine during pregnancy may increase the likelihood of infertility, birth defects, miscarriage, stillbirth, premature birth, fetal growth restriction, and sudden infant death syndrome. The rub with all the data is that women who drink more coffee than others nearly always differ from other pregnant women in many other ways also. For example, they are more likely to smoke. This report abstracted, from the *BMJ*, summarizes an interventional study by Bech et al showing that babies born to mothers who drink moderate amounts of coffee do not weigh less than those whose mothers drink decaffeinated coffee in the second half of pregnancy.

As far as caffeine is concerned, it does cross the placenta and quite easily so. Exposure to boluses of caffeine can certainly damage the fetal rat, but only when the comparable amount is 10 times higher than any human would ever ingest, even if they drank nothing but the most potent caffeinated beverage in a dose high enough to render them ill. In the 1980s, it was suggested that women who consume more than 1 equivalent of a cup of coffee per day were half as likely to become pregnant as women who drank less. Subsequent studies have debunked these findings, however. Nonetheless, early miscarriage is more common in women who drink substantial amounts of coffee in early pregnancy. This dose- dependent relationship between intake of caffeine before pregnancy and the risk of miscarriage suggests that a very high intake of caffeine prenatally is, in fact, unwise. The facts are, though, that caffeine consumption does not appear to make preterm birth more likely, and only 1 study has suggested a link with sudden infant death syndrome. The data from the latter study could not be replicated.

The US Food and Drug Administration has been advising women to avoid or limit the intake of caffeine in pregnancy since 1980. The randomized controlled trial by Bech et al might lead to a revision of this advice, at least with regard to the effects of caffeine on birthweight. We do need a larger, similarly designed, trial to show whether observational studies are right in suggesting that high caffeine intake increases the risk of stillbirth.

To close this commentary, here is a question related to therapeutics. Many of us know adults who claim they cannot swallow a pill. The query is, however, at what age can we confidently say that children should be able to swallow pills? The answer comes from a recent report by Meltzer et al.[1] It appears that at around age 6 one should expect a child to be able to satisfactorily swallow a pill, even without significant prior training or experience. In an observational study of youngsters age 6 to 11 years, some 91% swallowed a tablet using an ordinary cup or a patented pill cup. If you are not familiar with a pill cup, it is a novel device. When tilted into the child's mouth, water washes through a trap into the back of the throat carrying a pill with it, therefore, reducing pill swallowing to a one-step procedure, which may facilitate the learning of tablet swallowing. In order to use the device, fill the pill cup with water just below the pill-trap level. The tablet is placed in the well near the top of the cup. A child is merely told to drink the water in the cup, allowing the tablet to fall into their mouth and to be swallowed along with the water.

Thus it is that even some of the youngest among us can do what some of the oldest among us cannot do: swallow a pill effectively.

J. A. Stockman III, MD

Reference

1. Meltzer EO, Welch MJ, Ostrom NK. Pill swallowing and training in children 6 to 11 years of age. *Clin Pediatr.* 2006;45:725-733.

Analgesic effect of watching TV during venipuncture

Bellieni CV, Cordelli DM, Raffaelli M, et al (Univ of Siena, Italy)
Arch Dis Child 91:1015-1017, 2006

Aims.—To assess the analgesic effect of passive or active distraction during venipuncture in children.

Methods.—We studied 69 children aged 7–12 years undergoing venipuncture. The children were randomly divided into three groups: a control group (C) without any distraction procedure, a group (M) in which mothers performed active distraction, and a TV group (TV) in which passive distraction (a TV cartoon) was used. Both mothers and children scored pain after the procedure.

Results.—Main pain levels rated by the children were 23.04 (standard deviation (SD) 24.57), 17.39 (SD 21.36), and 8.91 (SD 8.65) for the C, M, and TV groups, respectively. Main pain levels rated by mothers were 21.30 (SD 19.9), 23.04 (SD 18.39), and 12.17 (SD 12.14) for the C, M, and TV groups, respectively. Scores assigned by mothers and children indicated that procedures performed during TV watching were less painful ($p < 0.05$) than control or procedures performed during active distraction.

Conclusion.—TV watching was more effective than active distraction. This was due either to the emotional participation of the mothers in the active procedure or to the distracting power of television.

▶ Who would have thought that watching TV would induce anesthesia? But then again, take a good look at many youngsters who are watching the boob tube. They look zombie-ized, truly spaced out sometimes. In this report, 69 children matched for age and sex underwent venipuncture for routine clinical purposes. The youngsters were 7 to 12 years of age. They were randomly assigned to having the venipuncture done without distraction, having the venipuncture performed while their mother interacted with them to attempt to distract them, or having the venipuncture performed while watching an age-appropriate cartoon on TV. At the end of the session, the child was asked to score the pain experienced on a scale from 0 (no pain) to 100 (maximum pain). The cartoons won hands down.

More than one maneuver has been tried to minimize pain associated with a heel stick performed on a newborn. Generally massaging a baby's leg for two minutes before a heel stick to obtain blood samples is both safe and does help reduce the pain response. A study was undertaken to document this. Pain was assessed utilizing the neonatal infant pain scale. Respiratory rate, heart rate and oxygen saturation along with cortisol concentrations were measured from blood samples. Both the pain score and the heart rate were higher after heel stick in babies who are not massaged.[1]

Other studies have suggested that audio/visual distraction can be a good source of pain relief. Cohen et al[2] observed that 4- to 6-year-old children watching a popular cartoon series felt less pain when undergoing certain technical procedures. Most settings that have used cartoon watching have involved children receiving immunizations. A good cartoon is twice as good as a mother in producing high-quality distraction and pain relief. I saw this phenomenon in action when observing our 18-month-old grandson having his first hair cut . . . not a whimper as he was bedazzled by a cartoon as the clippers clipped away.

Next up we will probably see cartoons going head to head against topical anesthetic creams such as EMA and EMLA MAX. Chances are that such a study will not be sponsored by a drug company, however. Warner Brothers, on the other hand, may be looked to for grant support.

J. A. Stockman III, MD

References

1. Jain S, Kumar P, McMillan DD. Prior leg massage decreases pain responses to heel stick in preterm babies. *J Paediatr Child Health*. 2006;42:505-508.
2. Cohen LL, Blount RL, Panopoulos G. Nurse coaching and cartoon distraction: an effective and practical intervention to reduce child, parent, and nurse distress during immunizations. *J Pediatr Psychol*. 1997;22:355-370.

Meconium and neurotoxicants: searching for a prenatal exposure timing

García JAO, Gallardo DC, i Tortajada, JF, et al (Univ Children's Hosp "Virgen de la Arrixaca," Murcia, Spain; Inst of Chemical and Environmental Research, Barcelona; Univ Children's Hosp "La Fe," Valencia, Spain)
Arch Dis Child 91:642-646, 2006

Background.—Exposure to organochlorine compounds (OCs) has been a subject of interest in recent years, given their potential neurotoxicity. Meconium is easily available and accumulates neurotoxicants and/or metabolites from the 12th week of gestation.

Aims.—To determine whether neurotoxicants, specifically OCs, could be detected in serially collected meconium, and to compare the results with those obtained in cord blood samples.

Methods.—A sample of cord blood and three serial stool samples were analysed in 10 newborns. Pentachlorobenzene (PeCB), hexachlorobenzene (HCB), polychlorinated biphenyls (PCBs), dichlorodiphenyl trichloroethane (p,p'-DDT) and its metabolite dichlorodiphenyl dichloroethylene (p,p'-DDE), and hexachlorocyclohexane isomers (α-, β-, γ-, and Δ-HCH) were analysed by gas chromatography.

Results.—From serial stool collection and analysis in newborns, there was an increase in the concentrations of HCB, p,p'-DDE, PCBs, and β-HCH between the first and last stools of the newborn. Levels of DDT diminished as pregnancy progressed. Concentrations in cord blood were positively associated with concentrations in meconium for p,p'-DDE and β-HCH.

Conclusions.—Meconium is a very useful instrument for the investigation of fetal exposure to neurotoxicants; serial collection and analysis of meconium should estimate the timing and degree of in utero exposure of the fetus to neurotoxicants. Analysis and interpretation of neurotoxicants in meconium results is a complex process. Measurement in meconium of a wide range of neurotoxic substances should facilitate early identification of harmful exposures, and enable rehabilitation and instigation of preventive measures.

▶ Exposure assessment for environmental neurotoxicants is not a simple matter, particularly when it comes to infants, toddlers and children. For this reason, novel methods are urgently needed to help us solve the controversies surrounding what are important and what are not important environmental exposures. Meconium, the first greenish feces of a newborn, has been used to some extent to analyze for cocaine to reveal maternal abuse, cotinine to indicate maternal smoking, and pesticides to show fetal exposure. Xenobiotics are assumed to enter the meconium in bile and/or are swallowed in amniotic fluid. Meconium is reported to accumulate starting between the 12th and 16th week of pregnancy, and as a sticky substance, its contents remain fairly stable over the months in utero, reflecting exposures from the second trimester of pregnancy right through the end of delivery. The advantages of studying meconium are pretty straightforward: ease and the noninvasive nature of collection. Furthermore, the analytic sensitivity for many compounds is better than when using urine or cord blood samples.

In the report of Ortega Garcia et al, we see that the investigators have divided meconium sampling into 3 periods: 0-10 hours, 10-24 hours, and 24-48 hours after birth. Concentrations of some environmental contaminants such as PCBs, hexachlorobenzene, and beta-hexachlorocyclohexane increase from the first meconium stool to the third, perhaps enabling the timing of when certain of these neurotoxicants first expose themselves to infants in utero.

It is a shame that the authors of this report did not measure fat content of their meconium samples to be able to express lipid soluble chemicals on a lipid basis. This is a study waiting to be done. Such a study would help us to compare the concentrations of neurotoxicants with previous studies on maternal concentrations of the same chemicals. In a very limited prior study, cord blood concentrations of dioxins turned out to be in the same range as those in meconium when both were expressed per microgram lipid.[1]

Current information on fetal or neonatal concentrations of environmental chemicals is very patchy, because for ethical and technical reasons, samples are not easy to obtain. Thus, all efforts to find novel tools for this research are valuable, including if it means studying infants' first poops.

To read more about this interesting topic, see the editorial by Ostrea et al.[2] Toxins seem to be around us everywhere, even in the places in which we provide care. Wastewater flowing out of hospitals is potentially dangerous stuff, for example. Out of a total of 38 samples taken from the main sewer of a French university hospital over a two-year period, 31 samples were positive in at least one microbiological assay of genotoxicity. Samples taken on a Monday and during periods of low rainfall were most likely to show evidence of toxicity. Which of the many thousands of chemical compounds released from hospitals are to blame is yet to be established, but researchers rate anticancer drugs showing up in sewage and antimicrobials as prime suspects.[3]

J. A. Stockman III, MD

References

1. Abraham K, Päpke O, Gross A, et al. Time course of PCDD/PCDF/PCB concentrations in breast-feeding mothers and their infants. *Chemosphere*. 1998;37:1731-1741.
2. Ostrea EM Jr, Bielawski DM, Posecion NC Jr. Meconium analysis to detect fetal exposure to neurotoxicants. *Arch Dis Child*. 2006;91:628-629.
3. Jolibois B, Guerbet M. Hospital wastewater genotoxicity. *Ann Occup Hyg*. 2006;50:189-196.

Continuous pralidoxime infusion versus repeated bolus injection to treat organophosphorus pesticide poisoning: a randomised controlled trial
Pawar KS, Bhoite RR, Pillay CP, et al (Giriraj Hosp, Pune, Maharashtra, India; B J Med College, Pune, Maharashtra, India)
Lancet 368:2136-2141, 2006

Background.—The role of oximes for the treatment of organophosphorus pesticide poisoning has not been conclusively established. We aimed to assess the effectiveness of a constant pralidoxime infusion compared with repeated bolus doses to treat patients with moderately severe poisoning from organophosphorus pesticides.

Methods.—200 patients were recruited to our single-centre, open randomised controlled trial after moderately severe poisoning by anticholinesterase pesticide. All were given a 2 g loading dose of pralidoxime over 30 min. Patients were then randomly assigned to control and study groups. Controls were given a bolus dose of 1 g pralidoxime over 1 h every 4 h for 48 h. The study group had a constant infusion of 1 g over an hour every hour for 48 h. Thereafter, all patients were given 1 g every 4 h until they could be weaned from ventilators. Analysis was by intention to treat. Primary outcome measures were median atropine dose needed within 24 h, proportion of patients who needed intubation, and number of days on ventilation.

Findings.—100 patients were assigned the high-dose regimen, and 100 the control regimen. There were no drop-outs. Patients receiving the high-dose pralidoxime regimen required less atropine during the first 24 h than controls (median 6 mg *vs* 30 mg; difference 24 mg [95% CI 24–26, p<0.0001]). 88 (88%) and 64 (64%) of controls and high-dose patients, respectively, needed intubation during admission to hospital (relative risk=0.72, 0.62–0.86, p=0.0001). Control patients required ventilatory support for longer (median 10 days *vs* 5 days; difference 5 days [5–6, p<0.0001]).

Interpretation.—A high-dose regimen of pralidoxime, consisting of a constant infusion of 1 g/h for 48 h after a 2 g loading dose, reduces morbidity and mortality in moderately severe cases of acute organophosphorus-pesticide poisoning.

▶ You will not see a study like this performed in the United States, and we are thus grateful to our colleagues in India for doing the study because organophosphate poisoning, while not common here, does occur. The Indian study is the first randomized trial that includes large doses of pralidoxime, and the findings suggest that higher doses would be superior to the lower-dose intermittent bolus that is commonly used worldwide. Please be aware that in Asia, these data are particularly important because that part of the world is where most of the pesticide poisoning worldwide takes place. Such poisoning accounts for about two thirds of suicide deaths in many parts of Asia. Intentional ingestion of organophosphorus pesticides has been common for the past 40 years in countries across Southeast Asia.

The data from this report will be important to those here in the United States who work in emergency departments. Atropine and pralidoxime represent the treatments of choice for organophosphate poisoning. We are fortunate that we can afford these drugs. Pralidoxime is expensive, and the high-dose treatment regimen suggested in this report runs about $400 for 2 days of administration, which is far beyond affordability in rural parts of the world. Less expensive sources of pralidoxime are needed to relieve the heavy burden of the cost of treatment of organophosphorus poisoning.

On a peripheral topic, each year, one of the large healthcare providers operating here in the United States (UnitedHealth), publishes its rankings of the healthiest and most unhealthy states. To find the report, you may want to go to the UnitedHealth Foundation web site.[1] The 2006 edition of America's Health Rankings shows Minnesota at the top of the list of the healthiest states. Minnesota has been among the top two states since 1990. Vermont was ranked second in 2006, the same as in 2005. Vermont moved up in the rankings from eighth to second in 2001. New Hampshire is number 3, followed by Hawaii, Connecticut, and Utah. Louisiana is 50th as the least healthy state, while Mississippi is 49th. South Carolina, Tennessee, and Arkansas complete the bottom five states. From 1990 to 2006, Minnesota has held the number one state position for 11 years of the publication of America's Health Rankings. While it still holds the number one position, the large difference between Minnesota and the average state has fortunately declined in the last several years. Minnesota's strengths include ranking first for a low rate of cardiovascular deaths, a low premature death rate, and a low percentage of the uninsured population. It is also in the top 5 states with a low percentage of children in poverty, a low infant mortality, a low occupational fatalities rate, a low motor vehicle death rate, and a high rate of high school graduation. Minnesota's biggest healthcare challenges are a prevalence of obesity of 23.7%, limited access to adequate prenatal care with just 75.9% pregnant women receiving adequate prenatal care, a violent crime rate of 297 offenses per 100,000 population, and a high prevalence of smoking at 20.0% of the population.

Louisiana has been listed as 49th or 50th ever since the rankings were first produced in 1990. The state ranks well for ready access to adequate prenatal care with 82.8% of pregnant women receiving adequate care and few poor mental health days per month with 2.7 workdays lost in the previous 30 days. It ranks in the bottom five states on 6 of the 18 measures with a high prevalence of obesity, a high occupational fatalities rate, a high percentage of children in poverty, a high infant mortality rate, a high rate of cancer death, and a high premature death rate. It ranks in the bottom 10 states for eight other measures.

J. A. Stockman III, MD

Reference

1. 2006 Overall America's Health Rankings. United Health Foundation Web site. Available at: http://www.unitedhealthfoundation.org/ahr2006/findings.html. Accessed June 21, 2006.

Characteristics of Children Receiving Proton Pump Inhibitors Continuously for Up to 11 Years Duration

Hassall E, Kerr W, El-Serag HB (BC Children's Hosp/Univ of British Columbia, Vancouver, Canada; Baylor College of Medicine)
J Pediatr 150:262-267, 2007

Objective.—To characterize those pediatric patients who receive long-term proton pump inhibitors (PPIs) and to determine the safety of long-term use of PPIs in this population.

Study Design.—Patient databases were screened for long-term PPI use, defined as more than 9 months of continuous prescription, between 1989 and 2004.

Results.—The median duration of PPI use in the 166 patients in the study group was 3 years (range, 0.75 to 11.25 years). A total of 80 patients used PPIs for 3 to 11 years duration; 35 of these for more than 5 years, and 15 for more than 8 years. Mean age at initial prescription was 7.8 years. At least 1 gastroesophageal reflux disease (GERD)-predisposing disorder was present in 79% of the patients; the major disorders were neuromotor (in 66%) and esophageal atresia (in 14.5%). No GERD-predisposing disorder was present in 35 patients (21%). Endoscopic findings included hiatal hernia in 39% and histologically proven Barrett's esophagus in 4.8%. Omeprazole was used in 90% of the patients; lansoprazole, in 7%. Six adverse reactions seen in 4 patients were potentially related to PPI (nausea and diarrhea, skin rash, agitation, and irritability).

Conclusions.—Children with underlying GERD-predisposing disorders compose the majority of long-term PPI users. Few adverse reactions to these drugs occur, and discontinuation of the drug is seldom indicated. These preliminary data suggest that PPIs may be efficacious and safe for continuous use for up to 11 years' duration in children.

▶ PPIs have become the mainstay of management of both children and adults with reflux. They are used not only in the short term for allowing an esophagus to heal, but also in the long term for maintenance of remission of reflux symptoms. Whereas the safety of omeprazole has been shown for adults given the drug for extended periods, safety data on prolonged use in children had not become available until this abstracted report by Hassall et al. One can see that not only do PPIs work, but they are also safe for continuous use up to 11 years in children, the longest period so far observed. Because reflux in some patients never resolves, it is likely that many will require the use of this pharmacologic class of drugs forever.

It should be relatively reassuring that PPIs can be used indefinitely. However, this does not mean that it is unnecessary to have more information about what happens with their long term use. Gastric acid is important in the gastrointestinal (GI) tract. It helps to absorb iron, for example. Some have suggested that infants and toddlers on PPIs for extended periods are at greater risk for the development of iron deficiency, and it is worth screening for this problem. We do not know the long-term consequences of achlorhydria on vitamin B12 levels or on the absorption of certain other essential nutrients. Life is full of unintended consequences.

While on the topic of drugs and chemicals, a number of chemicals related to medicine are named after colors. The background on how certain chemicals have received their names is quite interesting. In 1859, Gustav Kirchoff and Robert Busen invented a method for detecting the light spectra that substances produce when they are heated. They used the Busen gas burner, which has a very hot flame with little luminescence, to discover elements whose names reflect the color of the resultant light:

- Caesium—(Kirchoff and Busen in 1860) from the Latin *caesius*, grey-blue, usually referring to the eyes.
- Rubidium—(Kirchoff and Busen, 1861) from the Latin *rubidus*, red, describing a facial flush.
- Thallium—(William Crookes, 1861) from Greek *thallos*, a young olive green shoot.
- Indium—Ferdinand Reich and Hieronymus Richter, 1863) from Greek *indikon*, indigo.

From the article, "When I use a word: colourful metals"[1]:

Chlorine gas is green (Greek *chloros*); iodine vapor is violet (Greek *ion*). Platinum shines like silver (Spanish *plata*), and orpiment (*aurum pigmentum*), arsenic trisulfide (gleams like gold; the Greek for orpiment was *arsenikon* (Hebrew *zarnik*). Gold (arabic zarqun) also gives us zirconium, from the golden mineral zircon. Like chromium (Greek *chroma*, color), rhodium (rhondon, a rose), and praseodymium (prasios, leek green also vomitus), vanadium may get its name from its attractively colored salts - vanadis was the beautiful Norse goddess, Freya or one of her attendants. One of the most colorful elements, iridium is named after the rainbow (Greek *irius*) and pale bismuth (German *Wismut*) may mean "white mask."

So that's the skinny on all the metals that are colorful.

J. A. Stockman III, MD

Reference

1. Aronson J. When I use a word: colourful metals. *BMJ.* 2007;334:205.

Prepubertal Gynecomastia Linked to Lavender and Tea Tree Oils

Henley DV, Lipson N, Korach KS, et al (Natl Inst of Environmental Health Sciences, Research Triangle Park, NC; Univ of Colorado School of Medicine, Denver; Pediatric Endocrine Associates, Greenwood Village, Colo)

N Engl J Med 356:479-485, 2007

Most cases of male prepubertal gynecomastia are classified as idiopathic. We investigated possible causes of gynecomastia in three prepubertal boys who were otherwise healthy and had normal serum concentrations of endogenous steroids. In all three boys, gynecomastia coincided with the topical application of products that contained lavender and tea tree oils. Gynecomastia resolved in each patient shortly after the use of products containing these oils was discontinued. Furthermore, studies in human cell lines indicated that the two oils had estrogenic and antiandrogenic activities. We conclude that repeated topical exposure to lavender and tea tree oils probably caused prepubertal gynecomastia in these boys.

► See how you would handle the following case of a child who also presents with gynecomastia. You are seeing a 14-year-old boy as part of his annual physical examination. You note that he has bilateral breast enlargement. On careful questioning, the youngster also acknowledges that he had some discharge from his breast over the last several months. There are no other physical findings. The present history indicates that the youngster is also being seen by a psychiatrist for management an obsessive-compulsive disorder. This was unsuccessfully managed with sertraline (50mg/d), and now the patient is undergoing treatment with risperidone (2mg/d). Just how far should you go in working up the gynecomastia and galactorrhea?

There probably is little need to spend a lot of money evaluating this youngster's gynecomastia and galactorrhea. Although few studies have been done in children, in adults, risperidone has been shown to cause a marked and sustained increase in serum prolactin levels in a sizeable proportion of patients. In fact, the prevalence of hyperprolactinemia among young women taking risperidone for at least three months (mean dosage, 4-5mg/d) was 88% in one study.[1] Recognize, also, that case reports of increased prolactin blood levels and galactorrhea have been described after the administration of SSRIs such as fluoxetine, sertraline, fluvoxamine, or sitalopram. The problem appears to be caused by a serotoninergic-mediated inhibition of dopamine neurons at the hypothalamic level, exerting a tonic inhibitory control over prolactin release.[2] The problem with risperidone and SSRIs is a dose-dependent one and reversible upon withdrawal of the offending drug.

J. A. Stockman III, MD

References

1. Kinon BJ, Gilmore JA, Liu H, Halbreich UM. Prevalence of hyperprolactinemia in schizophrenic patients treated with conventional antipsychotic medications or risperidone. *Psychoneuroendocrinology.* 2003;28:55-68.
2. Holzer L, Eap CB. Risperidone-induced symptomatic hyperprolactinemia in adolescents. *J Clin Psychopharmacol.* 2006;26:167-171.

The Attitude of Physicians Toward Cold Remedies for Upper Respiratory Infection in Infants and Children: A Questionnaire Survey
Cohen-Kerem R, Ratnapalan S, Djulus J, et al (Univ of Toronto)
Clin Pediatr (Phila) 45:828-834, 2006

Over-the-counter cold remedies are widely used for symptomatic relief of upper respiratory tract infections. The safety of these drugs is not well established in infants and their efficacy is questionable. Our aim was to study the attitude of family physicians and pediatricians toward the use of cold remedies in infants and children. A questionnaire was sent to 400 family physicians and 100 pediatricians randomly selected across Ontario. The overall response rate was 53.2%. Sixteen percent of family physicians recommended cold remedies for infants 0 to 6 months of age compared to 4% of the pediatricians (P = 0.01). For infants 6 to 12 months of age, the difference between pediatricians and family physicians persisted (14% and 38% of, respectively; P < 0.001). Despite that cold remedies are not proven to be effective and some safety issues are associated with their use in the pediatric age group, physicians still recommend them. Continuing medical education programs should address the issue.

▶ Based on all currently available information, one would expect very different findings in this report. A systematic review of over-the-counter cold remedies has unequivocally shown that they are of highly questionable effectiveness and are associated with safety concerns when used in children.[1] A double-blind, randomized controlled trial also showed that there was no symptom relief between cold remedies in preschool children.[2] Nonetheless, in this study of Canadian generalist physicians and general pediatricians, a significant proportion were willing to recommend cold remedies in young children. Pediatricians compared with family physicians, however, were less likely to do so. An interesting aspect of this report is that many physicians readily admitted that they were "treating the parent rather than the child" or that "parents would have got it (the remedy) anyway."

Medications containing pseudoephedrine, phenylephrine, brompheniramine, chlorpheniramine, or diphenhydramine are not without their side effects, some of which can be serious and even deadly. They are best left on the shelves of pharmacies when it comes to tiny tots. If these ingredients are not bad enough, many over-the-counter cold medicines also have some alcohol in them. This commentary closes with a who-dun-it related to a youngster with a high blood alcohol level. You receive a call from the parents of a 4-year-old that the child has begun to act in a weird manner. He is clumsy and giggly. You immediately see the youngster in the office, and it appears as if he may be drunk. A blood alcohol is 0.9. The parents swear that they do not drink, and they have no alcoholic beverages in their home. What question should you ask them that may give a clue to the etiology of this child's intoxication? Query the parents whether they have begun to use an alcohol-based hand sanitizer. Such sanitizers have been documented to be a cause of alcoholic intoxication.[3] Back in 2006, the Maryland Poison Center, for example, was called about a 49-year-old, usually calm prison inmate, who was described as being "red-eyed, looney, combative, and intoxicated, lecturing everyone about life." Other inmates and staff reported seeing this prisoner drinking from a gallon container of Purell Hand Sanitizer. The inmate's blood alcohol level was markedly elevated. It was later confirmed that he had not consumed any other form of ethanol or other illicit substances. The patient was treated with fluid repletion and haloperidol, with no complications.

The Centers for Disease Control and Prevention has recommended that before and after having any direct contact with patients, healthcare workers use an alcohol-based hand sanitizer or wash their hands with an antimicrobial soap and water. Such alcohol-based hand sanitizers are now ubiquitously found in common work sites and in the home. Alcohol-based hand sanitizers are formulated as low-viscosity rinses, gels, or foams. They contain 60% to 95% alcohol or isopropanol. Ethanol has greater activity against viruses than does isopropanol, and the ethanol-based formulations are used much more commonly here in the United States than are the isopropanol-based formulations. They are sold under trade names such as Avagard D, Avant, Nexcare, Prevacare, Germ-X, and Purell. Many of the ethanol-based sanitizers also contain small amounts of polypropylene glycol or isopropanol.

Please be aware that alcohol-based sanitizers should be kept out of the reach of children. Realize, also, that given the high alcohol content of such sanitizers, they do represent a potential fire hazard. It appears that airport security folks are not aware of this problem because many passengers seem to get aboard planes with small amounts of hand sanitizers. They are as potent an accelerant as lighter fluid, the latter banned as a carry-on item.[4]

J. A. Stockman III, MD

References

1. Schroeder K, Fahey T. Should we advise parents to administer over the counter cough medicines for acute cough? A systematic review of randomised control trials. *Arch Dis Child*. 2002;86:170-175.

2. Clemens CJ, Taylor JA, Almquist JR, Quinn HC, Mehta A, Naylor GS. Is an antihistamine-decongestant combination effective in temporarily relieving symptoms of the common cold in preschool children? *J Pediatr.* 1997;130:463-466.
3. Doyon S, Welsh C. Intoxication of a prison inmate with an ethyl alcohol-based hand sanitizer. *N Engl J Med.* 2007;356:529-530.
4. Emadi A, Coberly L. Intoxication of a hospitalized patient with an isopropanol-based hand sanitizer. *N Engl J Med.* 2007;356:530-531.

Subject Index

A

Abdominal pain
  chronic, depressive symptoms and, 147
  functional, wireless video capsule for
    evaluation of, 145
  opiate analgesics in, effect on clinical
    evaluation, 148
Acetaminophen
  aminotransferase elevation in healthy
    adults receiving 4 grams daily, 142
Activated partial thromboplastin time
    (aPTT)
  prolonged, evaluation in children, 66
Acute chest syndrome, in sickle cell
    disease
  daytime pulse oximeter measurements
    and, 55
  lung function and, 56
Acute lymphoblastic leukemia
  effect of acute exercise on neutrophils in
    survivors, 463
  hypertension in, 445
  6-thioguanine vs. 6-mercaptopurine for,
    toxicity and efficacy, 439
ADHD (see Attention-deficit/hyperactivity
    disorder)
Adolescents
  anorexia nervosa in, fluoxetine
    treatment after weight restoration,
    16
  attention-deficit/hyperactivity disorder
    in, long-term atomoxetine
    treatment for, 357
  back pain in, algorithmic approach, 328
  cardiovascular risk factors in,
    brachial-ankle pulse wave velocity
    and, 225
  childhood maltreatment and health
    consequences in, 309
  deaths in juvenile justice residential
    facilities, 22
  depression in
    interventions in primary care, 346
    as predictor of sexual risk behavior,
      348
  disordered eating prevalence in a
    multiracial/ethnic sample of female
    high school athletes, 18
  lumbar disk herniation in, trends in,
    333
  meniscus tears in, results of operative
    treatment, 334
  mucopurulent cervicitis in, empirical
    treatment as chlamydial infection,
    13

sexual activity and contraception in
  immediate use of DMPA vs. bridge
    methods with later initiation,
    pregnancy rate and, 4
  patterns of oral contraceptive
    pill-taking and condom use, 3
  prevalence of unwanted and unlawful
    sexual experience reported by
    Danish adolescents, 19
  reported consequences of oral vs.
    vaginal sex, 1
smoking in
  changes in tobacco sources, 23
  health effects in adulthood, 488
sunburns, sun protection practices, and
  attitudes toward protection and
  tanning among, 1998–2004, 33
tuberculosis in, demographic and
  clinical characteristics, 264
weight gain in transition to adulthood,
  fast food consumption and
  breakfast skipping as predictors of,
  416
Adrenal insufficiency
  in children receiving high-dose inhaled
    fluticasone propionate, 135
Air pollution
  exposure in pregnancy, very low
    birthweight delivery incidence and,
    482
  infant deaths from 1989 to 2000 in
    southern California and, 481
  long-term exposure and incidence of
    cardiovascular events in women,
    483
Allergy
  alone or together with nonnutritive
    sucking habits, malocclusion in
    primary dentition and, 91
  cow's milk protein, umbilicus erythema
    as diagnostic sign, 144
  dental metal, palmoplantar pustulosis
    and, 92
  wheat, timing of initial exposure to
    cereal grains and risk of, 28
AMG 531
  for chronic immune thrombocytopenic
    purpura, 62
Aminotransferase
  elevation in healthy adults receiving 4
    grams of acetaminophen daily, 142
Aneurysm(s)
  intracranial in children, clinical
    characteristics, 211
  syndromes caused by mutations in the
    TGF-β receptor, 208

O

Obesity
  prevalence in survivors of childhood cancer, 447
  severe early-onset, congenital deficiency of the leptin receptor in, 425
  weight gain in transition from adolescence to adulthood, fast food consumption and breakfast skipping as predictors of, 416

Oligosaccharides
  prebiotic, use during first six months of life for reduced incidence of atopic dermatitis, 30

Opiate analgesics
  for acute abdominal pain, effect on clinical evaluation, 148

Opsoclonus-myoclonus syndrome
  rituximab as adjunctive therapy for, 455

Optic neuritis
  clinical features, MRI findings, and outcome in children, 473

Organophosphorus pesticide poisoning
  pralidoxime for, continuous infusion vs. repeated bolus injection, 504

Osteomyelitis
  acute hematogenous, changing patterns with emergence of community-associated methicillin-resistant *S. aureus*, 325
  vertebral, in cat-scratch disease, 323

Otitis media
  acute
    adherence to CDC treatment recommendations, 104
    antibiotics for, meta-analysis with individual patient data, 101
    predictors of pain and/or fever at 3 to 7 days for children not treated initially with antibiotics, 99
    trends in doctor consultations, antibiotic prescriptions, and specialist referrals for, 102
  chronic
    direct detection of bacterial biofilms on middle-ear mucosa in, 97
    tympanostomy tubes for development outcomes at 9 to 11 years of age and, 105
    otorrhea following placement, 107
  incidence after introduction of pneumococcal conjugate vaccine, 100

Oxygen saturation
  achieved vs. intended levels in premature infants, 397
  daytime measurements in relation to pain and acute chest syndrome episodes in sickle cell disease, 55
  trends immediately after birth, 397

P

Palliative care
  perinatal, for prenatally diagnosed lethal fetal abnormality, 408
  symptoms affecting children with malignancies during last month of life, 448

Palmoplantar pustulosis
  dental metal allergy and, 92

Pantoprazole
  for gastroesophageal reflux in children, dosage comparison, 152

Parvovirus B-19
  acute infection in hospitalized children, 275

Patent ductus arteriosus
  in extremely low birthweight infants, neurosensory impairment after surgical closure, 393

Pectus excavatum
  family study of inheritance of, 327

Pediatric hospitalists
  combined pediatric emergency department/inpatient unit approach in community hospitals, 312

Pediatric surgery fellowships
  compliance to the 80-hour work week restrictions, 289

Pediculosis
  hot air treatment for, 41

Pemphigus vulgaris
  rituximab and intravenous immunoglobulin for, 39

Periodontal disease
  maternal, risk of preterm birth with and without treatment, 395

Pertussis
  control in 2007 and beyond, 261
  epidemiology of hospitalized children with, effect of change from whole-cell to acellular vaccine in Canada, 260
  nonmedical exemptions to school immunization requirements and incidence of, 235
  prevalence in school-age children with persistent cough, 262

Phototherapy
  for neonatal jaundice, low-cost white reflecting curtains for increased effectiveness, 377

Author Index

A

Abdel-Latif ME, 392
Abdoh A, 107
Accadbled F, 334
Adams WG, 420
Adejuyigbe EA, 426
Adeodu OO, 426
Ahmed AR, 39
Aitchison TC, 371
Aladangady N, 371
Albert MH, 64
Alexander SW, 66
Alonso E, 141
Amer A, 37
Anand SG, 420
Annest JL, 302
Antonelli J, 256
Appelman CL, 99, 101
Arcement C, 175
Arnold SR, 325
Arslanoglu S, 30
Aryan HE, 211
Ashkenazi S, 247
Atkin JS, 41
Attia E, 16
Aung T, 472

B

Badra MI, 328
Bailey RC, 184
Bal MO, 119
Ballard RA, 400
Ballinger AB, 115
Balmaña J, 163
Balu L, 264
Barclay RL, 168
Barnhart DC, 406
Barr RG, 82
Barriga K, 28
Bass JL, 298
Basso C, 220
Batty GD, 75, 81
Bauchner H, 104
Baudouin V, 444
Baussano I, 491
Bax M, 341
Beal AC, 382
Bech BH, 499
Bell GJ, 463
Bellezza-Fontana R, 491
Bellieni CV, 501
Benavidez OJ, 202
Bennett PH, 422
Benzaquen H, 128

Berenholtz S, 316
Berhe T, 126
Beri D, 117, 137
Bertolami MC, 223
Bettinger JA, 260
Bhat R, 404
Bhoite RR, 504
Binder V, 64
Bishop MT, 359
Black RE, 415
Blakley B, 107
Bland RM, 280
Bloedon LT, 227
Blumenstein MS, 69
Boden JM, 187
Bonde E, 73
Bonsu BK, 254
Boyd JH, 55
Brady SS, 1
Braz RRT, 387
Brecelj J, 150
Breeze ACG, 408
Brenner R, 88
Brody DJ, 7
Buck JM, 467
Buckingham SC, 325
Buettner P, 296
Buncic JR, 473
Bussel JB, 62
Butow PN, 409

C

Callaghan WM, 388
Campbell MJ, 95
Campbell TF, 105
Candy DCA, 171
Cans C, 389
Carlin JB, 488
Cassard X, 334
Cassio A, 119
Cavacini LA, 39
Caveliers V, 155
Cefalo G, 450
Cereda S, 450
Cetin M, 445
Ceyhan M, 294
Chan G, 338
Chan L, 300
Chang DC, 470
Chang JJ, 309
Chang L-Y, 86
Charles MD, 272
Chen S, 165
Chen SY, 396
Chevalier I, 433

Chin RFM, 352
Chou S-C, 382
Clark HF, 269
Coates AL, 93
Coffey C, 488
Cohen-Kerem R, 509
Cokkinides V, 33
Collins S, 425
Conell C, 167
Connolly K, 359
Coory M, 409
Coovadia HM, 280
Corapci F, 76
Cordelli DM, 501
Corrado D, 220
Cotch MF, 476
Courneya KS, 463
Crawford TO, 364
Creswick HA, 327
Crist RA, 68
Croen LA, 391
Cross KP, 205
Cuchel M, 227
Curns AT, 270, 272
Cutter GR, 400

D

Dagan Z, 474
Dalton WT III, 23
Dalzell AM, 159
D'Amico D, 144
Dankert HM, 495
Dargaville PA, 402
Davies L, 50, 452
Davis JM, 84
Davis PG, 385
Deary IJ, 75, 81
DeBaun MR, 55, 59
de Borgie CAJM, 42
Debray F-G, 433
de Camargo B, 462
de Carvalho M, 387
de Haen M, 37
de Kleine MJK, 77
de Lorijn F, 173
Der G, 75, 81
De Schepper J, 155
De Serres G, 260
Devine OJ, 493
Devrim i, 294
Dhallan R, 314
Dietrich AJ, 345
Di Lallo D, 487
Dimmitt RA, 406
Di Napoli A, 487

529